"There is an urgent need for critical systemic sc
tural, and contextual forces shaping people's live
Family Therapy offers an essential transtheoretic
ers engage in transformative work, both in clinic

their communities. The authors skillfully distill complex theories into accessible, practical insights, demonstrating the power of critical thinking and intentional practice to create meaningful change. This is a vital read for family therapists ready to move beyond simply recognizing injustice and toward actively disrupting the status quo."

Leslie A. Anderson, *Assistant Professor, Family and Consumer Sciences, Morgan State University*

"Finally, a theory book students love to read! McDowell, Knudson-Martin, and Bermúdez provide conceptual and clinical resources to both reconsider and apply foundational systemic theories in a sociocultural context that expands therapists' abilities to serve clients from all backgrounds. They guide the reader to integrate third order thinking by engaging the complexities of societal systems, culture, and power influences on clients and the therapeutic relationship through case examples, reflections from practitioners, and reflexive questions. Therapists of all theoretical preferences will find themselves in this book!"

Kristen E. Benson, *PhD, Associate Professor, Department of Human Development and Family Science, Virginia Tech*

"By addressing concerns of isolation, individualism, and polarization, this third edition further equips systemic therapists to navigate today's social, cultural, and political realities. Its addition of socioculturally attuned assessment invites greater recursive reflection and integration of sociocultural realities in clinical practice and training. It is a valuable resource for those committed to socioculturally responsive practice and for educators preparing the next generation of systemic therapists."

Peter Rivera, *Associate Professor of Marriage and Family Therapy, Seattle Pacific University*

Socioculturally Attuned Family Therapy

Socioculturally Attuned Family Therapy, third edition, is a fully updated and essential textbook that addresses the need for marriage and family therapists to engage in socially responsible practice by infusing third order thinking throughout theory and clinical practice.

Written by leaders in the field, this book explores why sociocultural attunement and equity matter, providing students and clinicians with integrative guidelines and case illustrations applicable to practice. The authors integrate principles of societal context, power, and equity into 11 major family therapy models: Structural, Strategic, Experiential, Attachment, Narrative, Solution-focused, Collaborative, Cognitive Behavioral, Contextual, Bowen Family Systems, and Socio-emotional Relationship Therapy. Updates feature diverse voices describing creative applications of this framework, a new chapter on socioculturally attuned assessment, and expanded content on contemporary social issues such as social isolation, individualism, social inequities, and polarization.

This textbook remains essential reading for family therapists, counselors, social workers, and psychologists, as well as educators and supervisors wanting to apply a critical consciousness and third order thinking to their clinical and community work.

Teresa McDowell, EdD, is Professor Emerita of Marriage and Family Therapy and former department chair in Lewis & Clark's Graduate School of Education and Counseling. She is a licensed marriage and family therapist who currently serves as a social researcher, program evaluator, private consultant, and professional educator.

Carmen Knudson-Martin, PhD, is Professor Emerita of Marriage and Family Therapy at Lewis & Clark's Graduate School of Education and Counseling. She is an AAMFT clinical fellow, approved supervisor, and licensed marriage and family therapist. She is a founder of Socio-Emotional Relationship Therapy, which addresses the political and ethical implications of therapist actions on personal and relational development.

J. Maria Bermúdez, PhD, is Associate Professor of Couple and Family Therapy Program and Human Development and Family Science at the University of Georgia. She is an AAMFT clinical fellow and approved supervisor, and a practicing licensed marriage and family therapist. Her work is anchored in feminist-informed and culturally responsive approaches to therapy, research, community activism, and supervision.

Socioculturally Attuned Family Therapy

Applying Third Order Thinking to Theory and Practice

Third Edition

Teresa McDowell, Carmen Knudson-Martin, and J. Maria Bermúdez

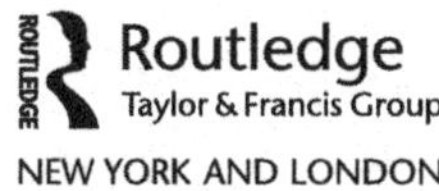

NEW YORK AND LONDON

Designed cover image: Getty Images

Third edition published 2026
by Routledge
605 Third Avenue, New York, NY 10158

and by Routledge
4 Park Square, Milton Park, Abingdon, Oxon, OX14 4RN

Routledge is an imprint of the Taylor & Francis Group, an informa business

First edition published by Routledge 2017
Second edition published by Routledge 2023

Library of Congress Cataloging-in-Publication Data
Names: McDowell, Teresa author | Knudson-Martin, Carmen author | Bermudez, J. Maria author
Title: Socioculturally attuned family therapy : applying third order thinking to theory and practice / Teresa McDowell, Carmen Knudson-Martin, and J. Maria Bermudez.
Description: Third edition. | New York, NY : Routledge, 2026. | Includes bibliographical references and index. |
Identifiers: LCCN 2025038241 (print) | LCCN 2025038242 (ebook) | ISBN 9781032797045 hardback | ISBN 9781032787367 paperback | ISBN 9781003493426 ebook
Subjects: LCSH: Family psychotherapy | Family assessment
Classification: LCC RC488.53 .M33 2026 (print) | LCC RC488.53 (ebook)
LC record available at https://lccn.loc.gov/2025038241
LC ebook record available at https://lccn.loc.gov/2025038242

ISBN: 978-1-032-79704-5 (hbk)
ISBN: 978-1-032-78736-7 (pbk)
ISBN: 978-1-003-49342-6 (ebk)

DOI: 10.4324/9781003493426

Typeset in Times New Roman
by KnowledgeWorks Global Ltd.

Access the Support Material: www.routledge.com/9781032787367

We dedicate this book to colleagues and students committed to a more just future through third order change.

Contents

Foreword to the First Edition (Fred P. Piercy) xi
Foreword to the Second Edition (Stephanie Brooks) xiii
Foreword to the Third Edition (Anne Prouty) xv
Preface to the Third Edition xviii
Acknowledgements xxii
List of Contributors xxiv

1 Socioculturally Attuned Family Therapy 1

2 Guiding Principles for Socioculturally Attuned Family Therapy 19

3 Third Order Ethics and Contextual Self-in-relationship 48

4 Socioculturally Attuned Engagement and Assessment 70

5 Socioculturally Attuned Structural Family Therapy 97

6 Socioculturally Attuned Brief and Strategic Family Therapies 118

7 Socioculturally Attuned Experiential Family Therapy 140

8 Socioculturally Attuned Attachment-based Family Therapies 163

9 Socioculturally Attuned Bowenian Family Therapy 187

10 Socioculturally Attuned Contextual Family Therapy 211

11 Socioculturally Attuned Cognitive Behavioral Family Therapy 233

12 Socioculturally Attuned Solution-focused Family Therapy 255

13 Socioculturally Attuned Collaborative-Dialogic Family Therapy 275

14 Socioculturally Attuned Narrative Family Therapy 300

15 Socio-emotional Relationship Therapy: An Example of Socioculturally Attuned Couple and Family Therapy 324

16 Socioculturally Attuned Praxis: Consciousness in Action 356

Index *382*

Foreword to the First Edition

Fred P. Piercy

This book is a timely gift to our field. McDowell, Knudson-Martin, and Bermudez offer us both the theory and practical guidelines we need to support equity in the face of sociocultural factors at play in all relationships. They explain *socioculturally attuned family therapy*, as a set of transtheoretical considerations that they apply to family therapies to support third order change. That is, they provide a way to understand and address sociocultural factors that promote and maintain unearned privilege, and misuses of power.

The authors explain that it is not possible for a therapist to be neutral in the face of power imbalances. Tolerance and acceptance are not enough. We must address the dynamic interplay between societal systems that privilege some over others. Uneven influence and opportunities can be, as the authors explain "based on social class, gender, race, ethnicity, languages, sexual orientation, age, nation of origin, abilities, and (even) looks." The authors show family therapists how they can integrate cultural attunement within a wide range of family therapy theories.

As a long-time author and editor, as I read this book, I reflected on the qualities that I value in professional writing. For example, does the author answer the "so what?" question. Why is a work important? What does it add to the field? This book's potential impact is easy to see. There is no more important issue in our field than how to provide culturally attuned therapy that appreciates the strengths of one's culture and family, identifies inequities, addresses inequities, and applies our family therapies in a manner that addresses these inequities.

As an editor, I also look for interventions that are theoretically grounded and brought to life through clinical dialogue, and practical exercises. McDowell, Knudson-Martin, and Bermudez do this in every chapter. They introduce each major model of family therapy, discuss its history and application, identify the enduring concepts of each model, then show how sociocultural attunement might be applied to each particular theory. I particularly liked their last chapter, that identified the steps in their approach that can be applied to any existing family therapy.

As for accessibility and tone, other editorial values of mine, McDowell, Knudson-Martin, and Bermudez have made difficult concepts clear, engaging, and eminently transferrable to practice. Also, in this era of political and societal bullying, the authors' approach doesn't shame or bully. They work with clients in a sensitive and kind manner that invites understanding and collaboration.

Perhaps the most important value in contemporary family therapy is cultural sensitivity. Indeed, the authors support greater cultural understanding, equity, and critical social conscientiousness. Their work is both impressive and important. I can see it transforming the way we practice family therapy, regardless of model. It is good that we are talking about social justice in our field. The authors operationalize this concept for family therapists. They provide an accessible, useful, affirming socioculturally attuned family therapy that examines sociocultural structures, supports relational equity, and thus social justice. McDowell, Knudson-Martin, and Bermudez' book will not only transform our practices and our clients but ourselves, as well.

Fred Piercy, PhD.
Professor Emeritus, Virginia Tech Family Therapy Doctoral Program
Blacksburg, VA
Past Editor, *Journal of Marriage and Family Therapy*

Foreword to the Second Edition

Stephanie Brooks

For more than 25 years I taught Introduction to Family Therapy to couple and family therapy students. In this course, students were invited to use culturally responsive practices, larger systems, power, and privilege to critique and modify family therapy approaches. How I wished for a textbook that provided a practical framework for navigating relational, socio-cultural, and political intersections in clinical practice. The first edition of *Socioculturally Attuned Family Therapy* generated excitement and stimulated the hearts and minds of couple and family therapists across identities, experiences, and philosophies. As the former Executive Consultant for the American Association for Marriage and Family Therapy Minority Fellowship Program (MFP), the concept of third order change helped to frame and name the MFP Fellows' commitment to social change. This was a clear signal that their work mattered, and they too had a seat at the table. It was moving to witness our professional community reflect on, recognize, and renew their personal and professional commitment to action inside and outside the therapy room.

Like the first edition, this contribution by Teresa McDowell, Carmen Knudson-Martin, and Maria Bermudez will forevermore shape how and what we think, practice, and teach about family therapy. The second edition of *Socioculturally Attuned Family Therapy* refines the guiding principles of the ANVIET approach and expands on how to facilitate change within and across embedded systems. The authors updated the chapters to include contemporary issues, added new references and for clarity restructured key graphic representations. Chapters 1 and 2 are significantly revised to include some of the most challenging health and societal issues we've encountered over the past five years such as COVID-19, climate change, and mental health. They shine a light on racism, trauma, power, and privilege how these matters promote and maintain structural inequality in the US. The introduction of *socio-relational determinants of health* is a timely analysis and further details our obligation to be socially responsible family therapists. These topics will without question influence our present and future work.

Several new features and chapters demonstrate the progression of McDowell, Knudson-Martin, and Bermudez' ideas about equity-based therapy. Chapter 3 includes their current reflections on third order ethics and self of the therapist. Chapter 15 is new, including a section focusing on third order thinking and third order transformative change across contexts such as community agencies, research and policy making. This chapter provides clear links and illustrations for socioculturally attuned family therapy and consciousness in action. The SERT model is comprehensively presented as an exemplar of an equity-based therapy approach. Finally, the authors invited our colleagues who are engaged in transformative work to share examples of how their work reflects third order thinking and change. The inclusion of over two dozen voices makes this book truly exceptional and elucidates for the reader how to think and practice equity-based therapy.

This book is a call for action. It will continue to generate dialogue about the future directions for couple and family therapy practice and the profession. The inclusion of C/MFT practitioner voices is a brilliant example of how to use your platform and harness community power to create a new reality of an equitable place.

Stephanie Brooks PhD, LCSW, LMFT
Dean of the College of Health
Cleveland State University
Cleveland, Ohio

Foreword to the Third Edition

Anne Prouty

I am thrilled to be asked to write the forward to the third edition of a book that has been one of the most important innovations in training our field has had this millennium. I have been training new therapists for over thirty years, a dream job that has enabled me to learn about family therapy across the United States and internationally. We need books that include voices of therapists working around the world. In my experience, systemic and relational therapists are universally hungry for perspectives that will help them help others, and we expect our models to be insightful, flexible, respectful, and current. Family therapy began as an endeavor to move beyond behaving as if mental health existed only within an individual to recognizing the inherent necessity of people's equitable and mutual interdependence for health and well-being. Growing into an ever more interconnected, global community is enabling the field of family therapy to explore, expand, challenge, and better reflect the people and communities we endeavor to serve, support, understand, and become. Family therapists are actively producing nuanced, challenging, insightful research and clinical work, but it takes time and dedication to immerse oneself. Whether we are new to the profession or experienced, we need pivotal textbooks whose authors have woven foundational ideas with cutting edge research and critical, innovative, clinical practice. *Socioculturally Attuned Family Therapy: Guidelines for Equitable Theory and Practice* has been a significant guide to action.

In the first edition of *Socioculturally Attuned Family Therapy*, McDowell, Knudson-Martin, and Bermúdez provided the field with ANVIET, a transtheoretical framework of guiding practices by which to enable third order change, a method by which family therapists could collaborate with clients to deconstruct and reconstruct people's uniquely embedded social systems, experiences, and possibilities. By applying their transtheoretical conceptualization of sociocultural attunement to many of the fields' models, their work provided scaffolding for family therapists to re-understand complex interdependent dynamics at intimately personal levels. McDowell, Knudson-Martin, and Bermúdez taught us a method that enabled consistent habits of mind to develop in our practice, and our evaluation of our practices in vivo. The addition of ANVIET guiding practices was an alteration that enabled our therapy models to resume relevance. The second edition of *Socioculturally Attuned Family Therapy* expanded to facilitating change across embedded systems, examined contemporary health and social issues, and included many global and richly described case examples whose authors brought the nuances of third order change to life. Centering the experiences of systemic thinkers, trainers, and practitioners from around the globe, readers were guided to step into many perspectives and learn how systemic thinking and practice can remain alive and must be consciously and continuously developed. I have experienced as a trainer that this emphasis on the necessity of continuous revision and development, third order change conceptualization, and socioculturally attuned practice strategies have enabled our students to see themselves and their experiences reflected in our profession's priorities and practices. This is essential if our field is to continue to grow and thrive.

Throughout the third edition of *Socioculturally Attuned Family Therapy: Applying Third Order Thinking to Theory and Practice,* McDowell, Knudson-Martin, and Bermúdez have added practice steps and integrated more of an emphasis on relationships being essentials for mental, emotional, and community health. They have updated discussions and included a lot of very current research and clinical references. For example, there is a new discussion hope and expectancy in solution focused therapy, a discussion on interpersonal neurobiology and experiential therapy, and a detailed and fascinating updated examination of the attachment research. But the most exciting updates are provided in the first four chapters of the book.

McDowell, Knudson-Martin, and Bermúdez have expanded their discussions linking equity-based practice, mental health, and relational well-being in chapter one, maintaining its international scope while including many family therapists' recent calls for social action and equity-based practice related to racial equity, anti-racist practice, attention to people's legacies of trauma, gender-inclusion, queer-conceptualization of family therapy, diverse social determinants of health, climate change, and social isolation. True to family therapy's core is a new examination of extreme individualism, and other practices that challenge people's social and relational connections and mutual responsibilities. Demonstrating that family therapists' work remains necessarily alongside people's lives and experiences and requires us to develop and refine our own critical consciousness to be of use to clients and communities.

Chapter two is also expertly revised and enhanced with an enriched discussion of third order thinking. McDowell, Knudson-Martin, and Bermudez review first, second, and third order learning before unveiling their new discussion of fourth-order learning and fourth order thinking, "shifting the focus to contemporary understandings of the nature of the universe…recognizing that humans are but one species among many." Thus, they have now opened the necessity of systemic and relational thinkers to move beyond human-centered conceptualization. Perhaps, enabling us to center nuanced, ancient supra-system conceptualizations, traditions, and responsibilities of highest order interdependence.

In chapter three the authors' discussion of ethics builds upon their work and offers new, liberating challenges to use the guiding principles of sociocultural attunement. The authors have expanded this chapter with a meaningful and helpful exploration of the social locations and histories of knowledges that have been centered in our ethics discourse. Indirectly touching on fourth order thinking, while then returning to challenge family therapists to recognize how these empowered and disempowered conceptualizations of ethics influence our clients' lives and our professions priorities.

McDowell, Knudson-Martin, and Bermúdez have created a new fourth chapter, "Socioculturally Attuned Engagement and Assessment." It is an exciting, practical, well explained guide that provides an appropriately challenging foundation for clinicians to better understand themselves. The process then guides the therapist to attune to the client's sociocultural context, carefully build an understanding of how their context is connected to their daily lives, and responsibly position therapy in relational and equitable values. McDowell and colleagues expertly walk us through forming a relationship and expanding our lens via five elements of the engagement process. Each of the elements are well described, thoroughly discussed, and humanized with a clear case example running through the chapter. Advanced clinicians can glean new ideas to enhance their work, their supervision, and their practice site's assessment practices. The trainer in me immediately saw how this chapter could provide guidance for building a relationally based, culturally attuned course for beginning therapists. The chapter culminates with a well-designed assessment summary.

As Jordan (1988) famously said, "*You can seize an idea with such force that it becomes a reality.*" This book remains a call to action. Third-order change and even stepping into fourth-order thinking is the future if we are to recognize and mobilize people's preferred ways of being, meaningfully and respectfully contribute to co-creating equitable relationships and social communities and being on this planet in this universe.

Anne M. Prouty Ph.D., LMFT
in private practice and
Assistant Professor of MFT, Seattle Pacific University, Seattle, WA USA
Professor of MFT, Daybreak University, Anaheim, CA USA
Former Editor-in-Chief (2001–2013), *Journal of Feminist Family Therapy: An International Forum*
July 19, 2025

Preface to the Third Edition

Our ideas have continued to evolve since the second edition of *Socioculturally Attuned Family Therapy: Guidelines for Equity in Theory and Practice* was published in 2022. In this third edition, we expand the concept of third order thinking and introduce some preliminary considerations of fourth order thinking. We integrate new ideas into each chapter, including advances in each family therapy model. There is a chapter on socioculturally attuned assessment in this new edition - a decision we made after discussing what we consider to be a lack of attention to family therapy assessment practices in graduate programs. We hope this will inspire greater congruence between formal assessment and the kind of treatment planning that is required in many settings and socioculturally attuned therapeutic practices.

We are witnessing an explosion in recent years of what we consider third order thinking and practice among colleagues who have published or otherwise shared their conceptual frameworks and practices. We are grateful to be able to showcase many of these innovators by including their voices in this edition. Their contributions provide examples of engaging in transformative praxis across multiple contexts, within and beyond family therapy, including work in communities, municipal and legal systems, medical systems, educational organizations, research, and policy making.

We use a variety of terms throughout this text to refer to sociopolitical identities. Contemporary preferred terms change quickly as the contested landscape of identity shifts. The freedom to self-identify, the potential power of claiming group identity, and the colonizing effects of being identified by others reflect the brutal struggle between structural equity and inequity. Given that this text will be used across disciplines, in different countries, regions of the US, and by diverse readers, by the time you read this text, some of the terms we use may be perceived as offensive and/or outdated. Even now, we move between terms in ways that are likely to feel dismissive, irrelevant, or uninformed to some readers. In numerous places across this volume, we advocate for *calling in* rather than *calling out* [see Loretta Ross, 2019; 2025], connecting rather than polarizing, and being patient with ourselves and others who are on a journey of becoming increasingly socioculturally attuned. We ask readers to engage with our intention to be inclusive, compassionate, and just, as we attempt to describe the complexities of diverse identities and social locations across and within cultural contexts.

As socioculturally attuned family therapists, we want readers to know who we are, our social locations, our intentions, our values, and some of our individual and collective stories in the field of family therapy. We have a lot in common. We are family therapy educators, supervisors, and clinicians with various types of professional experiences. All three of us are highly relational beings, dedicated to putting relationships first. We have shared our energy and creativity over the course of writing the first, second, and third editions of this text, struggling to make sense of how, as family therapists, we can all expand our work to support more just relationships. We have deeply valued the differences between us, which allows each of us to see with more than our own eyes. Following, we each share a few thoughts about our journeys thus far in the field of family therapy.

Teresa

Family has always been at the center for me. I became a family therapist in the 1980s. I remember walking around amazed, gaping at relationship patterns I was seeing everywhere. I couldn't pull myself away from a field that was teeming with energy, pushing to find new ways of creating change. I fell in love with counterintuitive thinking, with the MRI model, as well as structural and strategic family therapy. As the field developed I embraced solution-focused and narrative practices. Being active, intuitive, and imaginative—taking risks using experiential techniques—became central to my practice. I balanced the burden of trying to do therapy right with an entrepreneurial drive to think creatively.

A doctorate in liberation-based adult education helped me rethink family therapy and set the stage for challenging my own Eurocentric thinking, unexamined Whiteness, heterosexual and cisgender privilege, and middle-class legacy. The first half of my career I looked to family therapy to help me understand the world. The second half I searched beyond family therapy to find ways to understand and challenge unjust social and familial arrangements.

I enjoy reading and talking to creative thinkers. I have been in deep conversation about all things of interest with my son, Flynn, for the past three decades. Third and fourth order thinking emerged and became working concepts from our many talks. I have watched my son, Quentin, put shared ideas about equity to work in his role as an educational leader. My understanding of family deepened when my step-son, Rob, reconnected after being adopted as a child. I have seven grandchildren whom I love dearly. One recently became a family therapist.

I have witnessed tremendous growth in our field. The feminist critique revolutionized family therapy; however, there was a time when further ideas about social and relational equity were marginalized in classrooms, conferences, and journals. I was forewarned by my mentor to "let these ideas go" for fear they would harm my career. I had difficulty getting my first paper on racism and White privilege published until a journal accepted the work on the condition that I remove the word "oppression" from the manuscript. I shared concerns in the hallways at AAMFT conferences with colleagues who also had their presentations on critical social issues rejected.

Through the years, all of this has changed. We now have burgeoning conversations about colonialism, racism, social class, gender identity, sexual orientation, environmental justice, epistemic justice, body politics…ideas and practices are steadily advancing. I introduced third order thinking as defined in this text, in a 2015 American Family Therapy Academy (AFTA) brief. Over the past several years, these concepts have become common field language.

As our social and political climate changes, it may seem like our collective work in the field is being revoked, but I don't think so. There are too many of us, too many ideas, too many who are seeing what can't be unseen to erase these efforts. I believe the challenge at hand is to not get lost on the ground by insulating ourselves and giving in to political polarization. We need to keep our heads up, looking at systems at the broadest level, listening to those who see the world differently, and paying attention to how social and political rhetoric serves those with the most power and greatest resources.

Carmen

Before I came to this field, I taught family life education in high schools. I found myself fascinated by students who struggled, not by their "problem behavior," but by their stories of hurt, pain, and unfairness. Seeing students labeled as troublemakers, while misdeeds of "good" students (as I had been) escaped notice, heightened my curiosity about the systemic dynamics that create and maintain these inequities.

Then I moved to Iran. As a young woman of Scandinavian heritage raised on a farm in North Dakota, I experienced being on the outside and had to learn how to negotiate a social system organized so differently than I was used to. How did I buy groceries? How did I get from one place to another? Who could I trust? When the Tehran-American School hired me to teach family life education and psychology, I had to consider human behavior and relationships from perspectives different from my own. Later, living in Senegal and then teaching at international schools in Jordan and Costa Rica, I learned to see my North American world from the outside and to take apart and examine my taken-for-granted expectations. I experienced the privileges afforded to English speakers and US citizenship.

In 1983, I began to study family therapy as part of a PhD program in sociology. This was pure luck! Since then, I have focused on how the larger societal context operates in the moment-by-moment of therapy. New collaborators in each place I worked (Montana, Georgia, Southern California, and Oregon) stretched my thinking, and a diverse range of students and clients gave me windows into their worlds. As a White, monogamous cisgender, heterosexual temporarily able-bodied wife, mother, and grandmother, I am continually humbled by the limits of my understanding and the ease with which I am usually able to walk through this world. Yet I regularly witness the effects of societal inequalities. To me, promoting equitable relationships is both an ethical and clinical issue. Grappling with the intricacies of this work with Teresa and Maria has been exceedingly challenging and enriching. Despite ongoing assaults to the dignity, health, and well-being of all people and families, I am optimistic and uplifted by the burgeoning socioculturally attuned work in family therapy and elsewhere. Our shared efforts will always be an important work in progress.

Maria

I have been a couple and family therapist for over 30 years, and I consider myself a "purist." I graduated from two COAMFTE (Commission on Accreditation for Marriage and Family Therapy Education) graduate programs and have taught in two COAMFTE graduate programs. My studies have been strongly rooted in academic departments of human development and family science. What initially drew me to the field of family therapy was the non-pathologizing focus. Simple enough. But what fascinated me was the way in which family therapists think. I enjoy examining the multiple contexts of people's lives and seeing complex processes as they unfold. I greatly value all the family therapy theories and models, but being from Honduras, I was especially drawn to ideas that reflected my collectivistic, communal, and collaborative values, such as with postmodern and social constructionist approaches to family therapy.

Nonetheless, I did not fully immerse myself in diversity studies until I started teaching an undergraduate course called "Gender Roles across the Lifespan." I taught the course every semester for five years. It was life-changing, and learning from my colleagues in Women's Studies was enlightening and empowering. Learning critical theories helped me examine how structural, systemic, and relational dynamics shape our identities, social locations, and lived experiences. Learning from feminist scholars profoundly altered the way I integrated family studies and family therapy models and theories into the different aspects of my work. It was a paradigm shift that expanded my worldview and pushed me to deepen my understanding of diversity, social justice, and equity—professionally and personally.

I remember first being aware of disparities at a young age. Although I am from Honduras, I was mostly raised in Texas. During my childhood and adolescence, my mother and I would return to Honduras to see my father and my family there. We went four times; at age 4, 11, 15, and 19. Each time was impactful for me, especially given that this travel occurred during different stages of my development. Not only was it strange for me when people fussed over my fair skin and light blue eyes (awareness of my White privilege), I was extremely unsettled by seeing young children in the street, begging for money, selling gum and candy, and staring into the windows of the restaurants where we ate (awareness of my class privilege). It was confusing, and no one explained to me what was happening. I wasn't exposed to this in the US. Although my family in Honduras and the US was mostly "working" middle class, as I got older, I developed a sincere and deep gratitude and appreciation for our privileges. We had a house, reliable and consistent electricity, food, clean water, washing machines, a reliable postal system, good public education, new clothes and shoes, and a peaceful way of life. In 1970, we did not immigrate in the context of fleeing persecution or escaping violence, or financial distress. Instead, my mother, who learned to speak English in school and worked in an office as an accountant, brought us to the US for a "better way of life." My father, who was well regarded for his work as an auto mechanic, did not want to immigrate, but he conceded because of the opportunities that were not available for us there. Although I could not name what I knew, early in my life I learned about the effects of immigration, transnational families, colorism, language fluency, colonization, heteronormativity, and mixed documentation status.

What I later learned through my studies is that this "better way of life" is not accessible to everyone in the same way in the US or anywhere. The structural barriers and the trajectories of cumulative advantage and disadvantage lay the groundwork for the ways in which the "American dream" can be accessed and lived. The course of my life was altered by immigration, as it is for so many of us, almost all of us in the US. Although I am the only one of my siblings to obtain a college degree, largely due to their support and sacrifices, I would not have been in the position to influence others in the way I do today if my mother had not been in a position to change the course of our lives. As a consequence, I am greatly humbled and honored to co-author this book with Teresa McDowell and Carmen Knudson-Martin. I sincerely hope that how we describe our theorizing and apply our critical lenses to the practice of family therapy will help you, the reader of this text, critically evaluate and attune with a sense of urgency to the factors that shape our lives and our ways of working. It is time for another paradigm shift!

In Conclusion

Stepping out of what is familiar and trying something new takes a special mix of courage, excitement, and humility. As authors putting forth the new ideas in this and our last two texts, we have been immersed in that mix. We pass our work on to you now with the hope that you will have the courage to both use and challenge our ideas, that you will bear the humility of not always doing equity-based family therapy "right," and that you will join in our excitement about the future of our field.

References

Ross, L. (2019). I'ma black feminist. I think call-out culture is toxic. *The New York Times*, *17*, 1–2.
Ross, L. J. (2025). *Calling In: How to Start Making Change with Those You'd Rather Cancel*. Simon and Schuster.

Acknowledgements

We love this field and hold deep respect for all the family therapists and social scientists who advanced systems/relational thinking and practice before us. We would like to acknowledge the work of the many, many family therapy, family studies, psychology, social work, counseling, sociology, critical geography, public health, philosophy, education, history, global studies, and legal scholars, as well as others we reference throughout this text. Their collective efforts to understand and improve human relationships and societal conditions are incalculable. It is our privilege to build on their work as we simultaneously challenge ourselves to trust our own voices and experience. We set for ourselves a delicate balance between getting concepts "right" and telling the family therapy story through our own lens.

Along our different journeys, each of us was transformed by critical, feminist, and social constructionist scholars and activists. As the three of us discussed the third edition of this book and what it might accomplish, we continued to speak of the courage of our founders to question and transform the assumptions, practices, and ethics of mainstream mental health treatment; the wisdom of Bateson and other systemic thinkers who helped us see individual consciousness and behavior as part of a much larger whole; and the strength of the many feminist, anti-racist, LGBTQ+, and decolonising family therapists who have said, "enough!" In this new version of the text, we turn to those who are currently engaged in transformative work who share their voices—their experience and wisdom—by contributing to the text. We are deeply grateful, inspired, and informed by their praxes.

We are also deeply honored and grateful for the generative and equity-based work of Dr. Anne Prouty, who graciously agreed to write the foreword for this version of our text. She has been inspirational as a leader in diversity and social equity in family therapy, particularly through her devotion to inspiring socially just practices among the next generation of family therapists. Dr. Prouty has advanced the field of family therapy with research and writing on feminist-informed research, practice, and supervision. She continues to shape and influence graduate students to work at the highest level of rigor and integrity. Thank you, Anne, for writing the foreword for our book.

Each of us would like to acknowledge a few of those who supported us through the writing of this third edition. I, Teresa, would like to thank my children Flynn, Quentin, and Rob, and their partners, Alice, Lauren, and Janelle, for their support, including ongoing conversations that inspire new ways of thinking. I also want to thank my grandchildren Rooney, Ewan, Nina, Adina, Will, Elizabeth, and Lindsey, along with their children and future children who keep me active, engaged, and ever hopeful.

I, Carmen, thank colleagues Lana Kim, Jessica ChenFeng, and Olga Smoliak who continue to push me to further detail the processes of learning and practicing socioculturally attuned family therapy and the SERT model. I channel every day the lessons learned about working hard for what matters from my parents Phoebe and Nels Knudson. I am grateful to my husband John for understanding the life of a scholar-practitioner and his steadfast support. My children Chris and Kyara and their partners Melanie and Jerome continue to give me purpose and perspective, while my grandsons Ethan and Kai remind me why working toward a socially just future is so important. Thank you all for your love—and for reminding me to keep the fun and pleasure in living!

I, Maria, would first like to acknowledge my first professor in family therapy, Dr. Joe Wetcher. It is because of him that I fell in love with family therapy models and theories. I always hear him say, "If you are stuck with clients, then ground yourself in theory." You taught me to think critically, theorize, and have informed opinions. And thank you to my incredible community of brilliant feminist scholars who inspire me and remind me to stand in my power, especially Drs. Lorna Hecker (my first feminist professor and mentor who guided me in my first research project and encouraged me to publish), Anne Prouty, Katherine Allen, Elizabeth Sharp, Christi McGeorge, Desiree Seponski, Bertranna Muruthi, Luis Alvarez-Hernandez, Fausto Gomez-Lamont, Anisa Zvonkovic, and April Few-Demo, as well as colleagues, students, therapists, and activists, who, wearily, day in and day out, fight the good fight, doing the work of social and relational justice as *luchadoras en la justicia social*. And to my *bella familia*—my parents, Judith and Rene Perez, my devoted and loving husband, Romulo "Ronnie" Rama, to our amazing children, their partners, and our grandchildren. To my loving siblings and their spouses, my nephews and nieces, and their spouses and children. And to my dear lifelong friends… You know who you are. You all are my anchors and continuous source of support, joy, love, light, and encouragement. Thank you! I love you with all my heart and soul. And to the readers of this text, thank you for wanting to learn, grow, and walk on this journey with us as compassionate, committed agents of change. It's the only way forward.

Finally, we would like to thank each other (Teresa, Carmen, and Maria) for our unwavering support, professional collaboration, and friendship. We are not only colleagues, but through this journey, we have become sister-scholars. It is through the synergy of coming together to talk, listen, laugh, rage, challenge, question, and affirm that we were able to create, examine, and share the ideas presented in this book. For this, we are eternally grateful!

Contributors

We are deeply honored by, and grateful to our colleagues who have contributed to the second edition of our book (listed alphabetically). They are champions of third order thinking and change in family therapy and their respective disciplines.

Rhea V. Almeida, PhD, LCSW, developed the Cultural Context Model and has been a leader in liberation-based practice for more than four decades. She is also the director and founder of the Institute for Family Services. (Contributor of Text Box 2.4)

Tim Baima, PhD, LMFT, is in private practice in San Mateo, CA. He specializes in culturally sensitive relationship therapy, with interests in Whiteness, self-of-the-therapist training, and family play therapy. (Contributor of Text Boxes 3.1, 7.1 & 8.2)

Saliha Bava, PhD, LMFT, is a professor and MFT Program Director at Mercy University in New York and does private practice and organizational consultation. (Contributor of Text Box 13.1)

Stephanie Brooks, PhD, LCSW, LMFT, is the inaugural Dean of the College of Health at Cleveland State University. Her interests include MFT education and training, supervision, ADHD in Black couples, trauma, depression and addiction, and leadership. (Contributor of Text Box 10.1)

Jessica ChenFeng, PhD, LMFT, is Associate Professor of Marriage and Family Therapy & DMFT Program Chair at Fuller University in Pasadena, CA. Her interests include social contextual issues such as race, gender, migration, and spirituality. (Contributor of Text Box 16.5)

Manijeh Daneshpour, PhD, LMFT, is a professor and systemwide director of the Alliant International University Marriage and Family Therapy Programs. Her interests include issues of multiculturalism, social justice, third wave feminism. (Contributor of Text Box 16.2)

Justine D'Arrigo, PhD, is an associate professor at California State University San Bernardino. Their interests include the intersections of relational activism and therapy, navigating critical theory and poststructuralism, post-oppositional approaches to relationships and change, and exploring compositionism and curiosity in therapy. (Contributor of Text Boxes 1.2 & 13.2)

Elisabeth Esmiol Wilson, PhD, LMFT, is an AASECT-certified sex therapist, AAMFT-approved supervisor, and trained spiritual director. Her interests focus on socially just approaches to integrating couple therapy, sex therapy, and spirituality. (Contributor of Text Box 8.1)

Mario Fausto Gómez Lamont, PhD, is a licensed psychologist, practicing family therapist, and faculty member at the School of Higher Studies Iztacala of the National Autonomous University of Mexico (UNAM). He is part of the network of specialists in Gender Studies and Feminism at the Center for Research and Gender Studies at UNAM. (Contributor of Text Box 16.7)

Peter Fraenkel, PhD, licensed psychologist and associate professor at City University New York (CUNY). His reflections in this text are drawn from years of work with his graduate students at CUNY in which they developed, implemented, and evaluated a program for families living in homeless shelters. (Contributor of Text Box 13.3)

Marisol Garcia-Westberg, PhD, LMFT, is an experienced family therapy educator who is currently in private practice providing sex therapy. She has published numerous articles on equity, social justice, and activism. (Contributor of Text Box 3.3)

Shawn V. Giammattei, PhD, is a clinical psychologist with a group family therapy practice in California. He is the Associate Director of Mental Health for the Child and Adolescent Gender Center at UCSF, Benioff Children's Hospital, and founder of the Gender Health Training Institute and the TransFamily Alliance. He is a WPATH certified gender specialist and mentor. (Contributor of Text Box 14.2)

Lana Kim, PhD, LMFT, is an associate professor and program director of the MCFT program at Lewis & Clark College in Portland, OR. Her work has focused on culture and cultural identity, gender, couples therapy and parent–child relationships. (Contributor of Text Box 1.1)

Iva Košutić, PhD, is a scholar and social researcher. She is the author of numerous publications that support social equity and activism in, and beyond, family studies and family therapy. Much of her current work involves evaluation of social and health programs. (Contributor of Text Box 16.8)

Quentin R. McDowell, MA, is the Head of Mercersburg Academy, an independent secondary school in Pennsylvania. His work has primarily focused on educational leadership and organizational transformation. (Contributor of Text Box 16.4)

Hoa Nguyen, PhD, is an associate professor at Valdosta State University in Georgia. Her work draws from her Vietnamese immigrant family history of resettlement and rebuilding home in the United States post-Vietnam War. (Contributor of Text Box 2.3)

Elizabeth Oshrin Parker, PhD, is a family therapist and researcher. She has done research on a variety of topics including complex trauma, effects of discrimination on mental health, and quantitative research methodologies. (Contributor of Text Box 11.1)

Marcela Polanco is a Spanglish, Colombiana-Spanish and Immigrant-English speaker. She is interested in decolonial projects, including those that do not depend on the decolonial framework to address colonial power in everyday life. She is faculty at San Diego State University located in unceded territory of the Kumeyaay. (Contributor of Text Box 2.1)

Mudita Rastogi, PhD, LMFT, has an abiding interest in systemic intervention, gender, diversity, equity and inclusion, race, culture, ethnicity, multiculturalism, diasporas, global mental health, South Asian families, trauma, and intergenerational relationships. (Contributor of Text Box 2.2)

Fatma Arıcı Şahin, PhD, is an assistant professor at Kastamonu University in northern Turkey, with interests in couple and family therapy, feminism and gender studies, art therapy and creativity. (Contributor of Text Boxes 7.2 & 15.2)

Laurel Salmon, MS, LMFT, is the owner and operator of Ask Laurel, a mental health practice based in Nyack, NY, where she provides trauma-informed, socially just therapy and consulting services for youth, families, and adults. Laurel is also an adjunct professor in the Marriage and Family Therapy program at Mercy College. (Contributor of Text Box 14.1)

Dana Stone, PhD, LMFT, is an associate professor at Southern California State University in Northridge. Her work focuses on the multiracial experience and supporting early career therapists with marginalized aspects of identity in navigating the field of marriage and family therapy and counseling. (Contributor of Text Boxes 3.2 & 16.3)

Sally St. George, PhD, is Professor Emerita in the Faculty of Social Work at the University of Calgary. She is currently developing a new phase of professional life primarily focused on supporting others as they develop their work. (Contributor of Text Box 16.9)

William Turner, PhD, LMFT, serves as Distinguished Professor of Psychology and Family Therapy and Special Counsel to the President at Lipscomb University, Nashville, TN. His teaching and research interests are focused on African American family strengths and the intersections of hope, justice, policy, and faith. (Contributor of Text Boxes 5.1, 16.1, & 16.6)

Man-Tso Wei 魏滿佐 is a social work practitioner serving a diverse clientele at Earth Circles Counseling Center in Oakland, California. Informed by his Taiwanese heritage and queer identity, he is interested in how relational and societal processes impact individual and social belonging and well-being. (Contributor of Text Box 15.1)

Dan Wulff, PhD, is Professor Emeritus at the Faculty of Social Work, at the University of Calgary. He now invests in reading all those books he intended to read for many years and is writing about the things he most wants to write about. (Contributor of Text Box 16.9)

Toni Schindler Zimmerman PhD, LMFT, is a professor in the Human Development and Family Studies Department at Colorado State University. She has been acknowledged for excellence in community engagement and much of her work has focused on diversity, equity, and social justice. (Contributor of Text Box 12.1)

1 Socioculturally Attuned Family Therapy

Interconnecting cultural, economic, political, social, and environmental systems affect every aspect of daily life—how and where we live and die; what we have access to; our level of autonomy and respect; the influence we can bring to bear on others; the breadth of choices we have; our sense of value, safety, and security; our health and life expectancy; and the dynamics of our most intimate relationships (Browning & van Eeden-Moorefield, 2022; Knudson-Martin, 2024). These systems are mutually reinforcing in ways that maintain uneven landscapes that privilege some over others while also being in flux, at times yielding to transformative change.

↞↠

Attention to equity is vital to the practice of family therapy because unjust social and interpersonal relationships create and/or exacerbate mental health symptoms and relationship problems.

↞↠

Why Third Order Thinking is Important

Throughout this text, we refer to and expand our ideas about third order thinking (McDowell, 2015; McDowell et al., 2018, 2019, 2022) to illustrate why it is critical to attend to the larger societal context and issues of equity in therapy and to provide practical guidelines for doing so. Our job as therapists who prioritize client care and improving the lives of those with whom we work necessarily includes encouraging relational values of reciprocity, mutuality, and fairness as couples and families interact with each other (Knudson-Martin & Kim, 2023). The actions we take based on these shared values require awareness of our own positionality and accountability for how we conceptualize relationships and clinical concerns within sociocultural contexts (Lini & Bertrando, 2022).

Practicing from a third order perspective is more than making a choice to take a position. Supporting relational equity is a practical matter that must be considered in order for family therapy to be effective and successful (Knudson-Martin, 2013). There is no way to claim neutrality while working with the mental health and relational consequences of inequity. We either work to change oppressive dynamics or we help clients accept and adjust to what is unjust. In other words, failing to notice and/or to act can make us complicit in what is harmful and unjust, inadvertently helping to maintain inequity (Piercy, 2020; Watson et al., 2020). According to Watson et al., (2020):

> Given the fact that family therapists may unwittingly function as the best ally of an economic and political system that perpetuates institutionalized racism and class discrimination, we need to utilize a set of principles, values, and practices that are not just palliative or after the

DOI: 10.4324/9781003493426-1

> fact but bring forth into the psychotherapeutic and policy work a politics of care. Therefore, a strong call to promote and advocate for the broader continuum of health and critical thinking, preparing professionals to meet the challenges of health equity, as well as economic and environmental justice, is needed. (p. 832)

Our charge as systemic family therapists is to promote the health and well-being of all clients, across all sociocultural contexts. Third order, equity-based practice relies on our ability to situate problems within comprehensive contextual frameworks that include both common and idiosyncratic societal, systemic, and relational dynamics. Taking a multi-ocular view allows us to recognize institutionalized systems of privilege and oppression (e.g., racism, sexism, patriarchy, homophobia), alongside unique social positions (e.g., social class, positional status) and relational dynamics (e.g., differing levels of investment in the relationship, histories of relational injuries, the impact of adverse childhood experiences) that create and maintain power imbalances within relationships.

Family Therapy and Societal Context: A Brief Historical Overview

Over time, culture and societal context has become increasingly accepted as foundational to understanding and treating families (Falicov, 2015; Ho et al., 2004; McGoldrick et al., 2005; Piercy, 2020). Early family therapists were rebels who used new systemic perspectives and actually involved family members in therapy. Family therapy models emerged that were separate and unique from those in psychology and social work. As the field developed, so did ideas about cultural and societal context (Hair et al., 1996). Auerswald (1971) was one of the first to develop an ecosystemic approach to families, integrating community systems into practice. Early on in the development of structural family therapy, Minuchin and colleagues (1967) recognized the impact of poverty, discrimination, and oppression on family well-being. While not always practiced with the broader context in mind, structural family therapy's origins in structural functionalism encourage us to conceptualize the family as a social institution in systemic interaction with other social institutions. This includes an understanding of the potential impact of extra-familial forces and stressors on family roles and power dynamics.

Aponte (1976) built on these larger systems ideas, developing an eco-structural approach to working with families in the context of their communities. Others, including Wynne (1967) and Keeney (1979), argued for an ecosystemic epistemology that links open systems at individual, family, community, societal, and environmental levels (Hair et al., 1996). Imber-Black (1992) described families as part of multiple embedded systems within society. The feminist movement (e.g., Hare-Mustin, 1978; Luepnitz, 1988; Walters et al., 1988) shattered the view of families as apolitical, reciprocal systems by connecting intimate interaction to power dynamics in the broader society.

The argument that family therapists are in a position to create positive social change and should intentionally promote social equity is also not new. For example, in 1988 Goodrich et al. wrote:

> Whether intended or not, [family therapy's] impact on individual families … leads to an impact on our collective social life… This influence serves either to support or to change prevailing structures of belief and action regarding family life. Those of us who want this influence to be in the direction of changing prevailing structures must work to reform fundamental aspects of our professional field. (p. 180)

Several approaches routinely conceptualize and intervene across multiple systems in ways that support social and relational equity. Korin (1994) argued that critical conversations, based on the work of Paulo Freire, could be used to create emancipatory change. According to Freire (1970/2000), critical consciousness, or *conscientização*, can be raised through dialogue and reflection, which in turn leads to informed action. Social psychologist, Martín-Baró, along with his colleagues (1994, p. 40), built on this tradition arguing that "people must take hold of their fate, take the reins of their lives, a move that demands overcoming false consciousness and achieving a critical understanding of themselves as well as of their world and where they stand in it."

Rhea Almeida and colleagues (2007; 2018; in press) developed the cultural context model, which has been at the forefront of practice that helps clients better solve problems by understanding how societal systems affect their relationships. This approach is well known for using therapist-facilitated healing circles in which clients across societal contexts work together to raise each other's awareness of social positionality and coloniality in order to move toward empowerment and accountability. As early as 1994, Almeida began broadening the concept of intersectionality to include gender, race, class, sexual orientation and LGBTQ, abilities, and other identities. Charles Waldegrave, Kiwi Tamases, Flora Tuhaka, and Warihi Campbell (2003) have also been leaders in equity-based practice via their just therapy model that places context at the core of relational well-being. Just therapy and Narrative Family Therapy (White & Epstein, 1990) share roots in social constructionism. Societal context is highly relevant in these approaches as dominant social discourses shape not only how we think about ourselves, but how we interact with and think about others—the meaning we assign to all experience through language.

Feminist family therapy (Hare-Mustin, 1978; Prouty Lyness & Lyness, 2007; Silverstein & Goodrich, 2003) and socio-emotional relationship therapy (Knudson-Martin, 2024) are examples of approaches that regularly pay attention to how culture and societal systems create and maintain relational power imbalances that in turn create individual and relational symptoms. From as far back as 1998, McGoldrick and colleagues called for revisioning family therapy to address the effects of cultural, racial, sexual, and class-based inequity on families. The Galveston Declaration was developed in 2016 (Gosnell et al., 2017) to explore the transformation of family therapy toward values of pluralism, flux, opening space, and responsibility. Among other things, these values embrace multiple social realities, cultures and contexts, the emergence of new identities, restorative justice, and collective accountability.

In recent years, the field of family therapy has seen a burgeoning number of contributions to equity-based practice and calls for social action. These include understanding intersectionality (Almeida & Tubbs, 2020), centering decolonizing practices (Almeida & Williams, 2026), engaging in advocacy (Hodgson & Lamson, 2020; Holyoak et al., 2021), attending to global power dynamics and the impacts of war and collective trauma (Glebova & Knudson-Martin, 2023; Rastogi, 2021), working towards racial equity (Hardy, 2024; Watson, 2019), supporting Black Lives Matter (Kelly et al., 2020; Watson et al., 2020) and anti-racist practice (Kaslow et al., 2024), addressing collective legacies of trauma (Lee et al., 2023; Watson, 2024), engaging in transgender and gender diverse-inclusive therapy (Boe & Baldwin, 2023), advocating for LGBT-affirmative clinical training (McGeorge et al., 2018; McGeorge et al., 2021), reconceptualizing and queer-conceptualizing family therapy (Hartwell & Edwards, 2026), recognizing the impact of social determinants of health (Tambling et al., 2021; Waite & Nardi, 2024), and acknowledging the impact of climate change (Laszloffy & Twist, 2019; Watson et al., 2020). This movement has led to family therapists increasingly embracing the importance of developing their own critical consciousness, challenging dynamics of oppression, and advocating for social and relational equity (Golojuch et al., 2025).

Understanding of the processes by which larger contexts influence people's everyday experience and well-being is growing more nuanced. For example, studies of the sociopolitical nature of emotion show that power processes influence both *what* we feel and *whose* feelings are deemed to merit attention and care (Smoliak et al., 2022b). Attuning to the sociopolitical context of clients' emotion helps strengthen the therapeutic bond and makes visible complex interactions between power, vulnerability, and relational processes (Knudson-Martin et al., 2021). At the same time, practicing empathy can reinforce power differences if "helpers" assume their understanding is "true" without recognising that clients may accommodate the therapist and the process of therapy or without being accountable to how power is negotiated in the clinical setting (Smoliak & Knudson-Martin, under review).

Recent frameworks for considering the effects of sociocultural forces on daily lives recognize that the social structures that maintain racial, gender, sexual, and economic inequities (among others) interact with and support each other, and are *also* experienced and created (or recreated) personally as we interact with others (Bava, 2023; Falicov, 2014). As McDowell (2015) described, "while deeply influenced by macro embedded power dynamics, individuals within relationships still have choices and consider immediate local consequences of these choices" (p. 7). Though there is a tendency to see social locations as essential, stereotypic contexts, therapists must take a process view, looking at changes across time and place and complexities in how social identities are practiced (Hartwell & Edwards, 2026). For example, expressions of "soft" masculinities (e.g., showing feelings, vulnerability) in couple therapy sessions may collude with sexism to still maintain male dominance (Smoliak et al., 2022a).

Therapists are called to examine the coexistence and tensions between power and collaboration in clinical practice (Knudson-Martin, 2024; Ong, et al., 2023) and be responsible for the effects of their inevitable influence (Lini & Bertrando, 2022). A process view of how people interact with sociocultural contexts helps therapists be aware of the political (power) aspects of what we say and do. Therapists are called to develop stories of resistance as well as dominance, and "lean into the discomfort of uncertainty" so as to expand who and what is credited with knowledge and disrupt the influence of otherwise taken-for-granted power structures (Bava, 2023, p. 49).

Family Therapy in our Current Societal Context

No profession is separate from the larger societal contexts in which it practices and evolves. Today, in the third decade of the twenty-first century, the work of family therapy is profoundly impacted by fragmented social, political, economic, and physical environments that support some more than others, even as it becomes increasingly clear that well-being across all levels of life is interconnected (Argüello, 2023; Brock, et al., 2023). Four aspects of this context are especially relevant to socioculturally attuned family therapy: social isolation, individualism and the distant other, social inequities, and polarization—all of which have a substantial impact on health and well-being.

Social Isolation

In 2023, the US Surgeon General issued an advisory that identified loneliness as a serious public health issue due to its negative impact on physical and mental health (US Surgeon General's Advisory on the Healing Effects of Social Connection and Community 2023). The advisory pointed to structure, function, and quality as three core components of social connection. Structure refers to the number and variety of relationships we have, as well as how often we interact. Function refers to the degree to which our various needs are met by our relationships. Quality refers to the positive and negative aspects of our interactions with others. While all of these components are embedded in the practice of family therapy, the Surgeon General's call highlighted the connection between relational, physical, mental, communal, and societal well-being.

Across the world, the happiest and healthiest people prioritize relationships (Waldinger & Schulz, 2023); yet the surgeon general's analysis revealed that forming relationships is much more than an individual endeavor. It identified the need to develop "cultures of connection" that support relationships, including societal level factors such as how cities and greenspaces are laid out, how institutional policies shape everyday life, and how health care services are provided and researched. While loneliness and isolation have been increasing, the report found some groups more at risk than others, and that supports to nurture relationships and connectedness are not equitably available.

Individualism and the Distant Other

Most parts of the world report declines in social connectedness (Howe, 2023). What are particularly problematic are the individualistic assumptions that organize Western cultures and undermine relational values and resources—from within our most intimate relationships, to the workplace, social policies, and institutionalized practices (Bava & Greene, 2023, Jordan, 2022). This individualistic mindset shapes how problems are defined, studied, and addressed, reducing contextual matters to the individual level (Bermúdez et al., 2016; Wetzel, 2024). It is related to positivistic ontologies that favor knowledge derived from discrete objectified, quantified components that can be measured, rather than nuanced, interconnected socio-relational processes. This mindset, which distances practitioners from the people they serve, undergirds most current mental health practices, including couple and family therapy (Jordan, 2022; Wetzel, 2024, Whiting et al., 2024). With its systemic foundation and emphasis on working with relational processes, family therapy offers an expanded way to approach clinical practice. Yet, like mental health services more broadly, many therapists drift away from their systemic training, drawing instead on individualizing language and "empirical" concerns (Wetzel, 2024; Whiting et al., 2024).

The dominance of individualism obscures awareness of and responsiveness to how we are connected to our physical and socio-relational environments (Siegel & Drulis, 2023; Watson et al., 2020). It leads clients and therapists alike to view relationship matters as competing individual concerns and perspectives while de-emphasizing responsibilities to one another and our collective worlds (Fishbane, 2023; Knudson-Martin, 2025; Whiting et al., 2024). Socioculturally attuned therapists must be aware that atomistic thinking associated with White, heteropatriarchal Western culture was built into the concepts and professional ideals adopted by the family therapy field (Bermúdez et al., 2016; Jordan, 2022). We must look beyond the individual and family to include the larger society, a wider range of knowledge, and an ethic of care (Argüello, 2023; Knudson-Martin, 2024; Watson et al., 2020), while helping families serve as sites of belonging and healing in face of social inequities, stigma, and alienation (Hartwell & Edwards, 2026).

Social Inequities

Mounting research points to the impact of social, cultural, commercial, economic, political, and environmental contexts on our physical, mental, and relational health (Adler et al., 2016; Alves-Bradford et al., 2020; Mialon, 2020; Watson et al., 2020). These factors are typically referred to as social determinants of health. According to the US Department of Health and Human Services (*Healthy People 2030*), "social determinants of health (SDOH) are the conditions in the environments where people are born, live, learn, work, play, worship and age that affect a wide range of health functioning, and quality-of-life outcomes and risks." SDOH are most typically grouped into five domains: economic stability, education access and quality, health care access and quality, neighborhood and built environment, and social and community context.

Structural determinants of health refer to the mechanisms and power dynamics that are at the root of these inequitable conditions. These include laws and policies, governance, institutional practices, and worldviews, beliefs, values, and cultural norms (Heller et al., 2024). According to Heller and colleagues (p. 357), "structural determinants are derived from dominant societal values, beliefs and worldviews; reflect our histories; and can dynamically adapt to perpetuate—or disrupt—historical patterns of advantage and disadvantage." Social and structural determinants are produced and maintained by multiple interconnecting social, political, and economic factors that produce and maintain inequality and inequity. The results are stark contrasts in working and living conditions: gated communities vs. barred windows, private vs. public transportation, high-end grocery stores vs. food deserts, quiet vs. loud environments; long work hours in harsh environments vs. safe and comfortable work spaces; clean air vs. smog, lowland flooding vs. homes with a view, policing to protect vs. policing to control, concrete surroundings vs. natural landscapes, homes near outdoor malls and parks vs. homes near factories and trash dumps, and choice of provider vs. inadequate and fragmented public healthcare and services.

As family therapists, we tend to conceive of mental health and relational well-being as a matter of interconnected internal (e.g., cognitive, neurobiological) and relational (e.g., patterns of interaction, attachment) systems that are situated in longitudinal (e.g., families of origin, legacies of trauma) and latitudinal (e.g., societal positionality, social discourses) frameworks. While these ways of thinking are highly contextual in many ways, they can lead us to underestimate the significance of material realities and physical space (Cashin, 2014; McDowell, 2015; Soja, 2010). Likewise, we may not recognize the impact of SDOH on clients' abilities to seek and/or participate in treatment (Tambling et al., 2021).

•←→•

What we are calling *socio-relational* determinants of health refers to the impact of social and structural determinants on the interconnections between physical health, mental health, and relational well-being. Attuning to socio-relational determinants of health is central to our work as family therapists.

•←→•

While families are recognized as part of the social community and context, there has been little attention paid to the relationship between social structures, SDOH, and families. According to Deatrick (2017, p. 424), "the family is not typically theoretically justified and identified as central to social determinants of health." Yet, for those of us who work with families, the role close relationships can play in mitigating or exacerbating the effects of SDOH seems obvious. In fact, families and other important relationships play a significant role in amplifying and/or diminishing the positive and negative impacts of social determinants of health (Bergeron et al., 2020; Brock et al., 2023; Deatrick 2017). When family relationships are organized in ways that are isomorphic to unjust societal systems and structures (e.g., power-over relationships, male dominance), it can exacerbate the effects of discrimination and oppression on less powerful family members. On the other hand, when family members are able to socioculturally attune to each other, they are better able to resist and mitigate societal inequities and negative effects of social and structural determinants of health. In other words, when family members are aware of social structures and conditions that put them at risk, they are often better able to work together to navigate and buffer the effects. Relational inequities within families may compound and/or create negative determinants of health.

Polarization

Like the effects of isolation, ultra-individualism, and social inequities, increasing partisan polarization is further impacting physical, mental, and relational health (Fraser et al., 2022). There is evidence that polarization has led to an increase in stress, anxiety, and fatigue (Yousafzai, 2022), physical illness (Fraser et al., 2022), and relational conflict (Warner et al., 2021). While most families have found ways to navigate partisan differences, many others report mild to severe disruptions in their relationships. According to Yu and colleagues (2024), political incongruence and disagreements can create in-group vs out-group dynamics within families. Differences can also lead to family members making moral judgements about each other, even in the most everyday situations (Yu et al., 2024). There is also an affective component of polarization—an emotional dislike for the "other" (Kleinfeld, 2023). These dynamics may lead to difficulties accommodating and respecting differences in values and identity (Warner et al., 2021). Likewise, political differences may cause decreases in relational closeness, as well as greater conflict and stress—all leading to decreases in relational resilience (Afifi et al., 2020).

As family therapists, our concern is less about where individuals and families fall on the contemporary spectrum of political beliefs and more about the effects extreme partisanship, truth and morality stances, and polarization have on family and community relationships. This said, we recognize the very real impact of marginalization and discrimination that stems from and is supported by some politically fueled beliefs and practices. Social justice and identity politics are more than political differences to be debated, particularly for those who are routinely suffering the consequences of attempts to have their identities erased; living with constant threat of physical, emotional, and relational harm; enduring the cruel effects of not belonging in families and communities; and facing ongoing discrimination. Likewise, political and social ideologies that justify racial discrimination fuel the ever-growing chasm between the rich and the poor, exacerbating historically unequal access to achieving The American Dream (Armstrong et al., 2019). It can be difficult at times to navigate our complex contemporary landscape, remaining committed to social and relational equity without getting swept up and caught off balance by political diatribes.

While supporting social and relational equity is foundational to socioculturally attuned practice, we must also pay attention to our own potential to become polarized and moralizing in a political climate that seemingly demands us to choose "one side or the other." This includes the importance of checking our own, sometimes elitist—even "othering"—attitudes and beliefs by interrogating the role these play in maintaining inequitable social and economic systems. As socioculturally attuned therapists, it is important to recognize partisan polarization among ourselves and within the families we serve as situated within a much broader context of national and international power dynamics, including the relationship between income inequality and polarization (Gu & Wang, 2022). This allows us to better position ourselves to attune to each other and our clients and to help clients attune to each other in ways that can increase acceptance, understanding, and connectedness. We must guard against becoming polarized ourselves and challenge polarization between professional disciplines. In the words of Lorås and colleagues (2023),

> Failure to adopt an attitude of respect and humility toward our adjacent professional fields when cultivating our own preferred approach could result in an unproductive dichotomy. This might mean becoming too comfortable in our own camp, and at worst, believing in our own superiority. (p. 494)

What is Socioculturally Attuned Family Therapy?

What we have called *socioculturally attuned family therapy* (sometimes referred to as SCAFT), is a set of transtheoretical considerations that can inform new family therapy models and be integrated into existing ones. We use the term *sociocultural* to describe interconnections of societal systems, culture, and power. This includes not only shared meanings that define culture, but the dynamic interplay between societal systems that privilege some over others, resulting in uneven influence and opportunities based on social class, gender, race, ethnicity, language, sexual orientation, age, nation of origin, abilities, looks, and so on. Patterns that occur at individual, relational, and societal levels are recursive and continuous vs. discrete and unilateral. In other words, families impact community and society and vice versa.

Consider an example of a middle-class family that is eager to ensure their children excel in school, stand out in athletics and music, and demonstrate qualities of prosocial leadership. These efforts are aimed at maintaining or improving the social class of the next generation. This in turn reinforces the values, ideology, and cultural practices of those with the greatest influence in societal institutions to set these norms, e.g., those who are in positions to grant college scholarships and offer employment. In other words, the interconnection between societal systems, culture, and power supports hegemony, i.e., dominant cultural group control over major societal systems. Left uninterrupted, the routine practices, rules, and values of societal systems (e.g., education, government, professional associations, commerce) continue to benefit those with the greatest social influence.

↔

Sociocultural attunement refers not only to awareness of societal systems, culture, and power but to a willingness to pay close attention and be responsive to the experience of others.

↔

The worldview of those in non-dominant groups is often marginalized, creating what Fricker (2007) termed epistemic injustice. This includes those in centered, dominant groups routinely devaluing or dismissing the testimony of those in marginalized groups (Tatum, 1997). This is, of course, a central and intended outcome of colonial processes. Decolonizing practices re-center the expression, value, and locality of these lived experiences and collective ways of knowing (Almeida & Williams, 2026; Bermúdez et al., in review; Smoliak & Knudson-Martin, in review). Attunement infers being with others, bearing witness to their testimony, and helping them make meaning of their lived/social experience. This requires therapists to be acutely aware of colonial dynamics of which they are a part of by nature of their training, practice contexts, and cultural history. It is important to recognize the limits of our abilities to fully attune or "be at one" with clients. Attunement is not a single act, or reachable goal. It is an ongoing moment-to-moment process that occurs within the context of relationships.

Notice in Text Box 1.1 how Lana Kim describes attuning to clients within sociocultural context. Her description reflects the type of empathy and care toward others that is evident in contributions throughout this text. As Dr. Kim has expressed elsewhere (Kim et al., 2022), critical contextual consciousness and movement toward social justice require a relational approach. In other words, taking a critical sociocultural stance and being critical of others based on our evaluation of their social awareness are very different positions, with the latter contributing to an "us and them" relational framework that creates polarization rather than equity and inclusion.

Text Box 1.1 Lana Kim, PhD, LMFT

Lana Kim (she/her) is an associate professor and program director of MCFT at Lewis & Clark in Portland, OR. She identifies as a second generation Korean Canadian, cishet woman.

My teaching, clinical work, and scholarship seek to decenter dominant White, individualistic, middle class, cishet discourses and illuminate the ways in which these are privileged in our social structures and consequently marginalize other realities. I situate therapeutic problems in the context of who clients are and the inequitable societal ideologies and structures that produce problems. I seek to help trainees and clients draw these connections conceptually as well as translate these awarenesses into new relational ways of being with themselves and others.

I tend to conceptualize issues through the lenses of social constructionism and narrative therapy, but I work experientially in the therapy room. These models both relate strongly to socio-emotional relationship therapy (SERT), and as such, this model undergirds much of my practice.

I believe that in order to understand any clinical issue or aspect of human experience, you have to start with a deep curiosity about the person(s)' social identities, social locations, and their respective stratification within societal structures and how these relate to the problem. However, this is not a simplistic or linear process, as in order to attune to sociocultural context, one has to attend simultaneously to both larger systems as well as one's local, generational, cultural, and geographic context.

In my opinion, simply naming the dominant discourses or oppressive influences of the larger context in theoretical terms rarely seems to have a strong therapeutic impact. I find that bringing forth what narrative therapists would call "experience near" connections for clients that relate to the larger context evokes emotional responses within clients that enable them to viscerally "get" and engage with the significance of power processes and larger context influence in their lives.

I ask, listen, validate, and affirm. There is something so healing and empowering about having someone outside of your experience witness and say that it matters. This act of legitimizing another's experience can in and of itself be transformative. I also connect oppression and marginalization to larger social structures. Naming the impact that silence and marginalization has had on the problem and client(s)' experience as well as acknowledging that there are others who experience it too serves to counter the isolation that one can feel.

Beginning with the first session, I pay close attention to the dynamic power exchange happening within the system, assess the interaction in the context of larger systems, and track the relational impact. I try to bring the inequities into focus in the therapeutic conversation in a way that clients feel understood rather than blamed and then can start to see how it relates to larger societal structures beyond themselves.

I use positive connotation to name the relational intents I see from clients that are getting derailed by problematic discourses that persuade them to replicate patterns that don't serve the relational system. I help clients experientially connect to their own and one another's pain as well as validate strengths so they can feel motivated and empowered to resist harmful societal scripts and choose alternatives that better support their relational goals. I join with the system as a therapeutic partner by expressing my sense of belief in their ability to practice and live out preferred realities. I then help them claim, envision, and practice this change experientially in session.

I draw from my heritage and bicultural identity in both collectivist and individualistic cultures, but I tend to privilege relational values and ways of being in my work. I use a socioculturally attuned lens to understand my clients, get the problems they face, and facilitate transformative change.

Sociocultural Attunement and Common Factors

Common factors that affect change have received a great deal of attention in the helping fields, including family therapy (Karam & Blow, 2020). Debates have ensued regarding the relative importance of models, including the argument that common factors work through and enhance models (Sexton et al., 2004). While the same factors are not uniformly defined across theorists, they are frequently categorized as: 1) client and extratherapeutic factors, 2) therapist factors and therapeutic alliance, 3) hope and expectancy for change, and 4) the use of models and techniques. D'Aniello et al. (2016) encouraged family therapists to enhance common factors through cultural sensitivity and attunement. Following, we discuss how common factors are positively impacted by socioculturally attuned practices.

Client and Extratherapeutic Factors

Social location (i.e., intersection of identities such as race, gender, sexual orientation, and social class within specific local, social, and global contexts) determines many of the social and economic resources necessary to help solve problems. Socioculturally attuned family therapists pay close attention to the impact of identity within societal structures as well as standpoints that shape clients' experiences. Expanding the treatment system beyond an individual allows family therapists to more effectively intervene (Karam & Blow, 2020).

Consider a couple in their mid-60s in the US who identify as White, middle-class, and heterosexual. They enter therapy when the wife announces her intention to divorce. The husband begins the conversation by expressing his utter dismay at his wife's dissatisfaction with what he has experienced as a good marriage. From his perspective, they have had their share of problems raising kids, making financial ends meet, and getting along, but nothing he wouldn't expect. They have both worked and he has always respected his wife's right to make decisions on her own. From the wife's perspective, she has spent a lifetime accommodating a difficult man who seems to remain unaware of her experience, regardless of the number of times she tries to tell him he is controlling and dismissive. She reports a lifetime of mediating relationships between her husband and children, endless efforts to keep the peace in the family, and a desire to be on her own during the final stages of life. How could these perspectives be so different when the couple identifies as the same race, age, social class, and sexual orientation?

Understanding the complexity of gendered power dynamics and being aware of changing gender roles in the US are foundational to understanding this couple's differing perspectives and experiences. This includes awareness of the extratherapeutic factors that have affected their journey together (e.g., gender oppression, women's rights movement, male privilege, religious heritage). When we attune well to clients' social context, we get where they are coming from and are better able to join *with* them to craft compassionate, socioculturally attuned responses that promote equity and connection. Linking clients' felt experiences with inequitable societal patterns outside the relationship makes partners more receptive to change (Knudson-Martin & Kim, 2023). This clinical stance is similar to what Jessica ChenFeng described as *contextual differentiation* (Stone & ChenFeng, 2020)—awareness of and appreciation for how our own and others' thoughts and feelings are contextually situated, while also being able to separate oneself from them to envision other possibilities. Therapists are able to turn toward clients whose actions are hurtful to genuinely engage with them in facilitating change.

Therapist Characteristics and Therapeutic Relationship

Cultural awareness is core to the therapeutic alliance. Family therapists are expected to know themselves and to identify and work on their own cultural and personal biases in order to prepare for working with all families. Sociocultural attunement takes this expectation a step further. Socioculturally attuned family therapists must be able to take a multi-ocular view, simultaneously attending to 1) the complexities of societal structures and clients' social locations within those structures, 2) the significance of standpoint and worldview on individuals and relationships between individuals, 3) the nature of presenting problems as embedded within local, national and global contexts, 4) the impact of societal systems on power dynamics in all relationships, 5) the felt experiences and identities of clients in sociocultural context, and 6) how all of these factors influence themselves as therapists as well as the therapeutic relationship. Attending to the sociocultural context helps therapists accurately empathize with each member of the family and the family as a whole, which in turn enhances therapeutic alliance (Karam & Blow, 2020).

Within-system alliance, e.g., the alliance and bond between family members as well as their agreement on therapeutic goals and tasks, is also predictive of successful therapeutic outcomes. Anderson and Johnson (2010) researched the relationship between therapist–client alliance, couple alliance with each other, and levels of distress in the early stages of heterosexual couples' therapy. They found that when therapists formed stronger alliances with more powerful partners (in this case men), less powerful partners (in this case women) became more distressed. The opposite did not hold true. Men did not become distressed over therapists forming initially stronger alliances with their female partners. The authors suggested this outcome challenges the belief that when therapists are not able to join with all family members equally, they should form an alliance with the most powerful and/or distant family member. This practice, which is intended to keep families in therapy, seems to be contraindicated as it reinforces unjust social arrangements among adults. It makes sense that those in less powerful positions would become concerned and disheartened, perceiving therapists as maintaining the status quo and/or contributing to relational inequity.

In short, the therapeutic alliance is impacted by power dynamics in a societal context. Socioculturally attuned family therapists must be able to assess the nuances of power in relationships (Knudson-Martin, 2024), connect intimate relationships to larger social forces, and navigate their roles in ways that support relational equity. This includes improving within-system alliances by encouraging attunement of more powerful members to the experiences, feelings, and needs of less powerful family members (Knudson-Martin & Huenergardt, 2010).

Socioculturally attuned family therapists integrate multiple knowledges, including disciplinary, interdisciplinary, and non-disciplinary knowledge. Disciplinary knowledge draws from family therapy theory, models, and techniques. Interdisciplinary knowledge includes sociology, economics, political science, and other areas of study that inform how we conceptualize families in societal context. Non-disciplinary knowledge honors Indigenous knowledges, lived individual and family experiences, children's knowledge, non-Western knowledge, and the multiplicity of lifeworlds. Non-disciplinary knowledge is key to practicing from an anti-colonial stance that embraces ways of knowing that are not informed by formal education and instead rely on the wisdom of people and their local knowledge.

Expectancy for Change

Families come to therapy seeking relief from emotional and/or relational problems that they tend to define as residing in an individual. Family therapists help families view problems relationally (Karam & Blow, 2020), broadening possibilities for change. This allows families and therapists to set the agenda for change together in solvable terms. Clients sometimes enter therapy at the will of others, such as child welfare institutions and the justice system. Societal institutions may expect family therapists to serve as agents of social control by influencing families to change in what is considered prosocial ways. Care must be taken not to unintentionally recreate unjust social arrangements. Socioculturally attuned family therapists ask questions such as, "Who is expecting change and why? What is my role in facilitating change?" And "How is my role contributing to maintaining the status quo of inequity and/or promoting social equity?" Whose agenda is being privileged and why?

Understanding the complexities of societal systems, culture, and power allows socioculturally attuned family therapists to identify opportunities for change. They recognize and support resistance that draws from and leads to resilience, which in turn inspires authentic hope. Consider a couple who entered therapy when Miguel became depressed. Miguel identified as Mexican American male and Sally identified as European American female. They met when working to support the rights of migrant workers and shared political and social ideologies. Miguel was the only Latino administrator at a utility department where he routinely experienced racism from colleagues and customers. He felt isolated in a White community, remaining there at Sally's request. Sally described herself as anti-racist, offering her activism and marriage to Miguel as "proof" of her commitment to social justice. The therapist noticed, however, that Sally rarely acknowledged Miguel's experiences of oppression and marginalization. Unraveling this dynamic, including the differences in their racial experiences and daily stressors, led to increased hope for change. The husband's depression lifted as the couple began routinely attending to acts of daily racism, considering together how to resist racism, and entertaining the idea of moving to a more supportive community.

Application of Models

As noted above, an understanding of common factors helps therapists work through and enhance the theoretical models and frameworks used (Sexton et al., 2004). Sociocultural attunement improves the ability to use existing models in ways that support social equity. Family therapy models enhance change by offering clients and therapists a coherent framework from which to understand and find relief from problems. They serve as road maps that can inspire hope and confidence in the therapeutic process. Most family therapy models are considered to be evidence-based. The models presented in this text have relied on research for their development; have been shown through research to be effective for a variety of populations and conditions; and/or have been demonstrated to be effective by a large number of practitioners. These models share one of the common factors that is unique to family therapy, i.e., disrupting problematic relational patterns (Karam & Blow, 2020). The primary purpose of this text is to offer conceptual clarity and practical guidelines for socioculturally attuned practice across family therapy models, enhancing their role in the change process. Integrating concepts and practices across models is also common among many practitioners, including those who are engaged in equity-based work.

It is important to note that the field is constantly changing and our thoughts are continuously evolving. In Text Box 1.2, Justine D'Arrigo describes the importance of remaining aware in the present that one will likely change in the future.

Text Box 1.2 Justine D'Arrigo, PhD

Justine D'Arrigo (they/them) holds a PhD in MFT and is an associate professor at California State University San Bernardino. They identify as White and queer with particular interests in intersections of relational activism and therapy, navigating critical theory and poststructuralism, post-oppositional approaches to relationships and change, and exploring compositionism and curiosity in therapy. (More of their work is described in Chapter 13.)

I think it is important to note that my thoughts a month or six months or a year from now will probably be very different. My ideas and the ways I work always feel in transition, which I think is characteristic of my life as a queer person as well. I hope I always feel "on the way" to knowing how to do this work, and hope I never arrive at a place where I feel like I know how. Being "on the way" to knowing keeps me ever reflexive on how I show up in this work.

What Follows

We are joined in this third edition of *Socioculturally Attuned Family Therapy: Applying Third Order Thinking to Theory and Practice* by voices of many others who are engaged in transformative practices and third order thinking across diverse settings. We collectively address the need to practice family therapy in ways that infuse diversity, equity, and inclusion throughout theory and clinical practice. This includes attention to societal systems that shape our daily lives at intimate, local, national, and global levels. A variety of family therapy theories and models are routinely taught in advanced educational programs and practiced by clinicians worldwide. We join those who struggle to teach these models while helping students and supervisees integrate critical social awareness into actual practice. As practitioners ourselves, we share the difficulties professionals face in realizing truly just practice without abandoning their theoretical foundations. The primary question that guides our work is: How do we continue to use the models we so value in family therapy in ways that integrate the impact of culture, societal context, and power as essential considerations in therapeutic change? The aim of this text is to bridge theory to practice, maintaining the integrity of established models while integrating a contemporary understanding of diversity and social justice.

In this first chapter, we argue for the importance of paying attention to how societal context and power dynamics affect mental health and relational well-being. Chapter 2 centers on the concept of third order thinking (McDowell et al., 2019) and highlights the relevance of third order change (McDowell, 2015) in socially transformative practice. This includes defining societal systems, diversity, and socially just practice, and introducing ANVIET (attunement, naming, valuing, envisioning, and transforming) as a transtheoretical set of socioculturally attuned guiding practices. We contend that third order change occurs when families are able to recognize the impact of societal systems on their relationships, envision relationally equitable alternatives, and take liberatory action toward change that is transformative.

In Chapter 3, we explore contextual self-of-the-therapist and the application of third order thinking to the ethics of everyday practice, as well as some of the complexities and tensions involved. We highlight that attending to societal systems, power, and equity is core to ethical practice because these forces directly impact mental health and relational well-being. We also consider some of the tensions involved in doing this work. Chapter 4 focuses on socioculturally attuned assessment—how to expand the lens to "get the lay of the land" in which our clients' clinical concerns are embedded. We emphasize assessment as part of forming a therapeutic alliance that counters inequities and creates a shared understanding to guide the direction of therapy and the potential for third order change. This includes strategies to "map" how material realities and social-relational determinants of health impact the formation and meaning of clients' problems and potential solutions.

In the chapters that follow (Chapters 5–15), we integrate principles of societal context, power, and equity into the core concepts of major family therapy models, paying close attention to the "how to" of change processes. In the final chapter (Chapter 16) we apply third order thinking and ANVIET practices to equity-based interventions across community, organizational, and governmental systems; family therapy education and supervision; international relationships, and environmental contexts. We highlight the work and wisdom of a number of colleagues who act as change agents within these various contexts.

The chapters on family therapy models offer variety in how concepts are explained and examples are offered; however, each follows a similar format. We introduce the model and then offer examples of its application and historical highlights. We do not attempt to offer a thorough overview of how to practice each therapeutic approach, but identify what we consider the most enduring concepts of each model. We then integrate principles of sociocultural attunement, relying on theories of societal systems and power that are particularly applicable to the family therapy model at hand. We offer guidelines for practicing the model from a socioculturally attuned perspective and apply these guidelines to a case illustration. As you go from one chapter to another, we invite you to become aware of the commonalities of socioculturally attuned practice across models, while also appreciating the richness and differing perspectives of each foundational family therapy model.

Limitations

There are limits associated with any perspective or practice framework. What we advocate for is no exception. The first is what we chose to include. We offer an overview of what we consider enduring concepts from each of eleven family therapy models. We did not attempt to include all models of family therapy. We have been deeply engaged in identifying enduring concepts across models in a field to which we have devoted most of our working lives. We are aware, however, that others may choose different concepts as primary in each of the models we present, or define these concepts differently. The second limit involves the decision to offer an overarching framework of each model rather than an exhaustive overview. This decision relies on readers accessing fuller historical and in-depth practice knowledge of each model from other sources. Finally, our ideas are still forming and changing. New ideas continuously emerge that deeply inform how we think about and do family therapy. Our hope is that this work, and the ways in which others are applying third order thinking to their practice, will serve as an impetus for you to add to this body of work in meaningful ways that are uniquely situated in your contexts. In each chapter, we invite you to respond to reflexive questions and hope that by engaging with these questions, they will stimulate other questions that lead to generativity and transformational processes.

Reflexive Questions

- How do you define equity? What does it mean for you to conduct equity-based family therapy?
- As a therapist, how can you examine the effects of *socio-relational* determinants of health and intervene in ways that are meaningful and useful to your clients?
- How do your social location and intersectional identities position you and your clients in ways that are impacted by space, place, and climate-based inequities? Was this apparent to you during the COVID-19 pandemic, natural disasters, or large-scale traumatic events, such as surviving war, organized crime, or community violence? What advantages or disadvantages did you and your clients experience during times such as these?
- Who is most likely to be attuned to others in any given system? Who has the privilege to not attune and respond to the needs of others?
- What does it mean for you to acknowledge the history of trauma-based structural inequity in the US and/or your country of origin?
- How does the influence of oppressive legacies (e.g., slavery, genocide, racism, misogyny, sexism, ableism, homophobia, colonization, xenophobia) influence your beliefs about what is normative, good, healthy, and best practice?
- How do the four sociocultural factors mentioned in this chapter—social isolation, individualism and the distant other, social inequities, and polarization—affect you and the people that you know?
- How are you currently attempting to denounce "othering" practices? What factors help support you in this endeavor?

References

Adler N., Glymour M., & Fielding J. (2016). Addressing social determinants of health and health inequalities. *Journal of the American Medical Association, 316*(16), 1641–1642.

Afifi, T. D., Zamanzadeh, N., Harrison, K., & Torrez, D. P. (2020). Explaining the impact of differences in voting patterns on resilience and relational load in romantic relationships during the transition to the Trump presidency. *Journal of Social and Personal Relationships*, 37, 3–26.

Almeida, R. (2018). *Liberation based healing practices*. Institute for Family Services.

Almeida, R., Dolan-Del Vecchio, K., & Parker, L. (2007). *Transforming family therapy: Just families in a just society*. Allyn & Bacon.

Almeida, R. & Tubbs, C. (2020). Intersectionality: A liberation-based healing perspective. In K. S. Wampler, R. B. Miller, & R. B. Seedall (Eds.), *The Handbook of Systemic Family Therapy*, (Vol. 1, pp. 227–249). Wiley.

Almeida, R. V. & Williams, J. C. (2026). Postmodernism, decolonial critiques, and liberatory praxis. In O. Smoliak, E. Tseliou, T. Strong, S. Bava, & P. Muntigl (Eds.). *The Routledge international handbook of postmodern therapies*, pp. 86–99. Routledge.

Alves-Bradford, J. M., Trinh, N. H., Bath, E., Coombs, A., Mangurian, C. (2020). Mental health equity in the twenty-first century: Setting the stage. *Psychiatric Clinics of North America, 43*(3), 415–428.

Anderson, S. R. & Johnson, L. N. (2010). A Dyadic analysis of the between- and within-system alliances on distress. *Family Process, 49*(2), 220–235.

Aponte, H. J. (1976). The family-school interview: An ecostructural approach. *Family Process, 15*, 303–311.

Argüello, R. (2023) The outside and family therapy: A perspective from the relational thinking of Gilles Deleuze. *Australian and New Zealand Journal of Family Therapy, 44*, 95–107.

Armstrong, J., Carlos Chavez, F. L., Jones, J. H., Harris, S. D., & Harris, G. J. (2019). "A dream deferred": How discrimination impacts the American dream achievement for African Americans. *Journal of Black Studies, 50*(3), 227–250.

Auerswald, E. (1971). Families, change and the ecological perspective. *Family Process, 10*, 263–280.

Bava, S. (2023). A relationally responsive world: The politics of collaborative-dialogic space and process for generativity. In H. Anderson & D. Gehart (Eds.). *Collaborative-dialogic practice: Generative relationships and conversations across contexts and cultures* (pp. 37–54). Routledge.

Bava, S. & Greene, M. (2023). *The relational workplace: How relational intelligence grows diverse, equitable, and inclusive cultures of connection*. ThinkPlay Partners.

Bergeron, G., De La Cruz, N., Gould, L., Liu, S., Seligson, A. (2020). Association between racial discrimination and health-related quality of life and the impact of social relationships. *Quality of Life Research, 29*, 2793–2805.

Bermúdez, J. M., Alvarez-Hernandez, L, Muruthi, B. A., Machado-Escudero, Y., & Lamont-Gomez, M. F. (equal authors) (under review). Decolonizing approaches to family science as intersectional Latinx and Caribbean scholars working toward third order change, *Journal of Family Theory and Review*.

Bermúdez, J. M., Muruthi, B. A., & Jordan, L. S. (2016). Decolonizing research methods for family science: Creating space at the center. *Journal of Family Theory & Review, 8*(2), 192–206.

Boe, J. L. & Baldwin, D. R. (2023). Socioculturally attuned systemic therapy with transgender and gender diverse families. *Journal of Systemic Therapies, 42*(2), 27–45. https://doi-org.library.lcproxy.org/10.1521/jsyt.2023.42.2.27.

Brock, R. L., Calkins, F. C., Hamburger, E. R., Kumar, S. A., Laifer, L. M., Phillips, E., & Ramsdell, E. L. (2023). Learning from adversity: What the COVID-19 pandemic can teach us about family resiliency. *Family process, 62*(4), 1574–1591.

Browning, S., & van Eeden-Moorefield, B. (Eds.). (2022). *Treating contemporary families: Toward a more inclusive clinical practice*. American Psychological Association.

Cashin, S. (2014). *Place, not race: A new vision of opportunity in America*. Beacon Press.

D'Aniello, C., Nguyen, H., & Piercy, F. (2016). Cultural sensitivity as an MFT common factor. *American Journal of Family Therapy, 44*(5), 234–244.

Deatrick, J. (2017). Where is "family" in the social determinants of health? Implications for family nursing practice, research, education, and policy. *Journal of Family Nursing, 23*(4), 423–433.

Falicov, C. J. (2014). Psychotherapy and supervision as cultural encounters: The multidimensional ecological comparative approach framework. In C. A. Falender, E. P. Shafranske, & C. J. Falicov (Eds.). *Multiculturalism and diversity in clinical supervision* (pp. 29–58). American Psychological Association.

Falicov, C. (2015). *Latino families in therapy* (2nd ed.). Guilford.

Fishbane, M. D. (2023). Couple relational ethics: From theory to lived practice. *Family process*, *62*(2), 446–468.
Fraser, T., Aldrich, D., Panagopoulos, C., Hummel, D., & Kim, D. (2022). The harmful effects of partisan polarization on health. *PNAS Nexus*, *1*, 1–10.
Freire, P. (2000). *Pedagogy of the oppressed.* Bloomsbury. (Original work published in 1970).
Fricker, M. (2007). *Epistemic injustice: Power and the ethics of knowing.* Oxford University Press.
Glebova, T. & Knudson-Martin, C. (2023). *Sociocultural trauma and relational well-being in the Eastern European context.* AFTA SpringerBriefs in Family Therapy. Springer.
Golojuch, L. A., Morgan, A. A., & Mittal, M. (2025). "As therapists, we get to be quietly subversive": A qualitative exploration of CFTs' social justice practices. *Journal of Marital and Family Therapy*, *51*(2), e70006.
Goodrich, T., Rampage, C., Ellman, B., & Halstead, K. (1988). *Feminist family therapy: A casebook.* Norton.
Gosnell, F., McKergow, M, Moore, B., Mudry, T., & Tomm, K. (2017). A Galveston declaration. *Journal of Systemic Therapies*, *36*(3), 20–26.
Gu, Y. & Wang, Z. (2022). Income inequality and global political polarization: The economic origin of political polarization in the world. *Journal of Chinese Political Science*, *27*(2), 375–398.
Hair, H., Fine, M., & Ryan, B. (1996). Expanding the context of family therapy. *The American Journal of Family Therapy*, *24*(4), 291–304.
Hare-Mustin, R. T. (1978). A feminist approach to family therapy. *Family Process*, *17*(2), 181–194.
Hardy, K. V. (2024). Some subtleties of whiteness in the workplace: Steps for shifting the paradigm. *Family Process*, *63*(1), 1–14.
Hartwell, E. E. & Edwards, L. L. (2026) Queer contextualized family therapy. In E. E. Hartwell & L. L. Edwards (Eds.). *Queer-contextualized family therapy: Toward radically inclusive theory and practice* (pp. 1–25). Routledge.
Heller, J., Givens, M. Johnson, S., & Kindig, D. (2024). Keeping it political and powerful: Defining structural determinants of health. *The Milbank Quarterly*, *102*(2), 351–366.
Ho, M. K., Rasheed, J. M., & Rasheed, M. N. (2004). *Family therapy with ethnic minorities* (2nd ed.). Sage Publications.
Hodgson, J. & Lamson, A. (2020). The importance of policy and advocacy in systemic family therapy. In K. S. Wampler, R. B. Miller, & R. B. Seedall (Eds.). *The handbook of systemic family therapy* (Vol. 1, pp. 729–751). Wiley.
Holyoak, D., McPhee, D., Hall, G., & Fife, S. (2021). Microlevel advocacy: A common process in couple and family therapy. *Family Process*, *60*, 654–669.
Howe, N. (2023). *The fourth turning is here: What the seasons of history tell us about how and when this crisis will end.* Simon & Schuster.
Imber-Black, E. (1992). *Families and larger systems: A family therapist's guide through the labyrinth.* Guilford Press.
Jordan, L. S. (2022). Unsettling colonial mentalities in family therapy: Entering negotiated spaces. *Journal of Family Therapy*, *44*(1), 171–185.
Karam, E. & Blow, A. (2020). Common factors underlying systemic family therapy. In K. S. Wampler, R. B. Miller, & R. B. Seedall (Eds.). *The handbook of systemic family therapy* (Vol. 1, pp. 147–170). Wiley.
Kaslow, N., Clarke, C, & Hampton-Anderson, J. (2024). Culturally humble and anti-racist couple and family interventions for African Americans. *Family Process*, *63*(2), 512–526.
Keeney, B. P. (1979). Ecosystemic epistemology: An alternative paradigm for diagnosis. *Family Process*, *18*, 117–129.
Kelly, S., Jeremie-Brink, G., & Chambers, A. (2020). The Black Lives Matter movement: A call to action for couple and family therapists. *Family Process*, *59*(4), 1374–1388.
Kim, L., D'Arrigo, J., ChenFeng, J., & Esmiol-Wilson, E. (2022). Relationality as a way of being: A pedagogy of classroom conversations. In A. Desai & H. N. Nguyen (Eds.). *Global perspectives on dialogue in the classroom: Cultivating inclusive, intersectional, and authentic conversations.* Palgrave McMillan.
Kleinfeld, R. (2023). *Polarization, democracy, and political violence in the United States: What the research says* (pp. 14–40). Carnegie Endowment for International Peace.
Knudson-Martin, C. (2013). Why power matters: Creating a foundation of mutual support in couple relationships. *Family Process*, *52*(1), 5–18.
Knudson-Martin, C. (2024). *A step-by-step guide to socio-emotional relationship therapy: A socially responsible approach to clinical practice.* Routledge.
Knudson-Martin, C. (2025). *The socio-emotional relationship workbook for couples: Closing the gap between the relationship you want and the relationship you have.* Routledge.

Knudson-Martin, C. & Huenergardt, D. (2010). A socio-emotional approach to couple therapy: Linking social context and couple interaction. *Family Process*, *49*(3), 369–384.
Knudson-Martin, C. & Kim, L. (2023). Socioculturally attuned couple therapy. In J. Lebow & D. Snyder (Eds.). *Clinical Handbook of Couple Therapy* (6th ed., pp. 267–291). Guilford.
Knudson-Martin, C., Kim, L., Gibbs, E., & Harmon, R. (2021). Sociocultural attunement to vulnerability in couple therapy: Fulcrum for changing power processes. *Family Process*, *60*, 1152–1169.
Korin, E. C. (1994). Social inequalities and therapeutic relationships: Applying Freire's ideas to clinical practice. *Journal of Feminist Family Therapy*, *5*(3–4), 75–98.
Laszloffy, T. A. & Twist, M. L. C. (2019). *Eco-informed practice: Family therapy in an age of ecological peril.* AFTA SpringerBriefs in Family Therapy. Springer.
Lee, A. T., Chin, P., Nambiar, A., & Hill Haskins, N. (2023). Addressing intergenerational trauma in Black families: Trauma-informed socioculturally attuned family therapy. *Journal of Marital & Family Therapy*, *49*(2), 447–462.
Lini, C. & Bertrando, P. (2022). Positional responsibility in systemic-dialogical therapy. *Journal of Family Therapy*, *44*, 339–350.
Lorås, L, Whittaker, K., Stokkebekk, J., & Tilden, T. (2023). Researching what we practice–The paradigm of systemic family research: Part 1. *Family Process*, *62*, 947–960.
Luepnitz, D. A. (1988). *The family interpreted: feminist theory in clinical practice*. Basic Books.
Martín-Baró, I., Aron, A., & Corne, S. (1994). *Writings for a liberation psychology*. Harvard University Press.
McDowell, T. (2015). *Applying critical social theories to family therapy practice*. AFTA SpringerBriefs in Family Therapy. Springer.
McDowell, T., Knudson-Martin, C. & Burmudez, M. (2018). *Socio-culturally attuned family therapy: Guidelines for equitable theory and practice* (1st ed.). Routledge.
McDowell, T., Knudson-Martin, C., & Bermúdez, J. M. (2019). Third-order thinking in family therapy: Addressing social justice across family therapy practice. *Family process*, *58*(1), 9–22.
McDowell, T., Knudson-Martin, C. & Bermúdez, M. (2022). *Socio-culturally attuned family therapy: guidelines for equitable theory and practice* (2nd ed.). Routledge.
McGeorge, C. R., Kellerman, J., & Carlson, T. S. (2018). Indicators of LGB affirmative training: An exploratory study of family therapy faculty members. *Journal of Feminist Family Therapy*, *30*(1), 1–24.
McGeorge, C. R., Coburn, K. O., & Walsdorf, A. A. (2021). Deconstructing cissexism: The journey of becoming an affirmative family therapist for transgender and nonbinary clients. *Journal of Marital & Family Therapy*, *47*(3), 785–802.
McGoldrick, M. (Ed.). (1998). *Re-visioning family therapy: Race, culture, and gender in clinical practice.* New York: Guilford Press.
McGoldrick, M., Giordano, J., & Garcia-Preto, N. (2005). *Ethnicity and family therapy* (3rd ed). Guilford Press.
Mialon M. (2020). An overview of the commercial determinants of health. *Globalization and health*, *16*(1), 74.
Minuchin, S., Montalvo, B., Guerney, B., Rosman, B., & Schumer, F. (1967). *Families of the slums: An exploration of their structure and treatment*. Basic Books.
Ong, B., Tseliou, E., Strong, T., & Buus, N. (2023). Power and dialogue: A review of discursive research. *Family process*, *62*(4), 1391–1407.
Piercy, F. (2020). The future of systemic family therapy: What needs nurturing and what does not. In K. S. Wampler, R. B. Miller, & R. B. Seedall (Eds.). *The Handbook of Systemic Family Therapy* (Vol. 1, pp. 754–771). Wiley.
Prouty Lyness, A. & Lyness, K. (2007). Feminist issues in couple therapy. *Journal of Couple & Relationship Therapy*, *6*(1/2), 181–195.
Rastogi, M. (2021). A systemic conceptualization of interventions with families in a global context. In K. S. Wampler, R. B. Miller, & R. B. Seedall (Eds.). *The Handbook of Systemic Family Therapy* (Vol. 4, pp. 3–32). Wiley.
Sexton, T., Ridley, C. & Kleiner, A. (2004). Beyond common factors: Multilevel-process models of therapeutic change in marriage and family therapy. *Journal of Marital and Family Therapy*, *30*(2), 131–149.
Siegel, D. J. & Drulis, C. (2023). An interpersonal neurobiology perspective on the mind and mental health: personal, public, and planetary well-being. *Annals of general psychiatry*, *22*(1), 5.
Silverstein, L. B. & Goodrich, T. J. (Eds.). (2003). *Feminist family therapy: Empowerment in social context.* American Psychological Association.
Smoliak, O. & Knudson-Martin, C. (under review). *Rethinking sociocultural attunement through a postcolonial lens. Family Process.*

Smoliak, O., LaMarre, A., Rice, C., Tseliou, E., LeCouteur, A., Myers, M., … & Velikonja, L. (2022a). The politics of vulnerable masculinity in couple therapy. *Journal of Marital and Family Therapy*, *48*, 427–446.
Smoliak, O., Rice, C., LaMarre, A., Tseliou, E., LeCouteur, A., & Davies, A. (2022b). Gendering of care and care inequalities in couple therapy. *Family Process*, *61*(4), 1386–1402.
Soja, E. (2010). *Seeking spatial justice*. University of Minnesota Press.
Stone, D. J. & ChenFeng, J. L. (2020). *Finding your voice as a beginning marriage and family therapist*. Routledge.
Tambling, R. R., Hynes, K. C., & D'Aniello, C. (2021). Are barriers to psychotherapy treatment seeking indicators of social determinants of health?: A critical review of the literature. *The American Journal of Family Therapy*, *50*(5), 443–458.
Tatum, B. D. (1997). *"Why are all the black kids sitting together in the high school cafeteria?" and other conversations about race*. Basic Books.
US Department of Health and Human Services. (2020, August). *Healthy people 2030*. https://odphp.health.gov/healthypeople.
US Surgeon General's advisory on the healing effects of social connection and community (2023). *Our epidemic of loneliness and isolation*. https://www.hhs.gov/sites/default/files/surgeon-general-social-connection-advisory.pdf
Waite, R. & Nardi, D. (2024). A call for health justice: Striving toward health equity at a community health center. *Family Process*, *63*(2), 502–511.
Waldegrave, C., Tamases, K., Tuhaka, F., & Campbell, W. (2003). *Just Therapy–a journey: A collection of papers from the Just Therapy team New Zealand*. Dulwich Centre Publications.
Waldinger, R. & Schulz, M. (2023). *The good life: Lessons for the world's longest scientific study of happiness*. Simon & Schuster.
Walters, M., Carter, B., Papp, P., & Silverstein, O. (1988). *The invisible web: Gender patterns in family relationships*. Guilford Press.
Warner, B. R., Colaner, C. W., & Park, J. (2021). Political difference and polarization in the family: The role of (non)accommodating communication for navigating identity differences. *Journal of Social and Personal Relationships*, 38(2), 564–585.
Watson, M., (2019). Social justice and race in the United States: Key issues and challenges for couple and family therapy. *Family Process*, *58*(1), 23–33.
Watson, M. (2024). Caste and Black intergenerational trauma in the United States of America. *Family Process*, *63*(2), 475–487.
Watson, M., Bacigalupe, G., Daneshpour, M., Han, W., & Parra-Cardona, R. (2020). Covid-19 interconnectedness: Health inequality, the climate crisis, and collective trauma. *Family Process*, *59*, 832–846.
Wetzel, N. A. (2024). Embracing the other: Revisiting the epistemological foundations of family systems therapy. *Family Process*, *63*, 17–33.
White, M. & Epstein, D. (1990). *Narrative means to therapeutic ends*. WW Norton.
Whiting, J. B., Wendt, D. M., Eisert, B. C., & Fife, S. T. (2024). I and thou in dialogue: Becoming more relational in couple therapy. *Family Process*, *63*, 1–16.
Wynne, L. (1967). Discussion of the "individual and the larger contexts." *Family Process*, *6*, 148–154.
Yousafzai, W. (2022). Political polarization and its impact on mental health: Where do we stand? *Khyber Medical University Journal*, *14*(1), 1–2.
Yu, B. Y. M., Lam, C., & Chan, C. S. (2024). All we need is love? Irreconcilable political incongruence in families after the 2019 social unrest in Hong Kong. *Political Psychology*, *45*(3), 643–665.

2 Guiding Principles for Socioculturally Attuned Family Therapy

One of the hallmarks of being a family therapist is the ability to discern relational patterns and draw connections within and across systems. We move from the most intimate relational dynamic to a focus on the individual, while simultaneously expanding our lens to track family patterns over time and place within complex societal and cultural systems. We also continuously bridge theoretical frameworks with actual practice, enabling us to intentionally think about what we do. So, what does all of this mean when trying to make sense of clients' concerns? What do we choose to pay attention to? What do we look for? What informs what we see? How do we work together with clients to consider ways of thinking and doing that will expand possibilities for desired outcomes? These questions invite us to take a metaperspective in thinking about how we think; about the difference our thinking makes in what we do to engage families in positive, sometimes transformative, change.

Third Order Thinking

Early family therapists developed a new way of thinking and practicing by viewing clinical problems as embedded within relational systems. This initial first order, general systems approach was influential in shaping the field and practice of family therapy, but was limited and relatively short-lived. It relied on a metaphor that reduced and compared complex human relationships to biological or mechanical self-correcting systems. General systems theory (e.g., von Bertalanffy, 1968) was challenged by feminist scholars who pointed out that family members often do not share the same level of relational power and cannot, therefore, be equally influential or accountable for how the system is created, maintained, or its interactional outcomes (Hare-Mustin, 1978; Hair, et al., 1996). Intimate partner violence (IPV) is perhaps the clearest example of this; repetitive patterns of interaction can be traced, yet partners do not share equal influence or responsibility for the abuse. This critique was followed by a call for second order systems thinking and practice (Anderson & Goolishan, 1988; Hoffman, 1981, 1985; Keeney, 1983) by which family therapists began viewing the interactions between themselves and family members systemically.

Second order thinking takes a metaperspective that recognizes families and therapists as part of therapeutic systems. The therapist's social position and contextual viewpoint affects how they understand and "know" families. Consider tracking a pattern of interaction among family members in which a more powerful partner is doing all of the talking; when the less powerful partner attempts to interrupt, they are quickly silenced. Now step back and add the therapist to the pattern of interaction. When you do so, you notice that the therapist is primarily looking at and asking questions of the more powerful partner. When the therapist attempts to interrupt, the more powerful partner talks over the therapist leaving both the therapist and the less powerful partner silenced. Second order thinking not only urges us to consider the impact of the therapist on the therapeutic system; it also opens the door to understanding the practice of family therapy itself as a potentially contested, polyvocal, situated process in which meaning evolves through interaction.

DOI: 10.4324/9781003493426-2

Yet another shift was ushered in by social constructionists who expanded the focus on social context and challenged the foundation of family therapy as uniquely relying on the metaphor of systems and systems theory (Dickerson, 2014). These critical, feminist, and social constructionist understandings of societal context and power have prompted a shift toward third order thinking that makes systems of systems more visible (McDowell, 2015; McDowell, et al., 2019). In this way of thinking, mental health and relational well-being are impacted not only by family but by societal systems at all levels, including complex interactions within and between systems (e.g., political, social, economic). Looking back at the example above from a third order perspective, you notice that both the therapist and the less powerful partner are female, and the more powerful partner is male. By ineffectively attempting to intervene, the therapist is worsening the situation; now neither female—even the professional therapist—is able to interrupt societal systems of male privilege and patriarchy that are being exhibited in the therapy room.

•←→•

Third order thinking includes and expands second order and critical thinking by taking a meta view of mental health, relational well-being, and the therapeutic endeavor itself as nested in complex and dynamic systems of systems that are continuously shaped by collective meaning-making, culture, and power dynamics. (McDowell, 2015; McDowell et al., 2019; McDowell et al., 2023)

•←→•

Thinking from a third order perspective changes how we make sense of everyday life by placing experience and interactions within societal context and power dynamics. It broadens our lens thereby increasing available information and ways of understanding situations, which in turn, provides more pathways for change. As with any perspective, this frames what we see, what we look for, and how we organize and make meaning of our observations. This inclusive and expansive way of thinking shapes what we can envision and co-envision with others.

We view this meta perspective as going beyond schemas to acknowledge multiple broader systems of thought, or cultural logics, and to hold these sometimes competing paradigms in the same space. For example, during an initial session we might view and punctuate patterns that allow us to determine a diagnosis while acknowledging that the mind we are categorizing is both within and beyond the individual being diagnosed (Siegel & Drulis, 2023). We might experience members of a family as discrete individuals while recognizing the non-discrete, continuous nature of humans in relationship to each other and their environment. We might acknowledge the ability to know others through observing and eliciting descriptions of their experience while realizing that knowing and meaning are being created and evolving through interaction, in this case therapeutic conversations. At the same time, we might recognize that we have at any moment but a snapshot of something in motion that is much more complex and that what we are seeking to know is at least in part unknowable.

While not labeled as third order thinking, similar processes are described across other disciplines and theories, including decolonizing theory (Laenui, 2006), critical geography (Soja, 2010), and liberation-based education (Freire, 1970/2020). For example, Paulo Freire (1970/2020) described those who are oppressed often feeling powerless to do anything but conform (first order thinking). Becoming aware of the dynamics of oppression that affect one's life provides insight into how unjust relationships might be challenged (second order thinking). Liberation becomes possible through increased awareness of societal systems and institutionalized power that privilege some by oppressing others. Third order thinking helps discover, or unveil, how systems of systems (e.g., economic, political, social) and social discourses create and maintain material and social inequities. Figure 2.1 provides a visual map for practicing socioculturally attuned family therapy

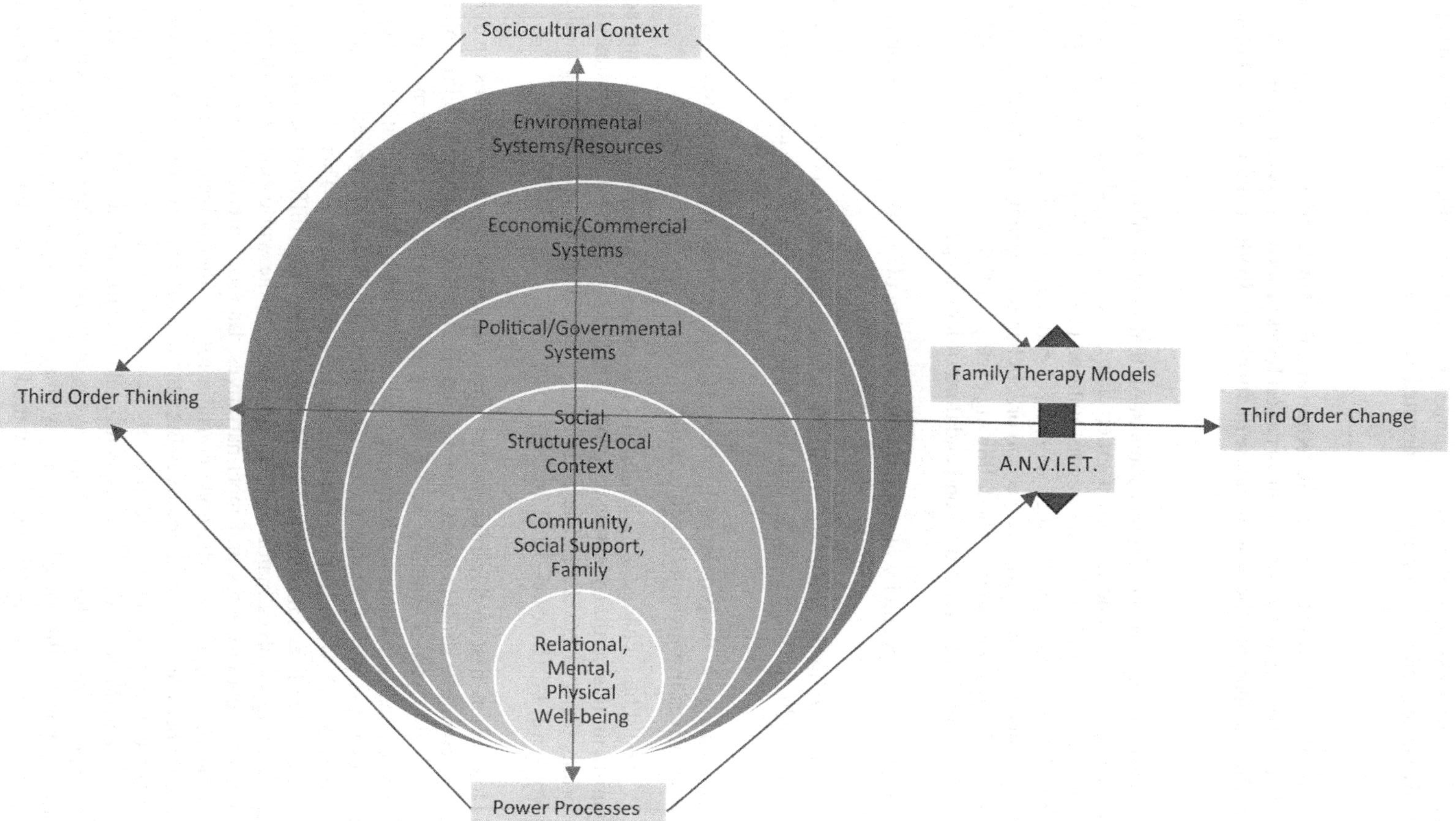

Figure 2.1 Conceptual framework for socioculturally attuned family therapy.

by conceptualizing first, second, and third order thinking within sociocultural context in ways that include power dynamics across multiple interconnected systems.

•←→•

Socioculturally attuned family therapists use second and third order thinking by applying a multifocal lens that can be expanded to view the broadest levels of societal systems and environmental contexts while magnifying the most intimate nuances of individual and relational dynamics.

•←→•

Third order thinking lays the conceptual foundation that guides third order change. A framework for considering first, second and third order change can be found in one of the earliest, groundbreaking annals of family therapy. Gregory Bateson (1972, p. 298) referred to logical types or *levels of learning* in *Steps to an Ecology of Mind.* Learning I and II correlate with what has become commonly understood as first and second order change. Learning III correlates with what we have defined as *third order change*. The following excerpt of Bateson's description of levels of learning shows a parallel with first and second and third order change.

> Learning I is change in specificity of response by correction of errors of choice within a set of alternatives.
>
> Learning II is change in the process of Learning I, e.g., a corrective change in the set of alternatives from which choice is made, or it is a change in how the sequence of experience is punctuated.
>
> Learning III is change in the process of Learning II, e.g., a corrective change in the system of sets of alternatives from which choice is made.
>
> Learning IV would be a change in Learning III, but probably does not occur in any adult living organism on this earth. Evolutionary process has, however, created organisms whose ontogeny brings them to Level III. The combination of phylogenesis with ontogenesis, in fact, achieves Level IV. (Bateson, 1972, p. 298)

According to Bateson, first level learning occurs when change is made but relationship dynamics and schemas (i.e., cognitive structures) remain the same (Bartunek & Moch, 1987). Possibilities for difference are limited to what is available within what he referred to as a set of alternatives; in other words, what can be imagined within a schema. Second level learning is change in the schema itself and resulting change in sets of alternatives. It focuses on the process level of relationships, creating new schemas (Bartunek & Moch, 1987). The rules of the system change. This allows relationships to be punctuated differently and members of a system to choose from different sets of alternatives.

Third level learning involves major shifts in how we see the world (Ecker & Hulley, 1996) through a focus on meta-processes and meta-narratives. Bateson referred to Level III learning as requiring a meta-perspective in which we consider sets of alternatives, leading to being able to choose not only between sets of alternatives but between schemas (Bartunek & Moch, 1987). When therapists target third order change, they are active and intentional, working in a space in which taken-for-granted assumptions are inspected, taken apart, and disrupted to reveal multiple perspectives and possibilities. This meta-perspective is in itself a paradigm shift, an epistemological repositioning in how we think and how we know what we know (McDowell, 2015). It invites us to re-examine the assumptions underlying clinical models and re-envision what is normal, natural, and possible (Hartwell & Edwards, 2026).

Expanded third order thinking integrates contemporary understandings of the nature of the universe (e.g., humans as a species, impact of the human species on the earth's environment, coevolution of plants and animals, the ubiquitous nature of life in the universe; c.f., Carroll, 2017). This includes recognizing humans as one species among many and challenging our species-centered perspectives (including a species that can debate the nature of reality and develop concepts such as social constructionism). While beyond what is typically practiced in family therapy today, a number of therapists and clients are exploring ontological shifts toward materialism (i.e., concerning the fundamental nature of matter), posthumanism (i.e., redefining relationships between human and nonhuman species), and beyond/post posthumanism (e.g., questioning the separation of human identity, Haroway's compost society) (Barraclough, 2023; Rhodes, 2021; Timeto, 2021).

First, Second, and Third Order Change

We often refer to first order solutions as "common sense," knowing their impact will be limited and make no real lasting difference in the way relationships are organized. For example, new parents who are arguing over who gets up at night with the baby might be coached to alternate, one taking odd days and the other taking even days. This might be helpful, but it rings of "common sense" first order change that fails to address the dynamics that prevented the couple from agreeing on this kind of obvious arrangement in the first place. Looking a little closer at the concept of common sense reveals the ubiquitous nature of the relationship between power and knowledge, i.e., the dynamic between dominant cultural worldviews or discourse and what we consider to be the natural order of things (Gramsci, 1971, McDowell, 2015). In other words, what we consider to be common sense is often dominant sense, bound by particular schemas.

•←→•

What is commonly understood as true or common sense often reflects the views, and maintains the privilege, of those with the greatest influence over its definition.

•←→•

Family therapists routinely target second order change, i.e., qualitative, discontinuous change that alters a system's rules, structure, and/or order (Watzlawick, et al., 1974). Second order change is said to have occurred when system rules and shared meaning change along with interactions. Compared to second order change, we often consider first order change as cursory since it does not alter the structure or rules of a system and maintains meaning frameworks or schemas. Second order change might involve addressing power dynamics that have been exacerbated and made more urgent by the couple becoming parents.

When purposefully considered and carefully sequenced, first and second order changes are both essential to the practice of family therapy. Second order shifts are followed by a series of first order changes within the new meaning-making schema and system rules. When new alternatives are created, everyday patterns of interaction shift as a result, which in turn support second order change. The new parents exemplified above might engage in second order change as they increase their attunement toward each other's needs and begin to share more equal influence. First order change such as alternating nights might then be a practical extension of this more foundational level change. First order change can be also important when a family is in crisis and needs stability. First order change is only a problem in therapy when it takes precedence or is present without attention to second and third order dynamics.

•←→•

Third order change expands possibilities and enables transformation.

•←→•

When therapists integrate sociocultural awareness into their approaches and open space for socially transformative change, they are engaging in third order change (e.g., cultural context model, just therapy, socio-emotional relationship therapy). When therapists engage in third order change, they help families connect their lived experience to broader systems of systems, raising awareness and questioning the impact of cultural norms, values, and societal power structures on relational dynamics and presenting problems. For example, the new parents mentioned above might now reflect on gender roles and gender equity, cultural norms embedded in systems of patriarchy across families and social institutions, as well as the impact of living in a capitalist society relative to social class and work demands.

Consider as another example, an intergenerational pattern of sons in conflict with their fathers. At a second order change level, a father might be encouraged to remember what it was like when he was a boy trying to please his father, feeling no matter what he did he could not live up to his father's expectations. This might soften his approach and increase his emotional attunement to his own son. If the therapist were to engage the family in dialogue or socioeducation about the bind in which fathers and sons often find themselves in patriarchal societies (e.g., sons being invited into patriarchy by their fathers who also insist on maintaining power over them), the family might be able to see how they participate in a widespread system that exacerbates unwanted conflict within the family. These types of revelations promote third order change that can be liberatory, releasing families from imposed societal structures and norms.

Principles of Socioculturally Attuned Family Therapy

As an interdisciplinary, transtheoretical framework, socioculturally attuned family therapy (SCAFT) supports the development of new models and builds on existing ones in ways that expand our abilities to understand the impact of societal systems and power dynamics on presenting problems and tailor interventions accordingly. Socioculturally attuned family therapists attend to how each family member's well-being is reflected in the ways relationships are organized, communication occurs, and decisions are made. They respect and integrate idiosyncratic perspectives and cultural values while simultaneously challenging oppression.

Following, we describe and relate principles of socioculturally attuned family therapy, emphasizing the concepts of third order thinking (McDowell et al., 2019) and third order change (McDowell, 2015). This includes how dimensions of power and societal context can be integrated into family therapy models to guide practices that support just relationships (see Figure 2.1).

Societal Context

Ecosystems include both living and nonliving organisms situated in space, place, and time. A family in rural Uganda awakens in a modest thatch-roofed hut to the sound of their farm animals—pigs, chickens, and goats—waiting to be fed. Their morning water must be boiled to drink the local tea. The air is clear, and the sun is reliably bright. Their beautiful tropical setting is rampant with malaria-bearing mosquitos. The economy suffers from a history of colonization, civil war, and global capitalism. Oil has been found beneath the ground, which signals social change as companies from China and the West begin circling. The family's ecosystem includes the entire context in which they are embedded, from the smallest insect to the largest landmass.

Societal context refers to the organization of human activity that emerges within and is dependent on all other aspects of ecosystems. A European American family wakes up in a small apartment in a large city in the United States (US). They hear familiar street noises and the sounds of neighbors arguing. The refrigerator holds nothing suitable for school lunches, so children are gathering coins from purses, pockets, and between couch cushions as the family cat looks on. A parent hurries the children, scolding the oldest for not making sure lunches were ready while grabbing an umbrella to walk the children safely to school against their objections. Clean water runs out of the tap, but the air is polluted. Buildings along the way are being remodeled as the neighborhood becomes gentrified, soon to be too expensive for the family to remain. Several miles away an African American family rushes to grab ready-to-eat breakfast bars as a father warns their only child to be in the car in 10 minutes or he will face having to walk to school. Fifteen-year-old James throws his iPad into a backpack that contains shorts and a t-shirt for after-school sports. He is worried that the Nike shoes he picked out for basketball might be too bright and will draw the wrong kind of attention from his teammates. James' mother is calling out spelling words they studied together the night before. They look forward to dinner out that evening. These families' morning activities and interactions have already been deeply shaped by differing incomes within their urban ecosystem.

•←→•

When we use the term societal context, we are referring to shared meanings that define culture, inform identities, and situate experience, as well as the dynamic interconnection of social systems that shape constraints and opportunities within specific spatial settings.

•←→•

The family in Uganda is headed by a 15-year-old girl, Dembe. Her maternal grandmother is alive but living on a separate family plot. She has two younger brothers and a younger sister. She is one of nearly half of the families in her village that are child-headed, most of whom lost their parents to AIDS. She and her 13-year-old brother, Jimiyu, are HIV positive. HIV/AIDs clinics have recently been closed due cuts in USAID funding, however antiretroviral (ARV) treatment is available at a hospital some distance from their home. Dembe must stay on the family land to protect the family belongings from those who might steal them when they are away seeking treatment or at school. Jimiyu has been challenging Dembe, siding with their late father's family who argues that the land and children should go back to the paternal clan as is customary when no adults are living. Dembe knows this will leave her and her siblings with nothing and refuses their interference, relying on Ugandan laws that protect the young family's right to their parent's property. Jimiyu has been yearning for items from the West, now increasingly advertised on city storefronts, the internet, and television. He recently accepted a pair of Adidas athletic shoes from a local NGO. Dembe is angry, fearing peers and extended family will be jealous and no longer help if they believe an NGO is supporting the family. Jimiyu is refusing his sister's and maternal grandmother's authority as women and elders.

Every moment of Jimiyu and Dembe's life is affected by the complex nature of sociopolitical and ecological contexts, including traditional gender roles affected by colonization, tribal and clan customs, Western NGOs, Ugandan government and laws, access to physical space and ownership of property, world economy, international power dynamics that influence the availability of ARV treatment, and so on. Societal systems are not simply benign organizational patterns that create a sense of wholeness. They are theaters where struggles for power, influence, and material advantage are acted out.

Social Structures

Third order change requires therapists to carefully examine the influence of social structures. Social structures include socioeconomic stratification, social institutions, and other large systems, which tend to reproduce processes that privilege some over others. Strategies that reproduce and reify these structures occur at all levels, including interactions within families. For example, Farrall and colleagues (2022) highlighted how the competitive nature of international economies and compounding inequalities impact parental aspirations, access to resources, and decision-making. Parents may feel pressured to protect and promote the well-being of children as they enter the contested social and economic terrain of adulthood by doing things like focusing on future occupations, arguing over grades and homework, and rewarding successful competition. These actions may, in turn, inadvertently contribute to reproducing social inequality.

•←→•

Social structures shape the meaning we make of our lives and relationships, the organization of our daily (even most intimate) interactions, the material realities in which we are situated, and the location and expression of our emotional, spiritual, and existential experiences.

•←→•

Social institutions include (among others) family and kinship, community, religion, social welfare and health care, education, economy, mass media, and government/politics. Social structures impose constraints and opportunities over possible individual, group, and institutional actions. Third order change is change in systems of systems within and/or across these social structures. For example, the US legal structures include laws for governing actions and systems for controlling law-breaking behavior, as well as avenues to protect civil rights and seek compensation for wrongdoing. Justice and protection are not, however, equally distributed among all citizens.

Social structures largely determine the material realities of our lives, which in turn deeply affect our well-being. The first US family mentioned above is also female-headed. Melinda is 35; her oldest daughter, Maya, is 15, followed by a 9-year-old daughter and a 6-year-old son. Melinda fled from a physically abusive husband and spent six months in a family shelter before finding a job and apartment. Her daily schedule includes working the night shift as an aide in a nursing home before coming home to help her children get to school. Despite the Equal Pay Act of 1963, as a White woman, Melinda makes approximately 80% of what a White man would make with a similar educational background, yet considerably more than most People of Color in the US (https://nwlc.org/resource/wage-gap-state-white-non-hispanic-women/). Systems of male dominance and patriarchy that promote and maintain violence against women have also deeply affected her family, and continue to be prevalent worldwide (Akhmedshina, 2020). The increasing focus on capitalism and the individual in the US has driven a trend toward warehousing the elderly, creating a greater need for professional caretakers (Esiaka & Adams, 2020), who are often underpaid in capitalist care systems (Nadasen, 2023). This provides Melinda with work, but work that is not highly valued in an ageist society that prioritizes productivity. Melinda must rely on her oldest daughter to help manage the family. When she enters family therapy because one of her children is failing in school, the therapist may pathologize Melinda for Maya's role as a "parentified child."

•←→•

Our relationships are shaped by context, but contexts are not neutral.

•←→•

All societies are plagued with social structures and institutions that promote and maintain unearned privilege, power imbalances, and misuse of power. Our interconnected identities—race, social class, age, sexual identity, gender, nation of origin, language, immigration status, looks, abilities, and other identity markers—shape our opportunities and constraints. People who hold greater social power typically have the strongest influence over the creation of social institutions, including their governing values, norms, and rules (Tatum, 2017). For example, in the US most universities and knowledge produced through universities privilege Western, Euro-centered cultural frameworks. Social welfare institutions likewise set expectations for family interaction and parenting based on dominant middle-class, Euro-centered cultural assumptions. As family therapists, we are in a unique position to analyze, navigate, disrupt, and intervene in these systems.

Culture

Another facet of socioculturally attuned family therapy is having an intentional and third order stance related to culture. Culture refers to beliefs, values, traditions, ways of being and doing, collective meaning-making, shared knowledge and attitudes, and conceptual frameworks for understanding the universe, including spirituality and religion. Culture is fluid and continually shifts as we collectively adapt to changing circumstances. In the example above, both Melinda and Dembe value their families and put the needs of others first. This is a cultural expectation for women in most societies. While it plays out differently in each cultural context, as women they are both struggling with patriarchy and both are deeply affected by global capitalism. Dembe holds cultural values of filial piety and respect for elders. This contributes to her conflict as elders in her father's clan, to whom she might have turned, no longer have her best interests in mind. Cultural traditions that once helped children in her situation now work against her as the dearth of resources leaves most of the country in need. When there were few children left without parents (there was no word for orphan in Dembe's native language prior to civil war and the AIDS pandemic) and clans had enough to share within tribal structures, children would have been protected when their holdings were turned over to elders, along with their care. In the US, Melinda personally cares for elders within a context that has created a growing demand for paid professional caretakers, but within a larger sociocultural context entrenched in ageism that devalues older adults. Maya and Dembe are both 15-year-old girls who love and support their younger siblings. They both spend time each day making sure their siblings are fed, sleep well, and follow family rules. What their dedication means and how it is valued or supported are vastly different across the cultural contexts of the US and Uganda.

James lives in the same city as Maya in one of the most prosperous countries in the world, yet their lives are quite different. James, also 15, gets annoyed with the constant attention of his parents, but knows he can rely on them for meeting the majority of his needs. He feels pressured to do well in school, as both parents are highly educated and expect him to maintain the family's social class advantage. Lately, his grades have been dropping as he spends increasing amounts of time in the privacy of his own room late at night gaming on the internet. When they enter therapy, the therapist fails to understand the nuances of internet addiction. She prioritizes Euro-centered cultural values of privacy and autonomy, subtly discouraging James' parents from insisting they have access to his room or limiting his access to the internet.

↔

It is generally agreed that culture is largely a social construction, a shared system of meaning-making and agreed-upon knowledge. What is often less clear, however, are the dynamics of power embedded in what we refer to as shared knowledge and meaning.

↔

According to Bourdieu (1986), those whose cultural practices are closest to dominant groups have the greatest advantage in society. This includes language, interactional styles, speech patterns, attitudes, and beliefs that can be instrumental in upward class mobility. Bourdieu used the term *cultural capital* to refer to the advantage of being able to navigate and mirror the culture of those in the center who have the greatest access to influence and economic advantage. In the US the most valued and centered cultural capital is that of White, middle and upper class, heterosexual, able-bodied, young to middle-aged men. Those most closely affiliated with this group secure lateral advantage while vertical advantage is secured via their legacies. Qualities associated with them tend to be considered markers of professionalism, while characteristics of People of Color and women are framed as too emotional or not professional enough (Hardy, 2022).

Consider top positions in corporate America. Most often these positions are filled by White men followed by White women who share the dress, language, and mannerisms of the White corporate world (Hardy, 2024). Those already established in the system maintain cultural capital by hiring others who are culturally like them, reproducing organizational culture. Cultural capital promotes social capital and social networks that reproduce individual, in-group advantage (Kaasa, 2019). In our example, the social capital necessary to move up in corporate structures provides entrance into social networks. This capital is the most valued currency in societal systems and social institutions, reifying the privilege of some and marginalizing others. This same dynamic is at play in most therapeutic settings.

Imagine, for example, the differences that are likely to occur in therapy for high and low-status clients. High-status clients are likely to have greater choice in where they go for services. They have greater access to a different therapist should they dislike their provider or feel uncomfortable in a particular context. In contrast, it is likely that stressors that exacerbate problems in the first place (e.g., inadequate transportation, lack of flexibility in work hours, economic stressor, language barriers) contribute to difficulties families with low status might have in even attending therapy. This in turn may be interpreted as low motivation for change by therapists in agencies that have strict "no show" policies. The currency of cultural and social capital also impacts the work of therapy (Garcia & McDowell, 2010). Think for a moment about how you might think and feel as you are getting ready to see someone who is a supreme court judge in couples therapy versus a single mother who has been court-mandated for parenting skills. How might this feeling affect your way of working with them?

The processes mentioned above are similar to colonial processes in which the culture and knowledge of colonizers is centered and imposed as superior. Colonization often relies on the meta-narrative that military strength, technological advancement, and scientific knowledge are evidence of a natural, linear progression of societies. Colonization is internalized, as those being colonized are compelled to assimilate and adopt colonizer language, dress, social practices, values, and beliefs.

Let's refer back to our example of the child-headed family in Uganda. Dembe and her siblings are Christians and benefit from the help of their church. They speak English and dress in Western clothes provided by church members in the US. Jimiyu is being inducted into the world market through media exposure to goods he has come to expect and view as superior but cannot afford. He is beginning to internalize Western values that privilege self over the collective, creating conflict between what he wants and what Dembe expects from him as a brother.

Colonization happens within societies as well. As therapists, we are often faced with externalized and internalized superiority and/or oppression (e.g., racism, sexism, classism, homophobia, ableism, ageism, nationism) in ourselves and in those with whom we work. Left unchecked, our own practices as family therapists can be oppressive and colonizing (Almeida & Williams, 2026; Almeida & Tubbs, 2020; Almeida, 2018; Almeida, et al., 2017; McDowell, 2015). For example, consider a family entering therapy because their three-year-old is having trouble sleeping in her own room. The therapist may inadvertently promote Euro-centered cultural values of independence and individuality if she simply assumes this is a problem that will result in long-term dependence or is a sign something is going wrong in the child's development. Wherever the child ends up sleeping, it is important that the therapist is able to help the parents think through their assumptions and how their concerns may be being influenced by dominant values with which they themselves may or may not agree. In Text Box 2.1, marcela polanco shares the central role decoloniality plays in her work.

Text Box 2.1 marcela polanco, PhD, LMFT

marcela polanco (she, her and hers) is a Spanglish, Colombiana-Spanish and Immigrant-English speaker. She is interested in decolonial projects, including those that do not depend on the decolonial framework to address colonial power in everyday life. She is faculty at San Diego State University located in unceded territory of the Kumeyaay. Her doctoral degree is in Marriage and Family Therapy, and her main topic of interest is Spanglish Decolonial Healing.

My everyday life, supervision, pedagogy, therapy, and research depart from the assumption that for the majority of the world, our experiences continue to be administered and controlled by Europe's modernity "universal" design, as disseminated through its authors, knowledges, languages, and settings since the conquest of the Americas. Although in English I trained in narrative therapy, I am no longer guided by knowledge and understanding organized as models in English to guide practices. This has sparked an interest in thinking, sensing, and doing through communal engagements guided by ethics, plurilinguality, forming coalitions, radical listening, or reception of stories. These vary as I continue to learn from people, families, and communities, including various decolonial projects outside of therapy and from various geo-histories.

I attune to sociocultural context and power dynamics through decoloniality. The decolonial project provides me with one possibility, among many others, to understand how our lives are embedded in modernity's design. I also identify and name issues through this lens. Coloniality is a tool for the analysis of how everyday lives are tied to modernity through its colonial matrix of power. This matrix disputes the control of four interdependent domains that shape our lives in the current world most of us live in: capitalism, eurocentrism, race/gender, and institutionalization. Coloniality helps me discern how our lives are not only tied to, but configured by, modernity's economic capitalist system, hierarchical categorization of identities through the ideas of race and gender, promotion of Eurocentric reason, evidence and scientific knowledge, and administered or governed by institutions and its policies.

I amplify and value what has been silenced and marginalized by making visible the coloniality of modernity's design. We can see its cracks and make these cracks opportunities for restitution. This not only means exploring coloniality within the context of people's lives who come to therapy, but also the therapist's life, family therapy as a profession, family therapy models, curriculums, educational institutions, and mental health providers of family therapy.

I interrupt unjust relationships and/or challenge unjust systems in my work from a geo-politics and body-politics perspective. For example, in decoloniality, we can locate practices, ideas, values, languages, and concepts in the particular contexts where they belong and the bodies who invented them. By doing so, we can no longer take these concepts for granted as the only and universal reality. By locating family therapy and its models within the location and bodies who developed our field, we can see more clearly that our field follows a particular genealogy, thus opening the possibility for the exploration of practices of people who come from other places and are generated from other genealogies.

I envision transformative change that supports relational equity and/or cultural democracy by supporting unlearning experiences that delink us from modernity's universalist promises. This means humbling English, European models, professions, the university, etc. to engage in possibilities for re-existence and co-existence in other languages, from other places, and by many other people. I approach and encourage transformative, third order change by incorporating decolonial projects that seek to delink from coloniality in the MFT curriculum and by engaging other than English languages to explore experiences of healing from modernity's fractures, with particular interest in Spanglish.

As mentioned throughout this section, all of these processes occur within global, national, and local contexts, highlighting the importance of taking a global perspective throughout our work. In Text Box 2.2, Mudita Rastogi shares her Systemic Integrative Framework (2020) that integrates a global perspective that pays close attention to pancultural, contextual, intersectional, and integrational aspects of identity, worldview, and just relationships.

Text Box 2.2 Mudita Rastogi, PhD, LMFT

Mudita Rastogi (she/her) has an abiding interest in systemic intervention, gender, diversity, equity and inclusion, race, culture, ethnicity, multiculturalism, diasporas, global mental health, South Asian families, trauma, and intergenerational relationships.

The Systemic Integrative Framework (SIF) emphasizes that systemic conceptualization and interventions must include an integration of a global perspective. We must include contextual and historical knowledge about communities and knowledge from the Global Mental Health (GMH) movement to be fully inclusive and culturally sensitive in our work as systemic family therapists. The body of work in the area of GMH focuses on inequities, differences, and diversity in thinking in families and communities across the globe, and especially for those who have connections across the diaspora due to their identity, immigration, displacement, and kinships.

Use of the SIF allows therapists and clients to pay special attention to the ongoing impact of sociopolitical events around the world (Rastogi, 2020). In a world of high connectivity, people are deeply impacted by events both locally, domestically, and even in far off locations. The SIF actively encourages practitioners, students, clients, and readers to examine the underlying assumptions of Euro-American frameworks and ask themselves how they can pursue a just approach, whether it is through validation of a different perspective, acknowledging the impact of unrelenting images of trauma on us, listening to stories of resilience, understanding the weight of political divisiveness on our psyches, and/or undertaking advocacy.

Client–therapist conversations are both an assessment and an intervention. Using circular and open-ended questions and the four domains of the SIF helps glean a multilayered picture of the client's worldviews (Pancultural), relationship to worldwide sociopolitical events (Contextual), past and present identities (Intersectional), and unique situation (Integrational). This process is cyclical and repeated in greater depth as therapy progresses. Clients' responses inform interventions and lead to deeper questions about their sociocultural context.

From the moment a client connects with me, I share that we will consider their challenges in the context of larger social realities and intersections. I use the SIF to guide the exploration of various areas of the clients' experiences. This might include proximal issues like difficulty finding a therapist who appreciates the nuances of the clients' culture all the way to traumatic feelings from having watched violence being inflicted on innocent civilians. I spend time in sessions linking the clients' responses to their presenting problems, relationship challenges, and larger systems.

I tune in keenly to the ways in which clients name, identify, and present themselves. I validate clients by saying something to the effect of: "You make an important point that this is not fair or benign. You are not imagining this. You were treated unfairly or what you witnessed is deeply disturbing. Sometimes, a lack of fairness comes from how institutions work, who yields power, commonly held beliefs about certain groups of people, or socialization practices, etc. This does not make it okay. If you would like, we can discuss your feelings of disempowerment (rage, sadness, fear, shock) a bit more today or in the future." Clients are encouraged to share stories of transgenerational adversities and are also gently challenged to identify their own blind spots and revisit them for fairness and accuracy, after which they are invited to repair what they can or make meaning of it.

The above process allows for new linkages and insights that sometimes relocate client challenges from within the individual and family, to societal processes. I help name the oppression and/or microaggressions that might not be voiced otherwise and encourage clients to do their own reflection and make connections around these issues outside the therapy room. Using the insights gained in the session, clients are encouraged to set goals that include not just personal care, transformation, and family changes, but social action, advocacy for self and community, and/or steps that impact larger systems. I also keep in mind that this is the client's journey, and it will progress at their pace.

As part of applying the SIF in diverse situations, the client-therapist-community systems are agents of third order change and are themselves transformed. From an SIF perspective, intervention is expansive, aspires to be sustainable, and includes change at all levels.

Outside of the therapy room, I have engaged in community work that can impact larger groups of people who might not have knowledge of or are unable to easily access mental health services and mentoring. I direct my research, scholarship, and community work towards third order change, such as interrupting injustice, reducing barriers, and increasing access to mental health services globally.

I identify as a systemic thinker, a teacher, a globalist, feminist, cultural interpreter, challenger, and a couple, marriage, and family therapy integrator. Being a wife, mother, daughter, sister, aunt, and friend are as important to me as my professional roles. I often describe myself as having two homes, namely the US and India, and am passionate about relationships in all corners of the world.

Relationships Between Species

There are significant differences in cultural perspectives and beliefs about the relationship between humans and other animals. These differences can have a significant impact on therapeutic processes. For example, as a Western therapist, I (Teresa) readily accept the view of pets as family members (Honeycutt, 2018) and often include them in conversations with families. I have welcomed dogs to join families in the therapy room, included pets in patterns of interaction and attachment, and recognized the importance of pets to individual and family resilience (Walsh, 2009a, 2009b). I was raised in a Western, Christian family and culture that views humans as superior to other animals and adopts a categorical view of non-human animals, i.e., distinguishing between those we keep as pets and those we eat; those we view as worthy of our protection and those we see as having little or no value. I found myself in a conversation with a Native American client who viewed animals in a very different way. She was deeply disturbed by precognitive dreams of death worsened by being visited by a white owl. Even though animals have symbolic and spiritual meaning in many cultures worldwide, my own speciesist view of humans as unique and innately superior to all other beings contributed to the risk that I would be "culturally sensitive" to my client's beliefs without recognizing multiple ways of knowing as equally possible and valid. As I struggled in the moment to navigate the situation, I met the risk the client had taken in sharing her local knowledge with a cultural outsider by also taking a risk by allowing myself to embrace the client's perspective as true. This opened space for both of us to authentically explore her situation. In retrospect, I realize I adopted a superposition.

Taking a Superposition

It can be difficult to reconcile competing paradigms, e.g., postmodern, modern, and critical perspectives, to effectively use them in family therapy practice. Metamodernism provides a broadened perspective of these and other ways of thinking that acknowledges their co-existence and the potential to create links between them (Dempsey, 2025; Gardner, 2016; Yousef, 2017). While the term metamodernism continues to center modern paradigms and postmodern critiques, we adopt an expanded definition that refers to taking a meta perspective in relation to all paradigms of thought or cultural logics. Cultural paradigms are widely accepted beliefs, assumptions, sets of ideas, and perspectives that define how we see the world. New paradigms challenge prevailing ways of looking at the world, often supplanting existing systems of thought (Kuhn, 1962). For example, at least in the Western world, modernism challenged prior paradigms (e.g., romanticism, supernaturalism) just as postmodernism challenged modernism. Condescending terms (e.g., animism, superstition, *espiritismo*) are often used to minimize, infantilize, and delegitimize non-Western, non-colonial, non-scientific systems of thought. Furthermore, the familiar phrase "we used to think…" reflects an assumption that humanity is making linear progress toward ultimate understanding. This way of looking at the world privileges contemporary Western (including modern and postmodern) thought by delegitimizing non-Western, non-colonial, Indigenous, local, spiritual, and traditional knowledge claims.

For us, taking an ontological and epistemological superposition allows us to simultaneously expand thinking in multiple directions to reflect on possibilities within, and relationships between, various systems of thought. This opens space to legitimize and participate within diverse ways of thinking and doing.

Power

Socioculturally attuned family therapists will also carefully attend to the matrix of power dynamics across contexts.

↞→

Power is a set of social processes by which individual and collective interests are determined.

↞→

Social context and relational equity are not add-ons but central to the development and maintenance of symptoms. In the previous chapter, we referred to a married, heterosexual woman entering therapy for depression. Locating the depression inside of her as an individual would likely limit her ability to think differently. Encouraging her to increase her physical activity and/or begin taking antidepressants, and offering a venue for her to express her feelings and concerns are important; however, imagine we include these potentially useful interventions but in the context of relationships and taking power into account. We help the couple develop an equal, mutually attuned relationship in which they both feel heard and connected (Knudson-Martin, 2024). They eventually share equal influence with each other as they negotiate to get their needs met within the relationship, as well as the social awareness to traverse a societal context that routinely privileges one over the other. Her depression vanishes.

Power dynamics are central to understanding emotional and relational well-being. While family therapists routinely explore emotion, we rarely contextualize emotion within social and relational power dynamics (Smoliak et al., 2023). Sociologists have found that those with influence and privilege tend to experience more negative emotions, including hurt, anger, guilt, and shame (Turner, 2007). Not getting what we perceive we deserve often results in negative emotions. For example, the third order nature of the Black Lives Matter Movement is often met with an angry backlash from those who fear their chances of getting what they expect and believe they deserve will be diminished, even if these expectations are based on a sense of entitlement and racial privilege.

Power processes not only inform *what* people feel, they also determine whose feelings are considered important, whose emotions are attended to, and who is considered worthy of care (Smoliak et al., 2022). Power thus works through emotion and can be replicated or transformed in therapy depending on the therapist's approach (Knudson-Martin, 2024, Smoliak at al., 2023). There is ample evidence that equality in adult relationships promotes individual and relational well-being, and analysis of nuanced power dynamics between couples has become increasingly sophisticated (Knudson-Martin, 2024, 2025). According to Knudson-Martin (2013) "the ability of couples to withstand stress, respond to change, and enhance each partner's health and well-being depends on their having a relatively equal power balance" (p. 6). She further contended that, "clinical change is hard to sustain unless therapists assess for and attend to the power processes underlying…relational dynamics." This calls for therapists to be able to assess and interrupt power imbalances rather than maintaining the illusion that one can be neutral in the face of relational inequity.

The analysis of power needs to extend beyond couples to include relational and social dynamics in non monogamous and polyamorous families. According to Jordan, et al. (2016), when working with polyamorous families, it is important to consider the complexities and interconnections between power within families, power between the therapist and family, and power without, i.e. between families and their social context. It may be difficult for monogamous therapists to fully attune to the stigma, social pressure, and discrimination that those who are polyamorous are likely to experience. It is important for therapists to scrutinize biases toward monogamy. Without this awareness, it is difficult to name, navigate, and interrupt problematic power dynamics when more than two people are in a committed relationship.

Power in the Practice of Family Therapy

Power dynamics have been theorized in a number of ways by family therapists over time (Young & Seedall, 2024). Early family therapists tended to view power as a pragmatic issue relevant to symptom formation and maintenance within family systems. Communications theorists (Jackson & Jackson, 1968) identified couple relationships as complementary or symmetrical. Complementary relationships were defined as those in which one partner was in charge and leading while the other was following. Symmetrical relationships were defined as those in which both partners wanted to lead, creating competition and escalating conflict. Nearly a decade later, Salvador Minuchin (1974) conceptualized power in families as vertical and horizontal through a focus on hierarchy and boundaries. Later, Cloe Madanes (1981) considered relational power imbalances as central to understanding and treating symptoms, the symptom itself being part of the power equation. Relational power dynamics were, however, not often placed in societal context. Hierarchical incongruencies and power imbalances were not routinely linked to systems of privilege and oppression until the feminist critique.

More recently critical social theories (e.g., critical race theory, intersectional feminism, queer theory, decolonial theory, critical geography, critical sociology) have been applied to broaden the understanding of and contextualize power in family therapy as relational and multi-directional (McDowell, 2015). Those with greater available resources are in positions to impose their objectives or will on others—whether directly or by default. For example, a parent often has a greater physical presence that can be imposed, as well as social power and financial resources needed by a child. The child can bring refusal to cooperate and emotional withdrawal to bear on the relationship, but a parent can deny the child movement within and beyond the home, withhold food and other wants or needs, and threaten or use physical and emotional pain to exert influence. Ultimately the child has the power of social institutions that protect children, but only if parents exert power that causes harm beyond what is allowed by law.

Descriptions of power mentioned above fall within a modern, structural functional paradigm. Postmodern approaches to family therapy attend to power in a different way, primarily based on the work of Michel Foucault (1972). What in the modern era was considered universal and natural came under further attack with the postmodern critique in which knowledge and power are seen as inseparable, i.e., what is considered knowledge depends on societal power relations. Power is not held, but enacted. According to this view, we don't possess power; power is constructive and generative as well as constraining.

Power is not simply coercive, but a productive organizing force in society and generated via interactional choreography. For example, power is produced when we get in line to ride a bus and admonish those who cut in front; when we enter a lecture hall and expect everyone to take a seat; or when we judge someone's overly casual attire at a wedding or funeral. This type of power results in policing ourselves and each other in order to create, shape, and conform to common, expected practices in societies and families. Take a typical, rather unnoticed family routine. All members of a family come to the table when called, sit and wait for the blessing to be said, pass food to others, begin eating using prescribed manners, and engage in lively conversation. Everyone knows what to do in this common social practice. If all family members don't come to the table, someone is designated to go and get them.

Power dynamics reverberate across all levels of societal systems and social structures, including our most intimate family relationships. Our face-to-face interactions are impacted by our access to power and resources on societal levels. Consider another family that gathers for dinner. When these children come to the table, they sit quietly out of the view of their father who often performs power through scowling or demanding silence. The mother attempts to mediate the effects of the father's exertion of power by predicting his needs, sending non-verbal cues to children if they complain about the food, and keeping dinner moving swiftly. This family performs a common social practice of having dinner together while reflecting broad organizing principles of their society in which women must be more attuned to needs and desires of men as men take on more authoritative roles; male privilege and dominance in the family mirrors social roles in which males are centered and dominant in government, business, religious, and other social institutions.

McDowell (2015) offered the following description that integrates modern, postmodern and critical understandings of power:

> Power is pervasive and unevenly distributed; systematic and idiosyncratic. Imagine power as everywhere shaping our collective and individual decisions about how to interact with each other across diverse contexts. We basically know what to expect within our cultural groups and familiar settings. We maintain social practices by policing each other and ourselves. Now imagine that power also pools up or thickens in some places; that some of us have more resources and greater influence to bring to bear in shaping singular and collective interactions. Collectively, those with greater resources and influence shape cultural practices and ideologies in ways that benefit their own group and maintain greater access to resources. Now imagine all of this in motion with those being threatened reacting to potential and actualized power by yielding, withdrawing, navigating, and/or pushing back… In other words, imagine a complex web of influence that is systematically designed to maintain power and access to resources of some over others but is also filled with idiosyncratic, highly nuanced power dynamics in local specific contexts. It is this type of complexity we deal with daily in the practice of family therapy. (pp. 6–7)

Decisions about Using Power and Influence

We are all deeply influenced by broad social power dynamics, yet as individuals within relationships, we still have choices about how to enact and/or garner influence with each other. We consider a plethora of immediate and long-term consequences of our actions. We may attempt to limit another's power over us by reducing their potential to overpower. At times we accommodate others to avoid harm or access power by proxy. We decide purposefully or inadvertently how to exert influence—what methods to use and how far to press. We evaluate the costs of persuading or demanding others bend to our will, calculating the nature and history of the relationship and how others are likely to respond.

For example, one of the partners in a same-gender couple demands the other come out to family and friends as their relationship moves toward the possibility of marriage. Has the situation become unbearable, warranting the risk of losing the relationship if there is a refusal to live openly married? Is the demand unreasonable, creating unwarranted risk or emotional stress for the partner who wants to move more slowly due to homophobia within their family? We also consider our own values and ideal selves as well as how we want others to see us. Was it difficult for the partner to make such a demand, as doing so goes against their view of self as a caring partner? Socioculturally attuned therapists must consider how multiple sources of power (and resistance to power) are part of the issues clients bring to us and our work with them (Young & Seedall, 2024).

Power and Resistance

Wherever there is oppression there is also resistance to oppression. Presenting problems can sometimes be identified as resistance to oppressive relationships. This can be imagined throughout the examples above: children run away or constantly fight with parents, a partner refuses to listen when feeling pushed by the other's demands, a family accommodates a domineering power figure but only in that figure's presence, a withdrawal into the safety and power of depression. Routine responses to being overpowered can become automatic, creating problems in future relationships. Resistance can, however, also create resilience and promote relational equality. For example, family members who learned to constantly accommodate an oppressive parent fine-tune their abilities to read moods, context, and nuanced power dynamics. The child who fights back develops the ability to speak out and weather conflict.

•←→•

When we miss power dynamics, we not only overlook the opportunity to build on resistance and resilience but risk inadvertently contributing to the problem.

•←→•

Less powerful persons can be pathologized and/or made to carry the greater burden for change when well-meaning therapists center their attention on simply removing symptoms of oppression. For example, it is not uncommon for a partner who is in a one-down position to feel dismissed by a more powerful and (therefore) less attuned partner. This may lead the one-down partner to common sense solutions such as repeating arguments and escalating in anger in attempts to influence the relationship. When the couple arrives in therapy, the therapist is faced with one partner who seems unreasonable and out of control (but is actually resisting being overpowered) and one who presents as cool and collected, even patiently enduring unreasonable wrath. In these situations, we may inadvertently reinforce relational inequity by resting our attention on calming the partner who resorts to screaming and nagging, seeing this partner's actions as the greater problem. If one of the partners is diagnosed, it is likely to be the one who is (actually attempting to be) out of control.

When we miss power dynamics, we also run the risk of missing what cannot be said in families. While this is often highly nuanced, the readiest example occurs where there is intimate partner violence. Hopefully, all family therapists now screen for violence, spending at least some time with each partner to offer opportunities for disclosure. Just as being overpowered can lead to angry outbursts, physical and emotional symptoms, and withdrawal, it can also lead to silence.

From Principles to Practice

Socioculturally attuned therapists sensitively apprehend and resonate with clients' social contexts (D'Aniello, et al., 2016; Knudson-Martin, 2024; Pandit, et al., 2014) while recognizing the limits of knowing, i.e., the incompleteness of their understanding, the evolving nature of what is knowable, and what remains virtually unknowable. Therapists must be vigilant to understand and consider the impact of intersecting social, historical, economic, religious, political, and cultural systems each time we intervene in a local "here and now" context. We must keep multiple systems levels in mind while considering the interaction between these systems, societal power processes, and specific family dynamics. In other words, therapists engage by continually connecting the dots between broad social levels and intimate and family relationships.

Socioculturally attuned family therapists continuously make the connection between power dynamics at larger social levels and problems at the most intimate relational levels. The concept of isomorphism is familiar to family therapists and can be used to understand the ways in which family systems reflect the organization of larger social systems in which they are embedded (Fishman, 2022). Sociologists refer to isomorphism as mimetic, normative, or coercive (DiMaggio & Powell, 1983). Families are affected by all three of these processes, i.e., they often mimic the organization, structure, and rules of larger social systems (e.g., patriarchy); follow social norms and values that govern institutions across societies (e.g., valuing hard work); and/or experience pressure from outside systems to conform to particular ways of being (e.g., parenting in socially sanctioned ways). From postmodern perspectives, families are thought to reflect and make meaning of their experiences through dominant social discourses. In turn, these discourses affect every aspect of life including how we feel and what we do.

Therapists working from a socioculturally attuned perspective need to be diligent not to inadvertently reproduce the status quo of societal context and power relations in the therapy process or in their work as advocates. Not noticing or intervening in relational inequity, failing to address sexism and racism, and practicing from White middle-class perspectives are just a few of the many ways we contribute to unjust systems. Likewise, taking a first-order, "us and them" stance in which we expect to create change by denouncing others, contributes to maintaining structural inequity via social, political, and relational polarization. Third space (Soja, 2010) can be created by engaging in critical dialogue and reflection (Freire, 1970/2000), imagining and supporting just relationships, and collaborating with families to create strategies for action that support third order change.

ANVIET: Transtheoretical Socioculturally Attuned Practices

Practicing socioculturally attuned family therapy requires us to infuse the practice of family therapy models with an understanding of how societal context and power dynamics contribute to mental health and relational problems. The transtheoretical goal of socioculturally attuned practice that supports equity can be integrated into interventions within all family therapy models using six practices to accomplish a central mission—to disrupt inequalities in social relationships that are largely invisible, taken-for-granted, or assumed natural and to open options for relational systems

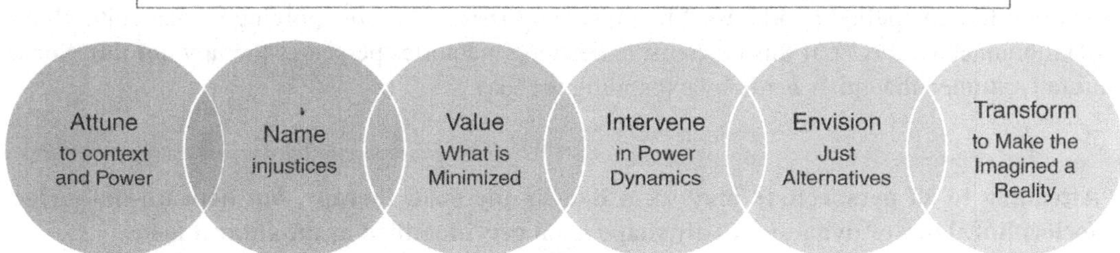

Figure 2.2 ANVIET: Sociocultural practices that promote third order change

that equitably support the health and well-being of all. Because awareness typically precedes action and transformation (Freire, 1970/2000), we present these practices in the order most likely to be effective: attune, name, value, intervene, envision, and transform. In actuality, they are interconnected and used in varying ways across each phase of therapy (Figure 2.2). ANVIET (attune, name, value, interrupt, envision, and transform) is an acronym for a transtheoretical guide for equity-based, third order practice.

Attune to Context and Power

Applying socioculturally attuned principles to each of the models described in this book means therapists intentionally attune to the connections between the larger social context and clinical issues from the very beginning of therapy. This is critical. A study of how therapists practice sociocultural attunement (Pandit, et al., 2014) found therapists internalized a guiding lens that led them to explore the connections between the emotions, behaviors, patterns, and ideas expressed in session and sociocultural processes. This lens prompted an internal dialogue regarding how societal discourses and power structures might underlie client behavior and expressions, as well as the therapist's own internal reactions. This guided what therapists reflected back to clients and the questions they asked in order to help create a sociocultural interpretation that resonated with clients' experience.

Sociocultural attunement occurred when clients appeared to feel understood; therapists "got" their sociocultural experience. When this happened "clients expanded their level of disclosure, showed more emotion, became more relational in conversation, and physically connected with therapists; i.e., nodding, maintaining eye contact" (Pandit, et al., 2014, p. 524). For example, when a therapist recognized and reflected a disabled woman's guilt because she could not care for her children "the way a mother should" as a sociocultural belief, the woman "began to tear up, nod, and share her struggles and fears about not being a "good mother" (p. 524). If clients did not resonate and instead avoided eye contact, disagreed, looked confused, changed the direction of the conversation, or told the same story again, therapists did not abandon their sociocultural lens. They modified their own responses, questioning/reflecting.

The goal of attunement is to not only understand the sociocontextual factors involved in a particular case, but to as much as possible apprehend a client's felt experience in that context—to be *with* them while maintaining humility regarding our ability to fully know another (D'Aniello, et al., 2016; Knudson-Martin & Smoliak, in press). A study of senior family therapists known for addressing social justice issues found they tend to be transparent with clients about what they see through their sociocultural lens, use inquiry rather than telling to bring these concerns to the foreground, and stay close to client experience when exploring sociocultural issues rather than using abstract concepts (D'Arrigo-Patrick, et al., 2017). Another study found that novice therapists often felt compelled to address "the presenting issues"'before applying a sociocultural lens (O'Halloran, et al., 2017). If this happens, underlying inequities persist as therapy unfolds. Socioculturally attuned therapists *begin* by expanding the lens.

•←→•

Attending to all perspectives may seem like simply good therapy, but beneath-the-surface sociocultural power dynamics easily shape what gets identified as the clinical focus.

•←→•

Socioculturally attuned therapists recognize and attend to how power dynamics are part of clients' experiences and are reflected in session. They do not allow more powerfully situated members to define the direction of therapy. As they help families explore problems, socioculturally attuned therapists are aware that not all voices in a relationship come from equal positions. For example, when a father says that the problem is that the mother and the boys fight, and the family seems ready to agree to this problem, socioculturally attuned therapists consider how power may be at play and invite other perspectives before determining the problematic sequence.

Name Injustice

In the process of "naming" we select some experiences or ways of knowing and directly or implicitly link them to possible feelings and actions (St. George & Wulff, 2014).

•←→•

It matters how we talk about clinical concerns.

•←→•

What therapists listen for, highlight, and name is not neutral and carries the weight of professional privilege (Bridges et al., 2022a, 2022b). When unfair or unjust circumstances and expectations are overlooked or minimized in clinical discourse, individuals are pathologized and clients blame themselves without connecting their troubles to larger conditions (St. George & Wulff, 2016). Socioculturally attuned therapists guide the conversation to name unfair or unjust circumstances and amplify voices whose experiences are likely to be silenced.

St. George and Wulff (2016) offered an example from their work in Canada. A middle-class biracial stepfamily sought therapy because their 16-year-old daughter had been caught lying and stealing. The parents had "developed a stern attitude of discipline using accusation, yelling, and punishment…as well as 'giving up' on their daughter" (p. 3). When the therapist attuned to the social context around this family's struggles, the daughter said she "didn't care what people at school said" and the parents described comments by co-workers and people at school that "mixed race families were always trouble" and "innuendos about blended families." Comments like these shamed the parents and led them to believe *they* were bad parents, exacerbating (or perhaps even causing) the family pattern of control and defiance. Naming the biases and the discrimination the family experienced expanded the conversation beyond the therapy room and enabled them to more thoughtfully address their responses to societal expectations and each other.

Value What is Minimized

Socioculturally attuned therapists acknowledge the worth of that which has been minimized or devalued in the dominant social structure and use these values and practices to promote healing (Knudson-Martin at al., 2020). By doing so, the therapeutic process begins to counter social inequities and sets the stage for transformation.

•←→•

Socioculturally attuned therapists develop special radar for ferreting out and highlighting strengths that dominant cultural and power processes mask.

•←→•

These include almost any strength associated with females or with cultures that place less emphasis on individuality and competition, such as caring for others, empathy, accommodating to preserve harmony, or prioritizing family and relationship bonds. They also include the skills and mindsets needed to survive with few economic resources or with physical disabilities.

Let's imagine a male client who sought help for depression. He has internalized an identity as "not assertive enough" and was recently overlooked for a promotion at work. He feels like a failure, like he doesn't fit. Rather than agreeing with the dominant culture assumption that what matters is that he learns how to better assert himself or promote the products he is selling, the therapist named the dominant value assumption and asks questions about other aspects of his identity, listening for and validating culturally minimized strengths.

Therapist: It sounds like there is a strong force for you to be assertive, to press your product, or stand up for yourself. I'm wondering about the other side—when you are there for others. Does that happen?

Client: I think I am there for others a lot. That's always been important to me, you know. But I need to learn not to do that so much, to be more aggressive.

Therapist: It seems like being there for others is a pretty important thing. Have you seen ways that that's been good in your life, or has made life better for others?

Validating this client's capacity and desire to support others countered patriarchal expectations that men should lead or dominate others. The therapy enabled him to feel good about himself, improve his relationship with his wife, and develop career goals that did not require him to discount the value of focusing on others. His depression dissipated.

Therapists also absorb dominant cultural values. The ability to recognize and explicitly value that which is socially marginalized or does not fit into dominant expectations requires reflective practices on the therapist's part. For example, an African American therapist presented a case in supervision. The client was a 28-year-old African American woman who lived with her mother and younger siblings and helped support them. The therapist initially defined the client's problem as a lack of maturity and differentiation from the family of origin, stating that she was sabotaging her own growth for the sake of the family. Despite her own identity as a Black woman, she evaluated her client through an individualistic lens promoted in academia and treatment systems (Whiting et al., 2024). A socioculturally attuned approach will explore and honor the client's ties to her family before automatically focusing on her autonomy. The therapist will be aware of how readily obligations to others are discounted in the broader culture and create space to value and reinforce them. She will be aware of how her own interpretations and responses may be skewed toward individualism as a dominant cultural value.

Intervene in Power Dynamics

Positioning therapy to disrupt oppressive power dynamics and support relational equity takes reflexivity and active intervention on the therapist's part (Jenks et al., 2024; Knudson-Martin, 2024). This does *not* mean that therapists need a directive stance toward therapy. Rather, they use their facilitative role to recognize when societal power dynamics are at play and use interventions that interrupt and challenge inequitable power while empowering clients to create ways to transform them. You will see many such examples throughout the case illustrations in this book.

Envision Just Alternatives

It is not enough to identify injustice or power inequities. Therapists need to provide space to imagine just relational alternatives. A task analysis found heterosexual couples dealing with infidelity *only* moved toward equity when therapists invited them to envision alternatives to gender stereotypes (Williams, et al., 2013). For example, they suggested enactments in which powerful partners initiate relational repair or asked partners to discuss what shared responsibility for maintaining the relationship would look like for them (an alternative to the idea that this is a woman's job).

When clients' social identities are marginalized, they may blame themselves for their problems– "I am lazy," "I have low self esteem," or "I have anger problems." Interventions into power dynamics will begin from the premise that these self-referents are examples of how persons located outside the dominant culture have been colonized by it (Bermúdez et al., 2024; Hernández-Wolfe, 2013; Jordan 2022). A socioculturally attuned cognitive behavioral therapist (Chapter 11) would help clients recognize the root of these thoughts, notice when they are being triggered, and envision a new response. A socioculturally attuned structural family therapist (Chapter 5) would explore the family rules and patterns around these ideas, help family members link these to the effects of social structures, and use enactments to envision alternatives.

Transform to Make the Imagined a Reality

Third order change results when what is imagined is made real. Socioculturally attuned family therapists collaborate with clients by being responsively persistent (Sutherland, et al., 2013). They keep bringing clients back to sources of strength and equity in their lives that enable their preferred vision of themselves. For example, in Boszormenyi Nagy's contextual family therapy (Chapter 10), socioculturally attuned therapists help people be intentional about their response to family and societal injustice, what they want to see going forward for themselves, their children, and posterity. They encourage and support clients' commitment and accountability to these ethical values, giving due credit and care to each other.

Socioculturally attuned family therapists help clients identify and solidify the changes they are making. They help clients see themselves as part of larger systemic processes and consider how others may respond as they make third order changes that resist dominant norms. They help clients develop social supports and strategies to sustain them, not only within their families, but in their communities and social networks. In essence, third order change is transformative, creating paradigmatic shifts and equity. In Text Box 2.3, Hoa Nguyen describes situating her work with queer immigrant families within sociocultural context.

In Text Box 2.4, Rhea Almeida offers another example, using cultural circles and ANVIET practices to move therapy from an individual endeavor to a community effort that helps clients consider the problems they are facing against the backdrop of intersecting sociopolitical processes. Participants envision alternative possibilities and support and hold each other accountable to making their transformative ideals real.

Text Box 2.3 Hoa Nguyen, PhD, LMFT

Hoa Nguyen (she/her) is an Associate Professor at Valdosta State University in Georgia. She teaches courses in diversity, inclusion, and social justice, and draws from her Vietnamese immigrant family history of resettlement and rebuilding home in the United States post-Vietnam War.

My work focuses on navigating the spaces between cultural and sexual identity, which is inherently embedded in social, economic, political, and environmental contexts. When considering the experiences of queer immigrants, their personal and relational problems are tethered to their social and cultural capital. Understanding the vital relationships and community in their lives serves as the groundwork for exploring possible insights, strengths, and opportunities. These communal resources are part of their survival in times of political and social strife. In particular, experiences of home and diaspora are complexified for queer immigrants whose lived experiences are rejected or erased by larger social discourses. At the root of this work is navigating the question: how can we create a sense of home and belonging for people of all sexualities, genders, and cultures?

I believe it is important to decolonize family therapy and become more attuned to the Western, individualistic lens that inevitably shapes psychotherapy. I attune in exploring dominant narratives that subjugate our clients' lives and work to construct possibilities that resist these marginalizing experiences. One such dominant narrative is the binary notion of gender, sexuality, and identity. For individuals and communities that exist beyond the binary, holding space for the complexity and in-betweenness embedded in their lived experiences is critical to challenge Eurocentric beliefs. By giving ourselves permission and legitimacy to live in the in-between spaces of culture and identity, we can counter these systems of oppression that dictate absolute thinking and ways of being.

Finally, I hope to bring into discussion the political, economic, and social injustices that are occurring in clients' lives. By naming these problems as contextualized within systems of power and oppression, clients are liberated from the blame and shame that are often produced through injustice, opening up other ways of being, other solutions, and other possibilities of seeing themselves and relating to others. Working with other professionals to disrupt the societal scapegoating of marginalized individuals is a key component of third-order cybernetics.

Text Box 2.4 Rhea V. Almeida, PhD, LCSW

Rhea V. Almeida (she/hers), director and founder of the Institute for Family Services, has been a leader in liberation-based practice over the last 4 decades.

I view liberation praxis, which is how I describe my work, as resonating with the "disruption" of coloniality. This endeavor involves disengaging with the status quo and erecting/installing instead knowledges and structures from border spaces. This is contiguous with providing families paths to disengage/disrupt the status quo in the spirit of healing and transforming lived experience embedded in oppressive spaces.

Liberatory healing today could not be more needed across sites and institutions, including schools, corporations, health and mental health institutions, and academic environments. That is, if there is a will to disembark from the project of coloniality and our collective moral compass of inhumanity.

Critical consciousness refers to awakening to the realities of the social and political order which are no longer viewed as unchangeable. Conscientización does not occur in a one-to-one individualized isolated context. It happens in community or healing circles as I call them. Using the graphic of Power, Privilege & Oppression, popular movies, songs, magazines, newspaper articles, and other forms of social media along with handouts/tools that reflect multiple intersects of social location, societal structures, and systems of inequity, the process of identifying and naming these lived experiences begins.

The path forward requires synthesis: simultaneous attention to multiple oppressions and privileges, linking public and private matters through dialogues and reflection. This process within a context and connection to people from varied backgrounds and complex lived experiences establishes the platform for identifying, naming and challenging trajectories of power, privilege, and oppression. Critical consciousness is an essential precursor to liberatory healing.

The process is a generative one in that the voices and lived experiences of dominance and those silenced and otherized are scaffolded. These conversations within the therapeutic space launch the imagination of interruptions and challenges of systems engaged/complicit in the evisceration of multiple lived experiences. This imagination of border spaces moves into action strategies through linking of collective connections.

An example of this process is that of Brianna, a Latina woman, working class, language challenged, single parent who was faced with Rosey, her daughter, being labeled ADHD and continuously receiving notes about her out-of-control behavior in the classroom. The school was relatively diverse with a larger percentage being White and middle to upper class. In bringing her daughter to therapy she was invested in aligning with us to teach her daughter to acquiesce to the school values and expectations of her behavior.

The problematized narrative by the school, and adopted by Brianna, did not occur in our space. Rosey was respectful, did not appear to have any behavioral issues but did appear to have difficulty reading at her grade level in our circle sessions. Upon receiving requested school documents, it became apparent that Rosey at the end of 3rd grade was reading at a 1st grade level. Throughout the second and third year of her behavioral problems in school, there was no remediation or testing of her reading skills. We recommended to Brianna that Rosey be tested with the goal of receiving some form of remediation. She was not convinced.

We explored her family of origin and her immigration stories from Costa Rica. She was raised by a single mother who made a living cleaning houses. Her father left when she was a toddler and she rarely saw him. She described a childhood of loneliness and deprivation–a childhood she would not want for any child, especially her own. She met her husband who lived in the US when he was visiting his family in Costa Rica. After a few years of a long-distance relationship, they married and she moved to the US. She was in the process of completing her GED when she became pregnant. Since the relationship was already turbulent, she did not want to have the baby. She got an appointment for an abortion and planned to have her cousin take her. On the day of the appointment, she was informed that her mother did not approve and therefore her cousin refused to take her. Her husband was an active alcoholic and did not care one way or the other. She went on to have Rosey. We had her engage in a ritual of letter writing to Rosey about the ambivalence of her pregnancy, ways in which she felt trapped with the pregnancy and ways in which her nurturing was inconsistent.

She participated and witnessed numerous sessions where others in the circle were addressing either their work or family situations that were oppressive and they were targeted in different ways, carefully crafting threads and plans to challenge and bring some accountability to their lives. After continuing in multiple critical consciousness sessions, with some members of the circle being in different systems of education, she moved from her belief that the school was a fair system that would not target her child to understanding the depth of this institution's targeting of her daughter. She came to understand her daughter's emotional acting-out as directly related to the school's reckless abandonment of her daughter's academic needs. Building alliances with various members of the circle, she was successful in demanding that the school test her daughter and provide her with an IEP necessary to provide the appropriate accommodations.

This shift in her standpoint towards institutions further allowed her to file for divorce from the father of her daughter who paid minimal in child support, yet bought a home with his lover, while she lived in a two-bedroom apartment with her daughter and mother. The economic benefit of this choice coupled with her daughter finally receiving the services she was entitled to exponentially altered her lived experience from the marginal space to which she was confined.

The process of identifying and naming processes and systems/institutions/people who create and sustain harm to others creates a space for imagining transformative/liberatory spaces. Once there is an imagined location bolstered by connections in community that amplify that vision, the process of personal evolution is inevitable, albeit at different speeds.

Summary

Socioculturally attuned family therapists *begin* by attuning to the societal and power contexts that surround and give meaning to the presented client concerns, as well as the sociocultural context of the therapy itself. Knowing therapy holds the potential to replicate and reinforce inequitable societal structures and discourses—or to challenge the status quo and invite more equitable possibilities—SCAFT therapists are attentive and intentional regarding the values their work represents. They therapeutically identify and name qualities and experiences dominant social systems overlook or minimize, especially those that resist domination and/or help maintain resilience in unjust circumstances. SCAFT therapists connect the dots between larger societal processes and what happens in the therapy room, developing interventions that disrupt oppressive power dynamics and support equitable relationships. They help clients envision third order change—just relational alternatives beyond the limits of dominant social discourses—and they help clients make what they envision real, transforming the ways they relate to each other and the larger society.

We conclude with a checklist of ANVIET practices (Figure 2.3). We encourage you to keep it handy. Look for how they are applied across contexts and in the models that follow in this book. As you pay attention to the many clinical examples, consider what they will look like in your practice, how you will make them yours, and what you will need to learn and develop to apply and advance these practices. Consider that each therapist will implement ANVIET practices through their preferred clinical models, social locations, and personal styles. We encourage practice and innovation. In the next chapter, we address third order ethics and self of the therapist issues that will be important as you immerse yourself in socioculturally attuned practices and make them yours.

- **Attune**: Understand, resonate with, and respond to experience within societal contexts.
- **Name**: Identify what is unjust or has been overlooked—amplify silenced voices.
- **Value**: Acknowledge the worth of that which has been minimized or devalued.
- **Intervene:** Support relational equity—disrupt oppressive power dynamics.
- **Envision**: Provide space to imagine just relational alternatives.
- **Transform**: Collaborate to make what is imagined real—third order change.

Figure 2.3 ANVIET practices checklist.

Reflexive Questions

- In your own words, how do you describe third order thinking? How does it lead to third order change?
- What does it mean to be able to connect the dots between individual and relational problems, power dynamics, and broader societal systems and environmental contexts?
- Who and what gives legitimacy to certain types of knowledge? How does this affect you personally and your practice professionally?
- Which social structures have the greatest impact on the families/clients/communities with whom you currently work?
- What advantages and disadvantages do you have based on cultural and social capital? How does this affect your work as a therapist and the persons with whom you interact in your practice?
- What do the spaces and places that you inhabit or frequent say about you, your social location, and your privilege and/or disadvantage? Are these spaces mostly similar or different from your clients?

References

Akhmedshina, F. (2020). Violence against women: a form of discrimination and human rights violations. *Mental Enlightenment Scientific-Methodological Journal*, (1), 13–23.

Almeida, R. (2018). *Liberation based healing practices*. Institute for Family Services.

Almeida, R. & Williams, J. C. (2026). Postmodernism, decolonial critiques, and liberatory praxis. In O. Smoliak, E. Tseliou, T. Strong, S. Bava, & P. Muntigl (Eds.). *The routledge international handbook of postmodern therapies*, pp. 86–99. Routledge.

Almeida, R. & Tubbs, C. (2020). Intersectionality: A liberation-based healing perspective. In K. S. Wampler, R. B. Miller, & R. B. Seedall (Eds.). *The handbook of systemic family therapy* (Vol. 1, pp. 227–249). Wiley.

Almeida, R., Dressner, L., & Tolliver, W. (2017). Decolonizing couples and family therapy: Social justice praxis in liberatory healing community practice. *Encyclopedia of couple and family therapy*. Springer International.

Anderson, H. & Goolishan, H. (1988). Human systems as linguistic systems: Preliminary and evolving ideas about the implications for clinical theory. *Family Process*, *27*, 371–393.

Barraclough, S. (2023). On becoming a counsellor: a posthuman reconfiguring of identity formation for counsellors-in-training. *British Journal of Guidance & Counselling*, *52*(6), 1054–1070.

Bartunek, J. & Moch, M. (1987). First-order, second-order, and third order change and organizational development interventions: A cognitive approach. *The Journal of Applied Behavioral Science*, *23*(4), 483–500.

Bateson, G. (1972). *Steps to an Ecology of Mind*. Jason Aronson.

Bermúdez, M., McDowell, T., & Knudson-Martin, C. (2024). Sociocultural attunement in family therapy. In K. M. Hertlein (Ed.). *The Routledge international handbook of couple and family therapy* (pp. 83–98). Routledge.

Bourdieu, P. (1986). The forms of capital. In J. G. Richardson (Ed.). *Handbook of theory and research for the sociology of education* (pp. 241–258). Greenwood Press.

Bridges, J., Vennum, A., McAllister, P., Balderson, B., Taylor, L., Lyddon, L. (2022a) Privilege awareness raising for couple and family therapists: A qualitative thematic analysis part 1. *Journal of Feminist Family Therapy*, 34(1/2), 38–66.

Bridges, J., Vennum, A., McAllister, P., Balderson, B., Taylor, L., Lyddon, L. (2022b) Clinical and training implications of privilege awareness for couple and family therapists: A qualitative thematic analysis part 2. *Journal of Feminist Family Therapy*, 34(1/2), 67–85.

Carroll, S. (2017). *The big picture: On the origins of life, meaning, and the universe itself.* Dutton.

D'Aniello, C., Nguyen, H., & Piercy, F. (2016). Cultural sensitivity as an MFT common factor. *American Journal of Family Therapy*, *44*, 234–244.

D'Arrigo-Patrick, J., Hoff, C., Knudson-Martin, C., & Tuttle, A. (2017). Navigating critical theory and postmodernism: Social justice and therapist power in family therapy. *Family Process*, *56*, 574–588.

Dempsey, B. (2025). *Metamodernism or the cultural logic of cultural logics* (3rd ed.). ACR Press.

Dickerson, V. C. (2014). The advance of poststructuralism and its influence on family therapy. *Family Process*, *53*, 401–414.

DiMaggio, P. J. & Powell, W. W. (1983). The iron-cage revisited: Institutional isomorphism and collective rationality in organizational fields. *American Sociological Review*, *48*(2), 147–160.

Ecker, B. & L. Hulley. (1996). *Depth oriented brief therapy: How to be brief when you were trained deep and vice versa.* Jossey Bass.

Esiaka, D. K. & Adams, G. (2020). Epistemic violence in research on eldercare. *Psychology and Developing Societies*, *32*(2), 176–200.

Farrall, S., Gray, E., Nunn, A., & Tepe-Belfrage, D. (2022). Global pressures, household social reproduction strategies and compound inequality. *New Political Economy*, *27*(4), 713–729.

Fishman, H. C. (2022). *Performance-based family therapy: A therapist's guide to measurable change.* Routledge.

Foucault, M. (1972). *The archeology of knowledge.* Routledge.

Freire, P. (2000). *Pedagogy of the oppressed.* Bloomsbury. (Original work published in 1970).

Garcia, M. & McDowell, T. (2010). Mapping social capital: A critical contextual approach for working with low-status families. *Journal of Marital and Family Therapy*, *36*, 96–107.

Gardner, L. (2016). Metamodernism: A new philosophical approach to counseling. *Journal of Humanistic Counseling*, *55*(2), 86–98.

Gramsci, A. (1971) *Selections from the prison notebooks of Antonio Gramsci.* International Publishers.

Hardy, K. V. (2024). Some subtleties of whiteness in the workplace: Steps for shifting the paradigm. *Family Process*, *63*(2), 488–501.

Hardy, K. V. (2022). The centrality of whiteness. In K. V. Hardy (Ed.). *The enduring, invisible, and ubiquitous centrality of whiteness* (pp. 3–33). Norton.

Hare-Mustin, R. T. (1978). A feminist approach to family therapy. *Family Process*, *17*, 181–194.

Hair, H., Fine, M., & Ryan, B. (1996). Expanding the context of family therapy. *The American Journal of Family Therapy*, *24*, 291–304.

Hartwell, E. E. & Edwards, L. L. (2026) Queer contextualized family therapy. In E.E. Hartwell & L. L. Edwards (Eds.) *Queer-contextualized family therapy: Toward radically inclusive theory and practice* (pp. 1-25). Routledge.

Hernández-Wolfe, P. (2013). *A borderlands view on Latinos, Latin Americans, and decolonization: Rethinking mental health.* Jason Aronson.

Hoffman, L. (1985). Beyond power and control: Toward a "second order" family systems therapy. *Family Systems Medicine, Winter*, 381–396.

Hoffman, L. (1981). *Foundations of family therapy.* Basic Books.

Honeycutt, J. M. (2018). Animals as family members. In J. M. Honeycutt (Ed.). *Communication diversity in families* (pp. 218–228). San Diego, CA: Cognella.

Jackson, W. J. & Jackson, D. D. (1968). *The mirages of marriage.* WW Norton.

Jenks, A., Adams, G., Young, B., & Seedall, R. (2024). Addressing power in couples therapy: Integrating socio-emotional relationship therapy and emotionally focused therapy. *Family Process*, *63*, 48–63.

Jordan, L. S. (2022). Unsettling colonial mentalities in family therapy: Entering negotiated spaces. *Journal of Family Therapy*, *44*(1), 171–185.

Jordan, L. S., Grogan, C., Muruthi, B., & Bermúdez, J. M. (2016). Polyamory: Experiences of power from without, from within, and in between. *Journal of Couple & Relationship Therapy*, *16*(1), 1–19.

Kaasa, A. (2019). Determinants of individual-level social capital: Culture and personal values. *Journal of International Studies*, *12*(1), 9–32.

Keeney, B. P. (1983). *Aesthetics of change*. Guilford Press.
Knudson-Martin, C. (2025). *The socio-emotional relationship workbook for couples: Closing the gap between the relationship you want and the relationship you have*. Routledge.
Knudson-Martin, C. (2024). *A step-by-step guide to socio-emotional relationship therapy: A socially responsible approach to clinical practice*. Routledge.
Knudson-Martin, C. (2013). Why power matters: Creating a foundation of mutual support in couple relationships. *Family Process*, *52*, 5–18.
Knudson-Martin, C., McDowell, T., & Bermúdez, M. (2020). Sociocultural attunement in systemic family therapy. In K. Wampler & R. Miller (Eds.), *Handbook of Systemic Therapies*, (Vol 1., pp. 619–637). Wiley.
Knudson-Martin C. & Smoliak, O. (in press). Relational disquiet as sociocultural attunement: Insights from affect theory. In C. Guanaes-Lorenzi, J. Gaete-Silva, M. Sesma-Vazquez, & K. Tomm, (Eds.). *Befriending relational disquiet*.
Kuhn, T. S. (1962). *The structure of scientific revolutions*. University of Chicago Press.
Laenui, P. (2006). Process of decolonization. https://www.sjsu.edu/people/marcos.pizarro/courses/maestros/s0/Laenui.pdf. Accessed September 26, 2024.
Madanes, C. (1981). *Strategic family therapy*. Jossey Bass.
McDowell, T. (2015). *Applying critical social theory to family therapy practice*. AFTA Springerbriefs in Family Therapy, Springer.
McDowell, T., Knudson-Martin, C., & Bermúdez, J. M. (2019). Third-order thinking in family therapy: Addressing social justice across family therapy practice. *Family process*, *58*(1), 9–22.
Minuchin, S. (1974). *Families and family therapy*. Harvard College.
Nadasen, P. (2023). *Care: The highest stage of capitalism*. Haymarket Books.
O'Halloran, E., Dunford, K., Kim, L., & Knudson-Martin, C. (2017). Learning to apply social justice: Studying SERT. Poster presentation. American Family Therapy Academy annual conference, Philadelphia, PA.
Pandit, M., Kang, Y. J., ChenFeng J., Knudson-Martin, C., & Huenergardt D. (2014). Practicing socio-cultural attunement: A study of couple therapists. *Journal of Contemporary Family Therapy*, *36*, 518–528.
Rastogi, M. (2020). A systemic conceptualization of interventions with families in a global context. In K. S. Wampler, M. Rastogi, & R. Singh (Eds.). *The handbook of systemic family therapy* (Vol. 4, pp. 3–31). Wiley.
Rhodes, P. (2021). Matter matters: Assembling life after Post-Milan. *Australian and New Zealand Journal of Family Therapy*, *42*, 351–360.
Siegel, D. & Drulis, C. (2023). An interpersonal neurobiology perspective on the mind and mental health: Personal, public, and planetary well-being. *Annals of General Psychiatry*, *22*(1), 1–20.
Smoliak, O., Al-Ali, K., LeCouteur, A., Tseliou, E., Rice, C., LaMarre, A., Davies, A., Uguccioni, B., Stirling, L., Dechamplain, B., & Henshaw, S. (2023). The third shift: Addressing emotion working couple therapy. *Family Process*, *62*, 1006–1023.
Smoliak, O., Rice, C., LaMarre, A., Tseliou, E., LeCouteur, A., & Davies, A. (2022). Gendering of care and care inequalities in couple therapy. *Family Process*, *61*, 1386–1402.
Soja, E. (2010). *Seeking spatial justice*. University of Minnesota Press.
St. George, S. & Wulff, D. (2016). Family therapy = social justice = daily practices = transforming therapy. In S. St. George & D. Wulff (Eds). *Family therapy as socially transformative practice: Practical strategies* (pp. 1–7). AFTA Springerbriefs in Family Therapy, Springer.
St. George, S. & Wulff, D. (2014). Braiding SCIPS into therapy. In K. Tomm, S. St. George, D. Wulff, & T. Strong (Eds.). *Patterns in interpersonal interactions: Inviting relational understanding for therapeutic change* (pp. 124–142). Routledge.
Sutherland, O., Turner, J., & Dienhart, A. (2013). Responsive persistence part I: Therapist influence in postmodern practice. *Journal of Marital and Family Therapy*, *39*, 470–487.
Tatum, B. D. (2017). *Why are all the Black kids sitting together in the cafeteria? And other conversations about race*. Basic Books.
Timeto, F. (2021). Becoming-with in a compost society—Harraway beyond posthumanism. *International Journal of Sociology and Social Policy*, 41(3–4), 315–330.
Turner, J. (2007). *Human Emotions: A Sociological Theory*. Routledge.
Von Bertalanffy, L. (1968). *General system theory: foundations, development, applications*. George Braziller.
Walsh F. (2009a) Human–animal bonds I: The relational significance of companion animals. *Family Process*, *48*(4), 462–480.
Walsh F. (2009b) Human–animal bonds II: The role of pets in family systems and family therapy. *Family Process*, *48*(4), 481–99.

Watzlawick, P., Weakland, J., & Fisch, R. (1974). *Principles of problem formation and problem resolution.* WW Norton.

Whiting, J. B., Wendt, D. M., Eisert, B. C., & Fife, S. T. (2024). I and thou in dialogue: Becoming more relational in couple therapy. *Family Process*, *63*, 1–16.

Williams, K., Galick, A., Knudson-Martin, C., & Huenergardt, D. (2013). Toward mutual support: A task analysis of the relational justice approach to infidelity. *Journal of Marital and Family Therapy*, *39*, 285–298.

Young, B. & Seedall, R. B. (2024). Power dynamics in couple relationships: A review and applications for systemic family therapists. *Family process*, *63*(4), 1703–1720.

Yousef, T. (2017). Modernism, postmodernism, and metamodernism: A critique. *International Journal of Language and Literature*, *5*(1), 33–43.

3 Third Order Ethics and Contextual Self-in-Relationship

Ethics are about what we do in everyday practice (Larner, 2015). When we think about ethics, we typically, and appropriately, think about reasoning. Shaw (2015) pointed out that ethics are, however, not only about rules and reason, but also about "emotions, intuition, and relationships" (p. 403). According to Shaw and Bagharamian (2022), ethics are inextricably linked to our relationships and the emotions we experience through connection with others. It is through relationships that we are moved to care about what is just or unjust. Sociocultural attunement allows us to be more connected, more understanding, and to see things from broader perspectives. This adds ethical complexity while moving us to support just relationships. It also echoes what we ask of clients as we encourage them to attune to each other, explore their values, and act with relational accountability (Fishbane, 2023).

All of this—what we think we know, how we are moved to act, our values and intentions—are embedded in social and relational context. Our ethical decisions are based on how we make sense of things; how we identify meaningful patterns from vast amounts of information (Scher & Kozlowska, 2012), as well as our intentions. What we believe to be the right thing to do is situated in a complex web of beliefs, values, rules, and morals within cultural, societal, and environmental contexts.

Third order ethics requires us to expand our lens to include broader social, political, cultural, and economic systems and to embody social equity in our practice. We are called upon to integrate foundational, tried-and-true family therapy clinical practices and ethics with interventions and ethical decision-making that promotes equitable relationships in order to help solve everyday problems. In effect, responding to unjust social processes is an ethical issue that requires purposeful action (Wetzel, 2024; Williams et al., 2023).

Third order thinking brings to the forefront dilemmas that may otherwise be veiled. Expanding our understanding of individuals and families within cultural and societal contexts adds a layer of complexity to what it means to "do the right thing." For example, what do we do when clients' goals are at odds with what is just for all family members? How do we position ourselves when we believe honoring cultural values and beliefs contributes to oppression? How do we navigate the process of raising awareness when doing so may disrupt relationships? What is our role in encouraging clients to unveil taken-for-granted cultural assumptions and practices that are unjust and harmful to themselves or others? How do we navigate differences in cultural values and worldviews between clients and/or between ourselves and clients? Making these types of decisions requires us to not only be socially and culturally aware in general but to continuously consider how our own context shapes how we think and what we do. In effect, we are perpetually embedded in the process of ethical decision-making (Larner, 2015; Scher & Kozlowska, 2012).

DOI: 10.4324/9781003493426-3

Codes of Ethics

At the most basic level, ethical positioning is a stance in which one is clear about the need to engage with clients in ways that are consistent with ethical guidelines and principles. The code of ethics is a collective agreement about what is right or wrong to do as (Western) family therapists in order to protect the public and our profession. We typically think of ourselves and others as practicing ethically as long as we don't break our professional code of ethics. We tend to "notice" ethics when ethical dilemmas arise, which in turn leads us to carefully consider and consult others regarding the best course of action. While this is essential to professional practice, we agree with Larner (2015) that attending only to these types of dilemmas tends to eclipse the everyday nature of ethical decision-making. Everything we do—or don't do—reflects what we consider to be ethical and right.

There are nine standards in the American Association for Marriage and Family Therapy (AAMFT) Code of Ethics. It is noteworthy that the very first standard, 1.1 is Non-Discrimination. It reads as follows: "Marriage and family therapists provide professional assistance to persons without discrimination on the basis of race, age, ethnicity, socioeconomic status, disability, gender, health status, religion, national origin, sexual orientation, gender identity or relationship status" (AAMFT, 2015). Despite its primary position in the code of ethics, many students and licensed family therapists intentionally or unintentionally position themselves in ways that are not aligned with this standard. Rejecting this standard may be overt, involving a conscious choice due to conflicting personal codes of morality, values, religious beliefs, cultural norms, or biases (Priest & Wickel, 2011). For example, the statement "I don't believe I can work with same-sex couples because I cannot in good conscience support their union or marriage or help them work toward their clinical goals," is a stance that knowingly contradicts professional ethics and this non-discrimination standard. Failing to align with this standard may also be less obvious. In these cases, family therapists are not likely to realize they are engaging in discrimination. Examples include working harder with a high-status client than a low-status client; failing to acknowledge one's own racial, class, gender, or sexual orientation privileges; using Eurocentric models without considering cultural fit, and expecting women to take on the majority of emotional work in couple therapy.

It is not always easy to discern complex ethical dilemmas inherent to practicing socioculturally attuned family therapy. Consider AAMFT Code of Ethics Standard 1.8, which requires respecting client decision-making autonomy. At first glance, it is easy to agree that clients should make up their own minds about whether or not they divorce, how they arrange child custody, what family form they choose, and so on. On the other hand, what happens when we think beyond individual autonomy? What if one family member has decided to accommodate another due to a power imbalance, even though doing so contributes to mental health issues or somatic complaints? What about when we expect clients to be able to make and carry out "autonomous" decisions without factoring in varying social and economic constraints?

Third order practice embraces the collective commitment to professionally and ethically serve the public, while at the same time recognizing that all decisions are grounded in cultural values and assumptions within societal contexts. While codes of ethics are created in the spirit of protecting the client/patient, they reflect the cultural values of those who authored them. For example, the AAMFT code of ethics serves as a set of standards that are situated within and reflect common or dominant cultural values within a North American context, yet are considered universally benevolent. This can inadvertently lead to colonization when the code of ethics and best practices in North America are "transplanted" to other countries without consideration of cultural and societal context. Sociocultural attunement requires careful consideration of cultural biases and how those in dominant positions of power unevenly impact what is deemed ethical practice.

Practicing Third Order Ethics

Third order ethics involves reflecting on how we conceptualize what we consider to be ethical, as well as what we assume to be in the realm of ethics (McDowell et al., 2024). Ethics are by definition relational, however, a number of scholars in the field (Boszormenyi-Nagy & Krasner, 1986; Gergen, 2015; Hecker & Murphy, 2015) have used the term "relational ethics" to refer to the ubiquitous nature of ethics in our everyday relationships with clients (Larner, 2015). This includes a focus on meaning-making (Gergen, 2015) within societal contexts in which dominant cultural values are often accepted as right across the broadest and most intimate levels of relationships (Hecker & Murphy, 2015). When we are fully embedded in the societal and cultural contexts in which we work—that is, unable to step back and think about how we think—we risk being relatively unaware of everyday ethics. Gergen (2015) referred to this as first order morals. He argued that second order morality is possible when we are aware of how meaning is made between us on a relational level.

Hecker and Murphy (2015) added what we would consider a third order ethical position by taking a meta-perspective of relationships within context, which includes analyzing power dynamics at the broadest and most intimate levels. By taking a third order perspective, therapists are able to recognize ways in which dominant cultural standards and practices tend to better serve those with more social power (e.g., male, White, high SES, cishet). Socioculturally attuned family therapists are intentional about interrupting processes in which social power operates through those with more privileged social identities, who are often viewed as more credible and have greater influence over what is considered right and true. As Fricker (2007) noted, processes in which those with more power shape social meaning result in invalidating or minimizing the experience and "truth" of those with less power (e.g., People of Color, women, LGBTQ+, low SES, differently-abled, citizens of the Global South). Fricker referred to devaluing and dismissing non-dominant knowledge—in effect rendering it silent—as epistemological injustice.

According to Fricker, epistemic injustice includes both testimonial and hermeneutical injustice. Testimonial injustice refers to not having adequate credibility due to one's social location. Hermeneutical injustice refers to lacking interpretive resources to understand one's experience due to being part of a marginalized group. In other words, thoughts and experiences that are not part of dominant (or sometimes even public) discourses become further marginalized without language to express them or create collective meaning. As Fürst (2024) noted, however, it is important not to assume those who are marginalized or oppressed don't have ways to describe the phenomena they are experiencing. In fact, novel concepts that become part of conversations in the public domain (e.g., sexual harassment) often begin when previously silenced people explore their subjective experience. This has implications for family therapists as they help individuals explore and name experiences that are marginalized or dismissed by others, including other members of the family. It also has implications for how we think about relationships between therapists and clients. According to Lee and colleagues (2019, p. 29), "Epistemic injustice occurs when therapists implicitly and explicitly impose professional and institutional power onto clients."

Third order thinking includes thinking about how we think and the effects of our thinking on the lives of those with whom we work. We rarely consider our ontologies—how we view the very nature of being—when practicing family therapy or producing professional knowledge. Our ontological imaginations (Norwalk, 2013) are limited by what we "know" to be true within our accepted realities. Consider the gravitation of Western family therapists toward integrating advancements in neuroscience into our understanding of relational attachment. Contrast this with a relative lack of interest in the West in accessing the spirit world to help families. As you read these last two sentences, you may have found yourself thinking "but, neuroscience is real!" What we consider to be real is, in effect, filtered through an ontological lens.

Epistemology, which is closely tied to ontology, refers to what we consider to be legitimate knowledge, which in turn is determined in part by how knowledge is created and acquired. Consider the evidence-based therapy movement. Those models that have gone through a systematic research process that demonstrates desired outcomes are valued from a Western scientific epistemology (Harding, 2008). Contrast this with the knowledge of experienced family therapists who stay current with existing research, are informed by theory and guided by models or frameworks, yet go beyond this knowledge by using their clinical wisdom, embodied knowledge, and clients' perceptiveness to create a gestalt that guides the process in any given situation. This type of local knowledge, which is created through collaboration with clients (St. George et al., 2015), is often de-legitimized and pushed to the margins in favor of what can be more easily manualized and measured.

Consider further the very discourse of ontology and epistemology as outcroppings of Western thought and language, along with the colonizing effects of paradigms such as modernism and post-modernism (Almeida & Williams, 2026). Decolonizing efforts include resisting the universality of Western thought. Bermúdez and colleagues (in review) challenge this universality by emphasizing the inseparability of thinking and feeling, or *sentipensar* (Escobar, 2014), when engaging in third order thinking and change. In the words of these Latinx/Caribbean intersectional scholars, "in doing so, we uphold a pluriverse (plural universes) that includes the multiple world perspectives of our Indigenous and African ancestors and comrades." (p. XX). This stance embraces multiple ways of knowing, decentering the belief in the superiority of Western thought and science.

Rocky Robbins (as cited in McDowell et al., 2020), Native American scholar, researcher, and therapist, pointed to the lack of epistemological and ontological fit between Western, English language therapeutic approaches and Native ways of being. In his words, "Every attempt to tap into traditional Native American healing ways is an apocalyptic form of resistance against a White system that dominates every particle of the air we breathe." This includes "deconstruction of Christian colonization, delineated White surveillance, [and] imploded internalized Western cardinal virtues." Robbins' research has demonstrated the positive impact of traditional Native American healing practices, including "visits to tribal geographic origins, sweat ceremonies, sun dances, stomp dances, vision quests, work with medicine people, and communication with ancestor spirits" (pp. 56–57).

Ontological and epistemological flexibility expands our potential to move across and within diverse ways of understanding and working by thinking beyond limiting dichotomies and single systems of thought (Bermúdez, et al., 2024). As noted in Chapter 2, taking a superposition opens possibilities to consider, and at times simultaneously hold, multiple perspectives. It provides a potential pathway for decolonizing practices that dismantle and decenter "oppressive realities" in favor of diverse systems of thought. This can help us navigate potentially complex and sometimes contradictory ethical territory. At the same time, it requires us to recognize that any understanding or way of looking at things delimits and excludes alternative views. By its very nature, the act of focusing blurs what is outside our focus. Likewise, our knowing is limited by 1) what we can observe and make meaning of at any given moment, limiting our ability to comprehend that which is complex and ever-evolving, 2) the co-constructed and constantly emerging nature of what is possible to understand, and 3) that which is not knowable.

Contextual Self-in-Relationship

Third order ethics asks us to routinely inspect our assumptions, values, and preferred theoretical concepts and practices; to engage in continuous reflection about what we are doing and why.

↔

Third order ethics requires therapists to make clinical decisions with an eye toward societal and cultural context, including the impact of therapeutic interventions in relation to power and privilege.

↔

Text Box 3.1 Tim Baima, PhD, LMFT

Tim Baima, (he/him), PhD, LMFT is a family therapist in private practice. More of his work is described in chapters 6 and 7.

As a White, cis-gendered straight man, I am seldom required to be mindful of sociocultural context as I go about my day-to-day life. Over time, with intentional effort, I have become more attuned to the significance of sociocultural context, and the role of power and oppression in my life and the lives of others. However, in order to attune to sociocultural context in my work, I remind myself that I am deeply conditioned to be misattuned, unresponsive, and emotionally disengaged from sociocultural context. If I am going to be attuned to sociocultural context, I must be intentional about it.

The work I do to support third order change in therapy is first and foremost rooted in the work I do on myself. I do not believe it is possible to embrace third order thinking in our role as therapists alone. In order to be effective in facilitating third order healing and transformation, it is essential to commit to dismantle systems of oppression in every aspect of our lives, including in the most intimate spaces in our relationships and in our own hearts and minds. In my view, this commitment is a commitment of radical transformative love that nurtures spiritual healing and growth.

Doing so results in questions such as: Why am I favoring this way of looking at things? Where do my routine assumptions come from? Whose worldview do they represent? Whose interests are centered? In what ways does my approach to understanding and helping to solve problems marginalize or minimize some clients' perspectives and experiences? What role are my emotions playing? How do my ways of thinking reflect and reproduce dominant cultural values and practices? How is what I am doing and saying supporting equity and/or challenging what is unjust? In Text Box 3.1, Tim Baima shares insights about the importance of being intentional in this process.

Therapist Social Location

•←→•

Ethical positioning is not possible without self-reflexivity, critical social awareness, and the ability to support relational justice.

•←→•

Self-reflectivity and critical social awareness are especially important for those in structurally ascribed positions of power, including family therapists. Arguably, those who have the most social capital and ability to influence are most responsible for facilitating necessary and important changes that lend themselves to equitable and just practices (Almeida, 2018; Hernandez & McDowell, 2010). Socioculturally attuned family therapists need to develop contextual consciousness in addressing issues of gender, societal power, and culture in clinical practice (Stone & ChenFeng, 2020). This includes attending to one's own experience of privilege and oppression (McDowell et al., 2003) as well as the impact of one's own cultural background (Ellenwood & Snyders, 2006; Hardy & Laszloffy, 1995; Hardy & McGoldrick, 2008) and preferred ways of thinking. To successfully attune to clients within their social and cultural contexts, family therapists need to uncover and correct biases that contribute to social inequity and inadvertently support unjust relationships (D'Aniello, et al., 2016; Knudson-Martin et al., 2020). It is vital for family therapists to reflect on their heterosexist biases, and for heterosexual and cisgender therapists to examine their privilege (Adams & Benson, 2005; McGeorge & Stone Carlson, 2011; Nealy, 2008). Additionally, we must develop an awareness of how internalized oppression, such as internalized sexism and racism, operates within us to perpetuate patriarchal structures, White privilege, and androcentric norms (Ellis & Bermudez, 2021; Sharp et al., 2007). This process is ongoing. People, cultures, and societal systems are always changing. Attunement is a way of being in which we never fully arrive. We must humbly commit to ongoing reflexivity and growth.

Awareness of Power

Power dynamics are ubiquitous. We are often blinded by our own positions of power and the mechanisms that support our privilege. This occurs by simply failing to inspect and acknowledge the ways in which our epistemological frameworks marginalize the lifeworlds and experiences of others (Fricker, 2007). Mental health symptoms and relational problems may be outcroppings of ways of resisting oppression. By accepting at face value symptoms that result from subjugation, we risk contributing to oppression by defining those who express symptoms of inequity as the problem.

•←→•

Awareness of power is a critical first step in engaging in ethical practice, regardless of theoretical orientation.

•←→•

We must also attend to power *outside* the therapy room, relative to our communities and practice settings (McGoldrick et al., 2021). Not all therapists and supervisors are in a position to challenge systems in which families are embedded or in which therapy takes place. Supervisors from the dominant culture may be surprised to learn that supervisees may not be willing to challenge people in a system that exacerbates their vulnerability. For People of Color, women, those with disabilities, immigrants, etc., this vulnerability may always be present, regardless of the years of experience, educational degrees, or positions of power (Hernandez, et al., 2009). For example, Norma Scarborough (2017), a Black family therapist who had been a supervisor for over 20 years described how her knowledge was often dismissed by supervisees:

> I initially believed that an education in the field would place me on an equal footing with my peers… However, when working with dominant culture supervisees, I often found that my concepts and recommendations were challenged. I would be asked if there were articles or readings that would back up what I was telling them or they would check with their practicum instructors… Many of my supervisees had never seen or been involved with an African American supervisor or professor. Their experiences…were influenced by unexplored biases, prejudices, and stereotypes… I invited open discussion about anything they felt comfortable discussing. (pp. 39–40)

Challenging powerful people within a system has to be done carefully, always gauging and balancing risk and reward. While dealing with her own marginalization and biased teaching and supervisory evaluations (see Kreitzer & Sweet-Cushman, 2021), Scarborough had to remain "informative and compassionate" as she helped supervisees confront their privileged positions and "challenge their own worldviews," (p. 40). This is not just a personal issue. It is vital that we work together, sharing our power to collectively interrupt and transform harmful power dynamics (see Chapter 16).

Myth of Neutrality

Early on, therapists were expected to be "objective" and "neutral" to avoid contaminating or negatively affecting clients' clinical processes with their own biases, values, and assumptions (Tjeltveit, 1986). As described in the preceding chapters, therapists are neither neutral umpires nor ones who stand above the conflict; they take the side of each family member, being empathic and fair toward everyone while positioning their work to promote just relationships—a position similar to what Boszormenyi-Nagy and Spark (1973) called multi-directed partiality. Therapists today are called upon to recognize the values inherent in their clinical models; that what we choose to say and do inevitably has repercussions. These value choices have ethical implications that require reflection and intentionality (Knudson-Martin & Kim, 2023; Lebow, 2023). At a time in which families and communities are being stressed and pulled apart due to social inequities and political polarization, it is more important than ever that therapists connect and create bridges across disparate points of view; that we seek to be aware witnesses to injustice, using our positions of power "respectfully and with dignity" in ways that are helpful rather than hurtful (Weingarten, 2023, p. 31).

Feminist family therapists were among the first to challenge the myth of neutrality, pointing to ethical concerns surrounding the assumption that therapists can be objective. Early on, Betty Carter (1985, p. 78) argued that "You cannot not act out of your age, gender, sibling position, experience, belief system, and wisdom, or lack of it. Your only choice is whether to do this consciously or unconsciously." These feminists critiqued foundational notions of circularity, neutrality, and complementarity, arguing that these concepts do not address issues of power and control inherent in family life and therapeutic processes (Bograd, 1984; Goldner, 1985); that neutrality is far from neutral. In fact, because most therapists have the power to influence clients in significant and lasting ways, postmodern and critical feminists asserted that therapists must operate from a transparent value position (Knudson-Martin & Kim, 2023; Leslie & Southard, 2009; Melito, 2003). We must engage in ongoing, thoughtful, contextual self-reflexivity in order to take an intentional stance that supports relational values in equity-based practice (Fishbane, 2023; Hardy & Bobes, 2017). This is especially important in cultures such as the US, in which individualistic values promote competition and disconnection (Bava & Greene, 2023; Knudson-Martin, 2025).

Use of Power in Practice

Power inherent in the very nature of being an expert (i.e., role power as a therapist) does not necessarily ameliorate power based on social location. Therapists with less privileged social positions may need to use their power to gain credibility and influence when clients are unconsciously discrediting them or needing more leadership. For example, therapists who are young and/or Persons of Color may not be afforded the privilege of lowering their professional position of power when their structural and systemic levels of power threaten their stance as therapists and educators (Quek & Hsieh, 2021; Seshadri et al., 2023). It is at times necessary for people in less powerful social or structural positions (e.g., women, People of Color, or those with a particular disability or difference) to embrace and elevate their power in order to help clients achieve their goals. This is done carefully, with humility and confidence that therapists know how to use their power as leverage to help them be effective, credible, and compassionate.

Therapists must be able to maintain their positions as experts while addressing interactions in ways that encourage clients' accountability and change. Let's consider racism directed at Cecilia, a Latina therapist as an example. McDowell and colleagues (2003) described her experience in a paper working on racial awareness and taking anti-racist stances in therapy. Following is an excerpt (pp. 189–190).

Client: I always thought when you called someone Mexican that it was derogatory.
Cecilia: Why do you think that?
Client: I guess it's just the way people use it. I've always tried to use Hispanic because I thought it was much more proper.
Cecilia: When you use the word Mexican, what do you think of?… You are not going to offend me.
Client: It's like there are different classes. When I think of Mexican, I think of people in a lot of trouble, people who don't speak English, more straight from Mexico. When I think of Hispanics it could be anybody else.
Cecilia: So Mexican conjures up bad things for you.
Client: They are a different class of people.
Cecilia: So for you when you think of Mexican, the terms that come up for you are not as good as White.
Client: Yeah, mm-hmm.
Cecilia: So now that you know I am Mexican, (Cecilia used this term purposefully to challenge the client's view of Mexicans) what does that mean to you?
Client: No matter what race anyone is, it doesn't bother me. I'm not racist; the only thing that bothers me is when someone can't speak English. I think they are ignorant. I can't help it.
Cecilia: But I am still wondering, does the fact that you know I am Mexican, does that affect how you think of me?
Client: I don't think of you as Mexican. I think of you as Latina.
Cecilia: What if I would have called myself Mexican instead of Latina, would you have thought differently of me?
Client: No, I would have thought of you as Hispanic. The only people that fit my negative view of Mexicans are people I don't know. Everyone I have ever gotten to know doesn't fit the stereotype.
Cecilia: Once you meet someone that doesn't match the stereotypes—What do you do?
Client: Every Hispanic person I have ever met doesn't fit the stereotype.
Cecilia: This is very interesting. What is it like for you for us to be talking about race like this?
Client: I like it, I guess I'm not racist, but maybe I have a lot of misconceptions. I don't want that. My parents were very prejudiced.
Cecilia: So is it okay if we talk about this again as it comes up?
Client: Yes, I would like to get into the topic of race. Like I have always wanted to date cross racially but don't know how I would deal with my family.
Cecilia: Okay. We are learning together here. You are helping me understand also. We can work together on this.
Client: I'd like to talk to my family about it.
Cecilia: Yeah, race is a difficult thing to talk about. It seems important that we find a way for you to talk to your family about this.

The authors (McDowell et al., 2003) discussed co-author Cecilia's ability to regulate her own emotions while her client expressed overt racism toward her. They pointed out that the therapist was able to maintain an inquirer stance, slow the process down to allow space for the client to explore thoughts about race/ethnicity, and connect the client's (lack of) racial awareness to therapeutic goals. The therapist in this scenario had the knowledge, fluency, and self-awareness to challenge what was happening in the moment while leading a conversation that allowed the client to openly express and begin inspecting his racism.

Self-disclosure and Relational Engagement

Issues around therapist self-disclosure are complex (Roberts, 2005). Socioculturally attuned family therapists recognize these complexities and navigate self-disclosure in ways that allow them to use their identities to encourage equitable relationships in families. In the example above, Cecilia decided to disclose her Mexican heritage to help her client recognize racism and its effects. The decision to disclose was carefully timed to both maintain and leverage the positive relationship between the client and therapist. In Text Box 3.2, Dana Stone shares making decisions about self-disclosure and inspiring self-awareness as an educator and supervisor.

There are some aspects of our identities that are (correctly or not) assumed by clients and other aspects we have control over sharing. Abilities, sexual identity, gender, race, and age may be visible or invisible, confounding what is known or assumed about us as therapists. We have at least some choice (depending on our context) over how much and what we share about our life experiences. This is the topic most associated with training in self-disclosure. We ask ourselves questions like "Am I sharing this to help the client? How will it be helpful? How will it impact our therapeutic relationship?" and "How does self-disclosure fit into the model I am using?" But what about differences that put the therapist in a one-down position relative to the broader societal context? How are these decisions made when the therapist has a choice about whether or not to disclose an experience or social identity? What about when a pansexual, gay, or lesbian therapist is working with a homophobic client? Or with a family in which a teen is coming out to parents who are religious fundamentalists? When does the therapist disclose sexual orientation to show solidarity and ally with a client or some members of a family?

There are no simple answers to these questions. In the example above, Cecilia was able to engage the client in a discussion about race and, in the process, disclose her own identity because she was guided by her relational socioculturally attuned stance that invited questions based on curiosity and respect, while also using her role as a therapist to open questions related to race and

Text Box 3.2 Dana Stone, PhD, LMFT

Dana Stone (she, her) is an associate professor at California State University in Northridge, and identifies as a multiracial Black-white, cisgender female, hearing, temporarily able-bodied, heterosexual, and non-religious. Her work focuses on multiracial experience and supporting early-career therapists with marginalized aspects of identity in navigating the field of marriage and family therapy and counseling. More of her work is described in Chapter 16.

As an educator and supervisor, it is innate in me to foster connection with others by sharing parts of my identity, my journey in this field, and to invite students and supervisors to share parts of their stories with me and each other. I believe sharing of the "self" in this way levels the hierarchy. While I know that I hold power and privilege as the teacher or supervisor, I genuinely believe that students in my classroom and supervisees in the group offer so much and can "teach" each other in ways I cannot. I integrate conversations about power and privilege regularly to encourage ongoing critical engagement with the self.

equity. Cecilia was able to take this stance and make appropriate ethical clinical choices in the moment because she regularly engaged in critical self-reflection, becoming what Stone and ChenFeng (2020) called contextually differentiated.

It can be difficult to attune to the emotions of those in social positions that differ from our own. In fact, we often assume what we feel, or imagine ourselves feeling, in another's situation is normal without considering culture, relational power, or societal context. Exploring sociocultural context, including our own positionality, perspectives, and emotions relative to societal contexts, is vital to our ability to assess and analyze power dynamics on both broad social and intimate relational levels, and as much as is possible, take in and resonate with another's sociocultural experience. When one is contextually aware, it is possible to be in touch with one's emotions and use this information to guide relationally directed clinical responses that promote equity and third order change (Garcia et al., 2015). In socioculturally attuned practice and application of third order ethics, thinking relationally and thinking contextually go hand in hand (Hardy & Bobes, 2017; Kim et al., 2017).

Tensions in Socioculturally Attuned Practice

There are a number of ethical tensions we experience as we come to define ourselves as socioculturally attuned family therapists. At times, these tensions seem like irreconcilable differences. At other times, it seems perfectly compatible to take a both/and position. We encourage readers to not see these tensions as dichotomous, but as continuums or at times competing values and goals. While there are many tensions in ethical equity-based work, we have chosen to emphasize the importance of recognizing the ways in which societal systems constrain personal agency, helping clients grapple with decisions about resistance to oppression, honoring clients' perspectives and/or being culturally sensitive while challenging oppression, and using power to balance power. We do not attempt to offer universal solutions, rather we hope the following will help readers consider the complexities and prepare to make decisions involved in equity-based therapy.

Recognizing Societal Constraints on Personal Agency

Equity-based therapists are often in a position of reconciling tensions between encouraging clients' personal empowerment and helping them negotiate societal constraints that limit their agency (Edwards, 2026). Many of us fall into the trap of thinking everyone can choose a different way of thinking, being, and living. This is a privileged perspective that leads us to assume we all have (enough) choice. We often assume clients can achieve anything they put their minds to if they change their thoughts and perspectives, or assume responsibility for their situation and actions. This rings of the myth of meritocracy, which is a common belief that we can "pull ourselves up by our bootstraps" in order to overcome adversity, be successful, or achieve our goals. We can fail to acknowledge that all of us, to varying degrees, have social and structural constraints that block our agency. For example, worldwide, women and girls are still prevented from having equal access to education, safety, control, voice, leadership, employment, and equal pay. LGBTQ+ people live with the daily oppression of heteronormativity and homophobia. People of Color continue to experience the oppressive effects of colorism/racism, white supremacy, and internalized racism. Those who live on low income are often geographically limited without equal freedom of movement or access to food or employment opportunities (McDowell, 2015).

•←→•

Therapists help families identify strengths and tap into resilience, yet when the session is over, many return to oppressive contexts.

•←→•

It can be difficult and disconcerting to acknowledge the complexity of social position, inequity, and socioeconomic status. People reared in a privileged or even moderate income bracket are often oblivious to the struggles of those living on severely low incomes. Economic security buffers many of us against the real material consequences of limited or scarce resources (McDowell, 2015). For example, in a natural disaster, state of emergency, or crisis situation, wealthy individuals and families have greater access to resources that help buffer the crisis. The real life consequences of inequitable access are tangible and affect how we embody space, pursue or access resources, and both perceive and realistically gauge our choices (Brock et al., 2023). Furthermore, mechanisms of marginalization and oppression have a cumulative effect, placing those in the most disadvantaged positions at higher risk, which in turn creates greater disadvantage across the lifespan (Lei & Beach, 2023; Merton, 1988). Research from the COVID-19 pandemic showed that some families respond more effectively to these societal inequities and stressors than others (Brock et al., 2023). Therapists can help clients resist internalizing oppressions while navigating the effects and maximizing agency within constraining contexts. Therapists can also be allies for change by supporting clients' efforts to transform social arrangements within their spheres of influence, e.g., individual, family, community, broader society.

Case Example

Marty, a White middle-class lesbian family therapist landed her first job out of graduate school providing in-home therapy to primarily People of Color living on low income. She exuded positivity and consistently demonstrated the ability to deeply care about all of those with whom she worked. She had firsthand experience of marginalization, oppression, and microaggressions that stemmed from homophobia. She was nervous but excited to get to work, to help her clients change their lives. Marty engaged clients in hopeful conversations, drawing on a strength-based therapeutic approach.

Within a few months, Marty found herself feeling increasingly less competent, even dreading the work she had once been so excited about. After a particularly frustrating family session, she finally blurted out, "I just don't see what I am doing wrong! Why aren't my clients getting better?" Marty's supervisor asked her to explain what she meant by "getting better," as Marty's clients typically reported that therapy was going well. During the supervisory conversation, Marty was surprised to realize she held the assumption that anyone can change their social status if they overcome psychological and relational problems. She held unquestionable goodwill and an unwavering belief that clients have the strengths they need to overcome problems. What she hadn't realized is that the assumption she held about her work—that as a therapist she could help clients overcome poverty by encouraging individual and relational change—was not only naive but inadvertently blamed clients for their own oppression. With time and experience, Marty would begin to recognize her role in supporting clients in being able to both navigate and transform unjust systems within their families and communities.

Working with Complexities and Potential Costs of Resistance

Family therapists witness daily the mechanisms and impact of everyday resistance. According to Vinthagen and Johansson (2013), "everyday resistance is about how people act in their everyday lives in ways that might undermine power" (p. 2). Everyday resistance is not always easy to discern as it is often hidden or disguised, in some cases as mental health or relational symptoms. Socioculturally attuned family therapists pay close attention to the nuances of power and carefully scan for forms of resistance in order to locate what is unjust and help families move towards equity-based solutions.

There are many forms of resistance to abusive or subjugating power. Strategies include education about societal systems and power dynamics (Freire, 1970/2000), disloyalty or disobedience to oppressive systems, identity movements, coalition building to take collective action, engaging in revolution, and refusing to accept dichotomous thinking and choices (Heldke & O'Connor, 2004). Other types of resistance include yielding when the cost of overtly challenging is too high, withdrawing when situations are unbearable, and understanding how to navigate dynamics of power and oppression. Directly challenging oppressive and dominant systems can be risky. Potential costs include not being believed and/or being labeled as a problem (McDowell, 2004). These must be weighed against the likelihood of positive change.

Those with the greatest privilege take the least risk in speaking out directly to promote change in family, community, and societal systems. They are most likely to be believed and be able to influence change with the most modest personal consequences. Conversely, those most marginalized take the greatest risk, being less likely to be believed and potentially paying the greatest personal cost (McDowell, 2004). Another way to resist is to recognize and challenge how unexamined thoughts and emotions inadvertently maintain oppressive structures (Medina, 2013). Refusing to explore our own perspectives or those of others may be a fear-based reaction, particularly for members of dominant groups (D'Angelo, 2018; Goodman, 2011; Hardy, 2024).

Case Example

Consider Chloe and Deidra, a female African American couple in a small Southern town who kept the intimate nature of their relationship a secret from their families and church. If their therapist believed that openness is a mark of emotional differentiation and that the couple suffered from having to maintain their closeted position, she may have engaged the couple in discussions about "coming out" without recognizing the important role the Black church played in their lives and the importance maintaining the story that they are "just friends and roommates" may have been in their ability to access other important forms of support and resilience.

Honoring Perspectives, Being Culturally Sensitive, and Challenging Oppression

Clients' beliefs and preferred directions for therapy may seem in opposition to what is just. How do therapists honor client beliefs, values, and goals when we believe they may inadvertently support the client's own subjugation or the oppression of another? This goes hand in hand with considering the unintended consequences of raising critical consciousness, including disruption to family relationships as worldviews change. The goal of being culturally sensitive can obscure the distinction between what is acceptable and what is unjust; what should be supported as part of someone's culture and what should be challenged, even if culturally supported.

•←→•

Socioculturally attuned therapists honor clients' cultural values and personal perspectives while simultaneously challenging oppression.

•←→•

It is often difficult to discern when to be confident in knowing when to be transparent about what we see or think, when to be cautious, or when to make a direct statement that challenges or affirms a stance. Marisol Garcia-Westberg captures a thoughtful, tentative, and embodied stance about knowing in Text Box 3.3.

Text Box 3.3 Marisol Garcia-Westberg, PhD, LMFT

Marisol Garcia-Westburg (she-her) is a therapist and educator.

I don't feel that I am completely right about things. I know my thinking is limited, so I have to act accordingly. I don't want to ignore the silence and marginalization that abounds. I try to catch myself when I am in the minutia of the issues—when I am hyper focused on what happened. Then I pull myself out and stand on the sidelines, looking and feeling the whole. My intellect gets me far, but I can miss injustice and disempowerment if I don't suspend my thinking and focus on the energy in the room. My thinking can be biased, so I use my perception of energy to fill in the gaps. I am limited in identifying and naming issues by my biases, emotional wounding, and lack of awareness.

I encourage transformative change by working on my own emotional growth and being open to challenge and to being wrong; being willing to not abide by norms and rules which are put in place to keep injustice; understanding that systems of oppression will not be dismantled by following rules, and supporting those doing the same.

Receiving feedback from therapists can be important and helpful to clients (Sundit, 2011). Equity-based therapists view understanding of societal context and power dynamics as part of their professional knowledge, which like other professional knowledge, has the potential to help solve presenting problems and improve clients' lives. Honoring clients' choices seems reasonable enough, but it is not always easy when a therapist believes choices are harmful to clients or others. Can we truly respect clients' choices if we believe they are unjust? In the end, there are times when therapists must take a both/and stance, instead of an either/or. We can honor a family's way of knowing and doing, respect their choices and decisions, and question institutional and structural practices that negatively affect them, while still honoring the practices of the profession. We can help clients explore the nuances and implications of cultural practices knowing that taken-for-granted cultural assumptions are not always just, cultures are not monolithic, and oppression is routinely met with resistance in all societies.

Case Example

Thomas, an Asian heterosexual, middle class, male therapist entered therapy with a family that immigrated to the southern US from China. Thomas noticed during his initial meeting with Tina, a 45-year-old daughter, and her 81-year-old mother, Maylee, that Maylee was often sharp tongued and critical of Tina. Tina described being married, working in a demanding job, and caring for two teenage children in addition to caring for her aging mother. Thomas recognized the importance of intergenerational family life and shared Tina's value of caring for elders. The situation resonated with his having grown up with his own grandmother in his parents' home. As he listened to Tina, he reflected on what it must have been like for his mother, who was the primary caregiver to his paternal grandfather. Thomas noticed that Tina was reluctant to stand up to verbal abuse from her aging parent and found himself at a loss for how to help. Thomas got caught between the shared value of caring for and respecting elderly members of the family and the need to help his clients confront an unjust and abusive parent–child relationship. Thomas needed to be able to help Tina name this conflict and work with her to explore her options.

Using Power to Balance Power

Family therapists are in the unique and challenging position of facing competing dominant discourses and societally supported power dynamics that differently affect clients in the same family, often privileging some over others. Practicing from an equity-based perspective requires therapists to be both countering and collaborative, moving flexibly between the two in order to analyze power dynamics, connect and collaborate with all family members, and position themselves to be able to disrupt oppressive relationship dynamics.

•←→•

Socioculturally attuned therapists value all voices in the family, not allowing any voice to overpower that of others.

•←→•

Therapists must be able to challenge power to create opportunities for equitable relationships to develop. Consider adult children who are trying to impose or dictate what they think their parents must do in their final years. If an aging parent is able to make choices, their voice must be heard. The therapist must intervene when the loudest voice is not that of the one who is most negatively affected by decisions being made. The therapist is confronted with their own power. What does this mean for the therapist? A study of how equity-based family therapists use their power to promote equity showed that they regularly balance interventions that actively counter injustice, with maintaining a collaborative relationship (D'Arrigo-Patrick at al., 2016). These therapists tended to deal with their power by asking questions rather than telling, and being open and transparent as they used inquiry to help clients make connections about social issues that impact their lives.

Case Example

Kimberly, a White, young, cishet female therapist-in-training began working with a cishet, middle-class, White couple. The wife, Amy, had persuaded her husband, Kurt, to enter therapy after a particularly volatile argument. While they both reported that their relationship had never been violent, they agreed that the level of rage and conflict was not what either wanted or expected in their marriage. During the first session, Kimberly was careful to talk to both Amy and Kurt in order to ensure they both felt heard. She noticed, however, that Amy often repeated her complaints to Kurt, who routinely dismissed them. When Kimberly attempted to interrupt and redirect, Kurt dismissed her as well. Kimberly firmly adhered to her interpretation of a collaborative stance in therapy, not wanting to impose her agenda on clients. This stance left her deadlocked, unable to find a way to challenge the power dynamic that fueled the couple's conflict. Without a way to facilitate the therapeutic process and use her influence as an expert to challenge Kurt's more powerful position, Kimberly was unable to intervene to support Amy or help the couple develop a more just relationship.

Reflexive Praxis

Reflexive praxis involves critical reflection as an ongoing routine that informs and is informed by action. As socioculturally attuned family therapists, we have an ethical mandate to continuously increase our social awareness, understand ourselves within social and relational context, notice and make sense of our felt experiences, and critically reflect on our practices. While this idea may be readily endorsed, we need to make intentional efforts to create space and secure places where this kind of ongoing growth is a primary goal. Curling and colleagues (2023) offered a list of recommendations based on the Galveston Declaration (Gosnell et al., 2017), including social justice education, reflexive praxis, strategies for overcoming cultural and linguistic barriers, community outreach, rethinking existing models to ensure holistic care, empowering through collaboration, collaborative advocacy, and professional development and self-care.

It is more effective and increases our accountability when we work collectively by engaging in dialogue, sharing our actions and reactions, reflecting, and discussing the ethical and practical implications of how we practice. In the words of Robinson-Wood (2023, p. 25), "Existing consciously in community with others who push back against oppression is liberatory. In this communal space, we learn from, teach, and are accountable to one another."

(Re)-explore Our Own Sociocultural Experience

Most of us have been asked during our training to reflect on our own social locations, cultures, and family backgrounds. We have found it useful to repeat this process as we become more socially aware and advance in our understanding of sociocultural attunement. It is more helpful to complete these exercises with a partner or group willing and able to engage in socioculturally attuned conversations. Some tools useful for therapists as well as clients are critical genograms (i.e., Kosutic, et al., 2009), cultural genograms (see Hardy and Lazloffy, 2003), gender genograms (i.e., DeMaria et al., 2017); sexual genogram (i.e., Belous et al., 2012), family cartographies (i.e., McDowell, 2015), and life maps (Knudson-Martin, 2024). Jordan (2021) explored the ethical impact of colonialism and the responsibility, particularly for majoritized therapists, to take steps toward decolonizing or "unsettling" colonizing practices. It is important while completing these exercises to pay close attention to felt experience and what we imagine to be the felt experience of others. Many of these exercises are about our pasts, which is helpful, but we also need to pay close attention to our whole selves, our internalized beliefs, felt emotions, and actions in the present. This is best done in a collective.

Engage in Reflection and Dialogue

The more you focus on developing contextual awareness, the more you learn. Whatever your starting point, paying attention to how your personal experience and the experience of others meld emotion, power, and social meaning is intense and transformative (Knudson-Martin, 2025).

↞→

Rather than seeking to become "objective" by overcoming bias, developing socio-emotional awareness means attuning to the sociocultural context of your felt internal responses and responsibly using this emotional awareness in service of therapeutic goals. (Knudson-Martin, 2024, p. 277)

↞→

Make reflecting on your own contextual experience a regular practice. As Tim Baima said earlier in this chapter, it is important to recognize the workings of power and oppression "in every aspect of our lives, including in the most intimate spaces in our relationships and in our own hearts and minds." Since this involves learning to see what we have been socialized not to see, most of us have had few guides to this essential awareness.

We recommend *The Socio-Emotional Relationship Workbook for Couples: Closing the Gap Between the Relationship You Want and the Relationship You Have* (Knudson-Martin, 2025). This guide provides case illustrations, exercises, and illuminating dialogues that will help you explore how what you feel and do connects to your relationships and place in the world. Working through this book with your partner, a friend, or a group (or even on your own) will increase your shared awareness of the impact of societal experiences in your lives. As you do, you increase possibilities for yourself and enhance your ability to work with contextual issues in practice. You can help people see how their personal vulnerabilities and struggles are connected to societal valuations and power dynamics and do what you need to do to "maintain a vision of possibility and be a keeper of hope" (Knudson-Martin, 2024, p. 11).

Your process of reflection and dialogue should be ongoing. Use this book and the workbook described above as jumping off points. Read widely. If you are White, learn how whiteness has structured not only your life, but the lives of many other groups (e.g., Hardy, 2022). Learn about the experiences of people whose backgrounds and lives are different from yours. Stretch yourself to build relationships with people outside your usual comfort zone. Bring curiosity and a genuine interest in knowing them and their worlds.

Develop Communities of Practice

According to Morrison et al. (2022), embodying social justice in family therapy practice involves not only developing a theoretical understanding but also attending to our felt sense when presented with what is unjust. These authors described a process they engaged in to learn to embody a social justice perspective. In addition to developing a theoretical understanding, they worked as a group to critically observe family therapy sessions while noting and attending to felt sense, engaging in transformative discussion, and applying new understandings to their own practices. We suggest developing communities of practice as a way to not only embody relationally just perspectives, but to increase accountability and ensure we have collective guidance in applying third order ethics.

Wilson et al. (2023) offered another excellent example of working collectively toward just practice. They coined the term antiracist reflexivity to describe an ongoing lifestyle and communal practice which includes engaging in "trauma-informed, mindfulness-informed work rooted in relational process, intersectionality, and antiracism," (p. 32). They suggest reflexivity that goes beyond individual reflection as a collaborative and postmodern practice.

Engage in ANVIET Informed Supervision and Consultation

Socioculturally attuned family therapy supervision and consultation are vital contexts for raising awareness, reviewing practice, and exploring ethics. These activities invite all of us—supervisees and supervisors, consultees and consultants—to more fully explore the application and ethics of socioculturally attuned practice. Table 3.1 provides examples of how ANVIET can be used in supervision to guide discussions that explore contextual self-in-relationship, sociocultural attunement in working with clients, and sociocultural relational dynamics in supervision. This guide is also helpful for those seeking or offering consultation.

Conclusion

Equity-based family therapists are faced with difficult ethical decisions and tensions relative to our role in the change process. At times, this means challenging common cultural practices that are oppressive. It also requires us to find hidden strengths in all cultures that may have been minimized or marginalized. To engage in ethical socioculturally attuned family therapy, we must rigorously

Table 3.1 Application of ANVIET to contextual reflexivity in supervision.

ANVIET Guideline	*Questions regarding contextual self-in-relationship*	*Questions regarding client*	*Questions regarding supervisor–supervisee relationship*
Attune: Understand, resonate with, and respond to experience within societal contexts.	What is it like for you as a [specific social location] to interact with this client [specify social location]? What assumptions or ideas about [people in client's social location] do you bring to the therapeutic encounter? How might your social location influence what feels appropriate in this case?	What do you think it is like for this client to live as a [insert social locations] in this world? How do you think others in their community view him/her/them? How do they respond? What messages about what it means to be successful/a good [insert social role or identity] do you think this client may have received?	How may power differences in our social locations affect our supervisory relationship? How do each of our expectations regarding hierarchy and social worth/value affect how we relate to each other?
Name: Identify what is unjust or has been overlooked: amplify silenced voices.	What skills or qualities of the supervisee are likely to be discredited or overlooked in the dominant discourse? By others? By self? What skills or qualities in others may the supervisee tend to discredit or overlook due to influence of dominant discourses? What societal inequities has the supervisee experienced? How may these influence supervisee's approach to therapy?	What skills or qualities of the client are likely to be discredited or overlooked in the dominant discourse? By others? By self? What skills or qualities in others may the client tend to discredit or overlook due to influence of dominant discourses? What societal inequities has the client experienced? How may these influence how the client responds to clinical concerns? How they feel about themselves?	What skills or qualities discredited in the larger societal context need to be validated within the supervisory relationship? How might our supervisory relationship contribute to discrediting or pathologizing skills and qualities not valued in the dominant discourse? How may power differences between supervisor and supervisee silence voice and perspectives? How may these be nuanced due to intersecting social locations?
Value: Acknowledge the worth of that which has been minimized or devalued.	What societally overlooked values and characteristics does the supervisee wish to support in order to promote justice? What societally overlooked values and characteristics does the supervisee struggle to validate? How may these relate to internalized values of the dominant discourse?	What societally overlooked values and characteristics may client endorse when space is created for them? How may valuing societally overlooked characteristics support this client's well-being? How can the therapist intentionally validate the worth of what has been minimized or devalued in this case?	What societally overlooked values and characteristics do we need to value so that our relationship promotes justice? What will our supervisory relationship look like when we validate and enact qualities disvalued and discouraged in the dominant culture?

(*Continued*)

Table 3.1 (Continued)

ANVIET Guideline	*Questions regarding self-of therapist*	*Questions regarding client*	*Questions regarding supervisor–supervisee relationship*
Intervene: Support relational equity; disrupt oppressive power dynamics.	How may supervisee's internal responses to the presence of societal power dynamics interfere with their ability to intervene in oppressive power dynamics? What will help the supervisee have the courage to intervene in oppressive societal power processes?	What kinds of interventions will help clients interrupt power imbalances in their lives? How can the therapist create awareness of power dynamics when they are present in the processes between clients or in their descriptions of interpersonal dynamics? What is required on the part of the supervisor to insure that therapy does not replicate oppressive power dynamics?	What is required on the part of the supervisor to insure that the supervisory relationship does not replicate oppressive power dynamics? How can it be safe for the supervisee to identify and disrupt inequities in the supervisory relationship? How can the supervisory relationship respond to inequities in the workplace or larger context of therapy and/ or clinical concerns?
Envision: Provide space to imagine just relational alternatives.	How does supervisee/ therapist envision working with client in ways that promote justice (third order change)? How would they know? What will therapist's practice look like when guided by preferred values/ relational systems?	What will clients' relationships look like when they are able to enact more equitable relationships? How may clients' preferred values support more just relationships? What have you noticed that suggests your clients are able to envision alternatives to societal inequities?	How do the ways we discuss client cases make space for us to envision and support just relational alternatives? How do we envision our relationship with each other supporting justice in clinical practice and the larger mental health system?
Transform: Collaborate to make what is imagined real: third order change.	How is the therapist working in ways that promote justice and third order change? What does it look like? What enables the therapist to maintain focus on just relational goals?	In what ways are clients enacting their preferred, more just relational goals? What does this look like? What enables clients to maintain focus on their just relational goals? How does the therapist support this process?	How does our supervisory relationship support just relational goals? How do we recognize and encourage equity within our relationship and the larger clinical system? Who do we draw on for support?

examine our cultural assumptions, values, beliefs, and attitudes (Bermúdez, 1997; Hardy & Laszloffy, 1995). We must find ways to develop accountability systems that identify when we are actively or passively oppressive in our practices. This includes moment-by-moment awareness and self reflexivity in the process of therapy as we implement clinical models. In the following chapters we offer guidelines that help address tensions related to equity and illustrate the relational nature of socioculturally attuned practices across models.

Reflexive Questions

- What are the ways in which we can differentiate between what is common, yet oppressive and culturally endorsed?
- In what ways are we held accountable to recognize and support resistance to oppression? Where does our use of power, or refusal to use power, fit into this accountability?
- How can you honor—yet challenge—beliefs, goals, and values that you believe may inadvertently oppress another or contribute to a client's own subjugation?
- How can you navigate the potential consequences of raising social awareness among family members when doing so may disrupt relationships?
- How can we help clients explore the implications of taken-for-granted cultural practices and assumptions that are not just? How do you as a therapist know when a practice or relationship is unjust?
- How do we take an ethical stance that interrupts the dominance of one culture or subculture or group over another?
- How might your ethical decision-making reflect the values of the dominant system at the expense of those with less power?
- How do we support client autonomy (Standard 1.8), while not reifying what is unjust by witnessing oppression and not taking action? How are these decisions affected by the concept of autonomy within cultural and societal frameworks?
- How do we promote equity and fairness in relationships while acknowledging the impact of societal systems on personal agency?
- How do we honor our client's cultural values and personal perspectives while simultaneously challenging oppression? How do we address beliefs, goals, and values that may inadvertently oppress another or contribute to a client's own subjugation?
- What do we do when our client's goals are not equitable or clients don't share the goal of an equitable relationship? What are some ways we can navigate this type of dilemma?
- What is our ethical responsibility to clients when we raise social awareness among family members and, in doing so, may disrupt their relationships?
- How will you know if the larger context of therapy inadvertently replicates oppressive power dynamics? What ethical obligations do we have to address these issues? What are the potential costs of this type of resistance? What type of support do we need to pursue equitable and ethical positioning?
- How do the ways we conceptualize and discuss client cases contribute to inequity and/or make space to envision and support just alternatives?
- How do we integrate third order ethics into our preferred family therapy models and practices?

References

Adams, A. & Benson, K. (2005). Considerations for gay and lesbian families. *Family Therapy Magazine*, *4*(6), 20–23.

Almeida, R. (2018). *Liberation Based Healing Practices*. Institute for Family Services.

Almeida, R. & Williams, J. C. 2026). Postmodernism, decolonial critiques, and liberatory praxis. In O. Smoliak, E. Tseliou, T. Strong, S. Bava, & P. Muntigl (Eds.). *The routledge international handbook of postmodern therapies*, pp. 86–99. Routledge.

American Association for Marriage and Family Therapy (2015). *User's guide to the AAMFT code of ethics*. The American Association for Marriage and Family Therapy.

Bava, S. & Greene, M. (2023). *The relational workplace: How relational intelligence grows diverse, equitable, and inclusive cultures of connection*. ThinkPlay Partners.

Belous, C. K., Timm, T. M., Chee, G., & Whitehead, M. R. (2012). Revisiting the sexual genogram. *The American Journal of Family Therapy*, *40*(4), 281–296.

Bermúdez, J. M. (1997). Experiential tasks and therapist bias awareness. *Contemporary Family Therapy, 19*(2), 253–267.
Bermúdez, J. M., Alvarez-Hernandez, L, Muruthi, B. A., Machado-Escudero, Y., & Lamont-Gomez, M. F. (equal authors) (under review). Decolonizing approaches to family science as intersectional Latinx and Caribbean scholars working toward third order change, *Journal of Family Theory and Review*.
Bermúdez, J. M., McDowell, T., & Knudson-Martin, C. (2024). Socioculturally attuned family therapy: A global perspective. K. M. Hertlein (Ed.) *International handbook of couple and family therapy* (pp. 83–98). Routledge.
Bograd, M. (1984). Family systems approaches to wife battering: A feminist critique. *American Journal of Orthopsychiatry, 54*(4), 558–568.
Boszormenyi-Nagy, I. & Krasner, B. (1986). *Between give and take: A Clinical guide to contextual therapy*. Psychology Press.
Boszormenyi-Nagy, I. & Spark, G. M. (1973). *Invisible loyalties: Reciprocity in intergenerational family therapy*. Harper & Row.
Brock, R. L., Calkins, F. C., Hamburger, E. R., Kumar, S. A., Laifer, L. M., Phillips, E., & Ramsdell, E. L. (2023). Learning from adversity: What the COVID-19 pandemic can teach us about family resiliency. *Family Process, 62*, 1574–1591.
Carter, B. (1985). Ms. intervention's guide to "correct" feminist family therapy. *Family Therapy Networker, 9*, 78–79.
Curling, D., Osazuwa, S., & Bhandal, A. (2023). Navigating the ethical path: Nonmaleficence and cultural humility in psychotherapy. *Journal of Systemic Therapies, 42*(4), 60–75.
D'Aniello, C., Nguyen, H., & Piercy, F. (2016). Cultural sensitivity as an MFT common factor. *American Journal of Family Therapy, 44*, 234–244.
D'Arrigo-Patrick, J., Hoff, C., Knudson-Martin, C., & Tuttle, A. (2016). Navigating critical theory and postmodernism: Social justice and therapist power in family therapy. *Family Process, 56*, 574–588.
DeMaria, R., Weeks, G. R., & Twist, M. L. (2017). *Focused genograms: Intergenerational assessment of individuals, couples, and families* (2nd ed.).
DiAngelo, R. (2018). *White fragility: Why it's so hard for white people to talk about racism*. Beacon Press.
Edwards, L. L. (2026) Queer contextualized Satir family therapy. In E. E. Hartwell & L. L. Edwards (Eds.) *Queer-contextualized family therapy: Toward radically inclusive theory and practice* (pp. 73–94). Routledge.
Ellenwood, A. E. & Snyders, R. (2006). Inside-out approaches to teaching multicultural techniques: Guidelines for family therapy trainers. *Journal of Family Psychotherapy, 17*, 67–81.
Ellis, E. & Bermúdez, J. M. (2021). Funhouse mirror reflections: Resisting internalized sexism in family therapy and building a women-affirming practice. *Journal of Feminist Family Therapy*, 33(3), 223–243.
Escobar, A. (2014). Sentipensar con la tierra. Nuevas lecturas sobre desarrollo, territorio y diferencia. Medellín: Ediciones UNAULA.
Fishbane M. D. (2023). Couple relational ethics: From theory to lived practice. *Family Process, 62*, 446–468.
Freire, P. (2000). *Pedagogy of the oppressed*. Bloomsbury. (Original work published in 1970).
Fricker, M. (2007). *Epistemic injustice: Power and the ethics of knowing*. Oxford University Press.
Fürst, M. (2024) Closing the conceptual gap in epistemic injustice, *The Philosophical Quarterly*, 74 (1), 229–250.
Garcia, M., Kosutic, I., & McDowell, T. (2015). Peace on earth/war at home: The role of emotion regulation in social justice work. *Journal of Feminist Family Therapy, 27*, 1–20.
Gergen, K. (2015). Relational ethics in therapeutic practice. *Australian and New Zealand Journal of Family Therapy, 36*, 409–418.
Goldner, V. (1985). Feminism and family therapy. *Family Process, 24*, 31–47.
Goodman, D. J. (2011). *Promoting diversity and social justice: Educating people from privileged groups*. Routledge.
Gosnell, F., McKergow, M, Moore, B., Mudry, T., & Tomm, K. (2017). A Galveston declaration. *Journal of Systemic Therapies, 36*(3), 20–26.
Harding, S. (2008). *Sciences from below: Feminisms, postcolonialities, and modernities*. Duke University Press.
Hardy, K. V. (2024). Some subtleties of whiteness in the workplace: Steps for shifting the paradigm. *Family Process, 63*(2), 488–501.
Hardy, K. V. (2022). *The enduring, invisible, and ubiquitous centrality of whiteness*. Norton.
Hardy, K. V. & Bobes, T. (2017). Core supervisor competencies. In K. V. Hardy & T. Bobes (Ed.). *Promoting cultural sensitivity in supervision* (pp. 3–14). Routledge.
Hardy, K. & Laszloffy, T. A. (1995). The cultural genogram: Key to training culturally competent family therapists. *Journal of Marital Family Therapy, 21*, 227–237.

Hardy, K. & McGoldrick, M. (2008). Re-visioning training. In M. McGoldrick & K. Hardy (Eds.). *Re-visioning family therapy* (2nd ed.) (pp. 442–460). Guilford.

Hecker, L. & Murphy, M. (2015). Contemporary and emerging ethical issues in family therapy. *Australian and New Zealand Journal of Family Therapy*, *36*, 467–479.

Heldke, L. & O'Connor, P. (2004). *Oppression, privilege, and resistance: Theoretical perspectives on racism, sexism, and heterosexism*. McGraw-Hill.

Hernandez, P. & McDowell, T. (2010). Intersectionality, power, and relational safety in context: Key concepts in clinical supervision. *Training and Education in Professional Psychology*, *4*(1), 29–35.

Hernandez, P., Taylor, B., & McDowell, T. (2009). Listening to ethnic minority AAMFT approved supervisors: Reflections on their experiences as supervisees. *Journal of Systemic Therapies*, *28*(1), 88–100.

Jordan, L. (2021). Unsettling colonial mentalities in family therapy: Entering negotiated spaces. *Journal of Family Therapy*, *44*(1), 171–185.

Kim, L., Esmiol Wilson, E., ChenFeng, & Knudson-Martin, C. (2017). Toward safe and equitable relationships: Sociocultural attunement in supervision. In R. A. Allan & S. S. Poulsen (Eds.). *Creating cultural safety in couple and family therapy supervision and training* (pp. 57–70). AFTA SpringerBriefs in Family Therapy. Springer.

Knudson-Martin, C. (2025). *The socio-emotional relationship workbook for couples: Closing the gap between the relationship you want and the relationship you have*. Routledge.

Knudson-Martin, C. (2024). *A step-by-step guide to socio-emotional relationship therapy: A socially responsible approach to clinical practice*. Routledge.

Knudson-Martin, C. & Kim, L. (2023). Socioculturally attuned couple therapy. In J. Lebow and D. Snyder (Eds.). *Clinical Handbook of Couple Therapy* (6th ed., pp. 267–291). Guilford.

Knudson-Martin, C., McDowell, T., & Bermúdez, J. M. (2020). Sociocultural attunement in systemic family therapy. In K. Wampler & R. Miller (Eds.). *Handbook of systemic therapies* (Vol. 1, pp. 619–637). Wiley.

Kosutic, I., Garcia, M., Graves, T., Barnett, F., Hall, J., Haley, E., Rock, J., Bathon, A., & Kaiser, B. (2009). The critical genogram: A tool for promoting critical consciousness. *Journal of Feminist Family Therapy: An International Forum*, *21*(3), 151–176.

Kreitzer, R. J. & Sweet-Cushman, J. (2021). Evaluating student evaluations of teaching: A review of measurement and equity bias in SETs and recommendations for ethical reform. *Journal of Academic Ethics*, 1–12.

Larner, G. (2015). Ethical family therapy: Speaking the language of the other. *Australian and New Zealand Journal of Family Therapy*, *36*, 434–449.

Lebow, J. L. (2023). The importance of relational ethics. *Family process*, *62*(2), 443–445.

Lee, E., Tsang, A. K. T., Bogo, M., Johnstone, M., Herschman, J., & Ryan, M. (2019). Honoring the voice of the client in clinical social work practice: Negotiating with epistemic injustice. *Social work*, *64*(1), 29–40.

Lei, M.-K. & Beach, S. R. H. (2023). Neighborhood disadvantage is associated with biological aging: Intervention-induced enhancement of couple functioning confers resilience. *Family Process*, *62*, 818–834.

Leslie, L. A. & Southard, A. L. (2009). Thirty years of feminist family therapy: Moving into the mainstream. In S. A. Lloyd, A. L. Few, & K. R. Allen (Eds.). *Handbook of feminist family studies* (pp. 328–339). Sage.

McDowell, T. (2004). Exploring the racial experience of therapists in training: A critical race theory perspective. *The American Journal of Family Therapy*, *32*(4), 305–324.

McDowell, T. (2015). *Applying critical social theories to family therapy practice*. AFTA SpringerBriefs in Family Therapy, Springer.

McDowell, T., Fang, S., Gomez Young, C., Brownlee, K., Khanna, A., & Sherman, B. (2003). Making space for racial dialogue: Our experience in a marriage and family therapy training program. *Journal of Marital and Family Therapy*, *29*(2), 179–194.

McDowell, T. Knudson-Martin, C., & Bermúdez, J. M. (2024). *Socioculturally attuned ethical practice in family therapy*. In K. Brown (Ed.). AAMFT Systemic Ethics Textbook.

McDowell, T., Knudson-Martin, C., & Bermúdez, J. M. (2020). *Socioculturally attuned family therapy: Guidelines for equitable theory and practice* (2nd ed.). Routledge.

McGeorge, C. & Stone Carlson, T. (2011). Deconstructing heterosexism: Becoming an LGB affirmative heterosexual couple and family therapist. *Journal of Marital and Family Therapy*, *37*, 14–26.

McGoldrick, M., Hines, P. M., Garcia Preto, N., & Petry, S. (2021). Reflections on our efforts to help mental health agencies become more "culturally competent." *Family Process*, *60*, 1016–1032.

Medina, J. (2013). *The epistemology of resistance: Gender and racial oppression, epistemic injustice, and resistant imaginations*. Oxford University Press.

Melito, R. (2003). Values in the role of the family therapist: Self determination and justice. *Journal of Marital and Family Therapy*, *29*, 3–11.

Merton, R. K. (1988). The Matthew effect in science, II: Cumulative advantage and the symbolism of intellectual property. *ISIS*, *79*, 606–623.
Morrison, T., Ferris Wayne, M., Harrison, T, Palmgren, E., Knudson-Martin, C. (2022). Learning to embody a social justice perspective in couple and family therapy: A grounded theory analysis of MFTs in training. *Contemporary Family Therapy*, *44*(4), 408–421.
Nealy, E. C. (2008). Working with LGBT families. In M. McGoldrick & K. V. Hardy (Eds.). *Re-visioning family therapy: Race, culture, and gender in clinical practice* (2nd ed., pp. 289–299). Guilford.
Norwalk, A. W. (2013). Ontological imagination: Transcending methodological solipsism and the promise of interdisciplinary studies. *Avant*, *4*, 169–193.
Priest, J., & Wickel, K. (2011). Religious therapists and clients in same-sex relationships: Lessons from the court case of Bruff v. North Mississippi Health Service, Inc. *American Journal of Family Therapy*, *39*(2), 139–148.
Quek, K. & Hsieh, A. (Eds.) (2021) *Intersectionality in family therapy leadership—Professional power, personal identities*. AFTA Springerbriefs in Family Therapy. Springer.
Roberts, J. (2005). Transparency and self-disclosure in family therapy: Dangers and possibilities. *Family Process*, *44*(1), 45–63.
Robinson-Wood, T. (2023). Introduction to the special section: Holding hope: Antiracism and social justice. *Journal of Systemic Therapies*, *42*(4), 22–26.
Scarborough, N. (2017). When dominant culture values meet diverse clinical settings: Perspectives from an African American supervisor. In R. A. Allan & S. S. Poulsen (Eds.) *Creating cultural safety in couple and family therapy supervision and training* (pp. 33–42). AFTA SpringerBriefs in Family Therapy, Springer.
Scher, S. & Kozlowska, K. (2012). Thinking, doing, and the ethics of family therapy. *The American Journal of Family Therapy*, *40*(2), 97–114.
Seshadri, G., Pereyra, S., Quek, K., Chen, H. M., & Hsieh, A. (2023). Social location, power, and disadvantage: Experiences of MFT faculty. *Journal of Feminist Family Therapy*, 1–20.
Sharp. E. A., Bermúdez, J. M., Watson, W., & Fitzpatrick, J. (2007). Reflections from the trenches: Our development as feminist teachers. *Journal of Family Issues*, *28*(4), 529–548.
Shaw, E. (2015). Ethical practice in couple and family therapy: Negotiating rocky terrain. *Australian and New Zealand Journal of Family Therapy*, *36*, 504–517.
Shaw, A. & Bagharamian, M. (2022). Ethics and emotions: An introduction to the special issue. *International Journal of Philosophical Studies*, *30*(3), 193–201.
St. George, S., Wulff, D., & Tomm, K. (2015). Research as daily practice. *Journal of Systemic Therapies*, *34*(2), 3–14.
Stone, D. & ChenFeng, J. (2020). *Finding your voice as a beginning marriage and family therapist*. Routledge.
Sundit, R. (2011). Collaboration: Family and therapist perspectives of helpful therapy. *Journal of Marital and Family Therapy*, *37*, 236–249.
Tjeltveit, A. (1986). The ethics of value conversion in psychotherapy: Appropriate and inappropriate therapist influence on client values. *Clinical Psychology Review*, 6(6), 515–537.
Vinthagen, S. & Johansson, A. (2013). Everyday resistance: Exploration of a concept and its theories. *Resistance Studies Magazine*, *1*, 1–46.
Weingarten K. (2023). Called to repair injustice: Connecting everyday practices to societal phenomena, creating momentum for solidarity and change. *Family Process*, *62*, 6–34.
Wetzel, N. A. (2024). Embracing the other: Revisiting the epistemological foundations of family systems therapy. *Family Process*, *63*, 17–33.
Williams, M. T., Faber, S., Nepton, A., & Ching, T. H. (2023). Racial justice allyship requires civil courage: A behavioral prescription for moral growth and change. *American Psychologist*, *78*(1), 1.
Wilson, M., Rhee, J. Haughton, N., Maynard, P., & Robinson-Wood, T. (2023). A child–parent psychotherapy case vignette with discussion from an antiracist perspective. *Journal of Systemic Therapies*, *42*(4), 27–41.

4 Socioculturally Attuned Engagement and Assessment

Imagine you are meeting a client/family for the first time. You begin to attune to how they describe the issues that brought them to therapy. This description and the clinical goals you develop together are not neutral processes. What clients say and talk about will often depend on your questions and how you respond to what they share. Moreover, you become aware of how your assessment of clinical issues evolves while you and the clients form a therapeutic alliance and a shared understanding of how to approach their concerns. As a socioculturally attuned therapist, you recognize that your clinical choices regarding what to assess and how to frame "the problem" influence the possibilities that can arise in therapy. Acting upon these clinical choices is an essential part of ethical positioning toward equity and relational justice (Chapter 3, this volume, Knudson-Martin, 2024; Murphy & Hecker, 2020). Though assessment is ongoing as you and your clients learn more, what you look for and ask about in the early phase of therapy sets the framework for what follows.

In this chapter we describe a collaborative assessment process that enables you and your clients to "get the lay of the land;" connecting their clinical concerns to societal power processes and cultural contexts, and forming a therapeutic alliance to address those concerns. These guidelines help you and your clients view presenting issues from a third order lens, not in a checklist manner, but as a dynamic conceptual and practical process.

Forming Socioculturally Attuned Therapeutic Relationships

Building and maintaining relationships is central to how family therapists work (Karam & Blow, 2020). Sociocultural attunement is important in all interactions, even when more comprehensive assessments have to be set aside in favor of acute assessments of risk and immediate interventions for clients who enter therapy in crises. In fact, it is often the ability of the therapist to attune that facilitates secure pathways to safety (e.g., reducing the risk of suicide, escape from violence and abuse) and encourages clients' disclosure of urgent needs (e.g., housing, medical care).

↔

Every interaction counts, from the first phone call to the moment we say goodbye.

↔

We know that developing a connection is vital to engaging clients; however, a connection alone won't ensure you are off to a good start in the therapeutic process. Engaging is more than the clients and therapist feeling comfortable with each other. It is about clients feeling seen, heard, and known, and engaging in a process of developing a shared understanding. Engaging and attuning are also about envisioning what is possible. This is more likely to occur when we free ourselves

DOI: 10.4324/9781003493426-4

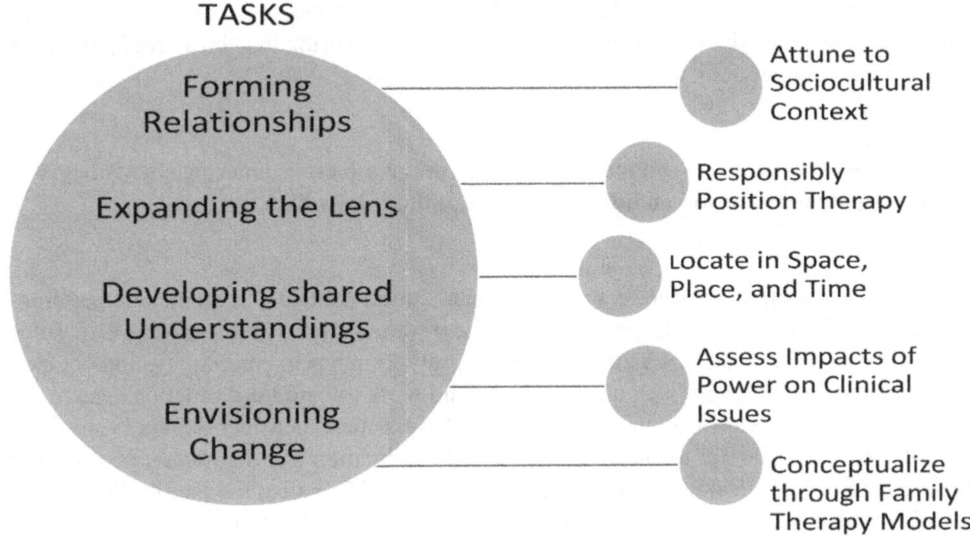

Figure 4.1 Tasks and elements of socioculturally attuned engagement and assessment.

from stuck positions and expand our lens to see the situation from a broader perspective. This creates space for new possibilities and previously unimaginable goals and solutions.

As shown in Figure 4.1, socioculturally attuned assessment occurs as you initiate the therapeutic relationship and set the foundation for your work together. This assessment includes the four tasks illustrated on the left: forming relationships, expanding the lens, developing shared understandings, and envisioning change. These are not linear "steps" to be taken. They are intertwined and collaborative interactions that may be well-received, contested, redirected, surprising, confusing, and/or affirmed. The goal is to move collectively with a sense of shared investment toward mutually envisioned change made possible by an expanded understanding of the problem's sociocultural context.

The question remains: What does a socioculturally attuned assessment look like in the session? How do we ensure that as we form relationships, develop shared understandings, expand the lens, and envision change, we do so in ways that integrate sociocultural context and support equitable relationships? The elements of socioculturally attuned assessment illustrated on the right side of Figure 4.1 serve as a guide. Though we will review them one by one, they are interconnected. In practice, you will likely go back and forth between them and experience assessment as a socioculturally attuned dynamic. As you do, you and your clients will develop a collaborative socioculturally attuned vision of their presenting challenges or goals and how their therapy will address them. This relational assessment process will also enable you to meet "standard" assessment objectives typically included in a systemic family therapy case conceptualization, including identifying urgent needs, resources, resilience, socio-relational determinants of health, family and community support, problem description, goals, etc. It also will provide a sociocultural context for interpreting and addressing diagnoses found in the DSM (*Diagnostic and Statistical Manual of Mental Disorders*) and relational concerns.

Elements of Socioculturally Attuned Assessment

Most clinicians collect "background" information on clients' social and cultural contexts, but few connect the dots between larger sociopolitical and cultural contexts and the individual and relational issues that are the focus (McDowell et al., 2019). We define socioculturally attuned assessment as a process in which you, the therapist, continuously bring in a third order perspective to make these larger connections visible.

As with drawings where you connect the dots to make a picture emerge, clients begin to see how the larger context is woven into the strands of their daily lives.

Think of this as a braiding process in which sociocultural contexts, interpersonal patterns, and physical and mental health are woven together in how we talk about problems and their solutions (St. George & Wulff, 2014). This emergent picture provides nuance, complexity, and compassion in how we understand and approach clinical issues and work toward third order change.

To illustrate the elements of socioculturally attuned assessment, consider Sophia as she begins to engage with the Carter family to create a picture of their situation and define the focus of therapy. At the suggestion of the school psychologist, Laurelle (aged 35), called the Family Center for help dealing with Brandon's (aged 9) and Logan's (aged 10) "disruptive behavior." She is also concerned that their older son Tyler (aged 15) is "noncommunicative" and "keeps to himself" and worried that her husband Nick (aged 35) seems angry and disengaged since being injured on a construction job nearly two years ago. In the initial intake, Laurelle identified herself as a Black African American, heterosexual, cisgender woman. She has been married for 15 years to Nick, a White, heterosexual, cisgender man. Laurelle is a Certified Nursing Assistant (CNA) and works as a home health care provider. Nick has been unemployed since his injury and was recently approved for Supplemental Security Income (SSI) disability benefits. Sophia (aged 27), a registered family therapy associate in her state, is assigned the case. Sophia identifies as a cisgender bisexual daughter of Romanian immigrants. She is partnered with a White heterosexual man who has two young children.

To set the stage for socioculturally attuned practice, Sophia asks who they consider family. She invites all of them to the first session and tells them this will enable them to explore the "bigger picture" together and decide how best to address their concerns. Like all case illustrations in this book, this example is based on a real case, however, identifying information and some details have been changed to protect confidentiality. Expanded treatment details for this case can be found in Knudson-Martin (2024, chapters 9–11). Excerpts of clinical dialogues from this book are cited in the case examples that follow.

Element 1—Attune to Sociocultural Context

As Sophia meets the family and begins to get to know them, she brings a third order lens that enables her to zoom out to reflect on the sociocultural context of this therapeutic encounter and be curious about the larger environment within which the Carter family lives. She brings with her an understanding that the therapeutic process itself is socially located and not neutral. She is aware that she does not know the unique experiences of this particular family, but is conscious that what they feel and do are not separate from how they are situated in time, space, and place. Sophia knows that larger systems support and value some more than others (Knudson-Martin, 2025). She will zoom in and out to connect these larger contexts to the family's lived experience.

Sociocultural Context of this Therapy

Mental health systems, theories, diagnostic systems, and how we, as clinicians, define our roles exist within larger social structures, economic and commercial systems (Nadasen, 2023), and cultural discourses. This means that despite personal values and commitments toward equitable and inclusive practice, couple and family therapists work in professional contexts that replicate social inequities, often without conscious awareness (Hardy, 2024; Roberts & Trejo, 2022). Sophia knows that institutional policies, diagnostic criteria, clinical practices, reimbursement structures, ideas regarding what it means to be professional, and where and how services are provided tend to reinforce health disparities based on racial, economic, gender, sexuality, and other societal influences (Robins et al., 2023). Challenging these inequities requires reflexive awareness and intentional practices that enable Sophia to be accountable for her impact on equity and well-being. This includes recognizing how professional and institutional systems tend to privilege individualistic frameworks that pathologize and stigmatize people whose experiences and values are marginalized within the dominant culture, and working from more relational, contextual and historically conscious models (Hartwell & Edwards, 2026; Waite & Nardi, 2024; Watson et al., 2020; Wetzel, 2024).

Before Sophia meets the Carter family, she is aware that although the mission statement at the Family Center emphasizes equity and inclusion, she—like others in her work setting more broadly—is not likely to readily live up to these values (Hardy, 2024). She pauses in a reflexive stance to ask herself questions about the sociocultural context of the therapy system itself, such as:

- What dominant cultural values surround this therapy?
- How are these values likely to affect what I notice and assess for?
- What is the physical/virtual location of the therapy? Who does this location and its accessibility benefit?
- What other systems are implicated in this clients' situation? (legal, educational, medical, employment, financial, etc.)
- How and why is this person/family identified as the patient/problem?
- What values are associated with how my professional role is defined? Whose interests do these values support?

Therapy with the Carter family is happening within a society structured around individualism (see Chapter 1, this volume). Though raised in an Eastern European immigrant family, the ways of thinking that Sophia learned as a psychology major and the clinical models she learned in graduate school were founded within Western culture. In order to receive reimbursement for the services they provide, clinicians at the Family Center must make individual diagnoses. Cultural and institutional pulls will direct her to take an "objective" position that will distance her from the members of the Carter family and skew what she looks for toward individual dysfunction and personal failings. It will be easy to implicitly blame the parents, especially the mother, for the children's troubles.

As she prepares to meet the family, Sophia wonders how difficult it will be for them to come to the Family Center. Even though the location was chosen to be more accessible to community members than a downtown site and extended hours are available, she is aware that getting to the appointment will take time, money, and coordination. She doubts Laurelle has flexibility in her work schedule, yet when the scheduler explained that the Family Center encourages in person meetings, Laurelle agreed, saying she wants what is best for her family. The Center has virtual options that Sophia and the family may decide to occasionally use if getting to the Center is onerous. They will balance the benefit of in-person work with relational processes with the challenges of getting to the session and the family's access to the internet. If privacy is possible, Sophia may also suggest some virtual sessions with individual family members or to include extended family.

The Carter family's therapy is embedded within the economics of health care. Their income is low. Nick is unemployed. Laurelle works in a physically demanding, low-pay job that includes medical insurance. Whether this insurance will cover the costs of the therapy will depend on individual diagnoses and how covered benefits are defined. For people without covered benefits, The Family Center offers a sliding scale for services, which often means being seen by less experienced clinicians.

The referral was made by the school psychologist. Sophia is curious how Brandon and Logan came to be identified as "problems" at school. She knows that students of Color are more likely to be labeled as "trouble-makers" and will expand her lens to explore their experience at school. By whom are they viewed as disruptive? What are they disrupting? As a result of Nick's injury, the family is also receiving federal disability benefits, which appears to have taken a long time for approval. Sophia wonders what it is like for Nick to be unable to work and what kind of conditions and opportunities Social Security benefits provide. She is not yet aware of other social systems that may be affecting the Carter family, but begins therapy interested in learning about them.

When the family arrives for their first session, they enter a world defined by the mental health system. As she introduces each of the children, Laurelle (mother) accommodates her perception of that system by repeating the behavioral and diagnostic terms the school psychologist used. Nick and the boys appear uncomfortable. He tells them to "quit fooling around and sit up" (Knudson-Martin, 2024, p. 191), a sign that he wants them to appear serious and respectful of this clinical setting and perhaps fears being judged by it.

Client's Sociocultural Context

Mindful that the inherent power hierarchy in this therapy setting may make trust difficult, Sophia seeks to facilitate a safe and supportive relationship with the family while simultaneously beginning to attune to their sociocultural context. She zooms in to ask each family member why they have come to therapy and what they hope will happen, then zooms out with questions that help her and the family see their struggles, aspirations, and possibilities within a larger context. For example, when Laurelle describes each of the children's problems, Sophia zooms in to reflect the exhaustion she heard in Laurelle's voice, "You've got a lot on your hands. It sounds exhausting" (Knudson-Martin, 2024, p. 187). When Laurelle resonates with this attuned response and says she's doing the best she can, Sophia expands the lens to bring forth the socio-contextual meaning around the exhaustion (dialogue from p. 288):

Therapist: (empathically) You're doing the best you can. [pause] When I talk to mothers, nearly all of them are exhausted and doing the best they can…but it never feels like enough—like they are somehow always expected to do more.
Laurelle: They're good boys. But I worry.

Rather than personalizing Laurelle's worry, Sophia uses contextual thinking to frame worry as a social process:

Therapist: You worry that they are being labeled as behavior problems? That people don't see the good in them?
Laurelle: Of course. Anything can happen out there!

Sophia introduces a question about the racial context of Laurelle's worry:

Therapist: Anything can happen—especially if you're Black?
Laurelle: (begins to tear up). They are so young. And already the school says they are trouble-makers!

While staying connected to Laurelle's statement that they are "good boys," Sophia names the inherent prejudice in the world in which the boys are growing up and Laurelle is parenting,

Therapist: You're doing your best to keep your boys safe—and enable them to grow into their full selves—in a world that doesn't treat everyone fairly, may not see the innate goodness in them. (Knudson-Martin, 2025, p. 288)

By explicitly bringing the socio-contextual nature of the clients' experience into the conversation, Laurelle begins to feel less judged and possibilities for how to understand and address their problems begin to expand. As Sophia engages with the family regarding their struggles and hopes, she continues her assessment and keeps in mind the following questions about the clients' sociocultural context:

- In what societal locations and contexts are clients embedded? How have these changed over time?
- How do each person's race and ethnicity impact their health, well-being, and relationships?
- What messages about gender, sexuality, and intimate relationships have each experienced and internalized? How are these reflected in their relationship patterns?
- How do factors such as education, socioeconomic status, race, immigration status, abilities, and economic situations impact access to resources, options, and personal and relational well-being?
- How do clients' age, abilities, religion, and other sociocultural factors impact client's sense of self, well-being, and relationships with others?
- How do social institutions (legal, medical, health, social services, etc.) impact clients' health, well-being, and relationships with others?
- How is the unique intersection of sociocultural factors and experience reflected in clients' identities, thoughts, feelings, and needs? How do these factors and experiences affect their sense of worth and belonging?
- To what extent are clients' options and decisions influenced/determined by their social contexts?

When Sophia asks Nick about his worries for the boys, he says they should "stay under the radar, not bring so much attention to themselves;" that he knows he should spend more time with them, but he's "in too much pain since the [explicative] accident." Sophia is curious about the sociocultural context of his response and asks him to say more about what "staying under the radar" means to him (Knudson-Martin, 2024, p. 191).

Nick: I used to get in trouble at school. I had a hard time focusing and being quiet in class. My dad's thing was "when you get in trouble at school, you get double at home!" I learned to keep it down—to stay under the radar.

Though Sophia will come back to the family of origin another time, she continues to expand outward. As she attunes to his hurtful relationship with schools, Sophia begins to connect the dots between his current responses as a father and his experience in larger systems (p. 192):

Therapist: (gently) School was painful for you. You don't want that for your boys.
Nick: They're smart kids. If I could make it through, they can too—if they quit acting like screwups!
Therapist: (slowly, softly) Being a screwup (breathes in and out) that hurts.

Nick: (softens his voice too) Yeah. [sighs] I felt that way a lot… I was a screwup—still am, I guess. [looks down]

Therapist: (still with an emotional tone) You worry you're not the kind of man—husband, father—you should be? Want to be? [Nick slowly nods] And you don't want that for Brandon and Logan. [Nick agrees].

Sophia's empathic response tells Nick she is interested in him, listening to him. Her choice of words begins to situate the therapeutic conversation within societal definitions in which Nick feels like "a failure in the eyes of the world" (p. 193).

Therapist: (softly) If Brandon sees himself as a screwup—or if others see him that way—that would say he's…?

Nick: That he's not good enough, not as good as everyone else—that he'll not make it.

Therapist: [tentatively] You feel you've not made it? That others look down on you?

Nick: And judge me—like I'm a second-class citizen because I can't work. (p. 194)

In this early stage of relationship formation, Sophia is beginning to see each family member individually and contextually, zooming in and out in her assessment. Though she is cautious, knowing it is not possible for her to fully apprehend their sociocultural experiences, she is responding from and communicating genuine interest in seeing through *their* contextual lenses. She is creating a therapeutic platform for further discussions of their sociocultural identities and the material realities within which they live. She wants to know more about their neighborhood and housing, what school is like for Brandon, Logan, and Tyler. She is curious about what it means to be biracial in these settings and the impact of larger gender, sexual, economic, and political systems. She wonders whether religion is important to them and what less visible differences may be involved.

Socioculturally attuned therapists know identity is more personal than simply an intersecting set of social locations or categories where people find themselves and/or others assign them or assume they belong. Sophia is interested in the "felt" identities of each member of the Carter family (Knudson-Martin, 2024).

•←→•

Felt identities are uniquely embodied social messages, patterns of belonging, and ideas about oneself and others that arise out of sociocultural experience.

•←→•

Sophia avoids categorical stereotypes and, instead, seeks to apprehend how personal felt experience gives meaning to the current situation.

Element 2—Responsibly Position Therapy

Clients make decisions about their own lives, but therapists are responsible for how their contributions influence which possibilities are enabled in the therapeutic process (Murphy & Hecker, 2020). Assessment needs to be based on awareness of how your own sociocultural context may affect what you see and your clinical choices—and how clients may frame their responses to you. Rather than replicating inequities built into social structures and ways of knowing, you are intentional about your clinical lens and how you use your influence. Responsible positioning means your assessment and subsequent clinical actions orient the therapy to all the contextual elements that impact the case so clients have options regarding how to position themselves toward each other and societal forces (Lini & Bertrando, 2022). To responsibly position therapy, consider the following questions:

- What are my felt social identities and social locations? What do these mean in relation to this particular client(s)?
- What are my assumptions/stereotypes about the social groups to which my client(s) identify and/or are categorized as being a part of?
- How do my positionality, assumptions, and values have the potential to reinforce inequalities and/or support equity?
- What values are implicit in the theories I will apply to this case?
- What values do I want to intentionally support?
- How will I navigate the tension I feel as I respond to multiple and contradictory stakeholders in this process?

Attention to Therapist's Sociocultural Position and Values

It is imperative that therapists attune to their own sociocultural position and values. If you are not aware of your own social locations, emotional reactions, and values, you are likely to either reinforce dominant cultural standards and inequities or reactively respond when these issues arise in session (García et al., 2015 Knudson-Martin, 2024). A thorough assessment needs to include awareness of your own sociocultural context as it relates to therapy. When Sophia reflects on her social identities, she realizes that she sees through the lens of someone who immigrated to the US with her parents when she was three years old. Though White, she has always felt like an outsider. As a young child, she quickly learned to figure out what was expected in social settings and followed these rules. In Romania, her grandfather "disappeared" and the family lost everything. Her parents came to the US seeking financial opportunity. Working hard was expected, no matter what obstacles they faced. Sophia realizes she has internalized negative views of people who don't seem able to "pick themselves up" when faced with setbacks, especially someone like Nick, who seems to feel "sorry for himself" and appears unaware of his privilege as a White male born in the US. She realizes she will need to attune to the sociocultural context of Nick's vulnerability (Knudson-Martin et al., 2021), while also exploring how heteropatriarchy and economic structures affect the Carter family in ways both similar and different from her own.

Sophia was always a "good," cooperative student. She is intrigued by Logan and Brandon, who smile and joke with her and their parents in ways she would never have done, and are reported as "disruptive" at school. She notes that Tyler seems connected to his younger brothers, but offers little about himself. Sophia knows that her own experience of keeping herself hidden stemmed from her family's experience that people outside the family could not be trusted, her sense of not belonging as an immigrant, and her confusion around sexual identity. She wonders what is going on for Tyler, what socio-contextual factors are involved, and how to engage with him.

Working with the Carter family brings up the complexity of parenting and Sophia's uncertainty regarding her own parenting roles. Knowing that in addition to a second shift of household labor women also often carry a third shift of caregiving and emotion work (Smoliak et al., 2023), Sophia is curious about how family and relational work is shared, or not, in the Carter family, even as she struggles with these issues in her own life. Awareness of her own emotional responses to social inequities can inform how to responsibly address them in her clinical work (Garcia et al., 2015).

Autonomy and responsibility for oneself and those you love are important values for Sophia and her family. As a socioculturally attuned family therapist, she appreciates the value of these qualities, but is also intentional in bringing a broader, more relational lens to her practice. While she resonates with clinical models that emphasize personal choice and accountability, Sophia also recognizes unfairness built into social norms, structures, and standards.

•←→•

She chooses words, questions, frameworks, and interventions that position her clinical work to counter these inequities by making social processes and patterns visible and helping her clients envision relationally just possibilities.

•←→•

Positioning Therapist's Role and Language

The use of the *Diagnostic and Statistical Manual of Mental Disorders* (DSM-5-TR, American Psychiatric Association, 2022) is an example of how Sophia is mindful regarding how she positions her professional role. The DSM categorization of symptoms has benefits, reassuring clients in many ways. Naming what they are dealing with can reduce uncertainty and distress and help focus treatment. A diagnosis may also be required to establish medical necessity to receive publicly funded services or reimbursement from health insurance companies. Nevertheless, the DSM does not adequately address the sociocultural or sociorelational contexts of symptoms.

> Use [of the DSM] can reinforce dominant cultural values and beliefs... Social inequalities and injustices may be concealed when clients' distress associated with social and economic inequalities, discrimination, and violence is framed as a personal or medical issue to be addressed with individually focused solutions.
>
> (Sutherland et al., 2016, p. 78)

Sophia seeks to position therapy systemically, orienting toward relationality and equity, while also drawing on scientific research that may benefit her clients (e.g., Larner, 2022). How she talks about diagnostic issues makes a difference. An analysis of couple and family therapy sessions when the focus was on diagnoses found that diagnostic talk tended to reinforce notions of the autonomous self, develop a pathological point of view, and medicalize solutions (Sutherland et al., 2016).

Though interested in possible diagnoses, especially in making sense of Brandon and Logan's behavior at school, Sophia actively positions against the risk of reducing her understanding of their experience to narrow stereotypic categories (e.g., Johnstone, 2021). For example, on a conference call with Brandon's teacher, she expands the conversation beyond the problems described in the referral (dialogue from Knudson-Martin, 2024, p. 213–214):

Teacher: Brandon is always up to something—egging another kid on, fighting ... anything but focusing on the lesson!
Therapist: It sounds like he has a lot of energy.
Teacher: He does! If only he could channel it into something productive.
Therapist: I'm curious what you've noticed about the positive aspect of that energy?

This question catches the teacher a bit off guard as it is not the usual story around Brandon. When he reflects on it, he says Brandon "has a good spirit" and "just wants to stir things up." Sophia is then able to engage the teacher in describing what that good spirit looks like and asks him to help her "keep an eye out for how Brandon uses his good spirit in a positive way" (p. 214). Countering a deficit characterization is important for any child labeled as disruptive or causing trouble, but is especially important for members of minority groups whose experience tends to be mislabeled and misunderstood in the dominant culture, including diagnostic categories (Johnstone, 2021).

Sophia realizes that the rules for success she learned were based on "habits of whiteness" that center Eurocentric values and ways of relating (Combs, 2022, p. 510). This includes how professionalism is defined (Hardy, 2022). Sophia has been socialized to believe that being professional means distancing oneself from emotion and maintaining the appearance of objectivity and rationality over relational connection. These dominating practices contribute to epistemic injustice; that is, when a person is not viewed as a credible source of information because their place in society is marginalized and/or when there is not shared language to name their experience because collective meanings are determined by those with the power (Fricker, 2007).

Sophia knows that how she uses herself and her emotional presence has the potential to perpetuate injustice or to mitigate some of its effects (Van Der Merwe & Wetherell, 2020). She positions therapy as an opportunity to value clients' voices and facilitate justice by seeking to apprehend their experience and helping them find words to name and understand it (Fürst, 2024; Johnstone, 2021). For example, when Sophia asks Tyler about high school, "he shrugs and says it is OK. The look in his eyes says it is not" (Knudson-Martin, 2024, p. 195). In an individual session, Sophia positions the conversation to center Tyler while acknowledging the differences between them and her lack of knowledge about his life.

Therapist: When I started high school, I was on the outside. I looked White, but as an Eastern European, I felt different and no one seemed to understand me. I don't know anything about your school or what that's like for you. But I'd like to understand.

As Tyler (whose skin is light brown) begins to talk, he describes a complex intersection of gender, race, and sexuality that confuses him.

Tyler: Black guys tease me for being a "White Dude" … The White guys joke about condoms and call me a "fag."

Tyler grows animated as he talks about these issues. Sophia focuses on socioculturally attuning to and giving voice to his experience:

Therapist: From what you said, when guys call you a "fag," it seems they are saying "you aren't masculine enough," not necessarily that they think you are gay. Is that right?

Tyler: Yeah. But I don't want to be a man like that. It makes me wonder if I am gay [pause]. It's OK if I am, but I just don't know.

Therapist: You'd like other options for how to be male—whether or not you are gay.

Tyler: Exactly!

As they talk about gender scripts, gender fluidity, narrow definitions of masculinity, toxic masculinity, alternative forms of gender expression, and how these may differ from sexuality, Tyler visibly relaxes and expresses less concern about needing to fit into one category or another. They acknowledge his parents' worries about him and agree to continue the conversation until he is ready to share his thoughts and feelings with them.

Element 3—Locate in Space, Place, and Time

Space (Soja, 2010) refers to the natural environment, as well as what is constructed within environments (e.g., homes, hospitals, parks, shopping centers, transportation). The spaces clients inhabit determine and reflect their access to resources such as employment, food, education, and medical care. Place is a related concept that refers to our sense of being within space, including the need for personal space, privacy, safety, and social interaction (Fitzpatrick & LaGory, 2000).

Family therapy can inadvertently dis-locate families, suspending them from the physical realities of daily life.

While our theoretical frameworks often make reference to time (e.g., family legacies, intergenerational patterns, narratives), they rarely consider the impact of space and place. Family therapy concepts (e.g., social discourse, family dynamics) can, in fact, act as seemingly autonomous webs of influence without connection to physical realities (McDowell, 2015). In addition, we typically meet clients away from where they live (either in our offices or online) in what Rhodes (2021) referred to as "non-places" (p. 358), further challenging our ability to understand their sense of place.

As Sophia engages with the Carter family, she seeks to tangibly see the spaces they inhabit and their sense of place in their home, their community, and the larger environment. She is aware of mounting research that points to the impact of our social, cultural, economic, political, and environmental contexts on our physical, mental, and relational health (Robins et al., 2023; Watson et al., 2020) and explores these in the Carter family's life. Sophia looks for and seeks to understand obstacles and challenges to well-being, but also to uncover and highlight relational resilience and resources (Brock et al., 2023; Walsh, 2016).

Place-ing Families and Therapy

After getting a sense of each family member's perspective on the presenting issues and hopes for therapy, Sophia asks the family if it is okay to step back a bit to get a broader picture. Knowing that a typical genogram, which asks questions about family members, names, ages, employment, education, illnesses, deaths, religion, relational dynamics, mental health, intimate partner violence, adverse childhood experiences, etc., results in a two-dimensional schematic that hints at, but is not grounded in space and place, she begins to sketch a critical/cultural genogram (Chapter 9, this volume; Glebova & Knudson-Martin, 2023; Hardy & Laszloffy, 1995; Kosutic et al., 2009) that adds multiple layers of sociocultural context to explore social location, migration, immigrant status, oppression, privilege, social class, race, gender, sexual orientation, historical setting, community factors, and so on. As Sophia helps the family consider and value the significance of their place and space over time on their relationships and well-being, she considers questions such as:

- What sociohistorical events are part of the family's timeline? How did their families make sense of them? How did these events impact family members and legacies?
- What aspects of clients' histories and current contexts are influenced by injustice and marginalization?
- In what ways do family members or their communities experience current or past sociocultural or political trauma?

- What sources of pride and shame are related to their cultures of origin and family legacies?
- What beliefs and dreams did their ancestors have? What were their messages about survival or success?
- How have family members been wounded by wrongs done by or to their people?
- How have family members been complicit in wrongs done by their ancestors?
- In carrying on family legacies, what values are important now? What sources of resilience may be drawn upon?

Laurelle's father was killed in the first Gulf War (known as Desert Storm) when she was a young child. She, her mother, and sister lived with her grandmother and aunt. They found a two-bedroom apartment in a "good" school district in the hope that Laurelle and her sister would have more opportunities. Nick lived with his parents and two siblings in a five-bedroom house located on the edge of a park. Nick and Laurelle met in high school. The dialogue below (Knudson-Martin, 2024, pp. 204–205) highlights how their attraction countered gender and racial stereotypes:

Nick: She sat next to me in biology. She was so smart and kept cracking these really funny jokes. [looks at Laurelle] She helped me write up my lab assignments. I'd probably have failed without her.

Therapist: You were attracted to her intelligence and wit.

Nick: Still am! It was like nothing could get her down. She always had a smile. [thinks] School wasn't much fun for me. Laurelle made it better and she didn't judge me.

Therapist: Laurelle, Nick says you made school better for him—supported him, didn't judge him. What attracted you to him?

Laurelle: Honestly, I wasn't at first. But then I started to appreciate that he wasn't so cocky like most of the guys. He wasn't a smartass. He treated me with respect.

Sophia expands outward, staying connected to them while beginning to locate their attraction in time and place:

Therapist: What was it like for you as a young Black woman in that school—over 20 years ago now—did you expect respect?

Laurelle: No. I didn't. And among teenage guys, I didn't see much respect for girls, period.

Therapist: So Nick didn't fit the stereotype—he didn't act like a [air quotes] typical teenage guy. [pause] Was it unusual in your school to date across racial lines?

Laurelle: There was some crossover. But we didn't really start out dating. It was more like support for each other. [looks at her body] I was kinda chubby. Boys weren't interested in me.

Therapist: You were surprised that any guy, especially a White guy, would find you attractive? [Laurelle nods]. And Nick, you're a White guy—from a more affluent family—how do you think it happened that you resisted those stereotypes about women?

Nick: Honestly [turns to Laurelle] don't get me wrong, I've always been lucky to have you—but I think it was partly an "up yours." I didn't like school, I didn't like authority, I didn't like my parents' snobbishness. I was looking to rebel.

Sophia helps them explore the impact of their social class and racial legacies. No one in Laurelle's family has ever owned a home. According to her mother, her father had hoped to use the GI Bill to go to college, but did not make it home from the war. Her mother's father, a Vietnam veteran, had also wanted to use the GI Bill to buy a home, but because banks redlined areas where

Blacks lived, he was never able to access these benefits (Agbai, 2023). In contrast, in the 1880s Nick's Norwegian ancestors took advantage of the Homestead Act (1862; National Park Service, n.d.), which gave them 160 free acres, provided they lived on and improved the land. Subsequent generations built on this to create generational wealth. When Nick's grandfather returned from serving in WWII, he was able to use the GI Bill to buy a home, which his parents subsequently sold to buy a bigger one in a "better" neighborhood.

Nick faces his unemployment, limited finances, and family roles through the eyes of someone raised to expect that resources will be available to him. Though he did not go college, through his father's connections he was able to get a good job in home construction and develop these skills. When the housing market crashed in 2008, Nick's parents helped him and Laurelle buy a small "fixer-upper" at a low price when the previous owners could no longer afford the payments and faced foreclosure. Laurelle approaches their situation through the legacy of strong Black women who did whatever was needed to survive. She does not expect to be respected or helped out. She is personally familiar with the idea that depression is for White women, "as an African American woman, we, in order to survive, historically, have learned how to wear the mask…to get through the day smiling" (Amankwaa, 2003, p. 312).

Laurelle and Nick's families exemplify the racial wealth gap in the US. According to Agbai (2023)

> White–Black racial inequality in wealth stands at $164,000, with Black households possessing $24,100 in net worth, while White households hold $188,200 (Bhutta et al. 2020). Homes owned by White households increase in value more quickly than those owned by Black families… Moreover, mortgages are more likely to become a financial burden for Black families, largely because of continued discriminatory and predatory lending practices. (p. 2)

This gap in material resources, which is structured into economic, political, and social policies and practices (Agbai, 2023), has consequences for physical, emotional, and relational health. It interacts with other inequalities such as gender, sexuality, nationality, ethnicity, abilities, etc., to affect the opportunities available to people, as well as how they—and others— perceive themselves.

For example, Laurelle did well in school and is a dedicated and dependable worker. When she graduated from high school, she wanted to become a nurse practitioner but lacked the financial and social capital to do so. Four years ago, she was offered a promotion to field manager and turned it down—in part because she did not trust her co-workers would respect a Woman of Color, but mostly because she did not think she could handle the increased workload along with her family responsibilities. Nick encouraged her to take the job. According to Laurelle, "We didn't talk about what I'd need from him to take on that responsibility—what would be different at home. It was like he wasn't affected—except by having more money" (Knudson-Martin, 2024, p. 271). Both Nick and Laurelle want the best for their sons. Now, even though Nick is at home during the day, old gender legacies guide their approach to parenting, with Laurelle contacting teachers and carrying the load of responsibility for how the boys are doing (Knudson-Martin & Mahoney, 2005; Smoliak et al., 2023). Laurelle also has serious health issues that cause her pain, but her sociocultural legacy tells her to keep going, while Nick's more entitled legacy seldom notices or helps take responsibility for her health.

Socio-relational Determinants of Health

As described in chapter one, "social determinants of health (SDOH) are the conditions in the environments where people are born, live, learn, work, play, worship, and age that affect a wide range of health functioning, and quality-of-life outcomes and risks" (US Department of Health and Human Services, *Healthy People 2030*). Some individuals, families, and communities benefit from positive and supportive factors, while others suffer negative effects of SDOH. Those with adequate income to live in safe neighborhoods, meet educational needs, and enjoy food security—those whose social locations place them at the center free from discrimination—do not experience the same type of stress, limited options, or risk as those at the bottom or in the margins.

Relationships may be negatively or positively affected by SDOH. Families can play an intentional role in mitigating harm by working together to navigate and buffer negative effects. The impact of SDOH may differ within families as well. In other words, the benefits or negative impacts are not necessarily evenly distributed. Most notably, relational inequities within families may compound and/or create negative determinants of health. The role of family is reflected in what we have termed "socio-relational determinants of health."

Sophia refers to Figure 4.2 to consider socio-relational determinants of health in the Carter family. These range from "upstream" factors such as environmental systems and resources, economic and commercial systems, and political and governmental systems, to "downstream" factors connected to these larger systems, such as social structures and local contexts and community and family social supports. All of these flow toward relational, mental, and physical well-being, which tend to be inequitably available. The effects on individuals, families, and communities perpetuate injustices in the larger upstream systems. While family therapists can and should participate in "upstream" interventions (e.g., advocacy for changes in policies and laws that focus on prevention), we are called upon daily to provide "downstream" interventions as we work with what are often the most vulnerable populations to understand and help mitigate the impact of these forces on mental health and intimate relationships.

↔

Socioculturally attuned assessments will inquire about the effects of social and relational determinants of health.

↔

Questions about SDOH should be part of discussions of family background, genograms, and sociograms. Activities such as structural/eco-maps and drawings can help identify the social determinants of health clients must navigate. Questions include:

- *Economic stability*—What financial resources are available to the client/family? What financial stressors are they facing? How secure is employment? How do workplace conditions and financial demands impact relational, mental, and physical well-being?
- *Education access and quality*—How available are educational resources? How do educational needs and backgrounds affect client/family well-being?
- *Health care access and quality*—How available is health care, what is the quality of care, and how well does it support the unique sociocultural needs of this client/family?
- *Neighborhood and built environment*—Where does this client/family live? What is their home like? What is their experience in the neighborhood? Is there clean air and water, greenspace, quiet, and safety?
- *Social, community, and family context*—Does this client/family experience a sense of inclusion and belonging? How much control do they have over their own life circumstances? Are support, acceptance, and friendships available to them?
- How do larger social, political, and economic structures, policies, values, and norms affect the above SDOH for this client/family?

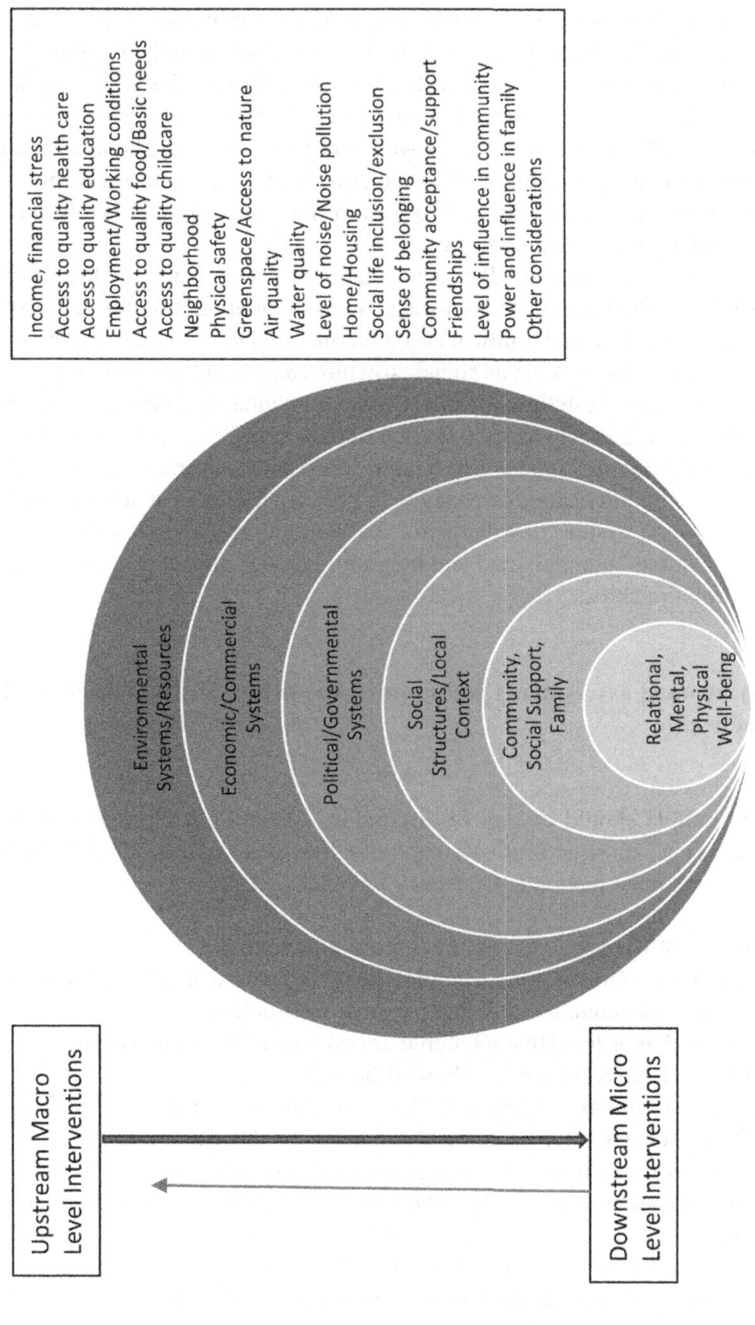

Figure 4.2 Systems impacting socio-relational determinants of health.

The compounding effects of SDOH create a social gradient of health. Those with greater resources and status live longer lives in better physical and mental health, while those with lower status and fewer resources have shorter life expectancies with greater physical and mental health problems (Alegría et al., 2018). Political economies impact health, including mental health (McCartney et al., 2019). In fact, there is evidence that those living in nations with high income inequality are more likely to experience depression (Patel et al., 2018). Likewise, several studies have correlated dollar increases in the US minimum wage with decreases in the rate of suicide (Ahern, 2020).

There is ample evidence that discrimination and oppression are detrimental to health. For example, race is a determining factor in the likelihood of physical illness, incarceration, addiction, and shortened life span (Jones, 2000), and LGBTQ+ youth are at greater risk for homelessness (Norman-Major, 2018) and suicide (Fulginiti et al., 2021). The negative physiological responses to discrimination are also well documented (Harrell et al., 2003). These processes are cumulative, leading to increased vulnerability of those who suffer a lifetime of structural inequality and discrimination (Dannefer, 2003; DiPrete & Eirich, 2006; Merton 1968).

The Carter family's health and well-being is related to a number of social determinants of health. They experience ongoing financial stress. Nick suffers from an injury caused by the physical nature of his previous work and shows symptoms of depression since becoming unemployed. Like many members of racially marginalized groups, Laurelle is diagnosed with diabetes and high blood pressure. She experiences recurring back pain that is exacerbated by her job as a home health care provider, for which her insurance company has denied surgery. The parents worry that the school system may be unfairly targeting Brandon and Logan (whose skin is dark brown like their mother's), and Tyler's social withdrawal appears related to a sense of not belonging and exclusion due to his race, sexual, and gender identities that don't fit the norm at his school.

To learn more about the environmental, social, and community factors in the Carter family's life, in a subsequent session Sophia helps them create a family cartography (McDowell, 2015). This tool is described in more detail in Chapter 7. Sophia gives the family a big piece of paper (you can also use poster board, dry erase board, or chalkboard) and marking pens, and invites them to draw a map of their town. She has them draw their house on the "map." She asks questions such as, In what part of the city is it located? Where do people with more money live? Those with less money? They identify the racial and ethnic nature of various neighborhoods. They add the location of schools, stores, public transportation, and parks. Where do friends and family live? What is their experience of living in this community? How do they get from one place to another? Where do they feel a sense of safety and belonging? What is their access to greenspace and clear air?

The Carter home is on the edge of a "good" school district. Most of the neighbors are White. It is a quiet neighborhood with well-maintained, moderate-sized homes. Theirs is one of the smallest. There are sidewalks, but no parks. Air quality in the summer is often poor due to higher temperatures and smoke from wildfires, which have become more common. The family does not feel accepted by their neighbors. The boys stopped riding their bicycles in the street after a neighbor on the cul-de-sac at the end of their street (incorrectly) told them several times that they were not allowed to ride there. The Carters have one car, which Laurelle takes to work unless Nick needs it for an appointment. Since they live in a suburb, grocery stores, medical care, and other amenities are several miles away. The boys take the bus to school. There is a city bus on a major street about eight blocks from their house, but getting to most places takes a long time and the parents do not feel comfortable allowing the boys to go on their own. There are parks and natural areas within an hour or two drive, but the family seldom has time for these excursions.

Sophia begins to apprehend how social determinants of health increase stress and challenge well-being for the Carters, especially related to time and logistical demands and a sense of belonging and inclusion. In the following dialogue (Knudson-Martin, 2024, p. 198), she helps them put words to the tensions and choices (or lack of them) they experience:

Therapist: You all feel a little [air quotes] less than in this neighborhood…you feel judged as… what? Less competent? Less valuable? Not good parents?…

Laurelle: It's hard to put words to, it's just a feeling, I guess—that we should be doing better. That we're not as good as them. [pauses] Nick always worked so hard, but not the "right" kind of work, you know. [pauses] Our boys are just as good as the other kids, but it's hard to keep up!

Therapist: (to Laurelle) And you? How safe and accepted do you feel?

Laurelle: (wry chuckle) I never expected to fit in. But this house was a good choice for our family, something I never expected. I'm grateful.

Relational Supports and Values

According to *Healthy People 2030*, relationship factors such as social cohesion and solidarity, social capital, social networks, and social support significantly impact health and well-being.

↞↠

Relational supports and values influence day-to-day interactions across and within all levels of social systems (e.g., families, communities, workplaces, governmental and educational institutions, health care).

↞↠

Assessing for and helping clients strengthen supportive relationships and social networks, and develop and effectively use social capital (Garcia & McDowell, 2010) are ways family therapists can intervene in SDOH.

- Do client's relationships mutually benefit and support each person?
- How are caring for others and emotional work valued in client's relationships and community?
- To what extent is responsibility for maintaining relationships shared within the couple/family? How are care and support extended in the larger community?
- What personal qualities and ideals do clients endorse that support loving, healthy, equitable relationships (even though these may be minimized in the broader culture)?
- To what extent do client's relationships/community enable them to withstand personal and social stressors and change?
- What sources of resilience have clients evolved out of efforts to resist power imbalances and societal inequities?

Laurelle's mother and sister live in a "poorer" neighborhood about 15 minutes away and stop by frequently. Care and support flow back and forth reciprocally between them, depending on who needs what when. Recently, Laurelle's mother's health has begun to deteriorate, and her sister is pregnant and on her own. While her family is a long-standing source of love and support, Laurelle is currently feeling an extra burden to be there for them, even while carrying most of the relational load in her household. On the other hand, Nick's family lives in a more affluent, gated community about an hour away. They seldom see them except for holidays or special events. Nick believes his parents are "racist" and treat his siblings' children better. Although his parents originally helped them finance their home, when Laurelle and Nick were not able to cover their bills following his injury, they borrowed from Laurelle's mother, who also has limited financial resources. The family does not appear to have other relational resources in the community, such as friends or church groups, or other social networks. Nick is isolated from everyone, even Laurelle and the boys, which exacerbates his feelings of uselessness and makes pain management difficult (Butler & Moseley, 2013).

Identifying and developing their relational resources will be an important focus of therapy. From the beginning of therapy, Sophia listens for relational aspirations that may be implicit or blocked by reactions to distress such as anger, fear, or hopelessness. For example, when Laurelle and the boys all describe Nick as angry and shut off from them, Sophia invites Nick's relational ideals by asking what it means to him that his family sees him as so disengaged, as though he doesn't care about them.

Therapist: I'm guessing that's not the message that you want to send to them—that you don't care about them.
Nick: I'm not me these days. It's hard—I know it's hard for them too.
Therapist: (softly) Tell them what you hope as you go through this time together.

This kind of conversation allows the family to name their caring for each other and to consider how they can support each other through the struggles they face. Sophia also recognizes caring work that usually goes unnoticed, especially when done by women (Smoliak et al., 2023), and raises questions about how they might want to share it. She notes many forms of resilience in the ways the three boys support each other and in the initial attraction between Laurelle and Nick, which was based on mutuality and resisting gender and racial stereotypes. Sophia plants seeds for discussions about how to engage Nick's family and refers Nick to a chronic pain education group that will help him feel less alone and enable a more relational response that focuses on what he has to give as well as what he needs (Knudson-Martin, 2024).

Element 4—Assess Impacts of Power on Clinical Issues

Power refers to social processes that determine whose collective and individual interests are served (see Chapter 2, this volume).

•←→•

Those with cumulative power determine what is important. Their interests are embedded in social structures, policies, norms, and everyday practices.

•←→•

These power processes influence what opportunities are available, how people view themselves and are judged by others, who notices others and accommodates them, and whose voice and interests are centered. Assessment of sociocultural context, responsible positioning, and location in space, place, and time all connect to power.

Sophia brings a third order lens to consider the effects of these power processes on each client's sense of self and expectations, the flow of power among family members and other people in their lives, and the impact of these on the clinical issues. To identify how power shows up in intimate and family relationships and personal health and well-being she considers:

- How much personal, interpersonal, and institutional power does each client experience as a result of their societal positions?
- How physically and emotionally safe are each client/family member with each other and in the community?

- How able are each client/family member to express and attain personal interests/goals?
- In what contexts do clients define what is "real" and/or are viewed as credible and knowledgeable?
- To what extent does a client's social power position lead them to organize around what matters to other(s) or expect others to accommodate them?
- How does one person's (or group's) sense of competence, optimism, or well-being come at the expense of another's physical or emotional health?
- How is one person's (or group's) financial security dependent on another's?
- How may client symptoms and/or problems be responses to their power positions?

Like all clinical assessments, the immediate physical and emotional safety of each client and those they could harm is the first power issue to address. This will help you determine what immediate action may be needed and whether family or couple therapy is appropriate. Meeting at least briefly with each individual helps identify what may not be safe to express with a partner or parent/caregiver present.

Sophia begins to track power from the outset, while simultaneously getting to know each family member, their hopes for therapy, and beginning to form relationships with them.

•←→•

Observations regarding power are most effective when directly connected to experience-near and in-the-moment processes.

•←→•

Sophia notices who attends to whom and whose interests and concerns are centered. She sees that Nick appears engaged only when he is speaking or his interests are addressed. In the example below (Knudson-Martin, 2024, p. 199–200), rather than make a judgment or pronouncement "from on high," she names what she is observing and asks the family about it

Therapist: (to the family) As we're talking, I notice that you all seem engaged and interested in what each other is saying; except Dad seems less involved. Is this how it is at home?
Logan: Dad mostly stays in his room.
Brandon: He just comes out to yell at us—he's mad all the time.

Sophia explores the two-way nature of their relationships:

Therapist: Dad says he wants some quiet. What are you wanting from Dad?
Logan: He could play with us.
Brandon: He could help us with homework. Tyler does that sometimes. And Mom when she has time.
Therapist: So you'd like Dad to be more interested in what you're doing? More involved? [Brandon and Logan enthusiastically agree]

Nick expects his family to attend to his interests, but does not attune to them. This is an example of how power structures in the larger society affect individual and relational well-being. Like most people, when Nick is asked whether he believes his interests should matter most, he says "of course not." He wants to be there for his family but has also internalized societal patterns and messages that say men's needs, time, and interests are more important. As Sophia explores this inconsistency, she gets in touch with Nick's shame that he is not able to live up to the power position expected of men;

a one-up position in relation to women and children. His sense of social failure is magnified since the accident, but it began as a child when he struggled with school. Nick learned that as a (White) man he is entitled to respect. He responds to being diminished in the larger society in ways that reinforce his power at home—at the expense of his relational interests. In this example (Knudson-Martin, 2024, p. 201–202), Sophia names the relational consequences of this power discrepancy:

Therapist: (to Nick) It's clear from what you've said that you love your children and are here, in large part, because you are concerned for them.

Nick: Of course. All three of my boys are very important to me.

Therapist: When you focus on [your] anger and misery, it's hard to show how much you care about them or pay attention to what they need.

Nick: Yeah. [sighs] yeah. But I *do* care.

Therapist: Laurelle, when pain and anger keep Nick from focusing on the children, how does that affect you?

Societal power processes tell Nick men should not need help. When Laurelle suggests ways to better communicate with the boys, Nick reacts with anger. She is left feeling alone as a parent, while carrying most of the responsibility.

Other societal power processes also affect this therapy, many of which show up when discussing the family cartography. As a mixed-race, lower income family living in a White middle class neighborhood, they are treated as less than. They do not feel comfortable with or supported by their neighbors. As a result, the boys come directly home after school and spend most of their time in the living room playing video games. They have little access to nature, exercise, or after school activities.

Financial stress is exacerbated by gender, economic, and social capital disparities that inhibit Laurelle's career aspirations. Racial disparities seem to have invaded their relationships with Nick's family and the emotional, relational, and economic support they might offer. Tyler's transition to high school is thwarted by oppressive sexual, racial, and gender structures that appear to organize relationships among the students. Racial biases may also be part of Brandon and Logan's troubles at school. Power disparities within the family make it more difficult to navigate the effects of these societal inequities. Social support is available from Laurelle's family—those with the fewest economic and educational resources—but power disparities limit the support and belonging available in the larger community and from other extended family members.

As hidden or not usually discussed power contexts are brought to the surface, the Carter family begins to see their concerns and hopes with a broader lens. Sophia applies this third order lens to conceptualize the case through a family therapy model. An overarching goal is to develop a shared understanding of the case that enables the family to envision possible changes that intervene in power processes to support relational justice, mutual well-being, and health.

Element 5—Conceptualize Through Family Therapy Models

Clinical models create additional focus for case conceptualization and treatment planning. Socioculturally attuned assessment connects the concepts that frame your clinical approach to the power and societal contexts of your particular case. The chapters that follow will help you apply the major systemic family therapy models through a third order lens. Table 4.1 gives a brief overview of a socioculturally attuned conceptualization of these models.

For example, if Sophia applies a socioculturally attuned *structural* lens, she begins with a view that healthy relationship structures support the optimal development of each member of the Carter family. She will consider how gender and racial norms and societal standards of success are part

Table 4.1 Socioculturally attuned conceptualizations of just relationships

Systemic Model	*Just Conceptualization of Health*	*Socio-contextual Considerations*
Structural	Relationship structure supports optimal development for all persons.	How do cultural norms, access to social and economic resources, and power influence interaction patterns?
Strategic	Circular patterns in the relationship support equitable power processes.	How may symptoms be resistance to societal power imbalances? How may hypotheses maintain or intervene in societal power processes?
Experiential	Relationship supports growth by liberating selves from destructive sociopolitical messages and expectations.	How do societal power differences limit open expression? How may sociocultural attunement to felt experience support shared resilience?
Attachment	Relational connections empower partners/family members to equitably support each other through life stresses.	How do societal gender/power processes affect emotion, expression of relational needs, development of relational bonds, and safety?
Bowen	Persons connect with family history and sociocultural contexts to build relationships and shared life choices from a differentiated sense of self.	How are personal biographies interwoven with societal relationships? How do societal power processes influence how differentiation is developed and expresed?
Contextual	Accountability and balance of fairness in current relationships transform the effect of past injustices and enable ethical future options.	How do past and current societal injustices affect the relational ethics, entitlement, and responsibility between partners?
Cognitive Behavioral	Awareness of contextual sources of thoughts and triggers enables relationship patterns that do not automatically follow societal norms and power structures.	How are personal and relationship schemas connected to societal schemas? Whose interests do internalized societal schemas represent? How are these replicated in relationship patterns?
Solution Focused	People choose and amplify solutions that expand possibilities for equitable, just relationships.	What forms of resilience and potential solutions can be drawn from legacies of the groups in which clients' identify? How might clients garner hope and envision possibilities based on past and present social movements?
Collaborative	Dialog includes and values each person's voice and creates space to imagine possibilities beyond taken-for-granted realities.	How do societal power process shape and limit what is brought to the dialog and whose interests are prioritized? What preferred ways of being are overlooked?
Narrative	Relationship narratives center just alternatives to dominant societal discourses.	How are dominant societal narratives embedded in partner's stories? Who has the power to determine which stories get told? How are alternative stories silenced?
Socio-Emotional Relationship Therapy	People develop relational options beyond the dominant discourse that enable them to navigate crises and injustices through mutual support.	How do social discourse, emotion, and relationship patterns converge in the moment-to-moment of therapy? How do these connect with societal context, power, and the Circle of Care?

Adapted from: Knudson-Martin, C. & Kim, L. (2023). Socioculturally attuned couple therapy. In J. Lebow & D. Snyder (Eds.). *Clinical handbook of couple therapy* (6th ed., p. 271). Guilford. Used with permission.

of interactional patterns at school and in the home. She notices how the family manages emotional distance and closeness. For example, Sophia might observe that Tyler engages to support his brothers, while Nick disengages and focuses on himself—a relational pattern that maintains a patriarchal power imbalance. Sophia will help the family develop a relationship structure that supports all of them, with the parents sharing care of their sons and responsibility for helping them deal with their troubles at school, rather than placing all this on Laurelle.

From a *Bowen* perspective, Sophia will help the Carter family develop just relationships based on differentiated selves. She will view misbehavior, anger, and depression as emotional reactivity to sociocultural contexts and family histories, and encourage family members to address these issues and their needs directly. Healthy differentiation will be based on equitable power processes. For example, Nick and Laurelle will differentiate from societal models that leave him emotionally disengaged and put relational responsibility and parenting on her. The family will support Tyler in differentiating from binary gender and sexual stereotypes and support Brandon and Logan in developing the emotional regulation necessary to navigate unjust social settings.

If applying *collaborative* practices, Sophia will seek to "create a dialogical relationship among family members that includes and values each person's voice and creates space to imagine possibilities beyond taken-for-granted realities" (Knudson-Martin & Kim, 2023, p. 270). Inequitable societal power processes, such as Nick's self absorption and delegation of parenting responsibilities to Laurelle, are resisted so they do not limit what is discussed or envisioned as possible. Sophia will invite the family to develop relationship models that work for them and overcome the effects imposed by dominant societal discourses (e.g., disruptive behavior, feelings of failure, limited sexual and gender options).

Application of a specific clinical model through a third order sociocultural lens—or systematically integrating several—helps create a shared understanding of the problem and direction for therapy.

•←→•

You can avoid one of the most common mistakes in assessment and goal setting— adopting a client's view of the problem and goals for change too quickly—by exploring the nature and context of the problem and expanding the lens through which the problem is viewed.

•←→•

Putting It All Together

Whatever systemic model you apply, your socioculturally attuned assessment frames how you and your clients envision change. As you put all the pieces together to create a plan for the therapy, the following overarching questions can guide your summary:

- How are client's presenting concerns reflections of their societal and power contexts?
- What stories of resistance and resilience are embedded in client's responses to their sociocultural context?
- How can this therapy join with clients to create the possibility of third order change?

These transtheoretical questions inform how you think about and approach the specific problems and co-occurring issues that brought your clients to therapy.

Figure 4.3 provides a suggested format for summarizing a socioculturally attuned assessment and treatment goals—to pull all the pieces together. In this format, you examine the presenting issues through a third order lens. You begin by identifying clients' sociocultural "group" memberships and felt identities and their impact on clients' relationships. You locate the client/family in space, place, and time and address the implications of these on physical, emotional, and relational

I **Therapeutic Context**
Consider the impact of the therapeutic context (e.g., agency expectations, limits on sessions, client access/ability to travel to sessions, reliance on technology, match between appointment availability and client work schedules, insurance requirements)

II **Group Memberships/Felt Identities**
Note group membership/identities (e.g., interconnected social class, ethnicity, race, gender identities, sexual orientations, etc.), and their impact on relationships.

III **Space, Place, and Time**
Situate families in space, place, and time. This includes socio-relational determinants of health (e.g., living situation, neighborhood, access to nutritional food, access to quality education, employment, and health care, safety, animals/pets, etc.; migration status; family/group legacies; extended family and friends; place of worship; intergenerational patterns; sense of belonging).

IV **Impacts of power on Clinical Issues**
Describe relational power dynamics in social context, including the impact of societal and relational power on problem(s).

V **Safety/Urgent or Immediate Needs**
Record risk assessments and the identification of urgent or immediate needs. Include action taken to ensure safety.

VI **Co-occurring Conditions**
Describe any existing conditions that impact the problem or should otherwise be considered/addressed (e.g., physical health problems, mental health conditions, addiction and/or substance use related issues).

VII **Model-informed Conceptual Description**
Use theoretical framework(s) to conceptualize and describe presenting concerns in ways that can help guide change (e.g., genogram, structural map, map of the problem, interactional pattern, socio-emotional relational dynamics, etc.).

VIII **Shared Description of the Problem**
Describe presenting concerns in a way that reflects shared understanding and language.

IX **Goals**
Develop and record goals. These should be expressed in ways that:

1. Support all family members
2. Resonate with the model(s) being used
3. Are congruent with the language of shared understanding
4. Reflect the expanded lens/new understanding of the problem
5. Ensure they are solvable
6. Encourage equitable relationships

X **Resources/Resilience**
Describe existing assets, values, relationship patterns, attitudes, behaviors, strengths that support goals.

XI **DSM diagnosis (if applicable)**

Figure 4.3 Example of assessment summary.

health and well-being. You address the impact of societal and relational power processes on clinical issues. Your risk assessment and identification of safety concerns, immediate needs, and actions to address them are informed by attention to socio-contextual power processes. You also identify other conditions that may impact the problem or need to be considered, such as other health concerns, addictions, and/or substance use.

Use a theoretical framework(s) to conceptualize and describe the presenting concerns. This gives focus and direction to guide the therapeutic process. As illustrated in the chapters that follow, apply socioculturally attuned principles to case conceptualization through a systemic clinical model(s). Summarize the description of the problem to reflect shared understanding and language between you and the client(s). Goals need to be developed and expressed in ways that:

- Support all family members
- Resonate with the model(s) being used
- Are congruent with the language of shared understanding
- Reflect the expanded lens/new understanding of the problem
- Ensure they are solvable
- Encourage equitable relationships

Identifying resources and sources of resilience, especially relational values and connections that can be built upon, is also important to an assessment summary that sets the stage for third order, often transformative, change.

Writing socioculturally attuned assessment summaries is, in itself, an intervention into individualizing, problem-focused ways of thinking that tend to support social inequities and inhibit relationality. Use clear language that is respectful and attuned to the life stages, societal contexts, and unique situations the clients experience. Avoid pathologizing terms. The writing process will help crystallize the expanded lens through which you and the clients now see the clinical issues they must navigate and how therapy will help. Write in ways that clients, if reading it, will find supportive and which inspire optimism and possibility for you, the therapist, as well as your clients.

Summary: Assessment as Foundation for Third Order Change

Each of the six socioculturally attuned practices (ANVIET) described in Chapter 2 support an assessment process through which you form relationships, develop shared understandings, expand the lens, and envision change (see Figure 4.1). From the beginning, you seek to **attune** to the client's sociocultural context. Awareness of your sociocultural location and the sociopolitical context of therapy helps you recognize and **name** what is unjust or minimized in the dominant culture and responsibly position the therapy to represent relational and equitable **values.** Guided by these values, the questions you ask and your responses to clients begin to **intervene** in societal power processes by expanding the lens and making power and sociocultural contexts visible. You set the stage for third order change by inviting clients to **envision** possibilities beyond what is usually taken for granted in society. As you create a shared understanding of the goals of therapy, you begin to **transform** client health and well-being and the options available to them.

Reflexive Questions

- How are you conceptualizing assessment from a third order lens? How is it similar or different from how clinical assessment is conducted in other approaches?
- How does this stance or approach align with your preferred model of therapy?

- How does using this approach to assessment align or contrast with the expectations of the place where you are practicing?
- When you think about your own sociorelational determinants of health, what does it say about your positions of disadvantage, vulnerability, and privilege? What aspects of these are visible or invisible to others, especially your clients or colleagues?

References

Ahern, J. (2020). Minimum wage policy protects against suicide in the USA. *Epidemiol Community Health*, *74*(11), 873–874.

American Psychiatric Association. (2022). *American Psychiatric Association Diagnostic and Statistical Manual of Mental Disorders* (DSM-5-TR).

Agbai, C. O. (2023). Wealth begins at home: The housing benefits of the 1944 GI bill and the making of the racial wealth gap in homeownership and home value. *SocArXiv Preprint*.

Alegría, M, NeMoyer, A., Falgas, I, Wang, Y. & Alvarez, K (2018). Social determinants of mental health: Where we are and where we need to go. *Current Psychiatric Reports, 20*(1), 1–20.

Amankwaa, L. C. (2003). Postpartum depression among African-American women. *Issues in Mental Health Nursing*, *24*, 297–316.

Bhutta, N., Chang, A. C., Dettling, L.J., & Hsu., J. W. (2020). Disparities in wealth by race and ethnicity in the 2019 Survey of Consumer Finances. FEDS Notes. Washington: Board of Governors of the Federal Reserve System, September 28, 2020, https://doi.org/10.17016/2380-7172.2797.

Brock, R. L., Calkins, F. C., Hamburger, E. R., Kumar, S. A., Laifer, L. M., Phillips, E., & Ramsdell, E. L. (2023). Learning from adversity: What the COVID-19 pandemic can teach us about family resiliency. *Family Process*, *62*(4), 1574–1591.

Butler, D. S. & Moseley, G. L. (2013). *Explain Pain* (2nd ed.). Noigroup publications.

Combs, C. (2022). Recovery from White conditioning: Building anitracist practice and community. In K. V. Hardy (Ed.), *The enduring, invisible, and ubiquitous centrality of whiteness* (pp. 509–527). Norton.

Dannefer, D. (2003). Cumulative advantage/disadvantage and the life course: Cross-fertilizing age and social science theory. *The Journals of Gerontology Series B: Psychological Sciences and Social Sciences*, *58*(6), 327–337.

DiPrete, T. A. & Eirich, G. M. (2006). Cumulative advantage as a mechanism for inequality: A review of theoretical and empirical developments. *Annu. Rev. Sociol.*, *32*, 271–297.

Fitzpatrick, K. & LaGory, M. (2000). *Unhealthy places: The ecology of risk in the urban landscape*. Routledge.

Fulginiti, A., Goldbach, J., Mamey, M., Rusow, J., Srivastava, A., Rhoades, H., Schrager, S., Bond, D., & Marshal, M. (2020). Integrating minority stress theory and the interpersonal theory of suicide among sexual minority youth who engage crisis services. *Suicide and Life Threatening Behavior*, *50*(3), 601–616.

Fricker, M. (2007). *Epistemic injustice: Power and the ethics of knowing*. Oxford University Press.

Fürst, M. (2024). Closing the conceptual gap in epistemic injustice. *The Philosophical Quarterly*, *74*(1), 229–250.

Garcia, M., Košutić, I., & McDowell, T. (2015). Peace on earth/war at home: The role of emotion regulation in social justice work. *Journal of Feminist Family Therapy*, *27*(1), 1–20.

Garcia, M. & McDowell, T. (2010). Mapping social capital: A critical contextual approach for working with low-status families. *Journal of Marital and Family Therapy*, *36*(1), 96–107.

Glebova, T. & Knudson-Martin, C. (2023). Clinical work with sociocultural trauma. In T. Glebova & C. Knudson-Martin (Eds.) *Sociocultural trauma and relational well-being in the Eastern European context* (pp. 103–115). AFTA SpringerBriefs in Family Therapy.

Hardy, K. V. (2024). Some subtleties of whiteness in the workplace: Steps for shifting the paradigm. *Family Process*, 00, 1–14.

Hardy, K. V. (2022). The centrality of whiteness. In K. V. Hardy (Ed.), *The enduring, invisible, and ubiquitous centrality of whiteness* (pp. 3–33). Norton.

Hardy, K. V. & Laszloffy, T. A. (1995). The cultural genogram: Key to training culturally competent family therapists. *Journal of Marital and Family Therapy*, *21*(3), 227–237.

Harrell, J., Hall, S., & Taliaferro, J (2003). Physiological responses to racism and discrimination: An assessment of the evidence. *American Journal of Public Health*, *17*(1), 76–89.

Hartwell, E. E. & Edwards, L. L. (2026). *Queer-contextualized family therapy: Toward radically inclusive theory and practice*. Routledge.

Johnstone, M. (2026). Centering social justice in mental health practice: Epistemic justice and social work practice. *Research on Social Work Practice*, *31*(6), 634–643.

Jones, C. P. (2000). Levels of racism: A theoretic framework and a gardener's tale. *American Journal of Public Health*, *90*(8), 1212–1215.

Karam, E. A. & Blow, A. J. (2020). Common factors underlying systemic family therapy. In K. S. Wampler, R. B. Miller, & R. B. Seedall (Eds.). *The handbook of systemic family therapy: The profession of systemic family therapy* (pp. 147–169). Wiley Blackwell.

Knudson-Martin, C. (2025). *The socio-emotional relationship workbook for couples: Closing the gap between the relationship you want and the relationship you have*. Routledge.

Knudson-Martin, C. (2024). *A step-by-step guide to socio-emotional relationship therapy: A socially responsible approach to clinical practice*. Routledge.

Knudson-Martin, C., & Kim, L. (2023). Socioculturally attuned couple therapy. In J. L. Lebow and D. K. Snyder (Eds.). *Clinical handbook of couple therapy*, (6th ed., pp. 267–291). Guilford.

Knudson-Martin, C., Kim, L., Gibbs, E., & Harmon, R. (2021). Sociocultural attunement to vulnerability in couple therapy: Fulcrum for changing power processes. *Family Process*, *60*, 1152–1169.

Knudson-Martin, C. & Mahoney, A. (2005). Moving beyond gender: Processes that create relationship equality. *Journal of Marital and Family Therapy*, *31*, 235–246.

Kosutic, I., Garcia, M., Graves, T., Barnett, F., Hall, J., Haley, E., Rock, J., Bathon, A., & Kaiser, B. (2009). The critical genogram: A tool for promoting critical consciousness. *Journal of Feminist Family Therapy*, *21*, 151–176.

Larner, G. (2022). Integrative dialogues in family therapy. *Australian and New Zealand Journal of Family Therapy*, *43*(1), 54–69.

Lini, C. & Bertrando, P. (2022). Positional responsibility in systemic-dialogical therapy. *Journal of Family Therapy*, *44*, 339–350.

McCartney, G., Popham, F., McMaster, R., & Cumbers, A. (2019). Defining health and health inequalities. *Public health*, *172*, 22–30.

McDowell, T. (2015). *Applying critical social theories to family therapy practice*. AFTA SpringerBriefs in Family Therapy. Springer.

McDowell, T., Knudson-Martin, C., & Bermúdez, M. (2019). Toward third order thinking in family therapy: Addressing social justice across family therapy practice. *Family Process*, *58*, 9–22.

Merton, R. K. (1968). The Matthew effect in science: The reward and communication system of science. *Science*, *159*, 56–63.

Murphy, M. J. & Hecker, L. L. (2020). Ethical and legal issues unique to systemic family therapy. In K. S. Wampler, R. B. Miller, & R. B. Seedall (Eds.). *Handbook of systemic family therapy* (Vol. 1, pp. 533–554). John Wiley & Sons.

Nadasen, P. (2023). *Care: The highest stage of capitalism*. Haymarket Books.

National Park Service (n.d.) The Homestead Act of 1862. https://www.nps.gov/home/learn/historyculture/abouthomesteadactlaw.htm

Norman-Major, K. (2018). Thinking outside the box: Using multisector approaches to address the wicked problem of homelessness among LGBTQ youth. *Public Integrity*, *20*, 546–557.

Patel, V., Burns, J., Dhingra, M., Tarver, L. Kohrt, B., & Lund, C. (2018). Income inequality and depression: a systematic review and meta-analysis of the association and a scoping review of mechanisms. *World Psychiatry*, *17*(1), 76–89.

Rhodes, P. (2021). Matter matters: Assembling life after Post-Milan. *Australian and New Zealand Journal of Family Therapy 42*, 351–360.

Roberts, K. M. & Trejo, A. N. (2022). Provider, heal thy system: An Examination of institutionally racist healthcare regulatory practices and structures. *Contemporary Family Therapy*, *44*(1), 4–15.

Robins, L. B., Johnson, K. F., Duyile, B., Gantt-Howrey, A., Dockery, N., Robins, S. D., & Wheeler, N. (2023). Family counselors addressing social determinants of mental health in underserved communities. *The Family Journal*, *31*(2), 213–221.

Smoliak, O., Al-Ali, K., LeCouteur, A., Tseliou, E., Rice, C., LaMarre, A., … & Henshaw, S. (2023). The third shift: Addressing emotion work in couple therapy. *Family process*, *62*(3), 1006–1023.

Soja, E. (2010). *Seeking spatial justice*. University of Minnesota Press.

St. George, S. & Wulff, D. (2014). Braiding socio-cultural interpersonal patterns into therapy. In K. Tomm, S. St. George, D. Wulff, & T. Strong (Eds.). *Patterns in interpersonal interactions: Inviting relational understandings for therapeutic change* (pp. 124–142). Routledge.

Sutherland, O., Couture, S., Gaete Silva, J., Strong, T., Lamarre, A., & Hardt, L. (2016). Social justice oriented diagnostic discussions: A discursive perspective. *Journal of Feminist Family Therapy*, *28*(2-3), 76–99.

US Department of Health and Human Services. (August, 2020). *Healthy People 2030.* https://health.gov/healthypeople
Van Der Merwe, H. & Wetherell, M. (2020). The emotional psychologist: A qualitative investigation of norms, dilemmas, and contradictions in accounts of practice. *Journal of Community & Applied Social Psychology*, *30*(2), 227–245.
Waite, R. & Nardi, D. A. (2024). A call for health justice: Striving toward health equity at a community health center. *Family Process*.
Walsh, F. (2016). Applying a family resilience framework in training, practice, and research: Mastering the art of the possible. *Family process*, *55*(4), 616–632.
Watson, M., Bacigalupe, G., Daneshpour, M., Han, W. & Parra-Cardona, R. (2020). Covid-19 interconnectedness: Health inequality, the climate crisis, and collective trauma. *Family Process*, *59*, 832–846.
Wetzel, N. A. (2024). Embracing the other: Revisiting the epistemological foundations of family systems therapy. *Family process*, *63*(1), 17–33.

5 Socioculturally Attuned Structural Family Therapy

The development of structural family therapy (SFT) by Salvador Minuchin and colleagues (1967, 1974; Reiter, 2018a) gave the field a way to map the organization of families and concisely describe their dynamics. This approach enabled practitioners to think about families as a unit and make sense of complex interactions. In SFT, families are understood as open systems that respond and adjust to the outside world (Colapinto, 2019). Presenting problems reflect and maintain family structures. SFT focuses on interactional patterns (Fishman, 2022) and the relative power of family members to influence these patterns. Structural family therapists recognize the inherent strength of families to positively adapt to changing circumstances. Therapeutic goals include restructuring interactions in ways that support the development of the family system and the well-being of all members. Structural family therapy was an early model that has continued to be developed (e.g., Fishman, 2022) and applied globally well into the 21st century to address a variety of issues (Dehghani & Bernards, 2021; Lo & Ma, 2022; McAdams, et Al., 2016; Pender Baum & Pender, 2023).

↞→

Socioculturally attuned structural family therapy invites families to consider third order change in how they organize their lives in relationship to broader societal contexts.

↞→

In this chapter, we highlight enduring concepts in SFT and demonstrate a link between family and societal structures. We illustrate how therapists can integrate principles of sociocultural attunement in assessing family problems and offer practice guidelines that can lead to third order change.

Primary Enduring Structural Family Therapy Concepts

Following are six concepts core to practicing SFT. The first three focus on how families are organized, including repetitive patterns of interaction, family and individual development, and family structure and hierarchy. The other three focus on interventions, including the importance of joining, challenging assumptions, and restructuring.

Patterns of Interaction

One of Minuchin's (1967, 1974) earliest discoveries was that families engage in repetitive patterns. Patterns are essential to daily functioning and living predictable lives. When patterns become rigid, however, they constrict the range of possible behaviors. Problems occur when families get caught

DOI: 10.4324/9781003493426-5

in patterns of interaction that they find unsatisfactory yet difficult to alter. Patterns interlock and repeat across situations. Even the most routine interactional patterns can reflect and reinforce broader problematic relational dynamics.

Think about a simple morning routine, (e.g., getting up, managing breakfast, getting ready for school, and going to work). Consider John, Emanuel, and their 16-year-old son, Max. John came from a White, upper-middle-class family. Emanuel's Mexican American family considered themselves working class. Max was adopted and is multiracial. John and Emmanuel share a business in which John takes the lead and serves as the "face" of the business while Emanuel manages the finances and personnel. John also attempts to take the lead at home, resulting in the couple arguing over tasks and struggling to negotiate differences. Now let's go back to the simple routine of getting up and getting ready for the day. Emanuel is the first one awake. He makes coffee and prepares breakfast for Max and John. When John gets up, he is anxious to get to work and calls out to Max to wake up. Max delays his response until John opens his door and yells "Get up now!" Max slowly gets ready for school and avoids eye contact with John when he sits down to eat. No one talks until John leaves for work. Once alone, Emanuel and Max enjoy a relaxed and playful conversation as Emanuel takes Max to school. Similar patterns of interaction occur across situations, leading the family to define Emanuel and Max's relationship as "close" and Max as "rebellious."

These repetitive, observable patterns of interaction are the basic unit of analysis for describing family structure (Fishman, 2022). Through observing repeated sequences of behavior among multiple family members, structural family therapists hypothesize about how a family is organized; who is in charge, who is aligned with whom, and the nature of individual, subsystem, and family boundaries. Exploring family members' thoughts and feelings that both inform and result from patterns of behavior provides information about family rules and roles as well as the impact of family structure on the well-being of each individual.

Family Development

Structural family therapists assume families evolve through stages of development. Each stage creates new demands and opportunities as family members strive to accommodate each other (Colapinto, 2018). This sometimes includes changes in members' multiple relational identities, e.g., parent, step-parent, spouse, oldest child, sibling, grandparent (Reiter, 2018b). The family must continuously accommodate the changing needs of its members as each grows and ages. The family must also accommodate changes in circumstances (e.g., economic shifts, illnesses, political climates, moves) through time (Minuchin & Nichols, 1993). A well-functioning family promotes and supports the development of all family members and can adapt to necessary changes. Family relationships or structures that limit the growth and development of children or adults are considered out of balance or problematic (Singer, 2024).

Structural family therapists do not take it upon themselves to determine ideal family structures per se, however, the link between how a family is organized and the development of its members guides decision-making relative to restructuring. Consider a family in which there were two White, heterosexual parents—Jim and Lacey. They had three adolescent children. The oldest was a 17-year-old girl, Laura. The second was a 15-year-old boy, Jimmy, and the third was a 13-year-old boy, Tim. Lacey worked as an administrative assistant to put Jim through medical school before staying home to care for their three children. She went back to work managing Jim's practice when all three kids began middle school. Once both parents worked full time, they relied heavily on Laura to cook meals and watch after Jimmy and Tim. Jim and Lacey bought Laura a car with the stipulation that she pick up her younger brothers and get them to sports events after school. The couple entered therapy when Lacey discovered Jim had an affair with a woman who worked at the hospital.

It was important to the family for Lacey to spend her time raising the children. She appreciated an upper-middle-class lifestyle and the status associated with being married to a physician. She was devastated by the affair, feeling vulnerable and angry. Jim allayed her concern with a promise that the affair meant nothing and would not happen again. This family structure privileged the developmental needs of the males, expecting females to play supportive roles. Jim's career was primary, and while the couple worked together toward his success, it was he who has been able to fulfill his developmental potential in a more powerful role. Lacey's development had been routinely compromised in favor of the development of all others in the family. Jim's affair highlighted the unfairness of the relationship, leaving Lacey increasingly disillusioned and resentful of the inequity between them. During therapy, it became clear that Laura was being ushered into a similar inequitable arrangement as a young woman. In her role as a sister, she was expected to place the needs of her brothers before her own, mirroring her mother's role as a wife who is expected to sacrifice her adult development for the sake of her husband's.

Family Structure and Hierarchy

The use of structure as a metaphor for describing this observable organization reflects Minuchin's early training as a physician who understood the human body as a system with an internal structure (Minuchin & Nichols, 1993). The observable interactional patterns in families that are referenced as a family's structure include who is close with whom (alliances), who sides with each other (coalitions), who is grouped together based on role and common interests, and age (subsystems), who has access to whom and what type of access (boundaries) and who has more or less influence over others (hierarchy).

Family maps are often used to describe, communicate, and track the way a family is organized. The map typically starts by drawing circles or using names, initials, or roles (e.g., mom) to indicate how close family members are to each other and their relative influence or power. For example, in the case described above, Jim and Lacey were both in a parental or executive subsystem and a spousal subsystem, however, they were not equal in power in either of these. A therapist might start the map addressing the structure of the spousal subsystem when Jim was having the affair and after the affair was over (see Figure 5.1).

Both maps acknowledge that Jim had more power in the relationship. The map on the left shows an open boundary between Jim and the woman at work with whom he had an affair. The map on the right of Figure 5.1 shows a solid line of disconnection once the affair ended. The individual boundary between Jim and Lacey shows more distance between them when Jim was having the affair. Now the therapist might add the rest of the family (see Figure 5.2).

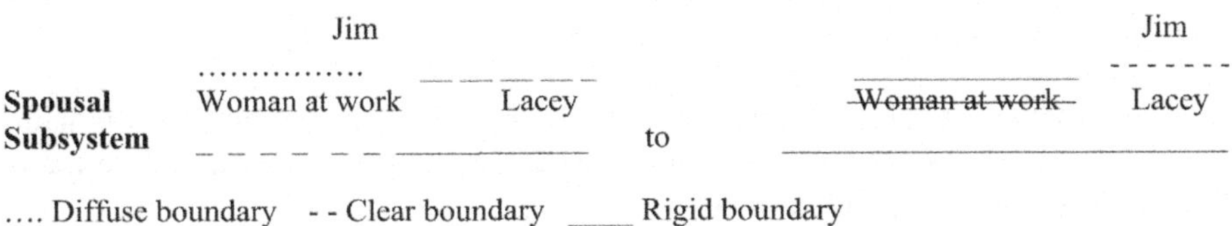

Figure 5.1 Boundaries within spousal subsystem when an affair is present.

Spousal Subsystem		Jim Lacey	
Parental Subsystem		Jim Lacey	
Sibling Subsystem	Laura	Jimmy	Tim

Figure 5.2 Entire family map including subsystems and how power influences subsystems.

The map in Figure 5.2 describes the family in the following way. Jim has more power than his wife/co-parent. The solid line beneath the subsystem demonstrates that Jim and Lacey kept their adult relationship as partners private and didn't share their relationship problems with their children. As parents, they each had different boundaries with the children. Lacey was more accessible to them than Jim, who maintained more distance. At this point, what we know about the family leaves some questions regarding the power dynamics among siblings. At first glance, it would seem that Laura, as the oldest child and the one who is responsible for helping her parents with the younger two kids, would be above her brothers in the hierarchy. The therapist would need to investigate further by asking to what extent her brothers listen to her, if her parents back her up, if she is in more of a supportive than authoritative role, and so on.

The therapist might have noticed that Mom and Laura had a close connection as the two females in the family. This might be considered an alliance between Mom and Laura. Upon further investigation, we might discover that Lacey and Laura frequently complained to each other about Jim's authority and undermined him when they thought he was being unreasonable. This would be described as a coalition between them against the father.

Joining

Structural family therapists recognize the necessity of joining with all family members in order to both challenge them and to invite them to consider alternatives. The family will only follow a therapist's directives and agree to be challenged if members feel connected to the therapist (Reiter, 2018b). Joining is an ongoing process throughout therapy, a relational commitment from start to finish.

↔

According to Minuchin, "Joining has nothing to do with pretending to be what you are not. It means tuning in to people and responding to the way they move you." (Minuchin & Nichols, 1993, p. 42)

↔

Joining requires the therapist to treat each family as unique. According to Minuchin, et al. (2014), joining is "a mindset constructed out of respect, empathy, curiosity, and commitment to healing" (p. 4). This can be difficult at times.

Think about working with a family in which a parent is emotionally and verbally abusive to a teenage child. It may be quite easy for many of us to identify and join with the child, but more difficult to genuinely join with the parent. The therapist must find a way to be equally respectful, empathetic, curious, and committed to the well-being of all family members in order to help them restructure the system. Structural family therapists join with families by using the family's language and reflecting the family's relational style (mimesis). They glean information about the family by becoming part of the system without getting caught in the system. Let's consider a family therapist getting caught in the system with Jim and Lacey's family described above.

Jim: It is tough working every day to support this family. Between office hours, hospital rotations, and being on call, I put in 70 hours a week! I don't think they really appreciate how hard I work to get everything this family needs and wants!

Lacey: Of course we do. This is not about how hard you work! How hard any of us work.

Jim: How hard ANY of us work? I'm the one out there busting my back…

Therapist: Clearly you work hard, Jim, but I think what Lacey is saying…

Jim (interrupts therapist): You know, Lacey, for once I would just like to see you…

[Therapist falls silent as she begins thinking how unfair Jim is being]

It is likely in the scenario above that while the therapist was trying to connect with all family members and ensure everyone felt understood, she got caught in the pattern of Jim dominating conversations and setting the terms by which discussions occur. The therapist was drawn into what was likely Lacey's experience of being overridden by Jim. In this way, the therapeutic system became isomorphic or parallel to the family system.

Challenging Assumptions

When families begin therapy they typically "know" what the problem is and often have an idea of what (and who) needs to change. They have tried a number of solutions based on their definition and understanding of the problem (Jackson & Landers, 2020). If the attempted solution would have worked, the family would most likely not seek help. Most clients expect help to come in the form of alternative solutions, not in alternative definitions of the problem. According to Reiter (2018b, p. 48) "Therapy is about increasing possibilities. The more families are certain the fewer possibilities are available."

Minuchin et al. (2014) asserted that the family's certainty in their definition of the problem works against change. It is up to the therapist to engage the family in co-constructing new ways of viewing the problem that will lead to different types of solutions. A mantra in SFT is "make sure you are solving the right problem." Too often, therapists accept the family's definition of the problem and get caught in attempting common sense and/or linear solutions. Below is an excerpt from a session with John, Emanuel, and Max in which the therapist gets caught in content, inadvertently increasing the certainty family members have of the problem.

John: The problem is that Max is having trouble growing up and taking responsibility.

Emanuel: He is a teenager! Your problem is you want everyone to be just like you!

John: I thought we agreed to focus on Max.

Max: (sighs and rolls his eyes)

Therapist: Lots of families worry about teenagers learning to take responsibility, and it is normal for teens to rebel a little. In fact, it is healthy!

While the therapist in this interaction attempted to normalize and smooth over the conflict, they were paying more attention to content (e.g., a teenager taking responsibility) than process (e.g., parents not acting as a team).

Structural family therapists introduce alternatives in how families think about problems. When problems are viewed differently, families are often able to see new possibilities and solutions. As mentioned above, the certainty of the problem, resulting in sets of solutions, is often the crux of how families get stuck. While early structural family therapists were more likely to determine a new framework and use their expert stance to get the family to accept a different reality (i.e., reframe), many contemporary therapists (Minuchin et al., 2014) see the process as one of co-construction. Let's continue with John, Emanuel, and Max to see how the therapist might have invited a new understanding of the problem.

Emanuel:	Yes, we understand that teenagers often rebel but Max is a good kid. John just expects too much.
John:	(rolls his eyes and looks away)
Max:	This is stupid!
Therapist:	As fathers, you expect different things from your son?
John:	I expect Max to act his age and take responsibility.
Emanuel:	He does. Max is doing great in school.
Therapist:	Max, it seems like your dads have different ways of looking at things. What's it like for you when they argue about you?
Max:	What do you think? I hate it!
Therapist:	John and Emanuel, how are you at being a team in other parts of your lives besides parenting? Your business? Your relationship?

Here the therapist moved the focus from Max to the parents working together. The therapist was trying out a new way to view the problem, inviting the family to see things differently. This effectively moved Max out of the role of being the problem. As long as there is a person designated by the family as "the problem," it is difficult to move out of linear, individual, common sense solutions in favor of relational, contextual change. In the example offered above, the therapist might have gotten caught in the view that Max was the problem because he was being rebellious, or that John was the problem because he was controlling, or that Emanuel was the problem because he failed to back up his co-parent. Accepting Max as the identified problem would have invited the therapist to get stuck where the family was stuck.

Challenging assumptions includes exploring family rules and expectations relative to family roles. The nature of assumptions is that they guide thinking, feeling, and interacting, often without being overtly discussed or intentionally considered. They operate without inspection, limiting alternatives. In the example above, John and Emanuel are operating from ideas they each have about how to be a good parent, who, if anyone, should be in the lead, what teenagers need from parents, what Max's intentions are, and so on. The therapist would guide enactments in which these assumptions could be identified, made overt, and intentionally altered or agreed upon. Following is an example of how a therapist might have challenged assumptions when working with Jim and Lacey in a couple session:

Therapist:	Jim and Lacey, would you tell each other what you hoped your relationship would be like—you know, when you first decided to marry? Lacey, can you start? Jim, while Lacey is talking will you please do your best to really listen? Then you will have a turn and it will be Lacey's turn to listen.

Lacey: I guess I thought we were going to be in this together. You know, me and you the whole way.

Jim: We are! We work together, live together…we're together 24-7! What more do you want?

Therapist: I want to make sure each of you understands what the other expects without interrupting each other. You have different ideas about what it means to be together through life. Lacey, can you say more about what you meant when you said "I thought we were going to be in this together?"

The therapist would continue to explore assumptions each holds about gender and power, paid versus family work, time together in contrast to making decisions together, the meaning of intimacy, and so on. The therapist would also explore family roles: What does each expect of a father, mother, husband, wife? Where were these ideas about roles formed? In what ways are expectations around family roles helpful or not helpful to the family as a whole; to each individual?

Restructuring

Enactments are a cornerstone intervention in SFT. A significant part of each session includes asking family members to talk directly to each other while the therapist pays attention to and helps shape interaction. Talking directly to each other in therapy offers families a new experience of purposefully rather than spontaneously interacting (Minuchin et al., 2014). The therapist can notice how they interact, watching for patterns that are problematic as well as those that work well. Enactments allow therapists to help families modify their interactions, set clear boundaries, better understand each other, and connect with each other emotionally. At first, the therapist is likely to want to observe even when communication escalates, is derailed by other family members, and/or reaches a stalemate. This provides important firsthand information about family dynamics. The therapist often comments on the interaction to help families take a meta-perspective of their relationships, i.e., learn to "talk about how they talk."

Therapists do more than observe and learn about family patterns through enactments. They interrupt, pause for interpretation, ask for emotional expression, and coach communication. They help distant family members come closer emotionally, help establish clear boundaries, and encourage members of subsystems to work together in part by using enactments. Butler and Gardner (2007) suggested five stages of enactments depending on the couple or family's ability to successfully talk directly with each other. When conflict is high and direct communication seems to do more harm than good, they suggest asking family members to talk through the therapist. When family members are able to communicate directly and the communication leads to solving problems, the therapist becomes less of a "go between," interrupts less often, and coaches interactions less. Below is an example of an enactment using the example above of John, Emanuel, and Max a little later in therapy.

Therapist: John and Emanuel, I am going to ask the two of you to talk directly about your vision of parenting together. What kind of team are you hoping to be? John, will you turn your chair to face Emanuel and Emanuel, will you start the conversation?

Emanuel: John, I want us to work together to be more understanding of Max.

John: I think we are understanding. Maybe too understanding.

Max: This is hopeless!

Therapist: For now, Max, I am going to ask you to let your dads talk. It can be tempting to interrupt them to help, but let's see how they do.

Max: I wasn't trying to help. It just drives me crazy when they do this.

Therapist: (turns away from Max and back to parents) Ok John, can you tell Emanuel what being a team looks like to you?
John: I think we should set rules and back each other up.
Emanuel: Yes, but you are setting the rules and then expecting me to follow them just like Max.
Therapist: So are you both saying that you want to set rules together and back each other up, but you want to really agree? Is that right?
Emanuel: (looking at therapist) Yes, but it can't all be on John's terms.
Therapist: Emanuel, can you look directly at John and say that to him rather than to me?
Emanuel: (looking at John). It can't all be on your terms.
Therapist: Emanuel, you also said earlier that you wanted the two of you to be more understanding of Max. Can you tell John directly what you mean?

The therapist in this scenario was unbalancing the system by offering Emanuel support in making his perspective heard by John. This temporarily disrupted the power dynamic in which John has more voice in the family. The therapist also unbalanced the system by ensuring the couple's interaction was not detoured through Max. Unbalancing is an important concept in SFT. It is assumed that the therapist has the necessary influence or power in the therapeutic system to direct interactions and can "lend" power to family members. Interrupting typical dynamics that stabilize conflict, such as detouring, is also a way to unbalance the system, opening possibilities for alternative interactions and solutions. Another typical unbalancing technique is to raise the intensity. Therapists can raise intensity in a number of ways including pressing the family to continue interactions at the point in which they typically stop and slowing down interactions to explore and express deep emotions.

Structural family therapists consider boundaries across all interventions. In the example above, the therapist worked on helping the family set a clear boundary between the parental and child subsystems by not allowing Max to interrupt his parents or help them out of their conflict. The therapist would not always have Max in the room, respecting the separation between spousal/parental and child/sibling subsystems. In the conversation above, Max being there gave the therapist the opportunity to block him from becoming part of the parental subsystem. In line with honoring the executive (parental and spousal) subsystem and the family's hierarchy, more conversations about fathering and about the couple's relationship would likely need to occur without Max present. Max, as a teenager, would also likely need to meet with the therapist alone from time to time to discuss his experience and prepare for how to talk to his parents about his needs.

Integrating Principles of Sociocultural Attunement

SFT can be practiced in ways that focus only on the interior of the family, with limited attention to sociocultural context. According to Williams et al. (2016),

> from the black feminist perspective, hierarchies exist beyond the family system that place individuals at a disadvantage. These include gender, race, political standing, and class. Structural Family Therapy fails to directly and explicitly address the overarching societal hierarchies that pressure family systems with prescribed roles and norms. (p. 42)

In this section, we integrate principles of sociocultural attunement into SFT by exploring connections between societal systems and family systems; between societal rules and structures and family rules and structures. This includes paying attention to how interactional patterns and power dynamics are reproduced across levels and settings in complex social systems.

Societal Context and Structure

•←→•

Socioculturally attuned structural family therapy expands the structural analysis of families to a structural analysis of families within societal structures.

•←→•

Socioculturally attuned SFT assumes that organizational patterns affect and are affected by all levels of interlocking systems, including families, communities, and societies as well as by social locations that intersect these systems (e.g., gender, race, social class, ability, sexual orientation, immigration status). Chappelle and Tadros (2021) offered an example of applying the tenets of SFT to societal contexts in order to better understand African American adolescents who have experienced poverty and trauma. In effect, they expanded the structural framework to understand how broader levels of systems impact the family. This is in keeping with using the metaphor of structure at a societal level to refer to systems of systems at a macro level. Repeated patterns of interaction among groups within and across social contexts, serve to create and maintain social stratification, patterned group relationships, and institutional organization. These systems are hierarchical, and access to influence and resources differ according to one's individual and group position in society.

The work of French philosopher and sociologist Pierre Bourdieu (1977, 1986) offers a bridge between our understanding of family structure and societal structure, family rules in relation to social rules, and the material world in relationship to the social world. Above all, Bourdieu viewed reality as relational, making many of his ideas helpful in linking family systems and social theory. Bourdieu's concepts of habitus, field, capital, and symbolic violence are particularly applicable to practicing socioculturally attuned SFT.

Enduring Patterns Across Contexts

Socioculturally attuned structural family therapists help families challenge limiting social scripts that maintain inequities (Eikers, 2023) to explore patterns of interaction that maximize potential and well-being for all family members. Social structures, like family structures, refer to patterns of interaction. Social and familial structures can be thought of as enduring repetitive interactions that both shape and are shaped by collective meaning-making and social arrangements (Vertovec, 2021). These patterns occur not only across contexts, but over time, contributing to transgenerational familial and social arrangements (Andina & Corvino, 2023).

According to Bourdieu (1986), it is within social space, or habitus, that we learn, internalize, and embody shared ways of thinking and doing, values, and beliefs. Habitus is a concept that expands our thinking beyond dichotomies to consider relationships between dualistic concepts; internal/external, objective/subjective, agency/structure, and personal/social. For example, a family may be concerned that a child is too shy. They attribute the behavior to an intrinsic quality of the child (internal). A family therapist is likely to look at the behaviors the family identifies as shyness, watching for patterns of communication and interaction that help make sense of these behaviors (external). At the same time, a family therapist may attribute the problem of identifying the child as shy (internal to the individual) to family dynamics alone (internal to the family) rather than considering how social dynamics including gender, culture, class, sexual orientation, race, and specific contexts influence behavior and patterns of interaction (external to the individual and family). In effect, family therapists must hold what is commonly described as internal and external in the same space, being most interested in the relationship *between* these conceptual frameworks.

Habitus refers to a combination of history and disposition within time and space (Ripoll, 2024) that shapes our thinking and guides our behavior in relationships. In effect, societal norms and expectations as expressed through social class, culture, and family contexts, together with our unique qualities, create dispositions. Dispositions are lasting but also changeable over time and transferable across settings (Bourdieu, 1986). This includes how we tend to think, feel, and act in various situations or relational fields. Take humor, for example, which is assigned to some people as an individual characteristic, yet relies on and is developed in habitus. Most "funny people" know how to read contexts well enough to predict what those around them might find amusing. In effect, humor is a relational dynamic at the crossroads of habitus and disposition within relational fields.

According to Maton (2014), "Habitus links the social and the individual because the experiences of one's life course may be unique in their particular *contexts* but are shared in terms of the *structure* with others of the same social class, gender, ethnicity, sexuality, occupation, nationality, region and so forth" (p. 52). In other words, while individuals and families are unique, they are also inseparable from the contexts and spaces (Ripoll, 2024) in which they exist. Habitus, or enduring patterned ways of being and doing, include family upbringing, past choices, social class, education, cultural norms, spatial setting, and much more; the sum of what makes us "who we are." This is both structured and structuring. In other words, our social context, history, and social location structure our thinking, attitudes, beliefs, emotions, and actions. At the same time, our patterned participation in society furthers the very structures that influence us. In fact, social structures become embodied through identity-based constructions such as gender, race, social class, ethnicity, and sexual orientation.

Let's consider Jim and Lacey from the example above as a case in point. Lacey embodies her social identity as a cishet (cisgender heterosexual), White, upper-middle-class female in many ways, including the way she thinks about her body and performs her social role. Her relationship to self and others is deeply influenced by her perception of a broader social gaze. She "watches her weight," gets her hair cut at an expensive salon, shops for clothes that enhance her "figure," participates in make-up consultations, and carries a designer purse. Jim does the same. He "keeps in shape" by participating in individual athletics, dresses in business casual sportswear when not at work, keeps his hair trimmed and face clean shaven, and wears designer eyeglasses. Jim's affair at work reassured him that he is still vital and attractive. The same affair leaves Lacey believing she has "lost her looks" (and the "pretty privilege" her looks have afforded her). Both Jim and Lacey inadvertently maintain their White privilege by adhering to the belief, and teaching their children, that race doesn't matter. Their attempts to conform to social expectations inadvertently contribute to social inequity by serving to maintain the status quo.

Group Relational Systems

Relational systems develop as groups differentiate from each other creating semi-autonomous spheres of action that over time become increasingly specialized. Power relations within and among what Bourdieu called "fields" serve to structure and shape patterns of interaction. Bourdieu (1977) used the term "doxa" to refer to the "rules of the game" within a field. These rules are typically not spoken or overt but assumed as if natural and inevitable. The rules limit the actions of agents within the field while benefiting those who know how the game is played. The positions we take in these fields, or relational systems, serve to maintain or disrupt power relationships; to keep the rules and power dynamics the same or change them. Agents in these fields use their positions, or power, to establish and enforce the rules which advantage them/their group. Take for example the highly contested ban on bilingual education in the US state of California. Native English speakers have the advantage in the field of education and professional positions over those for whom Spanish is their dominant language in childhood. This advantage is secured from preschool forward.

Bilingual education threatens this advantage by creating a more equal playing field; a change in the rules that would redistribute power. These contested social practices occur within physical space (Ripoll, 2024), such as the borderlands between Mexico and the US.

Power and Capital

•←→•

Family hierarchy and boundaries are directly reflective and impacted by power dynamics in society.

•←→•

From a structural perspective, power can be seen as connected to capital. According to Bourdieu (1986), economic, social, cultural, and symbolic capital all play a role in determining our degree of social influence and access to resources (Garcia & McDowell, 2010). Economic capital refers to money as well as capital that can be used to secure money without relying on one's own labor (e.g., investment capital). Social capital refers to social networks; relationships that provide opportunities to share resources and/or secure resources (e.g., insider knowledge of a job, reference letters for court, school, or employment). Symbolic capital is earned and unearned prestige (e.g., the title of "doctor," a high status family name, place of birth). These are all closely linked to cultural capital which refers to that which can be used to gain upward mobility (e.g., language and speech patterns, specific looks, dominant culture relational styles). Cultural capital is an important concept relative to power and equity, as those whose cultural practices are centered and dominant have an advantage, and those advantages are passed down transgenerationally (Roaldsnes, 2024). Those with the most influence and greatest resources tend to reproduce their group's advantage by privileging their own cultural practices (Furstenberg (2019). This influence and access creates lateral advantage for those most closely resembling and affiliated with dominant groups and vertical advantage through inheritance.

This social dynamic affects family dynamics. Consider a White family in which parents have transitioned from lower-class childhoods to the middle class by working hard, taking out student loans, adopting middle-class language and relational styles, and making sure they made connections that would provide them with as much advantage as possible. Now that they are stable in the middle class, they expect their children to enjoy and benefit from their work to secure economic and social resources. Let's imagine now that their teenager is spending her time with lower-class friends, not doing homework, and abusing substances. This is likely to be a problem for the family for many reasons, among them her squandering of the family's economic, social, and cultural capital.

Bourdieu's (1986) term *symbolic violence* refers to when social rules or practices (including family rules and practices) that support the superiority of one group (or family member) over another are misunderstood as inevitable. That is, when the superiority of one group over another is viewed as the natural order of things rather than socially constructed. This view is widely accepted and internalized by members of both groups. Bourdieu (1986) offered many examples of this including social class and gender relations. Relative to social class, those in the upper classes are often seen by all classes as smarter, more diligent, and superior to those in lower classes. This creates the illusion that social class largely depends on the character and effort of individuals. Now let's consider this dynamic relative to gender in family structure using Lacey and Jim as a case in point. The idea that Jim's career should come first and that his needs and comfort are more important reflects pervasive symbolic violence in most societies in which men are routinely privileged.

Symbolic violence occurs when constructions of male superiority are internalized by both males and females; when heterosexual relationships are seen as "normal" and homophobia is internalized; when industrialized societies are seen as "advanced"; when those who don't identify as male or female are seen as "other"; when whiteness is centered; and so on. This is not to say that resistance to these constructions doesn't exist or that those who are oppressed routinely don't realize inequity is not the natural order of things. In fact, family members who are marginalized or oppressed are often acutely aware of their experience even when uncertain of the broader social dynamics that inform family power dynamics.

Continuing with our example of Jim and Lacey's family, Laura is likely to feel conflicted; being pleased that her parents bought her a car while feeling slighted by her brothers' needs being prioritized over her own. The therapist would make covert rules overt, in this case bringing to light and challenging symbolic violence. This process would allow Laura and her family to identify the dynamics in which they are caught, make sense of their experience, and have more choices about what to do.

Third Order Change

Socioculturally attuned structural family therapists target third order change by engaging families in ways that raise awareness and question the impact of societal context on presenting problems. For example, a therapist might ask couples to speak directly to each other about what they learned about gender/race/social class/sexual orientation when growing up. This would include messages from parents, extended family, peers, and the media. As clients are coached to talk directly to each other about these influences, the therapist asks probing questions and offers opportunities for reflection that increase collective social awareness in the therapeutic system.

•←→•

The therapist is active and intentional, creating space where assumptions can be inspected—taken apart and disrupted—to reveal multiple perspectives and possibilities.

•←→•

This critical metaperspective is in itself a paradigm shift; a shift in how we think and how we know what we know.

Structural interventions are not limited to families and are often integral to transforming larger systems such as organizations, institutions, and communities. Consider the example William Turner offers in Text Box 5.1 in which he describes a community-level intervention that promoted structural change. In this example, Turner and his colleague were invited to promote racial integration by engaging community members across physical and social barriers to envision change and take steps toward transformation.

Text Box 5.1 William Turner, PhD, LMFT

William Turner serves as Distinguished Professor of Psychology and Family Therapy and Special Counsel to the President at Lipscomb University, Nashville, TN. His teaching and research interests are focused on African American family strengths and the intersections of hope, justice, policy, and faith.

There is a history of civil rights advocacy in Nashville, but the city has remained relatively segregated. Not only had it been segregated, but the government had actually built physical structures as barriers to integration. A new mayor in Nashville was interested in tearing down physical and social barriers and in an effort to do so, began visiting the many local colleges and universities. I happen to have two good friends at my university who are professors of conflict management and are African American attorneys. The three of us approached the mayor about doing something to help deal with social structure differences and barriers. She invited and funded our proposal to have table-talks where we brought people together from different backgrounds to have meaningful conversations for a few hours. The conversations were structured using conflict management rules. There could be no yelling at each other and facilitators at each table guided the conversation using a set of questions. The facilitators could deviate from the questions, but the conversations needed to remain civil. We began doing this in various communities around Nashville with great success.

The mayor then wanted to do something big and bold. Nashville had just built a beautiful new convention center. The mayor suggested having a day in which we invited the community to the convention center where multiple tables would be set up for conversations. We expected 300–400 people, but on the morning of the event, there were over 1000 who showed up from all walks of life—those from the wealthiest sections of Nashville to those who lived in the projects. It was a beautiful thing. We had meaningful talks followed by debriefing. We then developed a list of things we could actually do, and came up with a plan for how we would implement changes in the city.

Practice Guidelines

There are a number of important steps for practicing socioculturally attuned structural family therapy including, 1) revisioning the definition of family; 2) expanding the family map to connect the family to societal structures; 3) identifying societal influences on family power dynamics, rules, and roles; 4) encouraging families to explore and commit to equity-based relationships, and 5) helping families restructure to support developmentally appropriate relational equity.

1. Revisioning the Definition of Family

Socioculturally attuned structural family therapists flexibly and respectfully adopt clients' definitions of family. Minuchin and colleagues recognized that many different family members and important others may work together in parental subsystems to provide guidance and nurturing to youth. The structural approach has also been applied to a variety of family forms (McAdams, et al., 2016), challenging the assumption that adult (i.e., spousal) subsytems necessarily consist of two heterosexual, female/male gendered individuals (Diaz & Vitola, 2026). Socioculturally attuned structural family therapists must continue to challenge early norms and biases to effectively and ethically work with same and different sex, and same and differently gendered, couples as well as families of choice, polyamorous families, and consensually nonmonogamous persons (Diaz & Vitola, 2026; Gebel et al., 2023; Jordan et al., 2017).

2. Connecting Family and Societal Structures

Socioculturally attuned structural family therapists are familiar with the impact of worldview, family history, intergenerational dynamics, and social context on family functioning and the importance of attending to these in therapy. When they join with clients, they are exploring, attending to, and in some ways entering, a family's habitus. They are aware of the need to continually join throughout the process of therapy to ensure a deep understanding of each family's world. Socioculturally attuned structural family therapists map families within societal context, recognizing that family members go in and out of various social fields, which further influences their relationships with each other.

In our example of Jim and Lacey, Jim functioned daily in a medical field in which doctors are highly privileged and assigned significant relational power over patients and other staff. This, in combination with male and class privilege, affected the course of his affair with a nurse in his workplace. Belonging to the medical field provides economic, social, symbolic, and cultural capital that places Jim at an advantage in his relationship with the nurse at work and with Lacey. A socioculturally attuned structural family therapist would include these fields in the family map and understanding of family habitus. She would invite family members to explore how their individual positions in these social contexts affect their relationships, including the rules they live by as a family, as well as the unequal consequences members of the family suffer when they break a family rule.

3. Identifying Societal Influences on Family Power Dynamics

Socioculturally attuned structural family therapists look beyond the overt and covert rules of the family to understand their relationship to "rules" of various fields families inhabit. Consider our example of John and Emanuel who were raised in very different fields or contexts. Emanuel understood the intricacies of relational dynamics within lower-class, Mexican American communities. He knew the rules. When John entered this field, he was somewhat lost about what to do and how to be. Likewise, John grew up in upper-class fields that supported White privilege and dominance of White upper-class values, attitudes, and behaviors. When Emanuel entered John's world, he also didn't know all of the rules. This created complex and problematic dynamics for the couple. Their therapist would need to explore not only broad societal themes related to social class, race, and ethnicity, but also work with the couple to help them identify the "rules of the game" in each field they enter. This would ensure they can work together to navigate very different social situations in ways that they both feel supported as a couple. Rules within fields tend to support existing societal structures (e.g., taboos against talking about race support White privilege; believing those who have more are worth more supports existing class systems). Therapy is a place where these rules can be broken by making them overt, discussing their impact, and establishing greater agency over their influence.

4. Exploring and Committing to Equity-based Relationships

By connecting family to societal structures and identifying societal influences on family power dynamics, socioculturally attuned structural family therapists are poised to explore the impact and cost of relational inequity on individual and family well-being. Family members become increasingly aware of how societal dynamics affect their most intimate relationships as therapists initiate conversations that raise social awareness and expose power dynamics. These conversations include exploring the relational costs of power imbalances.

Back to Jim and Lacey. Jim enjoyed disproportionate power which allowed him to be more influential in setting the emotional climate in the home, meet more of his individual needs, and enjoy being accommodated by the rest of the family. When the costs of this power were carefully explored, it became clear to all (including Jim) that the children were closer to their mother and often resented their father. Jim had lost the respect of his wife and children, and the females in the family were routinely disempowered. This was very likely not what Jim and Lacey hoped for and may be in contrast to their stated values of raising strong children, supporting equal opportunity for their daughter, and Jim's desire to be close and revered by the family.

5. Restructure to Support Developmentally Appropriate Relational Equity

Socioculturally attuned structural family therapists share the assumption that families should be structured in ways that support optimal development for all members. Oppressive relationships and societal structures block equal opportunity for health and well-being, including individual and relational development. Influence and accountability must be balanced. For example, as children gain autonomy and influence, they are expected to become increasingly accountable for their actions and to consider the impact of their decisions on others. Parents may be in charge of most decisions but are expected to make decisions that benefit their children and consider the needs of the group. When one adult overpowers another, when the needs of one become routinely privileged over another, it is likely to create an imbalance that creates and maintains presenting problems. Addressing these imbalances and encouraging structural equity is central, rather than auxiliary, to treatment.

Case Illustration

Let's continue with our example of Emanuel, John, and Max. Emanuel was born in the US to parents who had migrated from Mexico without legal documentation/unauthorized. His early life was spent in the state of Arizona. When Emanuel was four his father was stopped for a traffic violation, was detained, and deported. From the time Emanuel was four until he was twelve, his father was deported to Mexico and returned to Arizona four times. The family finally made the decision that Emanuel and his mother would go to the state of New Mexico to live with his mother's sister. Emanuel's older siblings stayed behind as US citizens with jobs in Arizona. Emanuel rarely saw his father after that time.

John grew up in the state of Texas. His family owned a large, successful business. His father inherited the business from John's grandfather and succession of the business to John as the son and only child was carefully planned and executed. Emanuel and John met in college in New Mexico. After college, they moved back to Texas so John could run his family business. After John's father died, John liquidated the family business to start something new with Emanuel. This was an opportunity for the couple to move to Massachusetts where they would marry and begin the process of Emanuel legally adopting Max. Max was born in Texas. Max's biological father was White and in the military and his mother was Mexican, who was the young daughter of John's family's housekeeper. John's family's influence cleared the way for him to privately adopt Max as an infant.

The couple made the decision to be openly out as a married gay couple when they moved to Massachusetts. The business was put in both of their names and they bought a home together. They were able to openly parent together and developed a supportive community of friends and colleagues. Things went smoothly with John taking the lead in the business and Emanuel taking the lead in parenting until Max became a teenager.

Revisioning the Definition of Family

How we define ourselves and our relational patterns are deeply impacted by our (often unexamined) definition of family and how those around us define family. Many families experience the impact of being in committed relationships that are not defined or endorsed by others as legitimate. Relocating provided a supportive milieu for Emanuel, John, and Max to develop and grow as a family. Ideally, therapists not only affirm clients' definitions of themselves as families, but are able to raise awareness of the impact of social context on family relationships and help families navigate often complex, traditionally indoctrinated, politicized, and changing definitions of family across social and familial contexts.

Connecting Family and Societal Structures

The therapist working with John and Emanuel's family asked questions that raise social awareness in the therapeutic system. As the therapist analyzed the connections between societal and family dynamics, the family developed critical social awareness of the systems in which they were embedded. These conversations provided information that informed the process of mapping the family in societal context, which in turn provided direction for restructuring interventions. Following is an example of therapeutic dialogue between the therapist, Lisa, and the couple, John and Emanuel, that served to raise critical consciousness while assessing family in societal structure.

Lisa identified as a White, middle-class, bisexual, gender queer family therapist who had lived in Boston since childhood. Lisa had personal experience with homophobia, sexism, and cisgenderism. Lisa's own self-of-the-therapist work included critically examining how their interconnected identities provided privilege in some ways (White, middle-class, and living in a progressive city) and marginalization or oppression in others (bisexual, gender fluid). Understanding how societal systems and power dynamics impact their own life helped prepare Lisa to engage in critical consciousness with John, Emanuel, and Max.

Lisa: So John, you mentioned that when you and Emanuel first moved to the family property in Texas the two of you lived as friends. Can you talk more about that decision… how the decision was made?

John: My family is really conservative. By the time I met Emanuel, my parents knew I was gay, but I promised not to tell anyone in our hometown because of the family business.

Lisa: Who was most concerned about someone finding out and what were they worried might happen if others knew?

John: Mostly my dad. He had worked really hard to build the business. I think he assumed we would lose business if the community knew I was gay.

Lisa: What was that like for you and how did you approach Emanuel about your father's wishes?

John: I didn't like it, but my dad always called the shots. I told Emanuel it was something we just had to do if we eventually wanted the family business.

Lisa: Emanuel, can you tell John directly what it was like for you to be told to stay closeted in John's world? To have John and his father make this decision for you?

Emanuel: I felt so uncomfortable with your family anyway, John. They knew I didn't come from money. I'm not White. Plus, my being around seemed to just remind everyone that you are gay. I agreed because I love you, but I never felt like I fit in. I still don't.

John: Well you fit in as far as I am concerned. I wish you just wouldn't worry about my family. We left Texas, started a new life, sold the family business….

Lisa: So it sounds like the two of you are trying to talk about your differences in social class and race and how racism and classism have affected your relationship.

Emanuel: It is hard for us to talk about, but it has a big effect on us.

John: Really? I think we have done pretty well to overcome those kinds of prejudices.

Lisa: You have overcome a lot just to be a couple. At the same time, it makes sense to me that you, Emanuel, would notice the effects more. John, I know I am usually most unaware of the impact of my own privileges. This is much bigger than the two of you, but can we start by giving you some time, Emanuel, to really talk to you, John, about your experience?

This line of questioning eventually led John and Emanuel to better **attune** to each other and how their relationship was affected by broader societal structures. Increased social awareness prepared them to depersonalize differences and begin to work together to support each other and their son within an unjust society.

Identifying Societal Influences on Family Power Dynamics

By talking openly about racism, classism, patriarchy, and homophobia, Emanuel and John were better able to understand the dynamics in their own family. John tended to take the lead in major decisions, to be more demanding of Max, and to dismiss Emanuel's experience. Many therapists would connect this pattern to intergenerational dynamics and the socialization of males, but a socioculturally attuned structural family therapist would also identify this pattern as an inheritance of White, male, upper-class privilege. The process of raising critical consciousness through dialog and reflection would guide action toward liberatory change (Freire, 1970/2000, Korin, 1994). Following, Lisa **names** the inequities stemming from families of origin and John and Emanuel's social locations in the broader society.

Lisa: John, you mentioned that your dad made all the big decisions in your family. He even made the decision for you and Emanuel to live closeted in Texas. How do you make sense of this?

John: He was just the head of the household. I think men back then ran everything.

Lisa: Do you remember what that was like for you and your mom?

John: I hated it. He was always on me. I think my mom just checked out.

Lisa: Always on you?

John: He expected a lot. He put me in charge of running a whole section of the business when I was 15! If I complained he would tell me to "be a man." I thought he was going to have a heart attack when I told him I was gay!

Lisa: So being gay was not being a man?

John: I guess not.

Lisa: Working hard, not complaining, excelling at your job…what else does being a man mean? Being in charge of your family?

John: Yeah. He was just trying to help me grow up and be successful.

Lisa: Passing the baton? So you could be successful and in charge of your own family?

John: When you put it that way…

Lisa: How about you, Emanuel? What did your family pass down to you about being a man? Being in a family?

Emanuel: For us, family was everything. I learned you do what you have to for the family. My dad had to keep his head down…keep a low profile when he was in the states. My mom was strong and independent when he was gone but did whatever he said when he was around. It was confusing. I guess I sort of resented him.

Lisa: So even though your fathers both learned men should be in charge of the family, they had real differences in their power and privilege in the world. How do the differences in what you learned and the differences in race and social class impact the power dynamic in your relationship with each other? What messages do these dynamics send to Max?

A socioculturally attuned structural family map might look something like Figure 5.3.

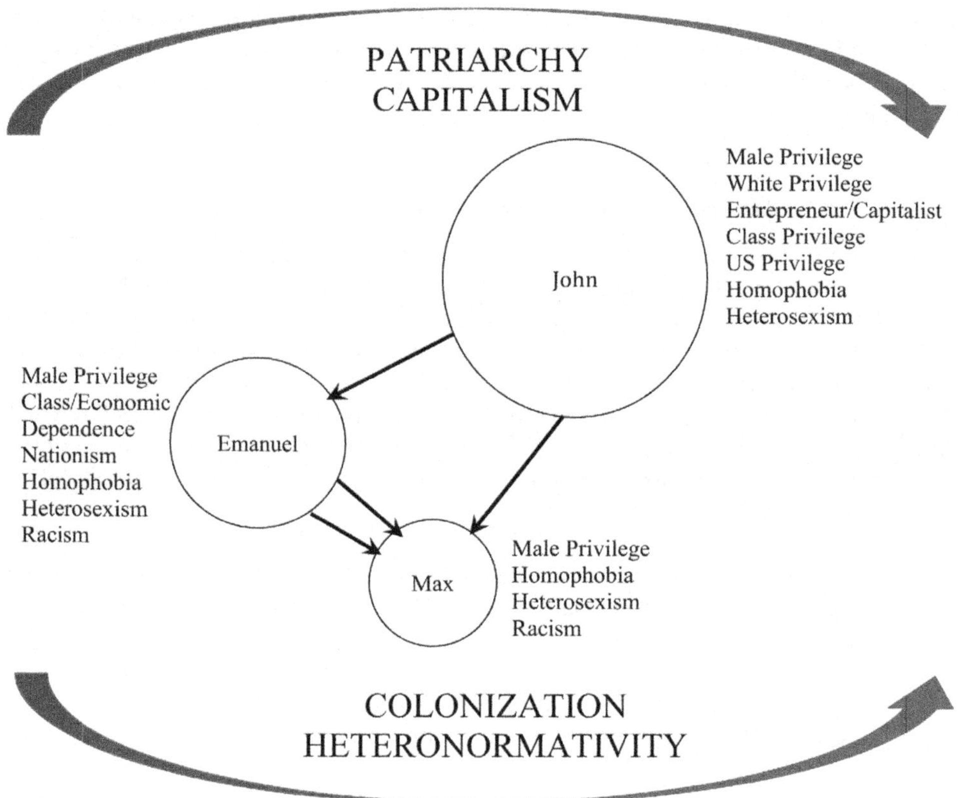

Figure 5.3 Example of a socioculturally attuned structural family map.

Exploring and Committing to Equity-based Relationships

Lisa **valued** all voices in the family as they helped the couple identify their egalitarian **values.** Emanuel and John described their ideal relationship as one in which they equally shared the responsibilities of running their business and parenting their son. They were committed to a fair and just relationship. At first, they saw the issues in their family being about personalities. Max was drawn to Emanuel because he was more patient and "laid back." John was a driven perfectionist who liked to be in control. Over time, what they viewed as internal dispositions were exposed as existing between the internal and external—between individuals and relationships, relationships, and societal context.

As Max grew up, he expected to enter adulthood in a family that prided itself on being democratic. This mirrored not only the values of the democratic society in which they lived, but the value John and Emanuel both placed on having a fair and egalitarian marriage. Emanuel and John wanted Max to become increasingly autonomous yet accountable to others. Their own fathers were in more powerful positions in the family and lacked the emotional and relational attunement they wanted in their intimate relationship as well as in their parenting. They also wanted Max to be socially aware and know how to challenge racism, sexism, classism, and homophobia. All three family members readily engaged in visioning changes in their relationships that promoted equity and closeness. This family had a multitude of strengths and experiences facing and overcoming oppression that could be jointly mobilized.

Restructure to Support Developmentally Appropriate Relational Equity

John and Emanuel were committed to dismantling the effects of patriarchy in their relationship. This included rethinking how to help Max "become a man." One of the ways Lisa **intervened** was by helping John find ways to connect with Max that did not rely on giving him advice or demanding performance. For example, Lisa asked John and Max to spend a session together in which they were guided in talking directly to each other and coached to communicate in ways that increased understanding between them. This included expression of feelings. John was also asked to spend time with Max between sessions. John had to learn to deal with anxiety surrounding letting go of control and to trust Emanuel as a co-parent and business partner. Lisa engaged John and Emanuel in discussions about power dynamics, social class, gender, and race to raise their social awareness and help them **envision** change. Lisa also worked directly with the couple to encourage them in direct communication, making certain Emanuel's voice was heard in the therapy process. John learned to listen more carefully and attune to his partner's needs and feelings. John also learned to seek out Emanuel's input on decisions after realizing that while he thought the relationship was equal, he often made unilateral decisions. Emanuel became more outspoken, disagreeing with John directly when needed rather than seeking the comfort of Max when he felt misunderstood by John. Lisa assigned homework in which John and Emanuel were to regularly meet to discuss the business.

Over time these structural interventions helped them **transform** their marriage from a patriarchal business model (typically supported in capitalist economies) to a more collaborative, team-driven model. They also began routinely checking with each other about parenting decisions. They both enjoyed individual relationships with Max that did not undermine Max's relationship with the other dad. Lisa openly talked about race, class, and culture with the couple and helped them talk with Max to better prepare him to resist racism and classism. Their increasing awareness prompted an interest in Max to engage in community activism. Overall, the family's hierarchy was realigned, and as a family, they became increasingly collaborative, valuing relationships over tasks and mutual involvement over control.

Summary: Third Order Change

Max, Emanuel, and John engaged in first, second, and third order change throughout the process of family therapy. In this case, first order change included things like asking Emanuel and John to spend one night a week on a "no-problems date." The therapist did not expect this type of common sense solution to change the relationship dynamics per se, but saw it as a step toward second order change in which the couple redefined their relationship as one that was closer and more equal. Second order change included Emanuel and John becoming more equal as parents and business partners and Max developing more balanced relationships with both of his parents. Third order change included an active decision by Emanuel and John to resist patriarchy in their relationships with their fathers and each other. This included challenging gender stereotypes that pressure men to be competitive versus cooperative, to be autonomous versus collaborative, and stoic rather than vulnerable. In the end, they were able to structure their family in more egalitarian and loving ways. This included becoming more aware and committed to dismantling multiple dynamics of oppression, including racism, sexism, heterosexism, and classism within their family and beyond. The family became fluent in discourses of liberation by taking a metaview of their relationships within a societal context. This expansion of relational options was liberating while holding each member accountable for unearned privilege and misuse of power in intimate relationships.

Text Box 5.2 Salvador Minuchin, MD

Salvador Minuchin (2017, p. 37), legendary family therapist, teacher, and social justice advocate argued that the person of the therapist is an instrument of change:

As I got more experience it became clear that the techniques by themselves weren't all that useful. It was therapists themselves who were the instruments of change, and to be effective, they had to recognize the way they were part of the system and the process in the therapy room, not just a neutral observer.

Many therapists today draw on multiple family therapy models and/or practice evidence-based approaches. Minuchin's words above do not negate the value of these models; they remind us that any clinical encounter is more than a set of skills and what we do is never neutral.

Reflexive Questions

- Consider a time when it was difficult for you to join with a client. What made it difficult to "attune to them and respond to the way they moved you," as Minuchin suggested?
- Describe the ways in which economic, social, cultural, and symbolic capital play a role in determining your degree of social influence and access to resources. How does this help or hinder you in your life and professional practice?
- If you were to expand your family maps (the one you grew up in and your current family now) to connect your family to societal structures, contexts, and spaces, what would the maps look like? How are the maps similar or different from each other?
- When you think of the optimal structure for a well-functioning family, what comes to mind? How might a socioculturally attuned lens inform your perspective?
- How can you work with families to help them restructure in ways that address power imbalances and support developmentally appropriate relational equity?
- How can you help clients move from mutual blame or narrowly defining their problem, to expanding their lens to view their problems as existing between the internal and external; between individuals and relationships and relationships and societal context?

References

Andina, T. & Corvino, F. (2023). Transgenerational social structures and fictional actors: Community-based responsibility for future generations. *The Monist*, *106*, 150–164.

Bourdieu, P. (1986). The forms of capital. In J.G. Richardson (Ed.), *Handbook of theory and research for the sociology of education* (pp. 241–258). Greenwood Press.

Bourdieu, P. (1977). *Outline of a theory of practice* (R. Nice, Trans). Cambridge University Press. (Original work published 1972).

Butler, M. & Gardner, B. (2007). Adapting enactments to couple reactivity: Five developmental stages. *Journal of Marital and Family Therapy*, *29*(3), 311–327.

Chappelle, N. and Tadros, E. (2021). Using structural family therapy to understand the impact of poverty and trauma on African American adolescents. *The Family Journal*, 29(2), 237–244.

Colapinto, J. (2019). Structural family therapy. In B. H. Fiese, M. Celano, K. Deater-Deckard, E. N. Jouriles, & M. A. Whisman (Eds.). *APA handbook of contemporary family psychology: Family therapy and training* (pp. 197–121). American Psychological Association.

Colapinto, J. (2018). Family development in structural family therapy. In J. L. Lebow, A. Chambers, & Breunlin, D. (Eds.). *Encyclopedia of couple and family therapy*. Springer International Publishing AG.

Dehghani, M. & Bernards, J. (2022). The effectiveness of structural family therapy in repairing behavioral problems and improving family functioning in single-parent families in Iran. *Journal of marital and family therapy*, *48*(4), 1040–1058.
Diaz, B. & Vitola, C. (2026) Queer contextualized structural family therapy. In E. E. Hartwell & L. L. Edwards (Eds.). *Queer-contextualized family therapy: Toward radically inclusive theory and practice* (pp. 26–49). Routledge.
Eickers, G. (2023). Coordinating behaviors: Is social interaction scripted? *Journal for the Theory of Social Behavior*, *53*, 85–99.
Fishman, H. C. (2022). *Performance-based family therapy: A therapist's guide to measurable change*. Routledge.
Freire, P. (2000). *Pedagogy of the oppressed*. Bloomsbury. (Original work published in 1970).
Furstenberg, F. F. (2019). Family change in global perspective: How and why family systems change. *Family Relations*, *68*(3), 326–341.
Garcia, M. & McDowell, T. (2010). Mapping social capital: A critical contextual approach for working with low-status families. *Journal of Marital Family Therapy*, *36*(1), 96–107.
Gebel, G., Griggs, M., & Washington, K. (2023). Evaluating structural family therapy from a nonmonogamy lens. *The Family Journal: Counseling and Therapy for Couples and Families*, *31*(1), 42–50.
Jackson, J. B. & Landers, A. L. (2020). Structural and strategic approaches. In K. S. Wampler, R. B. Miller, & R. B. Seedall (Eds.). *The handbook of systemic family therapy* (Vol. 1, pp. 339–364).
Jordan, L., Grogan, C., Muruthi, B., & Bermúdez, J. M. (2017). Polyamory: Experiences of power from without, from within, and in between. *Journal of Couple & Relationship Therapy*, 16(1), 11–19.
Korin, E. C. (1994). Social inequalities and therapeutic relationships: Applying Freire's ideas to clinical practice. *Journal of Feminist Family Therapy*, *5*, 75–98.
Lo, J. & Ma, J. (2022). The perceived helpfulness of structural family therapy in caring for Hong Kong Chinese families of an adolescent with intellectual disabilities: A qualitative inquiry. *British Journal of Learning Disabilities*, *51*, 440–449.
Maton, K. (2014). *Habitus*. In M. J. Grenfell (Ed.). *Pierre Bourdieu: Key concepts* (2nd ed., pp. 48–65). Routledge.
McAdams, C. R. III, Avadhanam, R., Foster, V. A., Harris, P. N., Javaheri, A., Kim, S., Kooyman, B. A., Joe, J. R., Sheffield, R. L., & Williams, A. E. (2016). The viability of structural family therapy in the twenty-first century: An analysis of key indicators. *Contemporary Family Therapy*, *38*(3), 255–261.
Minuchin, S. (2017, January). Systems therapy: The art of creating uncertainty. *Psychotherapy Networker* (pp. 37–38).
Minuchin, S. (1974). *Families and family therapy*. Harvard College.
Minuchin, S., Montalvo, B., Guerney, B., Rosman, B., & Schumer, F. (1967). *Families of the slums: An exploration of their structure and treatment*. Basic Books.
Minuchin, S. and Nichols, M. P. (1993). *Family healing: Tales of hope and renewal from family therapy*. Free Press.
Minuchin, S., Reiter, M., and Borda, C. (2014). *The craft of family therapy: Challenging certainties*. Routledge.
Pender Baum, R. L., & Pender, D. A. (2023). Using structural family theory in treating family conflict. *The Family Journal*, *31*(1), 35–41.
Reiter, M. (2018a). Salvador Minuchin, MD: Innovator and challenger. *Journal of Systemic Therapies*, *36*(4), 16–22.
Reiter, M. (2018b). Ten things I learned from Dr. Salvador Minuchin. *Journal of Systemic Therapies*, *36*(4), 46–56.
Ripoll, F. (2024). Overcoming the dualism between "society and space", with and beyond Bourdieu. *Progress in Human Geography*, *48*(3) 332–351.
Roaldsnes, A. (2024). Social capital and the intergenerational transmission of cultural capital: How parents' social networks influence children's accumulation of cultural capital. *Poetics*, *102*, 101873.
Singer, S. (2024). *Brief therapy for clients with challenging or unique issues*. Routledge.
Vertovec, S. (2021). The social organization of difference. *Ethnic and Racial Studies*, *44*(8), 1273–1295.
Williams, N. D., Foye, A., & Lewis, F. (2016). Applying structural family therapy in the changing context of the modern African American single mother. *Journal of Feminist Family Therapy*, *28*(1), 30–47.

6 Socioculturally Attuned Brief and Strategic Family Therapies

Brief and strategic family therapists introduced the idea that change can happen quickly. Change in one part of the system can create change in another part of the system and small changes can lead to more substantial, lasting change. Families are often viewed as trying to solve problems in ways that make sense but don't work, requiring therapists to think counterintuitively to intervene in family dynamics. Therapists using these approaches focus on the here and now, helping families change interactional patterns that inadvertently maintain the very problems they often wish to eliminate.

A number of important approaches to working with families fall under the broad heading of brief family therapy. These include the work of leading figures at the Mental Research Institute (e.g., Watzlawick, et al., 1967), the Milan group (e.g., Palazzoli Selvini et al., 1980), and Strategic Family Therapists (e.g., Haley, 1973; Madanes, 1984). As with many family therapy models developed in the second half of the twentieth century, brief models were based on Bateson's concept of families as systems (Jackson & Landers, 2020). The focus was on the family unit and tailoring interventions to specifically meet the needs of each family. Relatively little attention was paid to the broader social context. These approaches were originally influenced by Milton Erickson's counterintuitive approach to change (de Shazer, 1982; Haley, 1973) and have endured many rounds of influential thought including social constructionism. New approaches have emerged from these frameworks over time including queer-contextualized strategic family therapy that emphasizes embodied experience and the use of movement (Parrott, et al., 2026); Post-Milan approaches that incorporate social constructionism (Brown, 2010; Rhodes, 2012); systemic-family-individual (SFI) therapy (Codecá, et al., 2024); and other advances in Milan systemic therapy (Barbetta & Telfener, 2020; Fraser, 2020); as well as manualized strategic family therapy (Lockhart, 2024); and manualized brief strategic family therapy (Szapocznik & Hervis, 2020)).

⟵⟶

Socioculturally attuned brief and strategic family therapists promote third order change by factoring broad societal dynamics into possible hypotheses and interventions.

⟵⟶

In this chapter, we describe enduring concepts and practices related to brief and strategic family therapy. We illustrate how therapists can integrate principles of sociocultural attunement and offer practice guidelines. We then share a case illustration to demonstrate how integrating societal systems and attention to power can lead to third order change.

Primary Enduring Brief and Strategic Family Therapy Concepts

There are a number of tenets common across brief models, including a focus on the here and now, the assumption that change doesn't require insight and can happen quickly, and the idea that

DOI: 10.4324/9781003493426-6

small change can lead to bigger change (Nardone & Watzlawick, 2005). Early brief therapists highlighted that we *cannot not communicate* (Watzlawick et al., 1967). Even silence is a form of communication and communication may have more than one referent. Symptoms are sometimes viewed as metaphoric communication with interactional patterns around one problem, representing patterns around another less approachable problem (Madanes, 1984). For example, a family may complain of an adolescent repeatedly running away when in fact their unspoken concern is that one of the parents wants to leave the marriage. Strategic family therapists consider how families are organized using the metaphor of family hierarchy, but focus on power dynamics in ways that differ from structural family therapists.

In strategic therapy, problems are viewed as metaphors and/or resulting from incongruent hierarchies, or imbalances of power (Madanes, 1981). Those who carry the symptom are often resisting power dynamics that family members are unable to address. Interventions share the expectation that therapists will be active and carefully target directives to disrupt problematic relational patterns (Nardone & Watzlawick, 2005). While less common now in community agencies and private practice, therapeutic teams were sometimes used to form hypotheses, observe live sessions, and carefully design interventions for therapists to deliver during and/or at the end of sessions.

In this section, we offer enduring core concepts in the practice of brief and strategic family therapies. These include: 1) circularity and circular questioning, 2) viewing problems as attempted solutions, 3) thinking counterintuitively, and 4) assessing power imbalances. We describe what makes an intervention strategic, and emphasize the expectation that therapists be active agents of change.

Circularity

Patterns of interaction and thinking non-linearly remain hallmarks of the practice of family therapy. Brief and strategic family therapists used the term circular causality to refer to the idea that it is not necessary to discover where a problem started in order to find a solution. Each part of a pattern, or each action, is also a reaction, affecting and being affected by all surrounding actions (Watzlawick et al., 1967). Patterns can therefore be interrupted anywhere to create change. Later in this chapter, we will advocate for integrating analysis of societal-based power into circular thinking, arguing that therapists must be careful not to assume that family members have equal influence over the formation or resolution of problems or that families or family members are solely responsible for symptoms.

Circular questioning, introduced by the Milan team, provides a means of feedback while continually opening new possible explanations and views of the problem (Palazzoli Selvini, et al., 1980). The therapist asks questions to check out hypotheses about what is creating and maintaining problems. At the same time, family members are asked to share how they view relationships between other family members, as well as what they think others might think, say, or feel. This adds new information to their understanding of each other and the problems they face. The family not only hears about each member's views and experiences, but also what each assumes are the views and experiences of others. All questions reflect assumptions and answers confirm or deny hypotheses.

For example, if the therapist asks a family member, "When would your brother say this problem started?", they are sharing their assumption that there was a time when the problem did not exist and inferring that knowing the circumstances and timing of the problem's origin will help solve it. By asking one family member to assume the position of another, the therapist is adding information to the system (i.e., what one brother thinks the other thinks) while forming a hypothesis about why the problem is occurring. When the family member answers, "He would say it started soon after our mother died," the therapist begins to build a hypothesis that the problem is associated with the death of the mother. They then ask, "Who was closest to your mother?" hypothesizing that the problem is connected to the loss of a close relationship. When the client answers "None of us. In fact, we never felt we could live up to her expectations," the new information leads the therapist to rethink the hypothesis. It also leads the family and therapist to shift how they are making meaning of the situation together.

Hypothesizing is seen as suppositional, providing direction and making sense of problems relationally. Rather than seeking truth, therapists use hypotheses to guide treatment. Family members are invited to metacommunicate (communicate about their communication), which in turn, contributes to new ways of thinking and doing. Let's consider the example of the Bernadines, a White, middle class couple (Lily and Tom), who entered problem gambling treatment with their adult daughter, Mavis.

Therapist:	So Lily, I am wondering who you think is most concerned about Mavis's gambling?
Lily:	Well, I think Mavis is.
Mavis:	Really?!
Therapist:	If I were to ask you that same question, Mavis, what would you say? Who do you think is most concerned about the gambling?
Mavis:	Mom is—definitely! She's the one who calls me worrying all the time. She gets dad all worked up about it too.
Therapist:	So how would you describe their relationship? Mom and Dad's?
Mavis:	I don't know… I guess happy. Dad seems happy with their relationship. I'm not sure mom is. Maybe she wants him to be around more…pay more attention to what's going on.
Therapist:	And how do you think your mom would describe her relationship with your dad?
Mavis:	She would probably say they love each other, that all couples have to deal with differences, you know…the usual. She might say he is a grump no matter what she tries to do to make him happy (laughs and smiles at dad).
Therapist:	If your brother Mark were here, what would he say about your parent's relationship? (relational questioning)
Mavis:	He would take mom's side. I think he would say dad is kind of in his own world. Besides, Mark thinks I am a total loser!
Therapist:	So your brother would say mom is most concerned about the gambling and that dad is not as involved with things? How about your dad, who would he say is most concerned about the gambling?
Mavis:	Well, you can ask him, but he will say mom is.
Therapist:	Dad?
Tom:	I suppose Mavis is right. It really bothers her mom.
Therapist:	If mom were bothered less by the gambling would it still be a problem?
Tom:	Well of course. It's not like I don't care! Lily is just the most tuned in to it.
Therapist:	So mom, maybe they are saying you carry most of the worry? Is that how you see it?
Lily:	I suppose so.

In this brief exchange, the therapist was able to help the family identify a number of patterns, including how the family might be organized around the problem. Lily receives new information: that her husband and daughter believe she is most concerned about the problem. The family is offered a new idea: that mom is carrying most of the burden of the problem.

Problems as Attempted Solutions

Families are viewed as having the competence and strengths necessary to solve problems, however, there are times when solutions don't work and may become or exacerbate problems (Jackson & Landers, 2020). According to Watzlawick, Weakland, and Fisch (1974), there are three primary ways attempted solutions become or contribute to problems. The first is when families underestimate the need to take action. For example, a wife may complain that she does not have equal influence in her relationship with her husband, who in turn uses his power in the relationship to dismiss her concerns. This pattern continues until the wife leaves the relationship. The husband may then realize the need to respond, but responds too late.

The second type of attempted solution is when families overestimate the action needed to solve a problem. For example, a newly blended family comes into therapy because a stepfather is concerned that his adolescent stepson is not doing as he is told. When the therapist investigates, they discover that the son is doing well in school, observes curfews, does the majority of his chores, and is generally respectful to his parents. The stepfather is focused on the son's failure to pick up his room and to complete chores on demand, such as folding the laundry when asked. The stepfather's focus on minor non-compliance is inadvertently creating a problem, as the mother feels the need to defend her son, and the son withdraws from both parents. This overreaction to a minor issue adds to the tension in emerging stepparent–child relationships and exacerbates the power imbalance between the couple by highlighting the mother's lack of influence over the stepfather's unrealistic expectations.

The third type of attempted solution is when families repeat common sense solutions even when they exacerbate problems. Let's go back to the example of the Bernadines. Mavis (age 28) was having difficulty living on her own without the financial help of her parents. She worked at a minimum wage job and spent most of her free time in diners playing on electronic gambling machines. Tom and Lily worried about their daughter being evicted from her apartment, not having food, or being able to pay her phone bill. They were dedicated, as most parents are, to helping their daughter be successful and happy. They refused to give Mavis money to gamble, but when she needed money for rent or food, they felt compelled to help. They took over her phone bill to make sure they could always reach her, and she could call on them when she needed support. Providing financial support to encourage their daughter to be on her own is a common sense solution that is effective in some situations. In this case, parents were being held hostage by the gambling. They knew their daughter lost the money she needed, but didn't want her to face difficult consequences. Trying to help their daughter succeed and Mavis relying on financial support (which inadvertently supported gambling) became a pattern of attempted solutions that made the problem worse.

These attempted solutions rely on a specific point of view and can become redundant. In other words, the nonsolution can become a repetitive pattern, based on a way of looking at things. The therapist looks for and attempts to disrupt problem patterns by helping the family see and do things differently (Ray et al., 2019; Vitry et al., 2021).

Counter-intuitive Thinking

Brief and strategic therapies were influenced by Milton Erikson's counter-intuitive approach (de Shazer, 1982; Haley, 1973). Viewing problems from a counterintuitive lens can lead to creative solutions. How the family thinks about and defines the problem may be part of the problem, or at least keep them stuck and unable to discover a solution. In de Shazer's words (1982), "the therapist's worldview must help him [sic] see beyond the client's worldview. The therapist must see the client's problem from a different angle" (p. 21). In essence, the therapist reframes how the problem is understood, helping clients see it differently and lead them to different sets of solutions. According to Nardone and Watzlawick (2005), non-ordinary logic is key to unlocking the self-maintaining logic of most problems. They argued that "The strategic approach to therapy, linked directly to the contemporary philosophy of constructivism knowledge…is based on the assertion of the impossibility…of offering an absolutely true and definitive explanation of reality" (p. 38). It is precisely these many possible realities that open space for counterintuitive thinking.

Rather than being concerned about the cause of a problem, brief and strategic family therapists are interested in uncovering and disrupting what is maintaining the problem. The therapist must help families view problems differently in order to inspire greater options for change. Take for example a couple who entered therapy because a wife, who had the majority of power in the relationship, was unhappy about a husband who consistently acquiesced to her wishes. During the first session, the wife told the therapist they had come in so the therapist could get the husband to stand up to her. This couple was stuck in a self-defeating logic loop. The only way the husband was able to stand up to the wife was by refusing her demand that he do so. If the therapist accepted the client's position on the problem, they would worsen the problem by ineffectively trying to get the husband to be more assertive.

Therapists may define differences in family members' perspectives as being part of the problem (de Shazer, 1982). For example, one partner may insist that sharing emotion is primary, while the other views emotion as counterproductive. Joining with one view over the other typically leaves the therapist stuck as part of the system, attempting to use the same logic. A therapist would need to shift into a new level or type of solution. This might involve suggesting that it is not that one approach is better than the other, but the judgmental attitude each partner takes of the other that is problematic (Atkinson, 2005). This requires therapists to think beyond their own worldview about how problems should be solved. There are many ways of looking at what is true. A strategic therapist is most concerned with what works and what inspires hope for change (Haley, 1976). Haley was convinced that therapists need to help families construct problems that could be solved.

Incongruent Hierarchies

Like structural family therapists, strategic family therapists consider power dynamics and family hierarchy as central to presenting problems. According to Cloé Madanes (1981), "when one is dealing with a family…there is inevitably an issue of hierarchy because the participants are not all equal. They have status differences based on such issues as age, control of funds, and community-vested authority and responsibility" (p. 5). Madanes argued that all couples deal with issues of power and control as they typically divide areas of responsibility. She noted that family members have the potential to overpower each other, along with the potential to nurture and care for each other. Incongruent hierarchies occur when family members' influence does not match expectations for their roles. Consider a child who worries over and takes care of a parent with a drinking problem. Not only is the parent unable to consistently fulfill the role of caretaker and protector, but the child is placed in a position of taking charge of the parent. Unequal relationships between parents are sometimes balanced by one or more children siding with a one-down parent, but may also be balanced through symptomatic behavior (Madanes, 1981).

Take for example a cishet (cisgender heterosexual) couple in which the husband has more power to influence major decisions and sets the mood in everyday interactions. The wife accommodates him for the most part, but from time to time, she goes on spending sprees. She apologizes profusely when bills come in, but can't seem to stop. The husband is rendered helpless over his wife's spending, which he is unable to control. In this way, the symptom of overspending might be seen as serving to balance power in an unequal relationship. This perspective of power does not clearly differentiate overt power from acts of resistance to power. When therapists view the most symptomatic person in the family as the most powerful due to the symptom, they often overlook the symptom as a form of resistance to the non-negotiable power of another family member.

Therapist as Agent of Change

Brief and strategic models focus on the value of well-placed interventions that create change. Strategic interventions have become almost synonymous with the use of paradox, which has largely fallen out of favor, despite paradox being only one type of non-transparent intervention. Nardone & Watzlawick (2005) argued that there is no ethical dilemma when delivering non-transparent interventions because therapy is not a zero-sum game. The therapist has the best interest of the client in mind, and the therapist and clients win or lose together. There have also always been clear guidelines, including the imperative that interventions should never cause harm (Haley, 1980). Furthermore, paradoxical interventions must be win/win; helpful whether or not the family follows the directive.

What makes an intervention strategic is not that the paradoxical intervention is delivered in a non-transparent way, but the fact that it is specifically tailored to target and interrupt a problematic interactional pattern. The therapist is responsible for being active and directing the family, supplying interventions that create change within unique family and societal contexts. According to Haley (1980, p. 10), a useful theory "should guide a therapist to action rather than to reflection. It should suggest what to do." In fact, Haley placed the responsibility to create change squarely on the shoulders of the therapist. This mandate has changed over time to a greater reliance on collaboration between therapists and clients; however, the importance of therapists being active and accountable for intervening in problematic dynamics has endured.

Descriptions of the wide variety of strategic interventions are beyond the scope of this work and have been described in depth elsewhere. These include the Milan group's use of invariant prescription, paradox and counterparadox, therapy teams, and family rituals (Amorin-Woods & Selvini, 2023; Boscolo et al., 1987; Selvini-Palazzoli & Viaro, 1988); Haley's (1984) ordeal therapy and reframing techniques; and prescribing the symptom, pretending, seeing symptoms as metaphors and replacing their function (Madanes, 1981). The following examples are intended to give the reader a sense of typical strategic interventions.

Interventions range from direct and transparent to indirect with relatively hidden agendas. The obvious logic of some strategic interventions is apparent to the therapist and the family, or at least the adults in the family. Take for example, a common pattern between siblings and a parent. Joe (age 7) and Walter (age 5) fluctuate between playing well together and arguing. When the arguing gets loud and they start calling each other names, their custodial grandmother, Mary, enters the room to tell them to stop. If they don't stop, Mary raises her voice and sends them to their rooms. Mary is tired of the fighting and wants a new solution. The therapist asks Joe and Walter what they most enjoy and learns they especially love going with their grandmother to the dollar store, where they are allowed to spend three dollars each on anything they like. Mary agrees with the therapist to offer the money to each of them in a new way. Each week, she will exchange four dollars for 16 quarters. Mary is directed to place eight quarters in each of the two jars. Whenever she hears Joe call Walter a name, she simply goes to Joe's jar, takes out a quarter, and places it in Walter's jar. She does likewise when she hears Walter call Joe a name. If either child protests, they lose an additional quarter. This intervention interrupts the pattern of Mary intervening in sibling arguments while maintaining her role as a parent, ensuring that there will be no name-calling. Both children have control over keeping their money, and when they choose to spend it on name-calling it benefits the sibling whom they intend to insult.

The therapist might also offer a family an explanation without fully disclosing the reasoning behind an intervention. This doesn't necessarily mean the reason given isn't true, but the truth of the explanation is less relevant than the change in pattern. For example, a family enters therapy because their four-year-old is throwing fits several times a day. When she does this, her parents get upset with her and try to get her to stop, which seems to escalate the behavior. The therapist, after exploring all other potential causes for sudden disruptive behavior, discovers that the child did not throw tantrums until recently and shows concern that the child may have missed the important developmental stage in which young children learn they cannot control everything around them (i.e., "the terrible twos"). The therapist reassures the family that it is better for a four-year-old to go through the terrible twos than to go through them as a teen and encourages parents to make sure their daughter has at least one tantrum a day to get through this developmental stage as quickly as possible (strategic/paradoxical intervention).

The therapist and family carefully lay out exactly what is to happen when the child has a tantrum and how to insist on a tantrum if she hasn't had one all day. They rehearse prompting a tantrum during the session (presecribing the symptom). When they have to resort to prompting a tantrum, they are asked to sit together and have a cup of hot cocoa once it is all over. Prescribing the symptom creates a change in how the symptom is viewed, as well as each family member's action/reaction. Once you have voluntarily done something that you assumed was out of control, you are more likely to take a metaview that makes repeating the same behavior in the same old way nearly impossible.

Haley (1984) proposed that therapists help families abandon problems by creating "ordeals" that made problems too troublesome to maintain. For example, a family entered therapy after seeing a physician and learned that there was no medical cause for their 13-year-old's headaches, which had kept him out of school for several weeks. It was imperative that he return to school as soon as possible, but the family was uncertain what to do as the headaches persisted. The therapist explored developmental issues, problems at school, family dynamics, and so on, only to find that the boy's headaches seemed to center around some mild anxiety, which the solution of avoiding school exacerbated. The longer he was out, the more anxious he became about returning. In this case, the therapist elicited the help of parents and grandparents who were eager to see the problem resolved. Each of the adults agreed to be on call to spend one or two days a week in the school nurse's office. The school agreed that a parent or grandparent could sit with the student when he wasn't feeling well. This way, he would at least be at school, but never without someone to nurture him when he wasn't feeling well. The boy returned to school but not to the nurse's office, releasing his headaches to avoid the social embarrassment of having a parent or grandparent with him at school.

Integrating Principles of Sociocultural Attunement

Sociocultural attunement requires expanding practice beyond family systems to consider the relationship between families and society. The idea of circularity or that interactions occur in repetitive patterns, remains useful in challenging linear cause and effect thinking; however, the relative power family members have to create and maintain patterns must be taken into account. Likewise, it is important to understand parallel societal processes that promote imbalances of power and their impact on presenting problems. Socioculturally attuned brief and strategic therapists are called on to not only think counterintuitively but to think in ways that counter hegemony.

•←→•

From a socioculturally attuned perspective, symptoms are carefully considered to determine if and how they may serve as acts of resistance to unjust systems.

•←→•

Societal Context

Socioculturally attuned brief and strategic therapists are tasked with understanding how family interactions and the meaning of problems are impacted by culture and societal dynamics—the context beyond the individual family. Conceptualizing circularity and problem formation on a societal level can help therapists develop contextually informed strategic hypotheses.

Circularity in Context

Circular causality has been heavily criticized as promoting an assumption that problems are self-perpetuating and that all family members have equal opportunity to create change. Feminist family therapists challenged the assumption that family members have equal influence and that problems reside solely within families rather than reflecting power dynamics in the broader society (James & McIntyre, 1983). According to Goodrich and colleagues (1988),

> Circularity is another systemic construct that operates in women's disfavor. The idea that people are involved in recursive patterns of behavior, reactively instigated and mutually reinforced results either in making everyone equally responsible for everything or no one accountable for anything. (p. 17)

Haley (1980) actually voiced a related concern when he argued that "Systems theory, as it was applied to families, tended to describe participants as equals…a primary problem…is the way systems theory takes away individual responsibility" (p. 15).

Perhaps the metaphor of patterns as circular is itself a problem as it elicits a sense of equality and equidistance, like sitting at a round table at standard intervals. There is no one at the head of the table and everyone has the same amount of space. You can see and hear everyone equally. While the practice of continuing to track interactions until they loop back or "circle around" to the starting point remains helpful, in reality, patterns of interactions are more likely uneven, unequal, and asymmetrical; actions more or less voluntary, with participants having various levels of influence and choice across situations. Interactions are influenced by societal dynamics which afford greater power and influence in some families than others. Likewise, choices are often narrowed by social constraints, cultural norms, and power dynamics which limit actions and reactions.

Consider an Egyptian Muslim family in which an adult son, Omar, is unable to earn enough money to marry due to the country's long-term economic depression. He begins to stray from family and religious values in favor of hanging out and drinking alcohol with a group of peers who are in the same situation. He and his father, Achmed, engage in verbal conflict when he arrives home. His mother, Magda, attempts to intervene but is quickly dismissed by both males. The conflict escalates until Omar angrily leaves the house. Magda and Achmed then argue about how the situation was handled until Magda withdraws. Call to prayer calms and centers both Achmed and Magda who then come together in a loving embrace.

Culturally, Omar is expected to be a capable provider before he marries. Global economic disparities leave him caught between childhood and adulthood. He acts out in an adult way (e.g., drinking with friends) that leaves him paradoxically stuck in childhood (e.g., being scolded by his father). As a female, Magda enjoys economic rights and protection under Egyptian law, which interprets the Qur'an as guaranteeing those rights (Al-Mannai, 2010), yet like most women in the world, she has less power to influence men in a patriarchal society. Their religious beliefs and common cultural experience of being called to prayer five times a day serve as a source of resilience that helps them maintain connection in spite of conflict. This circular pattern is shaped by economic, religious, and cultural constraints and opportunities.

Problem Formation at a Societal Level

We must understand how societal dynamics contribute to problem formation and how some social problems are exacerbated by attempted solutions on a societal level. Consider financial aid from high-resource countries to low-resource countries. This makes good common sense to many of us. This aid ensures a positive political alliance and often enhances military strength that supports multiple government agendas. The countries receiving aid are hopefully in better positions to defend themselves through military force, build infrastructures, encourage trade, and lessen poverty. The dynamics of national lending and debt, however, create new problems. Those in power to disburse funds can do so in ways that benefit themselves, maintain their power, and/or support reforms that eventually fail. Low-resource countries can become increasingly indebted to powerful international lenders. This reinforces existing international imbalances of power (Soederberg, 2013). These common-sense solutions can have unintended effects at local levels. In this case, poverty, and the many emotional, relational, and health problems associated with poverty, may become increasingly difficult for families to overcome as governments must pay back their loans even when it means depriving families of basic needs such as safety, food security, health care, and education.

It is not uncommon for societies to under respond or over respond in ways that contribute to large-scale formation of social problems. For example, many societies significantly under respond to intimate partner violence, poverty, racism, homophobia, and other social problems. Failure to adequately respond leaves vulnerable family members and families most marginalized in society without protection and/or equal access to resources. The effect on families is widespread, contributing to many of the problems family therapists are only too aware of (e.g., medical problems, depression, anxiety, interpersonal conflict).

The work of Kabura described in Text Box 6.1 is an example of a brief, targeted intervention into a societal system. The intervention was tailored to fit a Ugandan cultural context by working closely with clan elders and religious leaders. The wisdom of clan elders and religious leaders is highly respected in the community. They are the first responders—one of the first to hear a complaint—when domestic violence occurs. These leaders integrated new knowledge of domestic violence into their traditional, cultural, and natural wisdom, which in turn informs their decisions on behalf of clan members. This intervention targeted a specific point in the pattern of interaction in the larger system in order to create change.

Kabura (McDowell & Kabura, 2016) sought to increase awareness of community leaders and accountability of those who commit domestic violence. This intervention did not directly address gender inequity per se, but made an important change that supported just responses to the outcroppings of inequity. Staff at Bishop Magambo Counselor Training Institute (BMCTI) in Fort Portal, Uganda reached out to local authorities and community leaders to raise awareness of domestic violence (e.g., signs of abuse, reporting abuse-related crimes, safety issues, the abuse cycle, procedures for referring to counseling). In Text Box 6.1 Kabura describes the impact of this strategic move.

Families are also influenced by cultural and societal contexts in their attempts to solve problems. Consider parents over-responding to children earning poor grades. Poor academic performance may result in fear, anger, and family conflict. These reactions are informed in part by economic systems that rely on education as a means of securing middle and/or professional class status. At some level, a second grader's poor academic performance threatens the family's and child's long-term economic security.

Text Box 6.1 Paschal Kabura, PhD

Paschal Kabura is a Catholic priest and founder/director of the Bishop Magambo Counselor Training Institute in the Kabarole District of Uganda. According to Kabura (McDowell & Kabura, 2016, p. 33):

If a husband beats his wife, the wife will likely go to her parents' home. Traditionally when a wife has gone to her parents, her husband has an obligation to appeal to her family and the clan elder in order to seek reconciliation. The husband is typically given a punishment and the wife returns to the marriage. Clan elders are now beginning to enter these situations with a better understanding of the abuse cycle. They are less likely to be deceived by the husband's show of remorse or promises to change. They realize all might not be well when a couple is in a "honeymoon stage." They are slower to move toward reconciliation and more likely to say things like "you tell us now that everything is o.k., but we need to go deeper into the cycle to get to the root of the problem." They are better able to recognize their own limits in solving this problem and are aware of how to refer clan members for help. Clan elders and religious leaders have significant leverage in referring families for counseling, helping to overcome the stigma associated with mental health issues. When sent by a clan elder or religious leader people are more likely to accept help. It is not unusual for someone to come to the counseling center at BMCTI saying "I did not think I would come here, but my elder told me this is what I need to do" or "My clan leader told me if I don't come here, he won't listen to me again." Clan elders and religious leaders sometimes consult directly with faculty and staff at BMCTI. In this way, these informal helpers are getting consultation for their work as well as opportunities to develop their skills without pursuing a degree. They can seek support when situations get complex. They are also empowered by borrowing the expertise of the center. For example, it is not uncommon for a community leader to say, "This is what Dr. Kabura has said."

Power

Strategic therapists carefully analyze power imbalances; however, symptom removal remains the primary goal (Madanes, 1981), rather than necessarily promoting relational equity. This may lead therapists to intervene in ways that mirror power dynamics and fail to help families consider more equitable and just alternatives. For example, many years ago, Teresa saw a family in which a teenage daughter and her mother got into chronic arguments. The father sometimes took the side of his wife and sometimes took the side of his daughter, typically being the one to make any necessary final decisions. As a then strategic therapist, Teresa asked the family to reenact the arguments in session and assigned the father the task between sessions of flipping a coin each time mother and daughter fought in order to decide whose side he would take. This intervention eliminated the pattern of mother and daughter fighting and father stepping in, but failed to address the societal dynamic of male dominance that maintained the father's one-up position in the family.

Post-Milan practice (Brown, 2010; Rhodes, 2012) emerged in response to the critique of the Milan group's lack of attention to power (e.g., Goldner, 1985, 1993; Hoffman, 1985) and the introduction of social constructionism. Therapists began being thought of as engaging with families to mutually understand problems within a societal context. Hypothesizing broadened to include social influences and analysis of power dynamics. As illustrated in Text Box 6.2, recent advances in

Text Box 6.2 Pietro Barbetta and Umberta Telfener

Pietro Barbetta and Umberta Telfener work at the Milan Center for Family Therapy in Milan, Italy. In the following excerpts, they (Barbetta & Telfener, 2020) describe important aspects of the ontological turn that embrace social constructivist thinking and acknowledge the very real consequences of inequity:

What is new in the Milan approach is a needed different attention to discrimination, poverty, social issues, and human rights. We are dealing with social issues such as marginalization, that is, what we systemics call out of order, and what the psychiatric discourse calls disorder. Our curiosity focuses on the social aspects that create discrimination and pathology, we are curious about the link between the institutional violation of human rights and new forms of pathology. (p. 11)

Systemic perspectivism moves people to exchange actions, discussing differences without disqualifying each other... We are interested in creating the conditions whereby the world outside is observed as a multiverse reality, with its own terms of engagement. It means that there are social ontologies: moralistic communities where a woman has to watch the way she dresses; oppressive institutions where a child can be psychologically abused; big companies where workers are forced to contribute to pollution under the threat of losing their job; criminal societies and terrorists who buy weapons from "regular" arms factories; criminal families (mafia) where loyalty is necessary to maintain appearances of normality; refugees who do not receive asylum in Europe, even though they come from camps and war. How can such realities be considered linguistic "constructions"? (p. 10)

the Milan approach (Barbetta & Telfener, 2020) include "the ontological turn," such as using lenses from different angles and positionalities to realize different points of view (epistemology), while maintaining awareness of realities that are beyond how we look at and talk about things (ontology); and "the corporeal turn," focusing on embodiment and embodied knowledge in a way that goes beyond biology, neurology, and psychology toward a gestalt that includes bodies and movement in relationship to social and political realities (Parrott, et al., 2026).

Societal Impact on Power Imbalances

In the earlier example, it didn't occur to Teresa that the symptom or pattern in which the family was stuck reflected an incongruent hierarchy on a societal level. Patriarchy and heteronormativity promote the assumption that sex and gender are conflated, dichotomous, and natural. Men and masculinity are more greatly valued and assume a one-up position in relation to women and femininity, even in societies such as the US that tout democracy and equality. At a societal level, men are more often the decision makers as was true in this family. By asking the husband/father to make an arbitrary decision about supporting either his wife or teenage daughter, Teresa was reinforcing the problem even while eliminating the symptom. She was also ignoring what may have been a form of resistance to male dominance by the mother and daughter.

Culture and Power

Family therapists often view culture as a matter of difference. Cultural competence is vital to ethical, effective practice, and therapists support cultural democracy by viewing all cultures as equally legitimate. There is a tendency, however, even among culturally competent therapists, to overlook the centering and dominance of some cultures over others, which potentially offers those in the majority culture greater social influence and access to resources (see chapters 2 and 4; Bourdieu, 1986).

•←→•

Culture affects how we attempt to solve problems, and what we consider intuitive or logical is often unexamined dominant cultural logic.

•←→•

For example, European Americans in the US tend to value independence and individuality. When a family enters treatment with a three-year-old who is having trouble sleeping on her own, it can be easy to follow the family's common sense logic of the importance of toddlers sleeping separately from parents. Common sense solutions (e.g., night light, door ajar, reward system) attempt to resolve what has been culturally framed as a problem. Family therapists might believe they are thinking "outside the box" when hypothesizing that the child's refusal to sleep alone is a function of family interactions (perhaps a problem in the couple's relationship) while failing to examine the expectation that healthy toddlers sleep alone privileges European American cultural dominance. The therapist in this situation would not necessarily discourage the parents from their goal, but could help parents put their decision in a cultural perspective.

Symptoms as Forms of Everyday Resistance

Everyday resistance is often overlooked as a response to oppressive power dynamics in families and societies. According to Afuape (2011), aspects of everyday resistance include the ways people always resist oppression; the ways we all struggle with contradictory positions and ways of responding to oppression that can coexist; the back and forward movement toward liberation that is forever shifting and changing; the place of our relationships and social circumstances in supporting or constraining movements in our preferred direction; and the possibility of being both oppressor and oppressed (p. 72).

•←→•

What we identify as problems might also be sites of everyday resistance, better understood as symptoms of power imbalances in society.

•←→•

For example, demonstrating depression may be both a genuine physical and emotional struggle and a way to resist an oppressive marriage or job. Strategic therapists notice this dynamic and hypothesize symptoms as exerting a type of power that can balance incongruent hierarchies. Practicing from a socioculturally attuned framework extends this idea beyond the family to link oppression to broader societal contexts. Women who are displaying depression as a form of resistance to a male partner's dominance are also resisting a much broader force of male dominance, which maintains this power dynamic in intimate relationships. A client showing depression or panic attacks in response to a workplace may also be resisting much larger issues (e.g., class privilege, racism, sexism) that promote and maintain unjust working conditions.

Resistance in the form of symptoms is also frequently overlooked as a site of resilience (McDowell, 2015). Consider a set of twins in a family in which a socially powerful parent is verbally and emotionally abusive. One twin argues back continuously and is labeled as a problem because she disrupts the family on a daily basis. The other withdraws, eventually relying on drug use to resist oppression. The first twin's behavior contributes to her resilience by helping her learn not to give up and to stand up even when under attack. The second twin resists by engaging in drug abuse, which is temporarily empowering within drug using contexts, but disempowering in the larger society (Stanton & Todd, 1982).

Third Order Change

Third order change occurs when there are shifts in how families see the world, allowing them to consider more possibilities for how to understand and negotiate their relationships. Socioculturally attuned brief and strategic therapists co-construct hypotheses with clients that include awareness of the impact of societal context on presenting problems. Raising social awareness helps families realize the impact of these broad social arrangements on their most intimate relationships and more directly and knowingly participate in dismantling incongruent hierarchies and relational patterns. This deeply impacts family rules and collective meaning-making.

↔

Third order change occurs in socioculturally attuned brief and strategic family therapy when families disrupt incongruent societal hierarchies in favor of adopting equity-based relational systems.

↔

Practice Guidelines

Practicing socioculturally attuned brief and strategic family therapy requires thinking beyond the family, broadening the circle of interactions and hypotheses to include power dynamics in societal context. Symptoms are viewed through a lens that considers their value as forms of resistance and symptom-free resistance is supported. Rather than being neutral observers who intervene to remove symptoms, therapists take a number of steps including; 1) broadening the circle, 2) thinking counterintuitively to counter hegemony, 3) including societal power imbalances in hypotheses, 4) affirming symptom-free resistance, and 5) intervening to support just relationships.

1. Broadening the Circle

Socioculturally attuned brief and strategic family therapists expand their view to **attune** to the interconnection of individual thoughts and behaviors, patterns of interaction, cultural lifeways, and societal dynamics. Consider the Bernadines mentioned above who presented with a gambling problem. Treatment for problem gambling is likely to include attention to biological (e.g., chemical changes in the brain, neuro-pathways), psychological (e.g., magical thinking, fantasies of the future), behavioral (e.g., gambling rituals), affective (e.g., emotional triggers), relational (e.g., attachment styles, family patterns around gambling behavior), contextual (e.g., financial issues, allure of gambling contexts), cultural/social (e.g., meaning of money, economic system, definition of success), and existential (e.g., illusion of control, beliefs around chance) considerations (McDowell & Berman, 2016). These areas are not discrete or dichotomous but deeply intertwined. For example, it is not possible to understand the meaning of money, the thought process around gambling, the family's reaction to problem gambling, or the allure of gambling contexts without understanding the society's economic system and cultural definition of luck and success. Even the dopamine released in the brain when taking a gambling risk is influenced by the economic system and the cultural value of wealth.

Circular questioning with the Bernadines from a socioculturally attuned framework that includes the larger context might continue as follows:

Therapist: I am thinking about why so often in families moms seem to carry most of the worry. Tom, what do you think most people would say if I asked them why women seem to worry a lot about everyone else?
Tom: I think most people would say that's just what mothers do.
Therapist: And what do you think they would say about fathers?
Tom: Well, I think most people would say fathers care a lot about their families too but just show it in different ways...working...doing things for the family.
Therapist: Mavis, if I were to ask your brother Mark the same questions, what would he most likely say?
Mavis: Well, Mark just stays out of things.
Therapist: Yes, of course, I notice he didn't come today (everyone laughs). But if you were to venture a guess, what might he say if he were here?
Mavis: I think Mark and I both go to mom when we need things because she is more likely to understand, so maybe she just knows us better and so worries more.
Therapist: Mavis what do you think your friends would say about the role of women being caretakers in the family?
Mavis: Most of my friends are not so interested in doing that. They want partners who will be more equal and to be able to do more of what they want to do.
Therapist: And your mom's friends? What might they say?
Mavis: I don't think they like it, but maybe they would say they are stuck being the ones who hold the family together. Most of them do a lot of making sure everyone else is O.K.—especially their husbands (laughs).

By broadening questions to include social discourse, the therapist was able to **name** and pursue gender and power dynamics within and beyond the family.

2. Think Counterintuitively to Counter Hegemony

According to Brown (2010), circular thinking must include therapists' awareness of their own beliefs and values as well as the impact of dominant social discourses on families and presenting problems. Being able to take a metaview of dominant social discourses and the dynamics of broad societal systems allows therapists to develop the critical consciousness necessary to think counter hegemonically as well as counter intuitively. We use the term hegemony to refer to mechanisms that maintain the status quo of unequal power distribution in society through social, political, economic, and ideological control. This includes, but goes beyond, the concept of dominant discourses to include laws, corporate and educational practices, social services, and so on. The therapist's critical awareness contributes significantly to how problems are framed and consciousness raising takes on a more central role in creating third order change. The therapist **values** sources of resilience and previously silenced voices of resistance. This is exemplified in the case illustration below as the family and therapist work together to raise critical consciousness in order to develop a hypothesis that is socioculturally attuned.

3. Include Societal Power Imbalances in Hypothesis

Socioculturally attuned brief and strategic therapy expand hypotheses to include societal power dynamics. Children typically have less power and responsibility than their parents. Power imbalances, however, are not part of the natural order of adult relationships. Viewing power imbalances as existing solely within the boundaries of families tends to pathologize individual relationships and limit how we are able to **intervene.** Consider a European American family in which there is an aging parent living with an adult child and two adolescent grandchildren. The rest of the family talks only to each other and frequently overlooks the grandparent when making plans. The grandparent is expected to go along with whatever decisions are made. This family is deeply influenced by a youth-oriented culture that devalues those who are no longer have social capital and power. If the grandparent is female and less than fully able-bodied, the power imbalance worsens as the family is likely to unintentionally act out the ageism, sexism, and ableism of dominant US society. The family enters treatment because the grandparent is having angry outbursts. If the therapist non-reflexively shares the worldview that older adults are worth less than younger adults and children, they are likely to view the grandparent's outbursts as a symptom of adjusting to old age rather than societal dynamics impacting the family.

4. Affirm Symptom-free Resistance

Resistance is a healthy response to oppression. Strategies for resistance may be quite varied, including withdrawing physically or emotionally, standing up and speaking out, yielding in order to get through oppressive situations, and trying to understand in order to navigate power dynamics (McDowell 2004). Socioculturally attuned family therapists are in a position to help clients **envision** ways to strategize against oppression in ways that don't cause them further harm.

Consider a firefighter who was the only female in her rural station. Her co-workers referred to her as an opportunity hire and excluded her from chances to perform. She was in a relationship with a man who shared the traditional gender role expectations of her family of origin and most of her community. She was referred to therapy by a physician after exhaustive tests could not determine a physical cause for her inability to swallow food. The therapist gathered information about all of the client's relationships before hypothesizing that the psychosomatic symptom was a metaphor of the client's resistance to being overpowered. The client and therapist began exploring dynamics in the client's life that she was "not willing to swallow." Identifying the oppression and attempts to resist oppression was a powerful consciousness-raising intervention. The client joined a group for women in male dominated workplaces that the therapist started after seeing many women in the community dealing with similar dynamics. Over time, the therapist, women in the group, and the client developed alternative approaches to resisting oppressive situations.

5. Support Just Relationships

It is not possible for a therapist to be neutral in the face of power imbalances (Knudson-Martin, 2013). If a therapist fails to address relational inequity, he unwittingly contributes to it by default. On the other hand, if the therapist encourages shared power, he may be criticized for promoting his own agenda. This would seem to be an impossible ethical bind if it were not for the fact that power imbalances often create and maintain the very symptoms the therapist and family are trying to eliminate (McDowell, 2015). From this perspective, the therapist is obligated to address what is harming the family. As noted above, therapy is not a zero-sum game (Nardone & Watzlawick, 2005). Shifting the power from the oppressor to the oppressed is not a successful outcome, as it maintains a power-over system that will continue to be problematic.

•←→•

Transformative action requires socioculturally attuned therapists to be aware of the impact of societal systems on all family members, including those who are acting in oppressive ways.

•←→•

Case Illustration

Tiana (age 16) comes to family therapy with her brother, James (age 10), and parents, Brandon (age 40) and Kisha (age 42). The family lives in a relatively safe middle-class neighborhood. All family members identify as Black, cishet (cisgender heterosexual), and able-bodied. Brandon and Kisha met 20 years prior while in college. Brandon grew up in a working-class family in which most of the men were in the building trades. Kisha's parents were upper-middle class and held important positions in the government. Tiana and James are both doing well in a private, Roman Catholic school. The family entered treatment with Ladonna, who works for Catholic Community Services. Ladonna identifies as a Black, cishet woman. She grew up living in relative poverty, however, her professional career now provides a stable middle-class income. The family explains to Ladonna that they are experiencing growing conflict.

During their initial visit, James responds to Ladonna's question about why the family came to therapy by resentfully stating, "My SISTER yells all the time." Brandon glances at James with a slight grin. Kisha interrupts with "There is too much fighting between everyone," glancing at James with a disapproving brow. The family describes a repetitive pattern of conflict. They offer a typical example in which Brandon makes a demand of Tiana (e.g., go close the door, fold this laundry), Tiana ignores her father, Brandon repeats the demand in an angry tone, James offers to do the chore ("I'll do it dad!"), then Brandon tells him to stay out of it and pursues Tiana, repeating his demand in an angry, physically threatening tone and posture. Kisha intervenes by asking him to calm down, while Tiana screams at her father as she withdraws to her room. Kisha tells Brandon that he can't just "boss her around! She is almost 17!" Brandon withdraws in anger until James comes and sits on his lap.

Broadening the Circle

The pattern of interaction described above seems relatively straightforward. At first glance, it appears to be a simple case of a teenager acting out and parents needing to agree on how to parent together as a team. Part of the problem, however, is that parents disagree on how strict to be with their daughter and Kisha disapproves of Brandon's approach. Brandon is not easily influenced by Kisha and despite her cautions, continues what Kisha considers overly aggressive parenting of their daughter. When Ladonna explores other areas of the parents' relationship, she discovers this is a pattern. Brandon is far more likely to influence Kisha than Kisha is to influence Brandon. Kisha frequently attempts to persuade Brandon to see her perspective, but is left feeling she is the one who must accommodate him.

Ladonna broadens the circle by exploring race, gender, and social class dynamics in society and how these dynamics impact this particular family. Expectations that Kisha will accommodate Brandon based on gender overshadow her coming from a higher social class background and are, in part, a response to the lack of respect Kisha knows Brandon experiences as a Black man in the broader society. For example, despite his competence, Brandon was not promoted as quickly from superintendent to project manager as his male counterparts in his White-dominated construction firm. Internally he is always on guard, careful not to upset others, knowing that men like him are often viewed by White people as dangerous. At home, he feels more entitled to relax his guard and expect obedience. Kisha wishes Brandon would treat Tiana less harshly, yet knowing he is often denigrated outside the home, she tends to protect his status in the family (Cowdery et al., 2009). Ladonna also explored differences in societal expectations, issues of safety, and avenues for success for Tiana and James as young Black women and men in the current US context.

Thinking Counterintuitively to Counter Hegemony

When family members' actions didn't attain the desired result, they repeated them anyway because they made sense. When Brandon made a demand of Tiana and she didn't comply, he continued with more of the same, repeating his demands more forcefully. Kisha repeatedly attempted to get Brandon to understand using the same arguments each time she was frustrated with how he was approaching their daughter. And so on, with each member of the family repeating the same type of common-sense response even though nothing changes. Thinking counterintuitively includes considering what message this problem pattern may be communicating and how the problem may be balancing an incongruent hierarchy.

↞↠

Thinking in ways that counter hegemony includes considering how family communication may reflect imbalances of power on a societal level.

↞↠

When Ladonna asks Brandon more about his concern over his daughter not doing as he asks, he explains that he "only asks her to do a few simple things!"

Ladonna: So you don't ask much of your daughter.
Brandon: No. Plus, what I tell her to do isn't difficult. Just keep the house up, help her mom with the dishes…
Ladonna: Really basic stuff.
Brandon: Yes, what I tell her to do is easy.

Ladonna recognizes Brandon's response as one that perpetuates female dependency and underachievement. She is especially concerned because she is keenly aware of the myth of the Black matriarch that can dismiss the ways Black women lack power (Hill, 2005). She goes on to challenge this societally informed belief.

Ladonna: Actually, that concerns me a little.
Brandon: What, that it's easy!
Ladonna: Well yes. Mom, what do you think Tiana is capable of doing?
Kisha: She is a pretty competent young woman. She gets good grades, is on the student council at school, helps me teach preschool on Sundays at our church. He's right. What we expect of her at home isn't much.
Ladonna: Tiana, is your mom right?
Tiana: I guess so. I just don't like being bossed around all the time!
Ladonna: I am wondering why your parents don't expect more of you. (Tiana rolls her eyes.) No, I don't mean more time or more tasks, but things that are harder to do…more fitting to your abilities. You are almost 17, right? Next year is your last year in high school…then what?
Tiana: I am going to college.
Ladonna: So Mom and Dad, what are you hoping she will learn from you in the next year before she goes to college?
Brandon: To be responsible so she can take care of herself.
Kisha: Well that, yes. And to be confident. She is a good person. I want her to hold onto herself and her values when she gets out on her own.

Ladonna continues to explore expectations for Tiana to be grown up; to take care of herself, make good decisions, and "stand up for what she believes in." Tiana agrees this is what she wants for herself and for her brother when he grows up. Brandon was stuck in a common sense, self-perpetuating cycle of asking less and less of his daughter in more and more demanding ways. He inadvertently undervalued his daughter's abilities and dismissed his wife's concerns and advice. He also used anger and aggression as a means to get what he wanted. Ladonna was thinking counterintuitively when suggesting parents ask their daughter to do more difficult tasks rather than doing less. If Ladonna would have simply encouraged Brandon to treat his daughter in a more developmentally appropriate way, (e.g., give her tasks for the week that she completes as she has time) she would be joining mom's voice and either be dismissed as another female in the therapeutic system or be demonstrating that she had more influence over Brandon's decision than did Kisha.

Ladonna was also setting the stage to counter patriarchy. Expecting too little of a 16-year-old daughter reflects low expectations for young adult females. Tiana was obviously capable of more adult contributions to the family. Ladonna engaged the family in discussions about what they wanted their daughter to be able to do as a Black female in society. Brandon agreed that he wanted his daughter to have the same rights and say in her life as men. This opened the door to talking about the couple's gendered relationships in which Brandon had more say than anyone else in the family and how this pattern inside the family might be exacerbated by racism that takes a toll on the whole family. Ladonna led the family in a discussion about how that came about, the cost to the family relationships, and what they envisioned instead.

Including Societal Power Dynamics in Hypothesis

The socioculturally attuned therapist working with this family began by asking questions that helped the family work with her to hypothesize how what was going on within the family reflected broader societal dynamics. The family was caught in an incongruent hierarchy found more generally in society and played out across many specific contexts in their lives. For example, Kisha and Brandon worked for the same company and had the same educational background. Both experienced being routinely marginalized by White peers, building customers, and company owners as the only two Black employees. The company was also highly organized around gender. The office employed only women, and only men worked in the field. While both Kisha and Brandon held highly skilled leadership positions in the company, the women in the office were frequently diminished and dismissed by male employees who (unlike Brandon) put off requests to complete paperwork, referred to getting "nag mail" from the office, and circulated sexist jokes.

Ladonna and the family worked together to develop a hypothesis that included a gendered power imbalance shaped by broader societal racial dynamics that left dad making unilateral decisions and exerting power. This dynamic cost dad some of his connection with his wife and oldest daughter. His use of aggression came at a particularly high price as family members sometimes accommodated out of fear. James joined dad's side, which also cost him closeness with his mother and sister and perpetuated the privilege sons sometimes have in African American households due to their lack of advantage in the larger society (Hill, 2005). Tiana needed to learn to stand up for herself in a context in which males continue to have greater privilege and expect women to accommodate them. Kisha and Brandon needed to learn, and demonstrate for their children, the ability to share equal influence in a world that marginalized each of them in different ways. This is in keeping with Madanes' (2006) reference to therapy as a place where resistance to the status quo can be acknowledged and supported (see Text Box 6.3).

Text Box 6.3 Cloé Madanes

Cloé Madanes is one of the developers of the strategic approach. According to her (Madanes, 2006):

Within each therapy client stirs a rebellious heart, a desire to challenge the status quo. Therapy is a forum for thoughts and feelings that are often considered to be unacceptable, antisocial, unsafe or dangerous to the morality and good order. (p. 6)

Affirming Symptom-free Resistance

The therapist in this situation affirmed the parents' desire to make certain their daughter was prepared for adulthood. This included, among other things, being able to take responsibility and complete difficult tasks independently. Ladonna, Kisha, and Brandon needed to guide Tiana in how to resist gender and racial oppression, including how to "stand up for what she believes in" as a young Black woman. She also affirmed Brandon's desire to be connected, Kisha's right to have equal say in what happens in the family, and the need for James to not have to take sides. Kisha, Brandon, and Tiana agreed on chores that were more challenging, would help prepare her for adulthood, and that she could fit into her busy schedule. This included helping her father change the oil in their cars, doing the weekly grocery shopping for the family, and giving her brother a ride at least three times a week.

Ladonna and the parents agreed to help Tiana practice asserting herself in effective and respectful ways. Dad agreed to make arbitrary demands of Tiana from time to time without the use of a loud voice or physically aggressive posture. Tiana agreed to respectfully decline or offer a time when she would be able to accommodate the request. Mom was then to review Tiana's efforts, coaching her as needed. Anyone in the family who noticed Brandan sharing power by thinking about others first, asking instead of demanding, or negotiating respectfully, was to warmly approach him and give him a kiss on the cheek. This strategic intervention prescribed the symptom but in ways that supported a shift toward greater connection and equality in the family.

Supporting Just Relationships

This family presented a relatively simple problem, but one that reflected a much broader social and family dynamic. By supporting just relationships, the therapist was able to help the family remove the symptom, but not without first recognizing the symptom as a form of resistance. In other words, the symptom revealed the *need* for third order change, while also providing strategic *leverage* for change.

Summary: Third Order Change

The family in the above illustration engaged in first, second, and third order change. Changing the types of chores Tiana was asked to do was a form of first order change. This intervention alone would not lead to second order or process level change, which is qualitative and discontinuous, altering the system's rules, structure, and/or order (Watzlawick et al., 1974). Changing the meaning of Tiana's refusal to comply with doing chores on demand from a form of rebellion to a necessary skill for adulthood led the way for second order change. Second order change included Kisha having more equal say in parenting and Tiana being supported by both parents in more developmentally appropriate ways.

Text Box 6.4 Cloé Madanes

Cloé Madanes stated the following at the end of a video recorded in 2008:

I have come to see that family injustice is the root cause of pathology and that for therapy to be effective, it must bring justice to the family. Sometimes injustice comes from outside the family and then the therapist must work on bringing justice from society to the family.

Third order change occurred in this family when there were major shifts in how they saw the world (Ecker & Hulley, 1996). The family was able to consider more possibilities for how to organize their relationships when they were able to take a metaview of gender, race, and power in society. This helped them realize the impact of these broad social arrangements on their most intimate relationships and to make more conscious choices about how they wanted to live. The therapist invited the family into third order change by working with them to develop a hypothesis that included awareness of the impact of societal context on the family's presenting problem. This, in turn, led to *further* second order change as they altered family rules about the meaning and impact of gender in relationship to influence and competence. We end this chapter with another quote from Madanes in Text Box 6.4.

Reflexive Questions

- How can taking a metaview of dominant social discourses and dynamics of broad societal systems help you develop the critical consciousness necessary to think in counter-hegemonic ways, as well as counter intuitively?
- What impact would having this metaview and critical consciousness have on you personally and professionally?
- If you were to think counter intuitively, how could this help you counter the effects of hegemony?
- Can you recall a time when you included power imbalances in your hypothesis of a presenting problem and in your analysis of what sustained it?
- What would it mean for you to encourage symptom-free resistance, for yourself and for your clients?
- What would it mean for you as a strategic family therapist if you were able to name the injustices coming from outside the family and work to bring justice from society to the family, as Madanes suggests?

References

Afuape, T. (2011). *Power, resistance and liberation in therapy with survivors of trauma: To have our hearts broken*. Routledge.

Al-Mannai, S. (2010) The misinterpretation of women's status in the Muslim world. *Digest of Middle East Studies*, *19*(1), 82–91.

Amorin-Woods, D. & Selvini, M. (2023). The influence of the Milan approach: Five decades of intergenerational change. A conversation with Matteo Selvini. *Australian New Zealand Journal of Family Therapy*, *44*, 108–121.

Atkinson, B. (2005). *Emotional intelligence in couples therapy: Advances from neurobiology and the science of intimate relationships*. WW Norton.

Barbetta, P. & Telfener, U. (2020). The Milan approach, history, and evolution. *Family Process*, *60*, 4–16.

Boscolo, L., Cecchin, G., Hoffman, L., & Penn, P. (1987). *Milan systemic family therapy: Theoretical and practical aspects*. Harper & Row.
Bourdieu, P. (1986). The forms of capital. In J. G. Richardson (Ed.). *Handbook of theory and research for the sociology of education* (pp. 241–258). Greenwood Press.
Brown, J. (2010). The Milan principles of hypothesizing, circularity and neutrality in dialogical family therapy: Extinction, evolution, eviction…or emergence. *The Australian and New Zealand Journal of Family Therapy, 31*(3), 248–265.
Codecá, L., Russon, J., & Selvini, M. (2024). The systemic-family-individual approach: The heritage and continuation of Mara Selvini Palazzoli's work in integrative psychotherapy. *Journal of marital and family therapy, 50*(3), 706–725.
Cowdery, R., Scarborough, N., Knudson-Martin, C., Lewis, M., Seshadri, G., & Mahoney, A. (2009). Gendered power in cultural contexts part II: Middle class African American heterosexual couples with young children. *Family Process, 48*, 25–39.
de Shazer, S. (1982). *Patterns of brief family therapy*. The Guilford Press.
Ecker, B. & Hully, L. (1996). *Depth-oriented brief therapy: How to be brief when you were trained to be deep–and vice versa*. Jossey-Bass.
Fraser, J. S. (2020). The evolution of a point of view: The enduring personal influence of the mental research institute. *Journal of Systemic Therapies, 39*(2), 51–63.
Goldner, V. (1993). Power and hierarchy: Let's talk about it! *Family Process, 32*, 157–162.
Goldner, V. (1985). Feminism and family therapy. *Family Process, 24*, 31–47.
Goodrich, T., Rampage, C. Ellman, B., & Halstead, K (1988), *Feminist family therapy: A casebook*. Penguin Books.
Haley, J. (1984) *Ordeal therapy: Unusual ways to change behavior*. Jossey-Bass.
Haley, J. (1980). *Leaving home: The therapy of disturbed young people*. McGraw-Hill.
Haley, J. (1976) *Problem-solving therapy: New strategies for effective family therapy*. Jossey-Bass.
Haley, J. (1973) *Uncommon therapy: The psychiatric techniques of Milton H. Erickson, M.D.* Norton.
Hill, S. A. (2005). *Black intimacies: A gender perspective on families and relationships*. AltaMira Press.
Hoffman, L. (1985). Beyond power and control: Toward a "second order" family systems therapy. *Family Systems Medicine, 3*(A), 381–396.
Jackson, J. B. & Landers, A. L. (2020). Structural and strategic approaches. In K. S. Wampler, R. B. Miller, & R. B. Seedall (Eds.). *The handbook of systemic family therapy* (Vol. 1, pp. 339–364).
James, K. & McIntyre, D. (1983). The reproduction of families: The social role of family therapy? *Journal of Marital and Family Therapy, 9*, 119–129.
Knudson-Martin, C. (2013). Why power matters: Creating a foundation of mutual support in couple relationships. *Family Process, 52*(1), 5–18.
Lockhart, E. N. S. (2024). Increasing transgender acceptance in religious families: A pilot study of manualized strategic family therapy. *International Journal of Systemic Therapy*, 1–34.
Madanes, C. (2008, December 11). *Part 2*. [Video file]. Retrieved on Feb 18, 2022 from https://www.youtube.com/watch?v=u6F_zKB7S9Y.
Madanes, C. (2006). *The Therapist as humanist, social activist, and systemic thinker: And other selected papers*. Zeig, Tucker, & Theisen.
Madanes, C. (1984). *Behind the one-way mirror: Advances in the practice of strategic therapy*. Jossey Bass.
Madanes, C. (1981). *Strategic family therapy*. Jossey Bass.
McDowell, T. (2015). *Applying critical social theory to the practice of family therapy*. AFTA SpringerBriefs in Family Therapy, Springer.
McDowell, T. (2004). Exploring the racial experiences of graduate trainees: A critical race theory perspective. *The American Journal of Family Therapy, 32*(4), 305–324.
McDowell, T. & Berman, E. (2016). *Best of both worlds: Integrating relational models into problem gambling treatment*. National Council on Problem Gambling conference, Tarrytown, NY, USA.
McDowell, T. & Kabura, P. (2016). Humanitarianism, colonization, and/or collaboration? Working together in Uganda and the United States. In L.L. Charlés & G. Samarasinghe (Eds.). *Family therapy in global humanitarian contexts* (pp. 27–37). AFTA SpringerBriefs in Family Therapy. Springer.
Nardone, G. & Watzlawick, P. (2005). *Brief strategic therapy: Philosophy, techniques, and research*. Jason Aronson.
Parrott, L., Alexander, P., Kawano, T. & Harrison, K. (2026). Queer-contextualized strategic family therapy. In E. Hartwell & L. Edwards (Eds.). *Queer Contextualized Family Therapy*, (pp. 50–72). Routledge.

Palazzoli Selvini M., Boscolo, L. Cecchin, G., & Prata, G. (1980). Hypothesizing— circularity—neutrality: Three guidelines for the conductor of the session. *Family Process*, *19*(1), 3–12.
Ray, W., Trappeniers, E., & Hale, D., (2019). Point of view matters: Seeing, hearing and acting in systemic practice. *Journal of Family Psychotherapy*, *30*(2), 61–75.
Rhodes, P. (2012). Post-Milan systemic therapy. In A. Rambo, C. West, A. Schooley, & T. Boyd (Eds.). *Family therapy review: Contrasting Contemporary Models*, pp. 136–140. Routledge.
Selvini-Palazzoli, M. & Viaro, M. (1988). The anorectic process in the family: A six-stage model as a guide for individual therapy. *Family Process*, *27*(2), 129–148.
Soederberg, S. (2013) The politics of debt and development in the new millennium: An Introduction. *Third World Quarterly*, *34*(4), 535–546.
Stanton, M. & Todd, T. (Eds.). (1982). *The family therapy of drug abuse and addiction*. Guilford Press.
Szapocznik, J. & Herivs, O. (2020). *Brief Strategic Family Therapy*. American Psychological Association.
Vitry, G., de Scorraille, C., Hoyt, M. (2021). Redundant attempted solutions: 50 years of theory, evolution, and new supporting data. *Australian and New Zealand Journal of Family Therapy*, *42*, 174–187.
Watzlawick, P., Beavin Bavelas, J., & Jackson, D. (1967). *Pragmatics of human Communication: A study of interactional patterns, pathologies, and paradoxes*. WW Norton.
Watzlawick, P., Weakland, J., & Fisch, R. (1974). *Change: principles of problem formation and problem resolution*. WW Norton.

7 Socioculturally Attuned Experiential Family Therapy

Joel, age 16, slouches in a chair in the therapy room with arms folded scowling at the floor. Joel's mother is animated as she explains her concerns about her son. Joel's father looks away, obviously frustrated with both his son and wife. Their therapist searches for ways to help the family express their thoughts and feelings to each other, with her own anxiety triggered by the family's fear that they cannot withstand hearing each other's true feelings. An experiential therapist in this situation moves toward the unexpressed emotion that the family seems to be avoiding, helping family members explore their inner worlds and express themselves to each other. Her goal is to make room for growth by encouraging family members to listen and have empathy for each other—to attune to each other. Discovering and sharing authentic experience shifts the way the family thinks, feels, and relates to each other. As a result, they become more connected, genuine, authentic, and flexible as they demonstrate the ability to tolerate individual desires, fears, anxieties, hopes, and dreams.

Experiential therapy emerged from existential humanism during the 1950s and 1960s and was developed primarily by Virginia Satir (1967) and Carl Whitaker (Napier & Whitaker, 1978.) Satir focused on communication and positive human potential, while Whitaker concentrated on the symbolic nature of family interaction. They were both charismatic, relying on their ability to be fully present to guide families into new and genuine experiences. Whitaker was well known for sharing stories from his own life and making playful, even absurd interventions that symbolized what was going on in the family and/or created temporary chaos to help the family reorganize without symptoms. The impact of Satir's use of self—her warmth, intuition, and authenticity—was sometimes referred to as magic (Banmen & Maki-Banmen, 2014). Many doubted the ability to reproduce experiential therapy as a model because it seemed to rely so heavily on the self-of-the-therapist rather than theory and technique. Nonetheless, Whitaker and Satir inspired generations of therapists to be hopeful and positive about human potential; to trust growth as an inevitable outcome of honest self-exploration and emotional expression, to rely on the transformative power of therapeutic experiences, and to use self-of-the-therapist in genuine and authentic ways.

The application of experiential ideas to therapy continues to expand. Today, in part in response to neurological findings regarding how the body responds to emotional pain and the role of affect in creating change, a growing number of integrative models incorporate an experiential approach to change (Hargrave & Houltberg, 2020; Johnson, 2019; Knudson-Martin & Kim, 2022; Taylor, et al., 2021; Zimmerman, 2018). Experiential techniques have also been integrated with specific family therapy models (Sohn et al., 2024) and widely used across models to engage children in family therapy (Barker et al., 2019; Dumont, 2008). Clinicians are also studying how to creatively utilize experiential interventions to bring a therapeutic presence to teletherapy (Heiden-Rootes et al., 2021; Taylor et al., 2021).

DOI: 10.4324/9781003493426-7

Third order change in experiential family therapy involves the family going beyond understanding each other within an intimate relational framework to awareness of the impact of societal forces on their experience and the experience of those around them.

•←→•

Third order change in socioculturally attuned experiential family therapy requires identifying, putting into words, sharing, and hearing felt experiences of the effects of societal power imbalances, such as marginalization, oppression, and privilege.

•←→•

In this chapter, we describe some enduring family therapy concepts and practices related to experiential family therapy and illustrate how therapists can integrate principles of sociocultural attunement into experiential approaches to broaden awareness of self and others in societal context. We argue that it is not possible to fully understand ourselves—how we think, feel, and act—without realizing the impact of culture, societal systems, and power dynamics on our everyday lives. To this end, we offer a set of guidelines for considering human potential within societal context and explore the role of power dynamics in emotion and emotional expression. We conclude with a case example that demonstrates these principles.

Primary, Enduring Family Therapy Concepts

The focus in experiential therapies is on each individual within a family system. Having multiple members of a family participate in therapy, including more than one generation, offers the therapist greater leverage for change and provides the family with greater continuity. The family system is seen as blocking or supporting individual expressions that drive self-actualization and growth, which in turn weakens or strengthens the family as a whole (Edwards, 2026). The approach focuses on the present, expecting change to occur through therapeutic experiences in the here and now. We have identified four enduring family therapy concepts associated with experiential therapies: 1) communication, 2) sharing emotions, 3) experiential interventions, and 4) therapist's use of self.

Communication

Experiential therapists help family members get in touch with themselves and communicate with each other in ways that are genuine and congruent. According to Satir (1967, p. 63), communication "includes all those symbols and clues used by persons in giving and receiving meaning." This includes verbal and nonverbal expression. It is not uncommon for people to communicate more than one message at the same time, prompting confusion in the message receiver. Accountability for communication is key. Experiential therapists interrupt attempts to send messages without taking responsibility for meaning. For example, one may say "I said I am not angry!" in a tone that clearly sends the message that they are in fact mad. The receiver is likely to believe the way the message is sent over its content but has no way to verify meaning. They are thereby stuck, unable to resolve conflict and difference.

Communication traps like this one derail authentic connection. Take John who won't tell his partner, Emily, what he wants, but becomes annoyed when Emily chooses a restaurant with a long line or goes to bed early on a night John feels amorous. When Emily questions John, he denies that he is unhappy yet remains quiet, withdrawn, and sullen. In a situation like this, an experiential therapist would encourage Emily and John to identify and accept their individual desires, hopes, anxieties, and frustrations, helping them put their thoughts and feelings into words. The therapist might ask the couple to demonstrate or communicate about their relationship through an experiential exercise. For example, she might ask them to sit back-to-back and talk to each other so their facial expressions can't be used to relay unclaimed messages. Or she might use a story from her own life, perhaps telling them about trying to understand what her preverbal toddler needs and how upset he gets when she guesses incorrectly.

Experiential therapy promotes democratic ideals of all family members deserving their own yearnings, choices, feelings, and needs, which they have the right and responsibility to clearly communicate. These approaches tend to expect communication and understanding to lead to agreement and the meeting of all family members' needs equally. However, while their attention to process can help facilitate more equitable interaction, there has historically been little direct attention to the relationship between power dynamics and communication in experiential approaches.

Processing and Sharing Emotions

Experiential therapists help people identify their emotions and then communicate them effectively. Consider Lars, a 70-year-old Norwegian American, Vietnam veteran, who is being cared for by his adult daughter, Vina. They come to therapy because Vina is "at her wit's end" with her father being cross and demanding. She agreed that he could move into her home, and she wants to be a good and caring daughter. She reports, however, that no matter what she does, Lars "refuses to be happy." During the therapeutic conversation, the therapist, Greta, notices a moment when Lars becomes quiet and puts his head in his hands.

Greta: Lars, what are you experiencing right now?
Lars: I am just listening. [looks up]
Greta: I noticed for a moment you looked down and put your head in your hands. What are you feeling as your daughter talks about you being difficult to please?
Lars: I don't know. Nothing.
Vina: That's the trouble dad! You don't care what I have to say.
Greta: Vina, how do you feel when your father turns away from you like that?
Vina: Angry! Hurt! Pissed off!
Greta: Lars, let's take a moment…I am going to ask you to help me here.
Lars: Okay.
Greta: (stands up, walks over to Lars and sits next to him.) Will you put your head in your hands and look down like you did a moment ago?

Lars follows the therapist's instructions and sits quietly.

Greta: (Lowers her tone and moves in close to Lars.) What are you feeling in your body right now? In your back, legs, stomach, heart, arms…
Lars: I don't know. I guess my chest is tight. (pause) Maybe I am having trouble swallowing.
Greta: So you're tight in your chest and throat. How about your head and hands?
Lars: I just want to disappear.
Greta: Your throat and chest get tight, and you want to hide…disappear. Can you name the feeling associated with that? Could it be hurt, anger, embarrassment, shame, disappointment, fear…?
Lars: (With heads still in hands) Maybe shame.
Greta: So shame…anything else (allows a pause)
Lars: Disappointment in myself.
Greta: (in a low and caring tone) That sounds really difficult, Lars—those feelings of being ashamed and disappointed in yourself.

Greta accepted that Lars had trouble accessing and naming his emotions. Vina was quickly able to identify emotions but not able to effectively share them in part because her father refused to listen and acknowledge hearing her. Feelings need to be both expressed and validated. Vina's frustration came from having to guess what her father thought and felt. She assumed he did not care when he reported not feeling anything. By slowing down the interaction, warmly supporting Lars while challenging him to identify and express himself, Greta was able to create a new experience. This moment of understanding would need to be followed and expanded over time for there to be the type of change needed for Lars and Vina to support each other in being their most authentic selves.

Greta did not address the context or power differences between Lars and Vina. Vina had a lifetime of being the daughter of a demanding and difficult father. She was a female and expected to be a caregiver who accommodated her father's wishes. Lars was a Vietnam veteran with untreated trauma and shame, which he held tightly inside. As a White cishet (cisgender heterosexual) male, he expected others to simply deal with his moods. He had never stopped to really think about his daughter's experience of him or the sacrifices she made to assume his care. Lars was a second-generation Norwegian American who was raised to keep his emotions intact and unexpressed. Military training and being socialized as a male in his generation strongly supported that mandate.

Satir (Banmen & Maki-Banmen, 2014) made the point that it is not just our feelings that are important but how we feel about our feelings. She argued that we are often disappointed in ourselves or ashamed of our feelings. We try to dismiss, change, or hide how we feel from others rather than fully exploring and expressing ourselves. This prevents our growth and leads to convoluted communication. Let's go back to the example of John and Vina. John struggles with telling Vina what he wants and also with how he feels when his needs aren't met. This is due, in part, to John wanting to please his daughter. He rejects his own needs to be the kind of person who puts his family's needs first. When this leads to his feeling irritated, frustrated, or disappointed, John is displeased with his own emotion and attempts to deny how he truly feels to himself and others. Vina then presses him to share his thoughts and feelings, eventually becoming frustrated herself. Now John is even more unhappy as his efforts to be selfless and please Vina have had the opposite effect.

Experiential family therapy highlights emotion without ignoring cognition. In fact, thinking, acting, and feeling are interconnected determinants of our experience. According to Connell, Mitten, and Bumberry (1998), "The goal of symbolic-experiential therapy is to provide an experience that flips the family's way of thinking. It must contaminate their way of perceiving reality and project them into a different way of interpreting and embracing life" (p. 2). Experiential therapists differ in their emphasis on helping clients connect their present emotions and experiences with the past. For example, Whitaker did not think clients needed to understand the current or historical cause of a problem to solve it, while Satir encouraged clients to become increasingly aware of themselves and to explore the lasting impact of childhood family of origin experiences.

Experiential Interventions

Experiential interventions are part of the process of therapy that unfolds as families talk about their situations, relationships, and experiences. The therapist takes the lead in structuring and guiding the therapeutic system toward growth that will resolve symptoms, rather than setting specific goals with the family at the beginning of the encounter. The therapist assumes positive outcomes will occur as a result of the therapeutic process; that given the right conditions, humans grow into their full, symptom-free potential.

Experiential family therapists take an active role in ensuring conditions for growth are met through identifying and sharing feelings and experiences. According to Napier and Whitaker (1978), "the therapist must win the battle for structure" while ensuring "the family takes the initiative for change" (p. 10). The therapist must be able to facilitate what happens in therapy, but the therapist must not be more motivated for change than the clients. It is the family's motivation that drives change. In other words, the therapist must be in charge of the process and engage fully as part of the therapeutic system without knowing the outcome of interventions.

Experiential therapists guide families through experiences that prompt awareness of self in relationship to others. Many forms of expression are available, including, but not limited to, movement, use of space and found objects, dance, drawing, and sculpting. Demonstrating rather than simply discussing family dynamics provides avenues for understanding through embodied experience and felt memory. Family sculpting is one of the most common experiential techniques (Papp et al., 2013). The therapist asks a family member to place others and themselves in the room in relationship to each other. For example, the therapist helps the sculptor decide where the family members are in relation to each other; who is in the middle and who is outside; who is turned inward and who is turned away; who is up on a stool and who is lying on the floor; and so on. She also helps the sculptor determine if someone should have a fist facing up, a hand facing out, or a head facing down, for example. No interpretations are solicited. Once all are "in place," the therapist moves from one to another, inviting the felt experience of being in the position each has been placed. The position of each person symbolizes the family dynamics from the sculptor's perspective.

Sculpting provides a way to begin to physically see how power, emotional distance, closeness, protection, and other reactions and relational dynamics are enacted. All are held in place in the family sculpture, listening to others' experiences from the positions they hold in the family. Family members do not always see the dynamics in the same way, and more than one sculpt can be completed to explore each other's perspectives. For example, consider a family in which the father often became loud, stood up, and moved toward his wife and children when he wanted his way. The therapist asked the family to engage in a sculpt of these situations, slowly and carefully exploring each family member's experience and emotions during these moments. When the sculpt was completed, the father sank into his chair in shock, stating, "I had no idea I was frightening them!" Even though he consistently relied on creating fear in those around him to get them to do what he wanted, it became clear through sculpting that he did not fully understand what their experience was like or the relational cost of his use of power.

Therapist's Use of Self

According to Roberts (2005), experiential therapy relies heavily on self-disclosure "as a way to mold shifting boundaries, help subjectivity to emerge, and add effect" (p. 51). This requires therapists to be diligent in dealing with their own self-awareness; their own emotional and relational health. Therapists must guide the therapeutic process while being open to experiencing therapeutic encounters. This includes being able to tolerate intense emotions in oneself and others. Consider entering a room with parents whose teenager had recently ended her life. Most of us would be filled with a sense of dread around the emotions we will encounter. Experiential work requires us to move in close to even the most painful experiences and honor the humanity of all involved. This is possible in part by viewing emotions as natural, helpful, and potentially healing. As Connell and colleagues (1998, p. 28) argued, "pain is not the enemy." From this perspective, attempting to help others simply feel better short circuits the growth process.

Experiential therapists are authentic, using themselves in a variety of ways. They might share a feeling they are having while in the room with a family, making a statement like "I am feeling some anger and I don't know where it is coming from. Is anyone feeling angry?" In this situation, the therapist points to what is already in the room, using their own experience and taking the kind of chance they expect clients to take. Experiential therapists might use images that come to them while sitting with clients to suggest the symbolic nature of family interactions. For example, a therapist might say, "I keep getting this picture popping in my head. I don't know if this makes sense or helps us at all, but I am envisioning the two of you in combat gear, dusty and tired, arm in arm coming out of a combat zone."

Likewise, they might use hunches to interpret things like family drawings (Dumont, 2008). Consider a family in which a 9-year-old boy is described by parents as being severely depressed. The therapist asks the boy and his 7-year-old brother to draw a picture of the family that includes each family member doing something while she talks with the mother and father. When the drawings are complete, the therapist notices the 9-year-old's drawing includes himself pointing at a rat in the corner while the rest of the family looks away. This prompts the therapist to turn to the family and ask, "who else feels depressed?" The mother looks at the father, who responds, "I do." Once the 9-year-old gets everyone to look at the rat, he is free to feel better, leaving the therapist in charge of helping his dad.

According to Edwards (2026), experiential therapists, particularly those working from Satir's model, which centers authenticity, must be aware of the incongruencies many clients are forced to live with due to homophobia, cisnormativity, racism, sexism, xenophobia, ableism, and gender essentialism. Edwards further suggested that therapists must be aware of their own moments of incongruence when hiding aspects of themselves based on similar social forces.

Interpersonal Neurobiology and Experiential Therapy

While a full discussion of neurobiology and experiential therapy is beyond the scope of this chapter, a brief mention may be helpful. Recent developments in neuroscience have been used to explain the effectiveness of Whitaker's symbolic-experiential family therapy (Roberts & Chafin, 2020) and the experiential approaches of both Whitaker and Satir (Bailey, 2022). Bailey (2022) applied Siegel's work on the triangle of well-being, or brain–mind–relationship, to experiential therapy by exploring key concepts of mind, integration, attunement, memory, and neuroplasticity. This integrative connection goes beyond the notion of a therapeutic alliance, to right-brain reciprocal non-verbal communication between therapists and clients (Schore, 2021). According to Schore, "the key clinical ability of the empathic psychobiologically attuned therapist is not to intellectually understand the [client] but to emotionally listen to and subjectively feel [them]" (p. 14).

Experiential therapists rely heavily on integrity, resonance, authenticity, and attunement; being fully alive and deeply interested in the families with whom they work. This resonance and warmth are foundational to being vulnerable and open to change. Siegel (2020) noted that it is this resonance that allows the human nervous system to connect and feel safe. Through resonance, attunement, exploring memory, and engaging in new and spontaneous experiences (Roberts & Chafin, 2020), experiential therapies have the potential to increase well-being by encouraging families to improve neural plasticity and increase neural and social integration.

This generative experience is relational and systemic, with one person influencing the internal state of the other (Siegel, 2019). Health is based on the ability to sense our connection to relationships and the environment (Siegel, 2023). According to Siegel, "modern culture is not promoting an integrative self, identity, or belonging" (p. 54). When guided by the dominant individualistic power-over value system, experience will reproduce neural pathways that support this view of the world and behavior; however, intentional expanded focus—such as that created by third order thinking—can evolve shared experience and corresponding neural systems that embody a wider sense of belonging, connection, collective meanings, and justice. In Siegel's (2023) words,

↞→↠

Opening our inner awareness to the reality of intraconnection might be the key that helps move us in an integrative direction as a human family on our fragile planet. (p. 266)

↞→↠

Integrating Principles of Socioculturally Attuned Experiential Family Therapy

Experiential therapy relies on humanist assumptions that given a supportive context free of barriers to positive growth, individuals and families can actualize their full potential. Social equity is paramount to individual, family, and group development across all contexts as it assures the widest access to that which promotes health and well-being (e.g., respect, inclusion, opportunity, affirmation of worldview, physical and psychological safety, access to education and health care, right to love whomever you choose, financial security).

Societal Context

↞→↠

Awareness of the impact of societal context on perspectives, feelings, and desires helps individuals and families take initiative to remove and/or better navigate barriers to growth.

↞→↠

Regardless of what is accomplished in therapy, many clients still face racism, sexism, nationism, homophobia, heterosexism, ableism, and poverty. These oppressive and marginalizing forces deeply affect physical, psychological, emotional, and relational health. Awareness of the impact of societal systems can, however, help us see which barriers are movable and how to navigate those that are not. This includes internalized "isms," the negative effects of socially supported relational power imbalances, and adherence to societal norms and expectations that are contrary to our well-being. Huft & Jonathan (2018) provided a pathway for addressing societal context by integrating feminist and experiential practice, in which:

> high value [is] placed on giving space for silenced voices in the therapy room. Therapists invite clients to engage in a transformational process that allows them to explore what voices have been allowed to be visible… The therapist helps the client identify in what ways the voices were systematically silenced, which allows the client to engage in consciousness raising. Ultimately, the goal is to liberate the client from oppressive beliefs that have forced them to reject or silence parts of themselves. (p. 294)

Experience and Broader Societal Context

Socioculturally attuned experiential family therapists recognize the importance of social awareness in the use of contextual self-of-the-therapist. Let's go back to our example in which the therapist, Greta, worked with Lars and Vina. Greta described herself as a second-generation German American. Greta grew up in a German enclave in Ohio, US. As is true for most family therapists, Greta worked extensively on understanding her own family background. For Greta, this included exploring the impact of her German American heritage. She explored her ability to identify, express, and elicit emotions. This included overcoming her initial discomfort in asking others to openly express feelings. Now let's imagine that Greta wants to become more socioculturally attuned, so she engages in additional work on her contextual self-of-the-therapist. This includes learning about the history of the civil rights movement in the US, exploring the impact of power dynamics on gender roles, understanding historical and contemporary identity movements, learning about the politics of war over the past century, and analyzing how societal systems such as patriarchy, social class, democracy, and colonization affect intimate family life.

As Greta becomes better able to understand herself in social context, she is able to help others, like Lars and Vina, explore how context shapes their feelings and experiences in relationship to each other. She recognizes how Lars' having a lifetime of White male privilege dovetailed into his stoic masculine, Norwegian attitudes, and wartime experience. Greta is now able to contrast this with Vina's challenge of being a respectful and caring daughter while maintaining her expectation of gender equality in all of her relationships, including her relationship with her father. Greta's personal and social awareness allows her to help Vina and Lars navigate the landscape of being a father and daughter in a specific societal and historical context. In Text Box 7.1 Timothy Baima describes how he approaches this kind of social awareness with clients while taking into account his own position as a White heterosexual male.

Text Box 7.1 Timothy Baima, PhD, LMFT

Timothy Baima is mindful of how his identity as a White, straight cis male from a working-class background is part of the clinical process and incorporates an experiential view of change into his systemic and attachment-based work (see also Chapter 8).

My clients have often been pulled into habitual relational patterns that undermine the very qualities in relationships they long for. I work to help them disentangle themselves from problematic patterns of relating and strengthen their bonds to one another by nurturing authenticity, attunement, responsiveness, and emotional engagement. I believe our connections to culture, power, and oppression are central to how we structure our lives and relationships. Therefore, commitments to see, acknowledge, and respond to power and subjugation both within oneself and in one's relationships are fundamental to forming bonds that allow people to be their whole authentic selves, and nurture themselves and one another. I appeal to my clients' hopes and dreams for their relationships. Often, they are misusing and abusing power in a desperate attempt to force the kind of relationships they long for, and it is only digging them deeper into a pit of isolation and emotional deadness. So, I crawl into the pit with them and talk with them about climbing out together.

It is tricky work to invite people to be their whole authentic selves when my social location as a straight White cis man makes it unsafe for so many people. Each client I work with will present me with new opportunities to grow in and through my relationship with them. Rather than assuming that I am trustworthy and thinking about how I "earn" my client's trust, I strive to become a more trustworthy person to them. I also discuss with clients how being a White straight cis man informs my view of the therapy process, and positions me in terms of what I may have a tendency to focus on in therapy and what I may miss (Watts Jones, 2010). It also provides an opening for me to ask clients how they identify in terms of race, ethnicity, gender identity, sexual orientation, social class, and religion. I share my perspective that culture is important, and that social power and oppression significantly affect people and relationships—sometimes in ways we do not even notice.

When I started addressing sociocultural themes in my work, I was afraid. At that time in my development, I was highly dependent on approval from others to bolster my own sense of self-worth. I especially craved affirmation and approval from clients with marginalized identities. I felt as if their approval affirmed me as being a good White person, a good man, and a good straight cisgender person. I became perfectionistic in my effort to address culture "the right way" and to say "the right things" during sessions. I was rather self-absorbed and came across as performative and cerebral, regardless of how much I genuinely cared for my clients. My focus on myself and my anxiety about looking ignorant or causing offense got in the way of being attuned and emotionally engaged. As I have learned to be nurturing with myself, I have become less dependent upon praise and affirmation from others for a sense of worth. I have learned that I can mess up in relationships and make amends. This has given me the freedom to move through my own discomfort and be curious, ask questions, return to conversations that were dismissed in previous sessions, and supportively challenge clients. I believe that as we allow ourselves to become more fully human and nurture our own growth with a balance of love and accountability, we are best positioned to guide our clients into the vulnerable spaces that will support their own transformation.

As described by Baima (Text Box 7.1), socioculturally attuned family therapists can also use self-disclosure to raise social awareness and support just relationships. For example, a socioculturally attuned family therapist might, at the right moment, share with a family her experience of watching her own father work so hard yet never enjoy the relationship connections he desired or her own struggle as a woman to balance being a mother with working. Another example might be a therapist disclosing how difficult it was to watch her brother come out as gay to parents who were confused and afraid of his sexual orientation. This type of disclosure can help normalize the experience and open conversations about social and contextual influences on families.

Experience in Community Context

While experiential interventions often attend to relational space within the family, the family's physical context and community are frequently overlooked as impacting experience. The context of community includes both space and place. Space can be thought of as the ecosystem, including all that is living and nonliving in a physical environment. Place refers to how we experience space. It is within a place that we meet our basic human needs for personal space, privacy, social interaction, and safety (Fitzpatrick & LaGory, 2000; McDowell, 2015). The spaces we inhabit, our sense of place, and our ability to secure our basic needs are highly dependent on societal dynamics of privilege, power, and oppression.

Socioculturally attuned experiential family therapists consider where families live, work, get medical care, shop, receive education, recreate, and so on relative to spatial justice. They recognize and address the consequences of dynamics of power and privilege on physical resources and community geography. McDowell (2015) proposed *family cartography* as a method for exploring the experience of families within a particular space and place. According to McDowell (2015), this is a way to "capture family life within the spaces family members inhabit in order to better understand the relationship between power, privacy, personal space, social interactions, safety, and

Table 7.1 Creating a family cartograph

	Sample Questions on How to Create a Family Cartograph
1	Describe the setting—physical environment, climate, town and neighborhood in which you live/lived/ grew up. (Map the territory.)
2	What kinds of social interactions are/were available to you in this setting? Where are/were you and your family able to go and not go in this setting? How safe do/did you feel? What level of privacy and personal space does/did this setting provide?
3	Describe the power dynamics in this setting. Include race, class, gender, sexual orientation, abilities, nation of origin, language and any other signifiers that are relevant. (Add these to the map using symbols.)
4	How do/did these power dynamics affect you and your family? In what ways do/did you and/or your family members participate in the oppression or marginalization of others? How are/were you and your family oppressed or marginalized?
5	Describe the home in which you live/lived. (Add to map as an excerpt.) What kinds of social interactions are/were available to you in and around your home? In what areas of the home did you spend the most time and why? Where are/were you able to go and not go in your home and why? How safe do/ did you feel in various spaces in your home? What level of privacy and personal space does/did this setting provide?
6	Who is/was in your family? Who has/had the most power? How is/was the power enacted? (Draw a map excerpt to show family.) How do these power dynamics reflect the broader power dynamics in your community?
7	What spaces on your map reflect sites of oppression? Describe the relationships in these sites. (Add oppression symbols to the map.)
8	Where are sites of resistance? Describe the relationships in these sites. (Add resistance symbols to the map.) How do/did you and/or your family resist oppression? Where, what and how do/did you learn to resist oppression?
9	What types of resiliency do/did you develop as a result of this geography? (Add resilience symbols to the map.)
10	What else would you like to add to the map?

Adapted from *Applying critical social theories to family therapy practice* (p. 63) by T. McDowell, 2015, New York, NY: Springer. Copyright 2015. Adapted with permission.

the problems presented in therapy" (pp. 61–62). Family cartographies can be used to illustrate and capture the context of a person or family's life. These maps do not need to be drawn to scale or use a predetermined legend. Rather, the therapist facilitates drawing a picture of the family's community, including neighborhoods, places of employment, relevant parks, places of worship and shopping, educational and medical resources, and sources of pollution, noise, danger/risk, and so on. Anything relevant to the family's daily lives can be included using symbols the family choses. McDowell suggested a number of questions that might be used to develop a family cartography of any period in a client's past or the present (see Table 7.1).

Once the community map is complete, the therapist can ask the family to draw their home within the community. This can include all rooms and outdoor spaces, how each room felt, who had the most influence or impact on the emotional "climate" in the home, and so on. This provides a physical reference for remembering and sharing experience and emotion. The exercise helps the therapist understand the experience of clients within a physical context while raising social awareness and relational insight among family members.

Cultural Attunement and Cultural Democracy

Socioculturally attuned experiential family therapists extend the humanistic value of each person having worth and deserving voice by striving for cultural democracy. The ideal of cultural democracy extends beyond acknowledging the heterogeneity of many societies to supporting the right of each group to its values, beliefs, and practices without marginalization or oppression by more dominant cultures (Košutić & McDowell, 2008). That said, all cultures balance individualism and collectivism. Likewise, all cultures generate and maintain both equity and oppression.

↢→

Practicing socioculturally attuned family therapy requires auditing what we assume is "good therapy" from a cultural perspective.

↢→

At a meta level, therapists must view each culture as equally valid and work within cultural frameworks to support the growth and well-being of all family members. This includes recognizing the tremendous diversity within cultural groups and families, along with challenging culturally supported power differentials. The practice of socioculturally attuned experiential family therapy includes asking questions such as: How do we understand the cultural context of emotion? How do we find ways for clients to express emotion to us and each other in culturally supported ways? What might it look like to be vulnerable within various cultures and groups? These questions help therapists reflect on the meaning associated with sharing thoughts and emotions directly with family members, which is often not prized or adaptive in all cultures.

For example, in many Asian cultures expressing one's own needs is counter to collectivist values that place the well-being of the group over that of the individual (Quek & Knudson-Martin, 2006.) Sharing one's feelings and needs may be viewed as placing a burden on others. According to ChenFeng and colleagues (2016), Asian Americans often carry "intangible loss" from generations of migration, loss of homeland, and marginalization in the host country. Each carries this burden on their own in "quiet fortitude" without leaning on others, not believing "that they should or could expect or ask for intimate emotional attention" (p. 5). Duty and loyalty to the family may be implicitly expected, while focusing on oneself may be viewed as selfish. A socioculturally attuned experiential therapist would need to work within this cultural framework to slowly acknowledge losses and "scaffold their movement towards vulnerability so that it did not leave clients feeling raw and unsafe" (ChenFeng et al., 2016, p. 5).

Consider Neeb, the aging father in a Hmong family who moved to the US after the Vietnam war. Like many Hmongs, Neeb left his village in the hills of North Vietnam to fight alongside the US. When the war was over, Neeb, his wife Me, and their daughter Kiab, took refuge in a midwestern US city. Their daughter, Luv, was born in the US. Luv now cares for her aging father. Neeb is not overtly demanding of Luv. He carries the burden of his past trauma in quiet fortitude. He is grateful that his children are thriving. Luv and Kiab are deeply grateful to their father and protect him from any additional burden after all he has lost and suffered. Kiab knows it is difficult for her sister to be the primary support for their father, but rather than stating this directly, she invites Neeb to spend more time with her family explaining how this would be good for her children. A therapist working with this family would need to share the deep respect for the father and the way the family quietly shares their burdens.

Greta, who has just walked out of a session with Lars and Vina, is now talking with Neeb, Luv, and Kiab for the first time. Neeb has been reluctant to leave his home for more than short errands. Greta is helping them renegotiate care for Neeb so Luv can meet her goal of completing a college degree.

Greta: Neeb, I see your daughters take very good care of you.
Neeb: I am blessed to have such wonderful children.
Kiab: We love him very much.

Luv: We are grateful to have a good father that would do anything for his family.
Greta: Yes, I can see that. Luv, you live with your father, or he lives with you?
Luv: Yes, we live together. My mother is gone so it is just us in the house now.
Greta: And you are in school? College?
Luv: Yes, I am getting a degree in advertising.
Greta: Neeb, now both of your children will have college degrees! Kiab, where do you live?
Kiab: I live close by with my husband and children. We are thinking father might like to come and stay with us some days when Luv is in school…

Many emotions and needs were expressed in this short exchange. The therapist noted that the father was well cared for. This complemented Luv as a caretaker and Neeb as a father who raised a loving daughter. The therapist also complemented the father by acknowledging the success of his children. Luv and Kiab acknowledged their father's sacrifice for them; the impact of war, migration, and loss by showing gratitude and respect. Kiab was able to indirectly tell her father that it would be helpful to Luv for him to allow her to care for him some of the time without stating that he was a burden on anyone. The family might move into expression of more emotion, but it would be done slowly and within the family's cultural language.

Power

Experiential therapy relies on a relatively democratic view of families. Though parents must have influence over children, therapy takes on a quality of treating all family members with equal respect and concern, making room for all voices. While this remains the goal, socioculturally attuned therapists do not assume all voices hold equal power.

Socioculturally attuned experiential family therapists analyze power dynamics from the broadest global to the most intimate family relationships.

Emotion and Power

Socioculturally attuned experiential therapists pay attention to how emotions are intrinsically connected to power dynamics and socio-cultural context (Turner, 2007; Pease, 2012). For example, negative emotion has been found to be associated with getting less than one's fair share (Turner, 2007). Consider a family in which one of three children routinely feels overlooked compared to siblings who excel in academics or sports. This child is likely to have negative emotions about parents, siblings, and/or self. Imagine the sibling who is amply rewarded for good grades gleefully running around the house. Let's now say the athletic child unexpectedly won a spot in the state finals—eyes wide and mouth dropped open, she lets out a shriek of delighted surprise—getting more than we expect leads to even more positive emotions. At the same time, the child who is routinely overlooked falls again into the background, feeling jealous, hurt, and/or devalued in comparison. In this case, the social valuing of success in sports during childhood overrides qualities and potential (e.g., kindness, other orientation, contemplative nature) of the child who withdraws.

Those with greater influence and power tend to experience more positive emotions, particularly when they see themselves as getting the respect and rewards they expect and feel they deserve. Those with less influence and privilege tend to feel more negative emotions, including hurt, shame, guilt, and/or anger. Shame and embarrassment tend to follow perceptions that we are at fault for not getting what we expect (Turner, 2007). Anger can result from viewing others as responsible for not getting what we expect and/or feel we have earned. Those who have less power may feel less worthy, while those with greater gender, race, or class privilege expect more and believe at some level that those who have less deserve less. Holding greater privilege and expecting more can lead to anger and frustration when others with less social privilege are afforded equal opportunities and access. Likewise, displays of anger can be used to maintain privilege through fear and/or threats, using one's privilege to negatively impact others. As Baima noted in Text Box 7.1, those with greater privilege may also misuse and abuse power in an attempt to force the kind of relationships for which they long and, instead, dig them deeper into isolation and emotional deadness.

Let's go back to our example of Lars and Vina. Lars has had a lifetime of male privilege. Even as a child, he experienced higher expectations being placed on him than on his sisters. These expectations sent him the message that, as a male, he was worth more and a greater investment to the family. The deference shown to him within the family (e.g., compliments for working hard, being excused after a meal while his sisters cleaned up) followed him through adulthood. Vina, on the other hand, received messages throughout her life that she was to accommodate and attune to others' needs. Lars uses cross and demanding behavior to get the attention he feels he deserves, but loses closeness and connection in the process.

Emotion and Resistance

According to Garcia, Košutić, and McDowell (2015) "emotions can fuel our social awareness and resistance to oppression...[and] prompt us to contribute, perhaps unwittingly, to oppression, [or]... intervene in our ability to see and resist oppression" (pp. 3–4). Power is reproduced in part through emotions that hold in place dominant systems of thinking, doing, and being. Emotions also contribute to resistance to oppression. Social movements are often associated with feelings such as anger over social injustice, love, and selfless solidarity.

•←→•

Feelings produced through processes of marginalization and oppression, as well as those that emerge from growing awareness of power structures, can mobilize us into action.

•←→•

This felt resistance is essential for social change, just as it is essential for interpersonal change. Consider a heterosexual couple who came to therapy with their only child, Laura (age 16). Laura and her father, David, frequently engaged in verbal conflict. Laura's mother, Kim, silently disagreed with David's strict fathering and experienced her own frustrations with his attempts to control their marriage. The socioculturally attuned experiential family therapist, Latisha, engaged the family in a sculpt. The family placed themselves in the room showing David with his finger wagging at Laura who is standing up to him. Kim was behind Laura, offering her support. As she was helping the family with the sculpt, Latisha asked what contributed to the father being in such a position of power. Along with personality and physical size, the family identified that he made most of the money. Latisha slipped one of the platforms she kept in her office under the father, raising his height in the sculpt as she continued to explore. Laura blurted out, "because he is the man and no one will stand up to him!" Latisha took out another platform, suggesting it represented male privilege. The family began to see how both women, mother and daughter, struggled against male privilege and the valuing of money-producing work over other types of work (e.g., running a family, school work, housework, relational work). This dynamic maintained the father's power but kept him from truly connecting with those he loves the most—his wife and daughter. Latisha continued to engage the family in exploring and expressing how societally supported power dynamics impacted their relationships and helped them all resist dynamics that were harmful to their growth as individuals and their connections as a family.

Connection and Equity

Power is highly nuanced and deeply impacts emotional attunement in intimate relationships. Knudson-Martin stated (2015):

> When power is not equal, the more powerful partner will be less aware of the other's experience. What makes it more complicated is that people in higher power positions generally are not aware of their power; they may not even realize that others are attentive to their needs or that their interests are dominating the agenda. On the other hand, people in less powerful positions are likely to automatically take into account the desires or expectations of the more powerful. People in powerful roles (i.e., teacher, employer, physician, husband) may take for granted that others accommodate them—or become distressed when they do not. (p. 16)

For example, children with an abusive parent often become highly attuned to the parent's feelings, reading footsteps, facial expressions, and voice tone for indications of mood. Those in power often lack awareness of the damage their power causes relationships. It is not uncommon for People of Color to point out how they must be knowledgeable and attuned to White people to be able to successfully navigate US society. White people (or those in the dominant group), on the other hand, may choose to go their whole lives without listening to the experience of People of Color (or those in the subordinate group) or learning about another culture (Tatum, 2017).

Imagine how paying attention to connection and equity might change the therapeutic process. For example, women often present as more emotionally expressive. In heterosexual relationships, emotional descriptions of needs are often repeated to male partners who in turn dismiss or pay cursory attention to requests. Experiential therapists work to help each partner understand and empathize with the other's feelings and needs. Consider viewing a female partner's emotional escalation as an attempt to influence a more powerful partner. She is bidding for connection and relying on empathy as a pathway to influence and/or as a way to prevent her partner from becoming upset. A socioculturally attuned experiential therapist would notice this and encourage shared power by helping the male partner learn to listen and attune to his female partner.

Third Order Change

•←→•

Third order change involves going beyond understanding each other to understanding the impact of societal contexts on our relationships, including how societal structures support the voice and welfare of some at the expense of others.

•←→•

Let's go back to Lars and Vina one more time. First order change might result if the therapist, Greta, were to help Vina explore her needs and set limits as a caretaker. Second order change might include Greta helping Lars and Vina understand their own and each other's frustrations, emotions, and experiences. Greater understanding and improved communication would help them both meet individual needs while negotiating a more satisfying relationship. Third order change would target understanding the broader societal context in which caring for an elder occurs. They would be able to name how caretaking and emotion work is devalued in US society and most often relegated to women. They would become more overtly aware of how their relationship is affected by societal power dynamics; the power difference between an older male father and younger female daughter. Lars and Vina would begin to recognize how male privilege and power erode the possibility for harmony and closeness in their relationship. Lars could become softer and more emotionally available in his later years, while Vina could become more empowered in her adulthood.

Practice Guidelines

Understanding the impact of societal systems on presenting problems increases therapists' ability to attune to client experience and tailor experiential interventions. Following are four guidelines important to practicing socioculturally attuned experiential family therapy; 1) honoring culturally relevant experience and expression, 2) encouraging awareness of self and other in context, 3) exploring relationships between power, emotion, and expression, and 4) promoting equity-based attunement and connection.

1. Honoring Culturally Relevant Experience and Expression

Every culture has rituals, traditions, and ceremonies that promote resilience and demonstrate collective values and beliefs. These serve many societal functions, including punctuating life cycle transitions, enhancing cultural norms, and/or solidifying religious beliefs. Most cultures have specific ceremonies for a person's birth, marriage, school graduation, initiation, coming of age, marriage, and death. These rituals offer insight into culturally informed beliefs about what is appropriate at a given age, for a specific gender, or a specific religion. Spiritual and religious beliefs and practices may be empowering and healing, and may also be harmful and sources of pain (Esmiol Wilson, 2018). Rites of passages may be formal (e.g., quinceanera, sweet sixteen party, or a debutante ball), or informal (e.g., such as rites for boys like joining a gang, fraternity, drinking alcohol, having sex, getting a driver's license, getting into a fight, or registering for Selective Services). There are also countless healing and cleansing rituals, meditation practices, and prayer rituals.

There are ample opportunities for therapists to **attune** to cultural rituals and traditions to help clients work through difficult transitions, problems, or merely connect with traditions they may have lost or forgotten. Asking clients if they have cultural, personal, family, and/or religious rituals, traditions, or ceremonies may help therapists have greater insight as to other ways of "being" in the therapy room that expands action oriented, creative, and sometimes non-verbal forms of expression. These processes can happen in person or via virtual sessions (Eppler et al., 2024).

It is also important for therapists to **attune** to the cultural nuances of nonverbal expression and communication and to honor those forms of expression in therapy. There are many ways in which our actions express culturally ascribed ways of being. How we use silence, touch, facial expressions, movements, embodiment, and physical closeness and distance all influence our gender and cultural expression. So often, therapists unknowingly adhere to androcentric, Eurocentric, and/or Westernized beliefs about what forms of communication and expression are privileged. Being open to learning and honoring multiple forms of expression is especially important for socioculturally attuned experiential family therapists. For many, connection and understanding can be best accessed with a glance, touch, or embrace. Clients need permission and the space to use all forms of expression that honor multiple ways of knowing, being, and relating to each other across cultural and relational contexts.

2. Encouraging Awareness of Self and Other in Context

Familiarity with societal systems and power dynamics is necessary to guide therapy in ways that attend to how the most intimate experience is affected by individual, relational, and societal systems.

•←→•

Socioculturally attuned experiential family therapists pay close attention to the impact of societal systems and the nuances of power that block the potential for growth in any and all family members.

•←→•

Those with greater societally assigned power are often unaware of the negative impact their power has on others. This creates pockets of stagnation for everyone involved. Consider David, a conservative Christian in a patriarchal family in which the husband/father is regularly accommodated by the wife/mother and children. While family members and the church expect him to be a spiritual leader, the father confuses this role with a *power over* stance in which he expects to make all final decisions and have his needs met first. He is unaware of the full impact of his actions as he experiences the positive effects of being accommodated without always knowing others are yielding or bending to his will. His wife and children feel routinely dismissed and forgo many of their own needs to meet his. It is relatively simple to see how the needs of the wife and children take a back seat, potentially limiting their growth and potential.

It is less clear that this dynamic also harms David, who is unaware of the increasing emotional gap or the growth limiting effects of being consistently accommodated by others. He is not challenged to put others first or to expand his faith by learning to truly serve, rather than control and "lead" the ones he loves. As he ages and turns toward his relationships for support and meaning, he is likely to be stunned and disappointed by the distance and resentment his behavior caused. Socioculturally attuned experiential therapists **name** inequities to help free *all* family members, including those in dominant positions, from the constraints of power imbalances, keeping in mind the well-being of all. In experiential therapy, naming arises out of the clinical process. Fatma Arıcı Şahin (Text Box 7.2) describes how using art can help clients recognize and name the sociocultural nature of vulnerable emotions.

Text Box 7.2 Fatma Arıcı Şahin, PhD

Fatma uses experiential approaches with a critical, social-contextual, and feminist perspective and incorporates various fields of art (music, dance, literature, photography, cinema, etc.) as tools/techniques that enable the expression of emotions. (See more of her work in Chapter 15.)

Using art in therapy is a powerful method that makes it easier for me to deal with sociocultural experiences. It helps create a safe and protective environment that enables people to share experiences through symbols that they would have difficulty expressing directly. Artistic expression often unwittingly and quickly reveals the implicit. In this safe environment, I can ask questions that help them give meaning to their sociocultural experiences through the symbols, and reach their vulnerable emotions underlying these experiences. Since the silenced and marginalized are often associated with counselees' most vulnerable emotions, I care about these emotions surfacing in a safe context. I create this safe space by reframing each partner's response to life challenges, both personally and in the broader context, as "a coping strategy," validating this way of coping while also making power processes visible by expanding counselees' interpretations of their revealed experiences with questions and reflections. Interpreting the here and now processes, which are also related to cultural issues, creates a fertile ground for change.

3. Exploring Relationships between Power, Emotion, and Expression

↔

Societal and interpersonal power dynamics may result in some family members being heard more loudly and/or accommodated by others, both in and out of the family. Those with less power may be emotionally demonstrative or shut down completely, preoccupied, or guarded.

↔

As therapists work to bring forth emotional experience in the room, they need to attend to power imbalances by helping more powerful persons attune and **value** the experience of those who are less powerful, working to avoid eliciting even more vulnerability from less powerful persons. When powerful persons become more attuned, they are also better able to respond in caring and relationally accountable ways. Understanding self and other in societal context increases the willingness of more powerful family members to step down from their positions and connect with others. Facing one's own privilege opens opportunities to be more accountable to loved ones, maintaining healthier interpersonal relationships.

Families must also be able to explore and support each other's experiences relative to power dynamics outside the family. Consider Sarah, who routinely experienced harassment from a male colleague at work. She and her husband, Nathan, entered therapy to find a way to deal with her growing anxiety and depression. Nathan told the therapist he had "tried everything short of beating [Sarah's colleague] up!" Sarah often came home distraught from being yelled at by her colleague or being the recipient of his unreasonable demands. Nathan responded to Sarah's emotional upset by becoming angry himself or telling Sarah what she should do. The therapist in this situation helped Nathan become more aware of societal dynamics around gender and to emotionally attune to Sarah. The situation at work and home were both embedded in gendered power dynamics, leaving Sarah with nowhere to turn where her experience and emotions could be validated. As Sarah and Nathan became more aware of gender and power, Sarah could take the lead (with Nathan's support) in reporting her colleague's behavior to Human Resources.

4. Promoting Equity-based Attunement and Connection

As the choreographer of the session, socioculturally attuned family therapists use themselves and their experience in the room to promote equity-based attunement among family members.

↔

Mutual attunement includes willingness on the part of everyone to pay close attention to each other's experiences, not only understanding but responding in ways that prioritize connection.

↔

Children may not feel heard or even have words for what they are experiencing. Less powerful persons with differing views may feel shut down in conversations and family decisions, or not even be able to articulate their experience, as there is no common language to legitimize their perspectives (Fricker, 2007). Socioculturally attuned experiential therapists notice when those in centered, dominant positions subtly dismiss the experiences of those with less power or those on the edges of family belonging, and create experiences that **name** their realities and **value** their voices.

Attunement infers attempting to be with others, bear witness to their testimony, help them make meaning of their experience, and walk next to them on their journey. In effect, we are **intervening** by inviting family members to socioculturally attune to each other. To do this, family members must be aware of the societal contexts that shape their lives and the impact of power dynamics on their relationships.

•←→•

Awareness must go hand-in-hand with the willingness and ability to tune in and effectively respond to each other.

•←→•

Consider a family living in the rural Midwest US in which Lou, age 14, who was assigned male at birth, is perceiving and experiencing himself as female. When Lou's family is out of the house, she tries on her sister's clothes and experiments with makeup. She shares this with no one, prays for her urges to go away, and is terrified of being found out. There is no one who talks about gender in her family or community; Lou just knows not to speak. When Lou is able to get access to the internet at school, she discovers she is not alone. She is not wrong because she has been assigned the wrong sex and gender. She now grows emotionally and intellectually alongside this liberating information, reaching out to others through the internet. Later, when she begins transitioning and decides to tell her family, they will need to socioculturally attune to her in order for the family to continue into the future together. Parents and siblings will need socioeducation about transgender identity and rights (Giammattei, 2015; Sorrentino, 2024). They will need to be able to listen to and empathize with Lou's silenced and marginalized experience. Her family will need to share emotion in ways that bring them together.

A socioculturally attuned experiential family therapist would facilitate this type of understanding and attunement within societal context. The therapist would interrupt microaggressions, such as parents asking what they did wrong. They would help the family challenge power dynamics that insinuate cisgender children are "normal" and **envision** acceptance and support for all children. As the family moves through this process, the therapist might encourage them to engage in a type of renaming ritual (Brown et al., 2010). Brown and colleagues (2010) described engaging in renaming rituals with African American youth who are "given a name at birth, and how during the struggles of childhood and young adulthood…may lose his/her way and need to be reminded of the name's significance to the community he/she belongs to" (p. 334). The ritual involves family and community sitting in concentric circles around the youth and stating aloud the meaning of the youth's name along with poems, songs, or other meaningful readings. In our case, Lou has an opportunity to stand before the community to affirm a new name that describes her journey and future. The therapist encourages **transformation** by asking supportive family and friends to gather to witness her journey by telling stories of her strength, affirming her identity through prepared statements, poems, and music; and standing to verbally and symbolically pledge their support.

Case Illustration

Emilio presented in therapy with sadness and confusion about his marriage. He and his wife, Mandy, had been married for 14 years. Many of those years had been difficult. He loved his wife, but she often got angry at him. He felt as though Mandy did not understand him or appreciate the efforts he made for her and their family and reported that most of their important discussions ended in heated arguments. He was a practicing Catholic, 32 years old, from the Dominican Republic. Mandy, who was European American, was from Dallas, Texas, and grew up Baptist. Both were college educated and wanted to raise their children as Christians. They shared values around family and education. Their therapist, Leah, was of bicultural descent. Her mother was from the

Northeast US and her father was Puerto Rican. Leah grew up in Puerto Rico and was fluent in Spanish and English. She shared her clients' experience of being from a mixed cultural family. Leah asked Emilio if he would consider inviting his wife to couples therapy given that most of his concerns centered around his marriage.

The therapist began by helping Mandy feel welcome. She focused on joining with her, asking about her life and background, and her hopes for the therapy. Mandy was forthcoming, but it became apparent that both Mandy and Emilio had difficulties expressing their emotions and did not openly discuss their thoughts or feelings. Mandy often responded with "I don't know," or "I'm not sure," and Emilio responded non-verbally, by just shaking his head yes or no, or lifting his shoulders. Leah saw that they were not able to fully express themselves in session. They seemed to be stifling their responses and emotions. Neither of them reported a history of violence, substance abuse, addiction, infidelity, financial distress, personal health problems, or any other individual and contextual issue compounding their marriage. Both had jobs they enjoyed, and their children, ages 4 and 6, seemed to be doing well. After the fourth conjoint session, the therapist asked if they were interested in trying an experiential and creative approach.

Honoring Culturally Relevant Experience and Expression

Given that both the therapist and Emilio were from a Latin/Caribbean culture, Leah asked if they would be interested in making a series of altars or shadow boxes for themselves as individuals and for themselves as a couple. "*Altares*," as they are called in Spanish, are personally handmade or assembled shrines or spaces that serve many functions, not only to spiritually honor deceased family members, but also as a way to express one's culture, relationships, and the things a person, couple, or family may value (Bermúdez & Bermúdez, 2002). *Altares* can be small movable shadow boxes, temporary shrines, such as those created for the Day of the Dead in Mexico, or more permanent shrines, such as those that occupy a small nook in homes to memorialize someone or something. Deeply rooted in Latino, Indigenous, Catholic, and Afro-Caribbean cultures, altar-making invites people to honor what they believe to be sacred, important, and meaningful, offering an opportunity to openly and publicly express those sentiments to others. In therapy, the process enables clients to express emotions and have an experience that generates a deeper experiential level of individual and relational growth.

Emilio and Mandy brought three large shadow boxes that they made from wood at home—one for each of them and one for them as a couple. They gathered things that were significant to them as individuals and as a couple and family (e.g., pictures, prayers, figurines, small objects such as a needle and thread, pictures from magazine clippings, small action figures, a perfume bottle, family pictures, candles, flags, small patches and awards, silk flowers, jewelry).

Encouraging Awareness of Self and Other in Context

Emilio and Mandy were able to talk about their shadow boxes as they created them. As they talked, the therapist was open and transparent with her experiences growing up in a bi-cultural home. She also explained that she was going to assume multiple stances in their process, such as catalyst, witness, coach, investigator, supporter, etc. Leah asked questions and made comments such as, "Tell me about the objects you brought in." "What does this mean to you?" "Where did it come from?" "What are your greatest memories about this?" "When did you become aware that this person/thing was important to you?" "As you look at your shared shrine/*altar*, what does this mean for you? Is there anything missing?" "What would you add or change?" "What do you want your spouse to know about this?" "What would others think if they saw this?" Asking questions helped

Mandy and Emilio discuss the thoughts, feelings, and meanings surrounding what they were doing. Having a creative and culturally relevant process helped them talk about issues such as culture, values, traditions, wishes, and fears in ways they had not been able to experience before.

Exploring Relationships Between Power, Emotion, and Expression

The process began by placing all of the pictures and objects on the table. They had a large grouping of matches, a wine cork and label, coins, rocks, plastic wedding bands, softball pictures, images of the beach, college memorabilia, concert stubs, and pictures of their children when they were born. They discussed the objects and pictures, then began to work together to place the images in the shadow box. As they worked, Leah asked about the influences that were instrumental in helping them remain strong as a couple, as well as the social forces that were negatively affecting their connection. These questions were difficult to answer; however, having the physical representation to reference helped Mandy and Emilio discuss what had caused them to drift apart and experience distance and isolation.

As Mandy and Emilio looked at their own personal *altares* and shared them with each other, they began to notice important differences and similarities in what they valued. Mandy began to cry when she noticed that Emilio had a cross with flowers at the center of his altar, along with images of his family and his country. Her images and objects reflected more about her hobbies and interests. When the therapist asked Mandy about the meaning of her tears, she said that she realized that he missed his family and the Dominican Republic and that she was sad that she had not been able to help him stay more connected to his culture and family back home. He reassured her that it was not her fault, and although it was true he felt isolated and lonely and missed his family, he loved her very much and that she and their children were his main priority.

Seeing their individual *altares* and being able to talk about them in an accepting and non-judgmental manner helped Mandy and Emilio express their emotions in new ways. With Leah's prompts, they were able to openly talk about the gender and cultural scripts, including how being socialized as a man had paralyzed Emilio, preventing him from talking about the helplessness he felt or his need to connect with his wife and family of origin more often and in meaningful ways. He missed sharing celebrations and honoring his cultural traditions. Although Emilio felt powerful in his day-to-day life, he felt as though Mandy held most of the power in their relationship because she spoke English with an American accent, was not an immigrant, and understood many more things about American culture.

Although Mandy spoke Spanish and greatly appreciated Emilio's culture, she admitted that she honored her traditions more with their children and often compared him to "American" friends who "seemed to have it more together." She also was able to talk about how she felt the need to "give" him more power by "letting him" make important decisions, manage their finances, and "let him" win fights so that he would not feel like less of a man. The process of having honesty, trust, and vulnerability enabled them to position themselves to begin to make the "couple *altar*" together. This shrine was a symbolic representation of who they are and who they aspired to be together as a couple and family.

The couple began to identify the many social forces blocking their potential. For Emilio, it was his pride and his inability to admit that he was fearful and worried about losing Mandy. For Mandy, it was primarily the social comparisons and not honoring Emilio's culture and his values. She realized that his values centered around his faith and family, and her values centered around material possessions, shared experiences, and traditions from her culture. They were able to talk about power dynamics between the Dominican Republic and the US that privileged Mandy's culture. Mandy's White privilege was a salient factor in their daily lives and relationship, which they had not found ways to openly acknowledge before therapy.

Promote Equity-based Attunement and Connection

After seeing all three *altares*/shadow boxes side by side, and having the experience of making them and discussing their multiple meanings, Emilio and Mandy were able to experience themselves-in-relationship in a different way. They became more attuned to one another, bearing witness to their testimony of pain, loss, regret, and their hopes for the future. The therapist guided them on this journey of self and mutual exploration and contemplation. By discussing social forces that were working against them, such as narrowly defined masculinity/machismo, immigration status, and rigid gender and cultural scripts, they were able to see how their different societal contexts shaped their lives and the expectations for their marriage and life together. Upon the completion of therapy, the couple was able to keep their *altares* as a reminder of their process of growth.

Summary: Third Order Change

In this case, Emilio and Mandy were able to engage in third order change by going beyond understanding each other to understanding the impact of their societal contexts. The global power dynamics and resource disparity between the US and the Dominican Republic shaped many aspects of their lives, including who had greater societal privilege, whose cultural practices were centered, and how they negotiated power dynamics relative to gender, language/accent, and race. Societal structures in the US supported the voice and welfare of Mandy at the expense of Emilio in some ways, and Emilio's male privilege supported his welfare over Mandy's in other ways. When they were unaware of how these dynamics shaped their relationship, they were more inclined to assign their problems to themselves and blame each other as individuals. By the end of therapy, they not only understood and appreciated each other's experiences more, but were able to come together to challenge oppressive societal forces on behalf of themselves, each other, and their children.

Reflexive Questions

- When thinking about your own *family cartography* as a method for exploring the effects of space and place on your family, what are the main things that come to mind? What would the map say about your context and how that influenced you?
- Experiential therapists make room for all voices, however, not all voices hold equal power. What helps you take into account broader sociocultural context in analyzing what gives or takes away your sense of power?
- What are some ways in which you have attuned to cultural rituals and traditions to help clients work through difficult transitions, problems, or connect with traditions they may have lost or forgotten? What were some emotional responses?
- When powerful persons become more attuned, they are also better able to respond in caring and relationally accountable ways. How does your social location help or hinder your ability to help others attune to those with less socially sanctioned power?
- Describe the ways in which you have, or would like to give meaning to the client's sociocultural experiences through symbolic, artistic, and creative interventions?
- If you were to make your own *altar*/shrine/shadow box, what things would you include that would reflect a symbolic representation of your life? Once you've made it, who would you show it to? What would they learn about you in the process?

References

Bailey, M. (2022). Science catching up: Experiential family therapy and neuroscience. *Journal of Family Therapy*, *48*, 1095–1110.
Banmen, J. & Maki-Banmen, K. (2014). What has become of Virginia Satir's therapy model since she left us in 1988? *Journal of Family Psychotherapy*, *25*(2), 117–131.
Barker, B., Cannell, C., Naylor, S., Pearl, K., Stewart, E., & Oka, M. (2019). Let's play: Using systemic and experiential techniques in the play therapy instruction of MFT masters' students. *The American Journal of Family Therapy*, *47*(1), 1–18.
Bermúdez, J. M. & Bermúdez, S. (2002). Altar-Making with Latino families: A narrative therapy perspective. *Journal of Family Psychotherapy 13*(3/4). [Reprinted in T. D. Carlson and M. J. Erickson (Eds.). *Spirituality and family therapy* (pp. 329–248). Haworth Press.]
Brown, A., Dimitriou, M. & Dressner, L. (2010). Rituals as tools of resistance: From survival to liberation. In B. J. Risman (Ed.). *Families as they really are* (pp. 328–336). WW Norton.
ChenFeng, J., Kim, L., Knudson-Martin, C., & Wu, Y. (2016). Application of socio-emotional relationship therapy with couples of Asian heritage: Addressing issues of culture, gender, and power. *Family Process*, *56*, 558–573.
Connell, G., Mitten, T., & Bumberry, W. (1998). *Reshaping family relationships: The symbolic therapy of Carl Whitaker*. Brunner Mazel.
Dumont, R. (2008). Drawing a family map: an experiential tool for engaging children in family therapy. *Journal of Family Therapy*, *30*, 247–259.
Edwards, L. (2026). Queer contextualized Satir family therapy. In E. E. Hartwell & L. L. Edwards (Eds.). *Queer-contextualized family therapy: Toward radically inclusive theory and practice* (pp. 73–94). Routledge.
Eppler, C., Bermúdez, J. M., & Cobb, R. A. (2024). Virtual altar making for grief and loss. In R. A. Cobb, *The therapist's notebook for systemic teletherapy: Creative interventions for effective online therapy* (chapter 33). Routledge.
Esmiol Wilson, E. (2018). From assessment to activism: Utilizing a justice-informed framework to guide spiritual and religious intervention. In E. Esmiol Wilson & L. Nice (Eds.). *Socially just religious and spiritual interventions: Ethical uses of therapeutic power* (pp. 1–14). AFTA Springerbriefs in Family Therapy, Springer.
Fitzpatrick, K. & LaGlory, M. (2000). *Unhealthy places: The ecology of risk in the urban landscape*. Routledge.
Fricker, M. (2007). *Epistemic injustice: Power and the ethics of knowing*. Oxford University Press.
Garcia, M., Košutić, I., & McDowell, T. (2015). Peace on earth/war at home: The role of emotion regulation in social justice work. *Journal of Feminist Family Therapy*, *27*(1), 1–20.
Giammattei, S. V. (2015). Beyond the binary: Trans-negotiations in couple and family therapy. *Family Process*, *54*, 418–434.
Hargrave, T. D., & Houltberg, B. J. (2020). Transgenerational theories and how they evolved into current research and practice. In K. S. Wampler, R. B. Miller, & R. B. Seedall (Eds.). *The Handbook of Systemic Family Therapy* (Vol. 1, pp. 317–338). Wiley.
Heiden-Rootes, K., Ferber, M., Meyer, D., Zubatsky, M., & Wittenborn, A. (2021). Relational teletherapy experiences of couple and family therapy trainees: "Reading the room," exhaustion, and the comforts of home. *Journal of Marital and Family Therapy*, *47*, 342–358.
Huft, J. & Jonathan, N. (2018). An integration of feminism into experiential psychotherapy. *The American Journal of Family Therapy*, *46*(3), 287–305.
Johnson, S. M. (2019). *Attachment theory in practice: Emotionally focused therapy (EFT) with individuals, couples, and families*. Guildford.
Knudson-Martin, C. (2015). When therapy challenges patriarchy: Undoing gendered power in heterosexual couple relationships. In C. Knudson-Martin, M. A. Wells, & S. K. Samman (Eds.). *Socio-emotional relationship therapy: Bridging emotion, societal context, and couple interaction* (pp. 15–26). AFTA SpringerBriefs in Family Therapy, Springer.
Knudson-Martin, C. & Kim, L. (2022). Socioculturally attuned couple therapy. In J. Lebow and D. Snyder (Eds.). *Clinical Handbook of Couple Therapy* (6th ed., pp. 267–291). Guilford.
Košutić, I. & McDowell, T. (2008). Diversity and social justice issues in family therapy literature: A decade review. *Journal of Feminist Family Therapy*, *20*(2), 142–165.
McDowell, T. (2015). *Applying critical social theory to family therapy practice*. AFTA SpringerBriefs in Family Therapy, Springer.

Napier, A. Y. & Whitaker, C. (1978). *The family crucible: The intense experience of family therapy*. Harper & Row.
Papp, P., Scheinkman, M., & Malpas, J. (2013). Breaking the mold: Sculpting impasses in couples therapy. *Family Process*, *52*(1), 33–45.
Pease, B. (2012). The politics of gendered emotions: Disrupting men's emotional investment in privilege. *Australian Journal of Social Issues*, *47*(1), 125–142.
Quek, K. M. & Knudson-Martin, C. (2006). A push towards equality: Processes among dual-income couples in a collectivist culture. *Journal of Marriage and Family*, *68*, 56–69.
Roberts, J. (2005). Transparency and self-disclosure in family therapy: Dangers and possibilities. *Family Process*, *44*, 45–63.
Roberts, T. & Chafin, M. (2020), Neuroscience and symbolic-experiential family therapy: Roots of [contemporary] psychotherapy. *The Family Journal*, *28*(2), 138–145.
Satir, V. (1967). *Conjoint family therapy: A Guide to theory and technique* (Revised ed.). Science and Behavior Books. (Original work published 1964).
Schore, A. (2021). The interpersonal neurobiology of intersubjectivity. *Frontiers in Psychology*, *12*, 648616. doi:10.3389/fpsyg.2021.648616.
Siegel, D. J. (2023). *IntraConnected: MWe (Me + we) as the integration of self, identity, and belonging*. Norton.
Siegel, D. J. (2020). *The developing mind: How relationships and the brain interact to shape who we are* (3rd ed.). Guilford.
Siegel, D. J. (2019). The mind in psychotherapy: An interpersonal neurobiology framework for understanding and cultivating mental health. *Psychology and psychotherapy*, *92*, 224–237.
Sohn, A., Zhao, J., & Tadros, E. (2024). Integrating structural and experiential family therapy in neurodivergent families: a case study. *Issues in Mental Health Nursing*, *45*(5), 477–487.
Sorrentino, D. (2024). *Transgender families*. Fulton Books, Inc.
Tatum, B. D. (2017). *Why are all the black kids sitting together in the cafeteria? and other conversations about race*. Basic Books.
Taylor, N. C., Springer, P. R., Bischoff, R. J., & Smith, J. P. (2021). Experiential family therapy interventions delivered via telemental health: A qualitative implementation study. *Journal of Marital and Family Therapy*, *47*(2), 455–472.
Turner, J. H. (2007). Justice and emotions. *Social Justice Research*, *20*, 288–311.
Zimmerman, J. (2018). *Neuro-narrative therapy: New possibilities for emotion-filled conversations*. Norton.

8 Socioculturally Attuned Attachment-Based Family Therapies

An infant makes soft baby sounds, gesturing excitedly with her hands. The child's father looks into her eyes, makes similar cooing sounds, and mirrors his daughter's gestures. The baby smiles and joins her father in their shared experience. This synchronous and reciprocal engagement is the essence of attachment. Attachment is an interpersonal neurobiological and social system that draws infants and caregivers together and serves to organize motivational, emotional, and memory processes (Siegel, 2020).

Attachment's importance was first identified by John Bowlby (1952) in a report to the World Health Organization on the effects of maternal deprivation on British children orphaned during World War II. At that time, the application of the theory tended to reify heteronormative and sexist assumptions that mothers are naturally bonded with their children and that care for children should be their primary role (Franzblau, 1999). Mary Ainsworth continued to build on the work of Bowlby [see Ainsworth et al., 1978] and their work greatly influenced the fields of child development and psychotherapy. Nevertheless, the value of bonds with other caregivers or the multitude of contextual factors that influence caregiving processes received little attention (Birns, 1999; Minuchin, 2002). Over the years, attachment theory has been more broadly studied and applied across the lifespan, elucidating the complex bonds between biology, emotion, relationship, and social context (Cozolino, 2016; Sabey et al., 2024; Siegel, 2020; van der Kolk, 2014) and even applying the theory to the relationships between animals and humans (Walsh, 2009) and with God (Esmiol Wilson, 2015; Esmiol Wilson et al., 2014).

Whether working with adults, children, or larger systems, attachment-based family therapies (ABFTs) focus on strengthening the connections that build and maintain relational bonds. They begin with the premise that "needing and receiving closeness and support is the essence of being human" (Greenberg & Goldman, 2008, p. 84). Among the best known attachment-based family therapies are emotionally focused therapy (EFT, Johnson, 2004; 2019), emotionally focused family therapy (EEFT, Johnson & Lee, 2000), attachment focused family therapy (Hughes, 2011), attachment-based family therapy (Diamond et al., 2014), and emotion-focused couples therapy (Greenberg & Goldman, 2008).

Attachment-based family therapy approaches for specific clinical issues and populations continue to be developed and tested. For example, recent ABFTs address sexual and gender minority young adults and their parents (Diamond et al., 2022), adolescents and young adults with suicide ideation and depression (van der Spek, 2023), emotionally focused parenting (Furrow & Palmer, 2024), using EFFT and play with preschool children (Willis et al., 2016), working with middle school aged children and adoptive families (Barbato et al., 2020), and parent education (Drain & Han, 2023). Related approaches draw on attachment-based principles that emphasize interpersonal neurobiology (i.e., Cozolino, 2016; Fishbane, 2013; van der Kolk, 2014) and the social

DOI: 10.4324/9781003493426-8

construction of identity and emotion (Knudson-Martin & Huenergardt, 2010; Knudson-Martin & Kim, 2023). ABFT practitioners are also identifying ways to work with relational bonds via telehealth (Edwards et al., 2025; Levy et al., 2021).

Supporting relational bonds is particularly important in the current sociocultural context in which the first decades of the 21st century have widened divisions among people, and in the US, the materialistic, consumer-oriented culture leaves people isolated, anxious, and polarized (Doherty, 2020; Piercy, 2020). In this societal context, Doherty (p. 43) argued, there is a need for "gluing" interventions that help people not only connect but invest in each other, both at the intimate couple/family level and with larger communities. Toward this end, some view attachment theory as a unifying theory that can be used as an underlying framework to inform clinical intervention (Johnson, 2019; Sabey et al., 2024; Seedall & Sandberg, 2020). "Interventions based on the power of relationships can be applied at various systems levels: friends, couples, families, communities, workplaces, environments, and even cultures" (Piercy, 2020, p. 754).

•←→•

Families engage in third order change when they are able to overcome sociocultural processes that inhibit attachment and enhance a sense of safety and belonging in complex webs of individual, relational, and societal contexts.

•←→•

Primary, Enduring Family Therapy Concepts

Sometimes people think of attachment primarily as a personal internalized model of relating. If early caregivers were responsive to us as infants, then we will engage with others from a secure base that enables autonomy and optimism (e.g., Ainsworth et al., 1978). If not, we approach life with caution or uncertainty. Individuals are assessed as being either securely attached, avoidantly attached, anxiously/ambivalently attached, or as having a disorganized attachment. While these categorizations are useful, rather than a static individual state, family therapists focus on attachment as a systemic relational *process* that occurs within sociocultural context, including oppressive contexts. Attachment processes can also serve to mediate and resist the impact of these contexts (Edwards, et al., 2026). ABFTs also recognize that attachment occurs across the lifespan; our need for each other is lifelong. According to Johnson (2019),

> Coregulation, rather than solo-regulation, is the baseline, normal, and most-efficient strategy for us as social animals… The attachment concept that we are better together, sharing the load and stress, seems to stand as a physiological fact rather than a sentimental statement. (p. 39)

In contrast to dominant Western culture that privileges autonomy, independence, and competition, attachment perspectives value relational needs and focus on processes around nurturing and giving care. The enduring family therapy concepts that follow help clarify the systemic, interactive nature of attachment: 1) focus on relational process, 2) intersubjective emotional regulation, 3) interdependence and responsiveness, 4) relational security and trust, and 5) change through emotional connection.

Focus on Relational Process

The above example of father and daughter illustrates the interactive nature of attachment. Let's call the child Mayuri. Attachment occurs *between* Mayuri and her significant caregivers. Mayuri has multiple caregivers. Her parents are divorced and share physical custody. They have arranged their work schedules so that each parent serves as the primary caregiver three days a week. On the days they are the primary parent, each drops off Mayuri at a well-staffed daycare for infants. How long she is at the daycare varies, but since each parent has some control over their work schedules, they seldom leave her for more than five or six hours. Both parents report confidence in the daycare providers, but experience a pull to get home to their child as soon as possible. They long to touch and hold her. Since family is important to them, they alternate Sundays with grandparents, sometimes leaving Mayuri with them and sometimes spending the time in gatherings with their large extended families.

The relational processes among Mayuri and her primary caregivers create shared meaning and experience from the moment of birth. Ed Tronick (2009), who studied the psychophysiology of emotional communication between infants and caregivers, emphasized that children are not passive recipients of adult action; rather, each actively changes the other. Staying with Mayuri and her father, let's imagine a situation similar to what Tronick's observational studies showed. As her father tries to put her to bed, Mayuri squirms and grasps his hair. She detects her father's fleeting angry facial expression and loud "Hey!" (even though it lasted less than a second). Mayuri grabs his hands and looks away. Almost immediately, father recognizes that Mayuri is distressed. He changes what he was doing and begins to soothe her, stroking her hair and speaking in a soft voice. At first, Mayuri remains turned away from him, but over the next 30 seconds, she begins to smile and look at him. When Tronick measured biopsychological changes in similar interactions, child and caregiver impacted the physiology of the other.

Whether working with parents and young children or adolescents or with adult relationships in family or community settings, attachment-based therapists (ABFTs) focus on the processes by which participants are emotionally accessible and responsive to each other. They look for how people handle their inherent relational needs. When attachment processes are working well, as with Mayuri, children learn that they can depend on others to be there for them, to notice their needs and respond in ways that affirm their experience. Parents will not always give children everything they want, and there will be conflict and disagreement in all relationships, but there will be a two-way flow of communication in which we listen "with an open mind and all of [our] senses" (Siegel & Hartzell, 2014, p. 82). We respond based on what was actually communicated, rather than automatic, predetermined, or disengaged. When this happens, we feel "felt" or attuned to, that we are not alone.

This interpersonal interaction shapes the neural processes by which our internal models of self-in-relation are encoded. When responses of significant others affirm our experience, we feel grounded and our sense of "self" is connected to something larger than ourselves. As with Mayuri, when there are ruptures to the immediate connection, they can be repaired. Adult experience is also emotionally present and appropriately available to children. Even at this very young age, Mayuri is learning that she has an effect on her father and can influence him and the other caregivers in her life. She learns to trust that she is safe and the world is predictable. She also learns to reciprocally attune to the needs and experiences of others (Tuttle et al., 2012).

From an attachment perspective, seeking and maintaining emotional contact is at the heart of healthy development. Isolation and loss are traumatizing. The need for responsive security-enhancing relationships continues throughout life (Knudson-Martin, 2012; Mikulincer & Shaver, 2012). The ability to move toward others in times of stress and crisis improves health and resilience (Taylor, 2002). Although adults are expected to set the tone with children, adult partners expect responsibility for the relationship to be shared (Johnson, 2019; Knudson-Martin, 2025). While early relational experiences shape an initial working model of attachment, new experiences continue to modify and elaborate internal attachment models (Johnson, 2004). Hurtful experiences of trauma, loss, stigma, and betrayal can move people from security to insecurity, while attuned, mutually supportive relationships can help heal old wounds.

Intersubjective Emotional Regulation

Human neural systems are designed to be interdependent (Cozolino, 2016; Fishbane, 2013). In order to develop, we must exchange emotion and information through what Cozolino called "the social synapse" (p. 19). Through the sharing of emotion, "we participate in the way each other's brains are built, how they develop, and how they function" (Cozolino, 2016, p. 87). The interactions between Mayuri and her father are not simply behavioral events; they are also emotional processes that connect daughter and father neurologically.

Mirror neurons enable people to share affective states (Siegel, 2020). They are specialized cells in the frontal lobes that permit us to viscerally apprehend another's emotional state and intentions. They let Mayuri's father register her distress and revise his response to her almost instantaneously. Attuned interaction between parent and child allows the parent's more mature brain to shape the child's developing one. The parent tracks the child's state and temporarily aligns with it. The child feels felt and her aroused state is calmed. Over time, a healthy pattern of arousal and inhibition, not excessive in either direction, is established (Siegel, 2020).

Clinical issues often relate to how people try to manage painful emotion without adequate emotional support. Efforts to regulate tender emotions, such as isolation or worthlessness, can be destructive. When a parent or partner (or therapist) is not attuned to our primary emotional states, words can seem empty, reinforcing a sense of being alone. In contrast, people with secure attachment histories are more able to regulate how they express emotion and respond to others with an attitude of acceptance, curiosity, and empathy (Hughes, 2009).

Interdependence and Responsiveness

When attunement and responsiveness are not present, the innate interdependence of relationships can be unsafe. Although Mayuri's parents, Rajan and Lakshmi, are able to provide a secure base for their daughter, they were not able to do so for each other. After their separation, Rajan discovered that he needed to orient toward his daughter's needs. He realized how out of touch he had been with Lakshmi's relational needs and experience. He had felt secure and independent in the world, but did not attune to his wife and did not know how to respond to her fear, sadness, and anxiety during their marriage and pregnancy. Lakshmi felt alone and misunderstood. She could not trust that Rajan cared about her or what she needed, and after a while, she disengaged from him.

The neuroemotional process of shared affect requires symmetrical power positions (Hughes, 2009). When roles are unequal, as between parent and child (or therapist and client), the more powerful persons (parents) must follow the child's lead and intentionally open themselves to taking in their experience. When parents communicate acceptance of their child's emotion, the child experiences mutual respect and love rather than shame or disgust (Trevarthen, 2009). As children experience their parents being sensitive and responsive to them, they develop reflective functioning that helps them make sense of their own experience and that of others (Hughes, 2011). When parents also communicate the impact of the child's behavior on them, this mutual intersubjective experience promotes relational security and trust that guides the child's life with others.

Relational Security and Trust

"Simply holding the hand of a loving partner can affect us profoundly, literally calming jittery neurons in the brain" (Johnson, 2008, p. 26). If one's working model of self and other does not anticipate safety, people develop other adaptive responses. It is a matter of survival. Porges' (2009) polyvagal theory helps explain the internal process. The vagus nerve connects the brain with other organs such as the heart, stomach, and facial muscles. It has multiple pathways. The usual instinctual response to a threat is to draw on the branch of the nerve that seeks engagement and connection to others. But when others are not expected to be safe, the other side takes over, shutting down these human connections. We may put up our guard, fight, or withdraw.

In our example, Lakshmi had originally felt safe with Rajan. However, because she had not always experienced safety with others, she was selective in whom she trusted and had learned to withdraw when people did not meet her needs. Rajan had been well-tended as a child but had spent many years depending on himself in a new culture where he felt an outsider. He had not learned to tune into or depend on others. Their three-year marriage did not provide Lakshmi and Rajan a secure base. Depending on each other for emotional support was difficult. Had either of them experienced physical or sexual abuse or other trauma, their dependence on each other might have felt even riskier. If one of them had been unfaithful, their sense of betrayal would likely have compounded the lack of safety and trust.

Change through Emotional Connection

Attachment-based family therapists (ABFTs) work by creating a safe environment in which people are able to experience new responses to vulnerable emotions. "As families learn to respond to one another in ways that are supportive and nurturing…attachment to other family members can gradually become more secure" (Willis et al., 2016, p. 1). ABFTs are active, present-oriented approaches in which experience is heightened through intersubjective dialogue, enactments, and/or play. This enables couples and family members to experience positive physical and emotional connections that actually rewire the brain.

The therapeutic relationship must demonstrate secure attachment qualities (Hughes, 2011; Johnson, 2019). Before couples or families can safely experience vulnerable emotions such as shame, loss, fear, sadness, desire, and longing for each other, the therapist must first attune to each person, seeking to understand and resonate with their underlying emotion. Therapists need to be open and genuinely engaged, including their experience of what clients present. They need to receive emotion openly and accept each person's experience. Even young children can learn to recognize how they affect others (Siegel & Hartzell, 2014) and use play to generate solutions that connect one another and develop empathy, intimacy, and self-worth (Willis et al., 2016). Throughout the process, therapists recognize and attune to clients' affective desires and help them safely experience positive connections with each other.

Integrating Principles of Sociocultural Attunement

Attachment theory is often used within Western psychology to promote autonomy and goal achievement, e.g., that a strong attachment bond decreases a child's need to stay physically close and enables exploration (Cassidy, 2008) or that an adult can "continue pursuing other goals without having to interrupt them to engage in actual bids for proximity and protection" (Mikulincer & Shaver, 2012, p. 260). The value of the relational bonds themselves can get lost. Though some are expanding the lens to consider the sociocultural context of attachment processes (Sabey et al., 2024; Siegel, 2020, 2023), AFBTs tend not to address societal influences or examine inequities in whose interests and values are being advanced. Therapists may miss contextual factors contributing to clients' problems (Edwards et al., 2026; Vatcher & Bongo, 2001) or help family members soothe vulnerable emotions that may more appropriately be viewed as injuries resulting from larger social structures and values (Smoliak et al., 2024). In this section, we consider the connections between attachment processes and sociocultural contexts, explore how societal power dynamics create disparities in whose experience is attuned to and understood, and consider third order change from an attachment point of view.

Societal Context

The ability to nurture attachment bonds is not just an individual or family problem. Like many family and child advocates (e.g., Edelman, 1980; 1987), Bowlby (1988) critiqued the failure of the dominant societal system to support relational bonds:

> [In the] world's richest societies…man and woman power devoted to the production of material goods counts as a plus in all our economic indices. Man and woman power devoted to the production of happy, healthy, and self-reliant children in their own homes does not count at all. (Bowlby, 1988, p. 2)

In a recent summit of attachment-based family therapists, presenters emphasized the influence of larger systemic factors and cautioned therapists against blaming parents for societal influences such as sociopolitical oppression, war, and socio-economic and cultural forces (Sabey et al., 2024). Co-author James Furrow stated:

> We understand the attachment system and the emotion system in context of culture and the ways in which questions of identity and insecurity are shaped by one's environment and experiences including racism and other forms of oppression…and then require a curiosity and humility to inform how we understand the role of attachment and emotion in this family's life together. (p. 1134)

According to attachment theorist Daniel Siegel (2023), "culture shapes how the brain learns to decode incoming information" (p. 27). Siegel identified the Western, and increasingly global, view of "an isolated, separate identity—the solo-self" as resulting in "disconnection from belonging… with individual, interpersonal, and planetary consequences" (p. 8). The narrow individualistic focus limits the integration of the mind necessary to make sense of a complex social world and ourselves (Siegel, 2020). In this view, the attachment processes foundational to health and resilience extend beyond individual families to experiences of belonging and trust in the larger society. They include the development of systemic empathy and compassion necessary to see oneself interconnected within a larger whole, as well as awareness of the impact of individualizing, materialistic cultural and power processes on emotion, sense of self, and relationships.

Dominant Culture Assumptions and Contexts

Dominant cultural assumptions and contexts affect how theory is interpreted and applied. Attachment is often viewed as a dyadic process without considering the role of other family members and social networks. We might assume that a child needs one primary caregiver. In fact, nonparental caregiving is either the norm or frequent in most societies (van Ijzendoorn & Sagi-Schwartz, 2008). In our example, Mayuri, whose grandparents immigrated to the US from India, is benefitting from access to multiple caregivers.

↞↠

Attachment processes between two people are always connected to what is happening with other family members, as well as friends, community members, social institutions, and societal norms.

↞↠

For example, Rajan's parents had at first been very angry with Lakshmi. They insisted he sue her for full custody and were willing to use their considerable financial resources to carry the cost of a prolonged legal battle. Confused, Rajan turned to the pastor of his family's Christian church. The pastor was able to prevail upon the grandparents to take a different approach. His support enabled Rajan and Lakshmi to overcome anger and cordially share primary parenting. Focusing too narrowly on the parent–child relationship or the couple dyad can overlook the need for support within the larger community, and may sometimes hold individuals responsible for conditions out of their control.

We may also unintentionally hold women responsible for relational change. For example, in a demonstration of emotionally focused therapy, the therapist helped a man get in touch with vulnerable emotions that he did not usually express. The therapist ended by suggesting that his wife could help him manage these feelings. Though significant attachment figures should *reciprocally* play this role for each other, research shows that clinicians regularly put the burden of change on women and expect them to calm men (ChenFeng & Galick, 2015; Loscocco & Walzer, 2013). Socioculturally attuned therapists could have interrupted this inequitable societal gender pattern by using the therapeutic relationship to encourage the husband to consider how his emotions might impact his wife and work with him to take responsibility for his emotion and response (Jenks et al., 2024; Knudson-Martin, 2024; see also SERT, Chapter 15 in this volume).

Warm personal styles might also be confused with attachment (Greenberg & Goldman, 2008). There are many ways loving and caring emotions can be expressed and experienced. For example, in Asian cultures expectations of "quiet fortitude" sometimes limit the direct expression of worries or concerns so as not to burden others (ChenFeng et al., 2016). If Asian partners or family members demonstrate a restrained emotional style, this does not necessarily mean less emotional attachment. Helping them share emotional vulnerabilities would still be part of an attachment-based approach, but therapists would first attune to each person's sociocultural experience around expressing emotion and work slowly and gently with them, appreciating and demonstrating respect for less demonstrative styles while helping intimate partners find a process that works for them.

For example, ChenFeng drew on her shared heritage with a second generation Taiwanese American couple to help the husband, Brian, emotionally engage with his wife Michelle (ChenFeng et al., 2016, p. 12):

Therapist: Brian, what did you notice that led you to initiate the conversation?

Brian: We got into an argument earlier that day and I noticed that I was upset about it. I kept thinking about it at work and wondered if it was impacting Michelle also… I guess… [looking down] I felt bad about my tone of voice since I know now how much that affects her.

Therapist: … And I also hear you acknowledging feeling bad. I know it's not typical for Asian American men to say things like that, especially with the experience you've shared about being put down in our American society; it's not easy to be open about what you're feeling… you're breaking out of gender expectations that our culture holds about being tough.

Michelle: Yeah quite honestly, I'm still having a hard time believing this happened, but I'm so happy. I feel really connected to Brian for the first time in a long time.

Ideals regarding appropriate enactments of autonomy and dependence vary widely across cultures and contexts. If parents in Japan complete a child's sentence, that might be considered a sign of positive attunement linked to a secure attachment style; the same behavior in the US would likely be viewed as intrusive and associated with an ambivalent attachment style (Rothbaum et al., 2002). In collectivist cultures, the hoped-for outcome of secure attachment would be a willingness to coordinate one's needs with others; nondisruptive actions that "keep the peace" might be a sign of trust and security. In Western societies, a secure person is typically viewed as one able to venture outward and take on independent tasks or roles.

Socioculturally attuned therapists would not be so quick to go along with cultural stereotypes or taken-for-granted expectations. They would, instead, help clients explore the relational consequences of cultural patterns. They would help parents consider what they would like their children to learn about engaging with others (e.g., Tuttle et al., 2012). For example, a Korean American couple brought their five-year-old daughter, June, to therapy because they were concerned that she was "disobedient and argumentative." As the therapist helped the parents attune to June's experience, they began to imaginatively take in what June was discovering about herself. Then the therapist helped the couple consider what "discovering herself" meant to them and how this fit with Korean and American ideas of how they wanted their child to relate. The therapist also attuned to the parents' shame around a "disobedient and argumentative" child, their sense that they were not good parents. After considering the sociocultural origins of their shame, the parents were more able to accept their daughter and take some pride in her independence while also clarifying which aspects of other-oriented behavior were important in their parenting.

Social Construction of Emotion

Neurobiological attachment processes are intricately intertwined with culture and context. From birth, the human brain is both internal and interpersonal, equipped to identify and feel the sensibilities of those around us (Trevarthen, 2009). What we feel is invited by particular social contexts. Rather than residing *within* an individual, emotions "link persons in the life of family and community" (Trevarthen, p. 56). When the Korean American couple above felt shame as parents, they were directly connected to a community of shared values and expectations that invited and gave meaning to their experience. Recognizing the contextual salience of emotion helps bring the larger societal context into moment-by-moment communication and interaction. As we'll discuss in more detail in Chapter 15, our body's emotional read includes the power context; what we feel is always related to our place in the social hierarchy (Cozolino, 2016; Smoliak et al., 2024; Wetherell, 2012).

Gender and Relational Needs

The need to feel "felt," and the security and validation that comes from feeling connected to significant others, is human. The creation of a gender binary that assigns people "male" or "female" at birth interferes with how relational needs are experienced, expressed, and heard (Fricker, 2007; Knudson-Martin, 2013). In most societies, attachment needs and behaviors are considered feminine. Characteristics associated with females are typically disvalued. Female experience is given less credibility and is less likely to be understood and validated (Fricker, 2007). Many quickly learn that demonstrating relational qualities is not masculine. Boys and men must either disown major parts of themselves or manage the conflict between their relational selves and societal gender discourse. Masculine stereotypes encourage them to externalize vulnerable emotions and blame and objectify others. Societal power structures shape an economy of emotion in which male needs and experiences are more attended to and validated (Smoliak et al., 2024).

Due to patriarchal influence on masculinity, many men are not socialized to have an other orientation, which has effects on their roles as intimate partners and fathers. Acknowledging emotional and dependency needs can be difficult. As in the example of Brian and Michelle above, socioculturally attuned therapists counteract these societal gender patterns by helping men own vulnerable emotions. They expect that men can and do nurture, and actively facilitate their efforts to do so.

This requires therapists to be in touch with their own socialized emotions and the gendered power context of their experiences, both within the therapy room and in their personal lives (see Tim Baima's description of his experience later in this chapter in Text Box 8.2).

Similarly, touch is a vital human need for everyone. It is connected to brain development and the ability to organize emotion (Johnson, 2008). Societal messages about sex and touch may limit this aspect of attachment. Sue Johnson, who along with Les Greenberg developed emotionally focused therapy (EFT), noted that "North Americans are among the world's least tactile people (p. 191)." Males, in particular, are culturally conditioned not to seek touch. Boys are held and caressed less. In adulthood, they may "funnel all of [their] attachment needs for physical and emotional connection into the bedroom" (Johnson, p. 192). People who do not feel safe to be emotionally vulnerable may seek what Johnson calls "sealed-off" sex that is focused on physical release rather than the relational bond. Their partners may feel used and objectified. Others may use sex as a way to find "solace," a way to feel reassured about attachment needs, especially when partners are not emotionally available. When sex is part of secure reciprocally attuned and responsive relationships, physical synchrony and emotional safety reinforce each other, and partners can relax into mutual pleasuring (Johnson, 2008). Cultural gender stereotypes and objectifying discourse around sex interfere with indispensable non-sexual touching as well as emotionally safe and loving sexual relationships. See Text Box 8.1 for an example of a socioculturally attuned approach to sexual issues.

Text Box 8.1 Elisabeth Esmiol Wilson, PhD, LMFT

Elisabeth Esmiol Wilson is an AASECT certified sex therapist, an AAMFT Approved Supervisor, and trained Spiritual Director. She describes herself as a White, cis gender, heterosexual, middle-aged mom and stepmom whose upbringing was rooted in an LGBTQ affirming, multiracial, multicultural, Episcopal church she attended with her single mother and younger sister in Kailua, Hawaii. Elisabeth's clinical and research interests focus on socially just approaches to integrating couple therapy, sex therapy, and spirituality, carefully taking into account the larger societal discourses and power structures and how religion in particular can be a factor that helps and hurts our mental, relational, and sexual health. Here she illustrates her socioculturally attuned attachment approach.

Abigail and Miriam originally came to me for sex therapy. They self-identified as a biracial, ecumenical lesbian couple with a shared history of sexual abuse. Both recently retired, they presented as very bright women with higher education degrees in psychology and religion. Interpersonally, they presented as a warm and playful couple with a great deal of love for each other. Abigail, who identified as White and Protestant, was sexually abused as a teenager by her uncle. Miriam, who identified as Latino and Catholic, experienced nonconsensual touch from a priest when she was a novitiate considering entering religious life as a nun. Both had experiences of disaffiliating from their non-affirming family of origin religious communities and finding an affirming, progressive Christian church they attended together. In therapy, I stayed aware of complexity and variety of different faith, race, culture, gender, and sexuality messages the couple had received through their families of origin as well as religious upbringings. I also attended to how power impacted mutuality in their relationship, and the impact of larger societal and religious messages on their current attachment issues. Finally, I explored how religious systems of inequity continued to impact their current faith and varying degrees of freedom they experienced in their expressions of sexuality and shared sexual pleasure.

I tend to name issues directly, using curiosity and open-ended questions to help hold the complexities, while attuning to the underlying emotions and power disparities and how these impact relational mutuality and secure attachment. We discovered that their differing theologies of atonement (reconciliation of God and humankind through Christ) deeply impacted their sexual pleasure. We explored questions such as "What is the impact of believing in an atonement in which forgiveness and reconciliation are freely offered on how you show up with each other emotionally and sexually?" We explored the impact of their sexual and religious abuse on their image of God and on how both continued to view the role of sexual pleasure in their relationship. "What differences do you notice in yourself as you move to understanding reconciliation as a relational process?"

I name not only the social injustice but the impact of the injustice, giving space for emotional processing and space to feel the impact of being silenced and marginalized. We explored both Miriam and Abigail's deep desire and sense of calling to participate in a shared spirituality, and the splitting and hiding that was historically necessary to even pursue that path. We explored how to honor their grief without further silencing the beauty of living in the fullness of their shared religious, relational, and sexual identities.

Sometimes my work includes challenging the messages of unjust systems that clients may have already physically departed from, but which nevertheless remain psychologically present. We slowed down their sexual scripts, exploring in detail the thoughts, images, and feelings that emerged in them as they moved through early, middle, and late stages of arousal. I encouraged Abigail and Miriam to interrupt these oppressive messages in the moment, sometimes in their own head, sometimes verbally with each other, slowing down their sensual and sexual experiences to create more space for congruent, accepting, pleasurable connection.

Part of my work with Abigail and Miriam included inviting them to envision a relationship model that they had never seen actualized. As I supported them in dreaming together, the process itself was transformative. Together they envisioned a spiritually connected, equitable, mutually attuned relationship, in which they were connected together to a larger religious community. While not all the folks they cared about supported their vision, Abigail and Miriam remained committed to modeling a kind of love that would support others like them to more easily envision a path toward relational equity and love.

Class and Attachment

The ways attachment processes are theoretically described and researched tend to reflect Western middle class values (Birns, 1999; Franzblau, 1999). Yet how people approach caregiving and receiving varies considerably depending on social structure and the future they are preparing their children to enter (Lareau, 2003; Tuttle et al., 2012). Working-class parents have less control over their schedules and less income for quality daycare than the example of Mayuri above. The dispositions and values any of us bring to parenting and intimate relationships reflect the structured social arrangements we inhabit (Lareau, 2003).

For example, Luellen and her children were referred to therapy after her oldest son, Darnell (aged 11), told a school counselor that his mother locked him in his room when he came home after curfew. To resonate with Luellen, a low income, African American woman raising her boys in a neighborhood where many young men join gangs or become victims of violence, the therapist needed to attune to how important it is to Luellen that her sons be obedient and follow the rules. This will also be necessary for them to safely negotiate racism and be successful in school. Independence and assertiveness, qualities often valued by White middle-class parents, may be risky in a world where Darnell could easily be judged as delinquent, defiant, or dangerous.

People nurture securely attached relationships across all socioeconomic strata (Birns, 1999). Members of economically disadvantaged groups often demonstrate considerable emotional resilience. For example, studies of children of Latino immigrants in the US show high levels of emotional well-being and social skills (Fuller & Coll, 2010). Nonetheless, stresses such as limited economic resources, space, and time affect the structure and organization of family life (McDowell, 2015). Differences in measures of attachment security between socioeconomic contexts can usually be explained by the degree to which social environments support attachment processes (Bliwise, 1999).

Hermeneutical Justice

A core premise of attachment theory is that people develop a coherent self-narrative when their experience is attuned to and relationally validated (Siegel, 2020).

•←→•

The ability to make sense of one's experience may be disadvantaged when dominant cultural meanings systematically limit who can express themselves and be understood.

•←→•

For example, incongruence and the resulting sense of isolation are commonly experienced by those who identify as gay and lesbian, transgender, or who identify outside the gender binary (Bernards et al., 2025; Diamond et al., 2022; Edwards et al., 2026). This is not simply a matter of parental criticism or rejection; it is part of the larger context in which the meanings of gender and sexuality are constructed. For example, Michael, who had transitioned from female to male about ten years prior, sought therapy because he was anxious about a forthcoming career change. He described positive relationships with his family and a stable marriage with a cis woman. Yet in this situation in which he would be developing another aspect of his identity and new kinds of collaborative work relationships, he was faced again with what Miranda Fricker (2007) called *hermeneutical injustice*, inequities in whose experiences are understood and given social credibility. This means that the dominant culture offered little shared understanding as a resource to support Michael's experience. According to Fricker (2007, p. 163), "it tends to knock your faith in your own ability to make sense of the world."

At the start of therapy, Michael was confused by his anxiety because he anticipated his new colleagues would be accepting. But acceptance is different than *being known*. Over the years, Michael had adapted to unremitting hermeneutic isolation by disengaging from his own emotional experience. His family, partner, and friends tried to understand but lacked collective meanings to activate mirror neurons to attune to him. Systemic obfuscation encouraged him to opt out of shared meaning-making that constitutes the self (Fricker, 2007). While outwardly friendly and socially involved, he kept an emotional distance, even from himself. Naming this as a societal problem rather than a personal deficiency helped Michael overcome some of the isolation and slowly experiment with steps he could safely take to attune to himself and others.

Hermeneutic injustice creates a lack of credibility (Fricker, 2007). People do not take in your experience as being possible or as making sense. Patricia Hill Collins (2000) described how Black women in academia and other institutions learn to survive in a system that only recognizes knowledge and experience consistent with dominant White male culture. Bermúdez and colleagues, as Latinx and Caribbean family scholars and therapists, have described experiencing the same (under review). From an attachment perspective, the isolation and assault to self are substantial.

Power

↞↠

Attachment is highly contextual and impacted by power dynamics, inclusion, and a sense of belonging at intimate, family, community, and societal levels.

↞↠

Expanding our lens beyond family puts relational bonds within systemic patterns that reflect and maintain societal power inequities (Edwards et al., 2026; Knudson-Martin, 2012, 2013; Medina, 2013). What we feel, who is noticed and attended to, and the likelihood that we benefit from attuned support, depend on social power processes that govern communication (Fricker, 2007).

Effect of Power on Emotion

Neural circuitry always registers our place in the social hierarchy (Cozolino, 2016; see also SERT, Chapter 15). The unfolding of emotion is interactive, taking into account both attachment and power contexts (Greenberg & Goldeman 2008). For example, Ben and Liz, a White cisgender couple in their 20s, with recent college degrees, sought therapy because of escalating anger and verbal assaults. Just looking at behavior, it would appear each contributes equally to the escalation. Each was using anger to protect relational vulnerabilities. But their gender and social class locations placed them in different power positions, with very different emotional consequences.

As a male from an affluent family with parents he described as warm and loving, Ben believed himself to be "open" and "giving." He valued his relationship with Liz but was blind to the ways he perpetuated systemic ignorance of, and inattention to, the experience of those with less social power (hermeneutic injustice). He expected to be taken seriously and have agency over his own life. When Liz questioned him about his activities or expenditures, anger—inseparable from his power and identity positions—just seemed to erupt. He would lash out at Liz, blaming her for not trusting him, questioning her judgment and knowledge, (i.e., "testimonial injustice" in which he does not take her voice or experience seriously) (Fricker, 2007).

Liz, also from a loving family, but one with limited economic resources, tried to be sensitive to Ben's interests. Her roots lower in the social hierarchy taught her that silence was often safest in new settings (Medina, 2013). Her safety depended on gathering information about her environment. Like others in one-down social positions, she was almost always aware of what Ben was likely to be thinking and feeling (Knudson-Martin, 2013). She not only wanted to understand his actions and choices, in her one-down position, she *needed* to understand. When Ben lashed out at her, she felt hurt and even more vulnerable. Her sense of dismissal and injustice motivated angry retorts.

The emotions Ben and Liz experienced are not just personal power dynamics between them; they reflect and maintain societal power imbalances. These persistent patterns are built into social structures and may not be obvious to participants (Wetherell, 2012). Therapists need a guiding lens that seeks to understand how a particular emotion is linked to larger societal power contexts (Pandit et al., 2014). Attending to power imbalances, such as between Liz and Ben, is important to creating safety in the therapeutic encounter. Socioculturally attuned attachment therapists will not ask Liz to express vulnerable emotions without first creating a context in which Ben is able to listen to her.

Effect of Power on Who Attunes

Supportive attachment requires reciprocal attunement; however, those with higher power statuses tend not to notice or attune to those with less social power unless they intentionally seek to understand and connect (Knudson-Martin, 2013). This usually is a question of *will* (Medina, 2013). Attunement requires a willingness to temporarily let go of one's own perspective and take in another's. Instead, power processes invite persons in dominant positions to expect subordinates to soothe and regulate their uncomfortable emotions. Ben takes Liz's attunement to him for granted until her questions seem to challenge his identity, autonomy, and/or authority.

Third Order Change

Third order change from an attachment perspective includes awareness of the sociocultural context of one's attachment responses. Persons in powerful positions tend to focus outward rather than inward, blaming others rather than self-reflecting (Greenberg & Goldman, 2008). Their anger, intimidation, or silence becomes a way to regulate others.

•←→•

Third order change is facilitated when powerful persons become aware of their social location and intentionally attune themselves to others.

•←→•

As in Ben's case, powerful persons need to experience their own vulnerabilities and open themselves to the experience of others rather than resort to control. People in one-down positions are likely to be silenced as they adapt so they can maintain safety and security. From an attachment perspective, Liz's eventual anger, rather than withdrawing, is an invitation or plea for Ben to engage. Instead of viewing her retorts as dysfunctional, it is also possible that they can be experienced as resistance to power. Tuning into the power context of her anger can raise useful awareness and self-reflection regarding how one wants or can respond to unjust circumstances (Garcia et al., 2015; Medina, 2013). As Ben and Liz become more contextually aware, his willingness to hear her anger and learn from it will be an important step.

Community and Empowerment

The impact of power on well-being extends to the community, the workplace, and the larger society. When people live in social contexts that affirm their identities and connections, they can be well and offer the best of themselves back to their communities. Prejudice, discrimination, and structural inequalities have an insidious effect, perpetuating objectification, commodification, and exploitation in the routine ways people treat each other (Collins, 2000). Countering these injustices through third order change is more possible when people build relationships with others who understand and support them (Almeida, 2019).

The Latino Health Access (LHA) in Orange County, California (Bracho et al., 2016) is an impressive example of collective empowerment. Participants in vulnerable low-income communities battle addiction, manage diabetes, stop violence, or improve children's health by building strong community and relational bonds. Their philosophy resists oppressive societal power processes "with a heart that feels love for our community and expresses that love through acts of solidarity" (p. xv). Grounded in science about the effects of societal inequities on health, but prioritizing the wisdom of the community, the project works through strengthening bonds and networks among neighbors. Everyone gives and everyone receives. Sarai, a *promotora* (community expert) who struggled with parenting and an abusive relationship summed up the positive impact of community bonds:

> When fear comes to me, I take a few steps back. Then I talk to others in the community and stop being afraid... We belong to each other. Every day we work to create and invite people to safe, protected spaces where they can be themselves, feel stronger, overcome their fears, and be part of the solutions.
>
> (Bracho et al., 2016, p. 67)

Models like LHA support family bonds within wider webs of relationships and use those bonds to construct new knowledge, resist injustice, and create transformative change (e.g., Collins, 2000).

Socioculturally attuned attachment-based family therapists promote third order change within families; however like the Latino Health Access project above, it is also important to address attachment processes in community and societal contexts. Working with schools to develop the capacity for empathy (Gordon, 2018), apply relational pedagogy (Reichert & Nelson, 2018), or implement a compassionate systems framework (Siegel, 2020) are examples of expanding the contexts for development of trust, belonging, and connection. Similarly, identities are formed and nurtured (or not) in workplaces; when these settings are structured to center and tend to relationships, people feel seen and relational connections replace isolation (Bava & Greene, 2023). At the societal level, policies and practices can help support care, connectedness, and well-being or they can work against them.

Practice Guidelines

•←→•

The goal of socioculturally attuned attachment based therapy is to develop relational connections that enable couples and families to equitably support each other in the face of life's stresses and injustices in order to engage in transformative action.

•←→•

We suggest the following five guidelines to help attachment-based therapies incorporate a socioculturally attuned approach that attends to power and societal context; 1) recognize power's effects on relational safety, 2) attune to the sociocultural nature of emotion, 3) accentuate relational needs, 4) initiate power-sharing through engaged enactments, and 5) consolidate equitable relational patterns.

1. Recognize Power's Effects on Relational Safety

When first engaging with individuals, couples, or families, socioculturally attuned therapists seek to understand how social power, the capacity to "influence how things go in the social world," (Fricker, 2007, p. 9) is reflected in how participants orient to each other and the larger environment. How likely is each to *feel felt*? Who attends to whom? How do gender and other power contexts affect responses to vulnerability? How might vulnerabilities stem from larger societal sources? How do these patterned responses create safety for some at the expense of others? To create an equitable foundation for therapy, therapists act to balance power in ways that support emotional safety for everyone. They take in each person's perspective without unintentionally allowing more powerfully situated members to define the direction of therapy.

2. Attune to the Sociocultural Nature of Emotion

Safety is enhanced as therapists actively **attune** to the sociocultural nature of each person's emotional experience (Knudson-Martin, 2024). Socially aware listening is facilitated as therapists attune to client emotion through a lens curious about how personal experience connects to larger societal discourses and power processes, such as the idea that women should not question men:

Therapist: It's so distressing when Liz questions you, almost as though she is questioning your judgment.
Ben: Yeah! Like she's putting me down. Like she doesn't trust me.
Therapist: What's that like for you? What might it seem to say about you as a man?

Therapists reflect an understanding and **name** client's sociocultural experiences, explicitly linking emotions, experiences, and processes with sociocultural context:

Ben: Nobody ever questioned my dad. I don't know why she is always questioning me! Who does she think I am?
Therapist: So, when Liz questions you, could it be that you feel like you're not much of a man in her eyes. You want her to look up to you. Am I getting that right? [David nods]. It makes sense to me that if you learned that men are supposed to be right, to be looked up to, it might be pretty uncomfortable if it feels your authority is questioned.
Ben: I'm not really like that you know–not one of those men who has to be the authority.

As clients identify the social contextual nature of their emotions and feel understood, like Ben, they are more able to reflect on themselves and others, which enables more connection and accountability to self and others. In Text Box 8.2 Tim Baima describes how he raises consciousness of power and intimacy issues, and how demonstrations of power may be tied to "socially unacceptable" feelings of vulnerability.

Text Box 8.2 Timothy Baima, PhD, LMFT

Attachment theory frames Tim Baima's understanding of healthy relationships and healthy autonomous functioning. Below he describes his approach to identifying and naming sociocultural issues with his clients, taking into account his identity as a White, straight cis male from a working-class background.

First, I believe it is my responsibility to take risks with my clients. I initiate conversations about sociocultural context even when I am uncomfortable and bound to be clumsy in my effort to do so. I have long abandoned the dream of phrasing every question with the eloquence of master therapists and have been pleasantly surprised to find that even a question such as, "Could race have had something to do with that interaction?" can be very effective as long as I have the courage to ask it.

Second, I use therapeutic self-disclosure to place my questions and comments in context. I might join with a privileged client by sharing ways I have similarly misused power related to my own unearned privilege. When I draw attention to possible manifestations of oppression related to marginalized identities I do not share, I may lead by acknowledging my position as an outsider. When I do so, I attempt to communicate that I understand that I am leaning into a topic I can never truly understand.

Third, I draw heavily upon Kenneth V. Hardy's (2016) Validation, Challenge, Request (VCR) intervention. For example, when I want to challenge a White partner to see how his defensive posture with his Partner of Color shuts his partner down, I may start by validating his desire to be connected. Perhaps he is even taking that defensive tone because he fears losing his partner. This type of validation allows the client to feel understood and cared for and more receptive to a challenge about how his tone is actually preventing him from getting the very connection he desires, and to a request to listen to his partner differently.

Finally, people with social privilege often use domination to avoid discomfort, inconvenience, and vulnerability. We may draw upon the power associated with a privileged part of self to compensate for the vulnerability and pain we feel in a subjugated part of the self. I see many clients who use their power to silence and dismiss important parts of themselves as well as their partners and children. These clients are often able to suppress their own internal world and control the people they are in relationship with, and then end up confused about how empty and alone they feel. When these clients recognize how domination over self and other restricts intimacy, they tend to become more receptive to learning how to let go of domination in order to embrace love.

I believe that love and intimacy are characterized by self-reflection and self-nurturance that facilitates growth. Therefore, reflecting on our relationships with unearned power, privilege, and oppression is an act of love towards ourselves and towards all those with whom we are in relationships. It is important to note that those of us with unearned power and privilege are far more likely to misuse and abuse that power and privilege not when we ***feel*** *powerful, but when we feel uncomfortable, afraid, insecure, or vulnerable. Often it is when hurt, abused, or subjugated aspects of ourselves are triggered that we compulsively draw upon our unearned power and privilege to navigate the inherent discomfort of such situations. Therefore, I believe that third order change must involve attending to both privileged and subjugated aspects of self (Hardy, 2016). Empowering ourselves or our clients in areas we have been traumatized, hurt, or oppressed, goes hand-in-hand with learning to abandon a dependence on domination rooted in our privileged parts of self.*

3. Accentuate Relational Needs

Dominant Western cultures minimize relational needs and, as noted earlier, increasingly leave people feeling isolated and focused on material concerns. Attachment-based therapists look for and highlight each person's relational commitments and **values.** They look for relational strengths already present, but which may be currently hidden or overlooked. This helps those in powerful positions be willing to attune to subordinates. A demanding and punitive father may be guided to express his love and concern for his acting out teenager. Angry teens may fear they are not loveable and long for acceptance. A couple divided by hurt may need help recognizing their dreams for love and understanding.

Identifying, **naming**, and focusing on relational needs creates a vision of what clients are working toward. As the therapist resonates with and gives voice to clients' relational foundations and dreams, they "feel safe enough to be in touch with their need for emotional connection and the positive intentions each held for their relationship" (Wells et al., 2017, p. 21). Therapists can then help clients access and express these hopes and commitments as they rebuild and develop their bonds. Individuals get perspective on how they want to engage in relationships and what to expect. Therapists may **intervene** to help clients consider how other family members, friends, work, community contexts, and societal discourses support (or not) their relational values and needs.

4. Initiate Power-sharing through Engaged Enactments

Socioculturally attuned ABFTs help clients choreograph engaged encounters that interrupt societal power dynamics and facilitate attuned connection. Similarly to socio-emotional relationship therapy (see Chapter 15), they **intervene** by inviting more powerful persons to listen and respond, express vulnerability, and take initiative in building relational connections. Therapists work with in-the-moment-process between clients, focusing on how they relate to each other and exploring the underlying sociocultural nature of emotion. Clients begin to see how they enact cultural stereotypes and power dynamics, as well as recognize when they experience connection and mutuality.

5. Consolidate Equitable Relational Patterns

As clients experience relational safety, connection, and reciprocal support, therapists heighten and expand the moment. They encourage clients to recognize what they did to build relationship and highlight the positive relational impact of these actions. In the process, clients are able to articulate ways they have "become more fair and reliable… to have a sense of shared accountability" (Wells et al., 2017, p. 24). Therapists help consolidate experiences of equitable commitment and relational investment and help clients **envision** how they will engage with each other and the larger society going forward. Socioculturally attuned therapists will have been attentive throughout to key persons and communities that support clients' **transformation** through evolving relationship bonds and identities.

Case Example

Jolene (31) was referred by her midwife following the birth of Matthew (5 months). The therapist, Norma (26), a Black family therapy intern who used female pronouns, invited Jolene's wife Lara (33) to the first session. Norma learned that the White, cisgender female couple had been married for five years, together for nine, and also had a 4-year-old daughter, Camilla. When Lara, a kindergarten teacher, gave birth to Camilla she took a year's [unpaid] maternity leave. Jolene, an advertising account manager, was doing the same now with Matthew, while Camilla was in preschool in the mornings and with Lara's mother in the afternoon. Jolene had looked forward to a special time with Matthew; instead, she was "losing it." She felt inadequate, incompetent, and ashamed. She was especially humiliated that Lara, who was diagnosed with multiple sclerosis (MS) when she was twenty, was a "natural" mother, despite coping with her MS, which included damage to the optic nerve, somewhat unpredictable balance, and occasional flare-ups.

Recognize Power's Effects on Relational Safety

As Norma began to get to know Jolene and Lara, she was interested in who was oriented to whom. The couple quickly described Lara as a "caregiver." Lara's accounts frequently included Jolene's perspective. Jolene appeared much less attentive and attuned, insisting that Lara focused too much of her time on friends and family that did not deserve her.

Lara: Like last weekend, my cousin needed a ride. Jolene was mad at me for doing that. I understand how she feels; she thinks I'm being taken advantage of.

Jolene: It's stupid! You never learn!

A pattern of unequal attunement continued throughout the session. Jolene was the beneficiary of considerably more relational care from Lara than she returned. Each woman had suffered childhood abuse and/or neglect and had worked to overcome the effects of these attachment injuries.

Lara trusted that Jolene loved her and minimized the hurt she experienced when Jolene did not tune into her. She was used to soothing Jolene, helping her work through her stresses. But when she tried to help Jolene in caring for Matthew, Jolene just seemed to get more depressed.

Jolene also described feeling betrayed when she discovered that Lara had coffee with Dillon, her "first love." It had been ten years since Lara had seen Dillon when she ran into him unexpectedly. They had coffee to "catch up." She did not tell Jolene about the meeting fearing that it would upset her. Norma recognized Lara's secretiveness as a reaction to Jolene's "disentitled power," common among victims of childhood abuse (Wells et al., 2017, p. 129). Although more prevalent among men, this kind of power does not stem from an overtly powerful position; it is often connected to feelings of worthlessness and unlovability. Yet their self-focus creates a power imbalance in the relationship.

Attune to Sociocultural Nature of Emotion

Norma conveyed a deep interest in knowing and "getting" each partner's experience through a sociocultural lens. Jolene was not stereotypically "feminine," but she internalized all the societal messages about "a good mother." When she did not always feel loving thoughts toward her baby, she felt like a failure. She could not tell anyone, especially when she had been so sure she had so much love to give. The more she felt like a failure, the more isolated and withdrawn she became. Norma reflected and validated the sociocultural nature of her experiences, linking emotion to relational and societal contexts:

Norma: All your life you've known you have so much love to give.

Jolene: [When my parents abandoned me] I was on my own. I knew all I needed was a chance. I knew I would be a good mother…I've been a good mother to Camilla.

Norma: Even though your mother couldn't be there for you, somehow you carried this idea with you, of a good mother…like a dream. Do you think your dream is similar to other women's?

Jolene: I think everyone knows what mothers are supposed to do.

Norma: When I talk with mothers, almost everyone seems to feel like they're failing in some kind of way. Women get a lot of messages about all that they're supposed to do—and how loving they're supposed to be.

Jolene and Lara had spoken at length about what good mothers they would be, how they would arrange donors, how they would manage child care. They did not speak of their fears, doubts, and vulnerabilities. This was not simply because of prior attachment injuries. It was also because women receive strong societal taboos regarding expressing and sharing these feelings (Knudson-Martin & Silverstein, 2009; Mauthner, 1999).

Norma also explored the extra pressure Jolene and Lara felt to represent the LGBTQI+ community as "good mothers" and how all these intersected with MS disability:

Lara: I have always kept going no matter what. When my uncle molested me, when I was bullied at school because I looked funny and didn't have the right clothes, I never told anyone. I didn't let myself care. When MS came, more of the same.

Norma: You've always had to keep going. It was all on you…and from what you've said, you always tried to make it easier for others.

Lara: I didn't want to make people uncomfortable. I didn't want to worry my mom. With MS, people don't understand. They might think I shouldn't be a mom [shrugs and smiles]. I have to keep smiling and doing my best anyway.

Accentuate Relational Needs

Norma helped the couple begin to see their relationship patterns and provided a relational framework through which to understand depression and repair power imbalances. She validated and built upon the positive connections already evident in the relationship.

Norma: I see the love—how much you each value your relationship… You've described patterns in which Lara is really focused on you, Jolene. I'm guessing that you want to be there for her, too [Jolene agrees]. What's happening now and how hard it is to not feel the way you want with Matthew, it might be a good time to find a way to make the back and forth more shared, to make the relationship a safe harbor for each of you. My hunch is that it will help the depression, too.

Positively framing the couple's commitment to each other and their family helped counter societal messages that they were "less than" and not entitled to care. Conversations that connected their family experiences to larger societal contexts helped remove personal blame and develop empathy for themselves and their caregivers' situations:

Norma: [to Lara] What do you think it was like for your mother…taking care of you on her own?

Lara: She was working all the time. She was working for us. If she knew what my uncle did, what I was going through… I couldn't do that to her.

Norma: It seems like you had a sense that your mother was carrying a very heavy load. Even then, it seems you might have known there was injustice there [Lara emphatically agrees]. Almost as though to the rest of the world your family wasn't very important.

Initiate Power-sharing through Engaged Enactments

Jolene and Lara adapted differently to emotional insecurity. Lara worked to calm others, while Jolene kept emotional distance, unaware of how much she depended on Lara for emotional stability. Jolene had survived by not letting herself feel vulnerable. In the incident with Dillon, she did not let herself feel what it was like to need someone; instead, she tried to control Lara's relationships. She had not developed the practice of taking in what others felt or reflecting on her own feelings. Jolene loved Camilla's bubbly 4-year-old laughter and felt good when she held Camilla close. With Matthew it was different. She was on her own most of the day and he didn't respond the way she expected. The more helpless she felt, the more unlovable and unworthy she felt. Lara was moved when she witnessed Jolene's vulnerability, but neither paid attention to Lara's relational needs.

Norma developed enactments that interrupted the couple's power imbalance and expanded attachment beyond a dyad. First, she asked Jolene to reflect on what she thought it might be like for Lara when she (Jolene) was having such a hard time with Matthew. This helped Jolene move away from self-focus that not only perpetuated the power imbalance but also maintained the feedback loop between isolation and depression (Knudson-Martin & Silverstein, 2009). In setting up the enactment, Norma first validated Jolene's despair, then drew on her love for Lara:

Norma: [to Jolene] It's so hard. You feel like a failure as a mother, as a person… I'm also wondering what it's like for Lara. You've said so clearly how much she means to you. What have you noticed? What's it like for her to see you so down?

Jolene struggled to have a response. She wanted Lara to tell her, but Norma stayed with Jolene, supporting her to imaginatively take on Jolene's experience:

Norma: You know her. "Hard for her," you said. What's hard?
Jolene: [Pauses. Looks at Lara, then shrugs]. Just hard, you know. I can't be easy to deal with!
Norma: You see that it must be hard for Lara. What do you think the hardest part is for her?

Norma gently persisted so that Jolene could have a successful experience of attuning to Lara. She resisted the temptation to simply ask Lara.

In a second enactment, Norma asked Jolene to share a fear that she had regarding Lara. Norma asked Lara just to hear it. This was very difficult for both women, but Norma wanted Jolene to practice vulnerability in the safety of the therapy room. After Jolene took the lead in expressing vulnerability–her fear that she was not loveable–Norma helped the couple process the experience, emphasizing both the emotional risk they took and the positive consequences. This set the stage for mutual sharing of vulnerability:

Norma: This is a hard time for all of you. You both need each other; you're both vulnerable. But Jolene's pain is easier to see. And I can understand, Lara, why you don't want to add to Jolene's plate right now. But I wonder if there is a way you could check in with each other and each share a vulnerability you're feeling? Agree that you don't need to try to solve it right then, just listen.

Consolidate Equitable Relational Patterns

Norma continued with enactments designed to help the couple risk an expanded level of emotional engagement. She persisted in paying attention to the balance of giving care and highlighting the positive aspects of their evolving relational bond. Though it can take considerable time to rework attachment traumas (see Johnson, 2002; Wells et al., 2017), Jolene began to feel better almost immediately and each week the couple reported a more secure bond. They said that the depression and the incident with Dillon were the best things that happened to their relationship. Their prior therapy had helped them develop personal responsibility, but they appreciated that this therapy validated their closeness. Instead of feeling like a set of diagnoses, they felt affirmed as mothers and partners. Conversations about mutual care and emotional support included considerable discussion about living with MS. The fact that Jolene wanted to share this part of her life was astounding to Lara. Jolene, who had always been "private," joined a support group for mothers and quickly became one of the organizers.

Summary: Third Order Change

First order change is "common sense" but does not change the systemic ways people engage with each other. Perhaps they learn some new communication skills or how to better manage symptoms. Jolene might have taken an antidepressant or discussed her experience with a therapist. Perhaps Lara would have learned more effective strategies to support Jolene through the depression. These potential steps would have been unlikely to stimulate second order change given the nature of the couple's attachment bonds with each other and their children. Their responses to each other would still reflect different adaptive responses to earlier attachment injuries. Jolene would still have received more understanding and care than Lara. Lara would have remained the competent one, able to look after herself and others, even while dealing with a chronic illness.

Second order change would have resulted in new ways of relating based on increased security. Their strengthened bonds would have decreased anxiety around parenting and supported more flexible boundaries outside the nuclear family. They would have been more able to share responses to MS, but understanding themselves in relation to the larger society most likely would not have changed. They would have still seen themselves as "survivors" creating a better life for their children. They would not have questioned societal messages about mothers. They would have not had a lens through which to see their experiences as part of societal patterns larger than their family. They would not have experienced transformation through being aware of the effects of injustice in their lives. They would not have seen how abuse, abandonment, lower socioeconomic status, disability, and their sexualities all intersected with limited credibility still accorded women, or how this limited their ability to know themselves and each other and to recognize their own worth (Edwards et al., 2026; Fricker, 2007; Medina, 2013).

Third order change for Jolene, Lara, and their children began with the willingness of a straight, single, African American intern therapist, to step away from her own knowing to as much as possible take in the sociocultural nature of Jolene and Lara's emotional experiences. As she took time to try to truly understand and to link her clients' experiences with their social locations and societal power, Lara and Jolene began to see themselves and the world around them through new eyes. They felt validated as never before. Norma's carefully choreographed enactments helped them transform an unequal power dynamic that had not only maintained previous attachment responses but also reproduced underlying societal messages of unworthiness. Their relatively quick transformation reflected the empowerment they felt as they began to see their experience as similar to others in their positions (Fricker, 2007; Medina, 2013). Jolene's leadership in a mothers' support group also enacted third order change as she and Lara began to see alternative possibilities and choices in their roles as women, mothers, and community members.

Reflexive Questions

- How can you, as an attachment based family therapist, expand the notion that attachment is not only a dyadic process, but one that often includes other family members, social networks, and norms?
- When considering your multiple positions of power within and across certain contexts, how do they influence who you attune to for emotional connection?
- How can you balance power in ways that support emotional safety for everyone?
- What are the ways in which you can identify, name, and amplify clients' relational needs so that family members and friends can be more in support of them?
- How do you know when your clients are experiencing relational safety, connection, and reciprocal support? What are the signs?
- How can you as an attachment-focused family therapist heighten and expand the moment and work toward envisioning and consolidating equitable relational patterns?

References

Ainsworth, M. D. S., Blehar, M. C., Waters, E., & Wall, S. (1978). *Patterns of attachment: A psychological study of the strange situation*. Erlbaum.

Almeida, R. V. (2019). *Liberation based healing practices*. Institute for Family Services.

Barbato, A., D'Avanzo, B., Vadilonga, F., Cortinovis, M., Lombardi, S., Pili, F., … & Visconti, A. (2020). Systemic family therapy integrated with attachment interventions for adoptive families. Development of a treatment manual. *Journal of Family Therapy*, *42*(4), 536–559.

Bava, S. & Greene, M. (2023). *The relational workplace: How relational intelligence grows diverse, equitable, and inclusive cultures of connection*. ThinkPlay Partners.

Bermúdez, J. M., Muruthi, B. A., Alvarez-Hernandez, L., Machado, Y., & Lamont-Gomez, F. (equal authors) (under review). Decolonizing approaches to family science as intersectional Latinx and Caribbean scholars working toward third order change, *Journal of Family Theory and Review*.

Bernards, J. C., Hunt, Q., Henriques, C., Bledsoe, A., & Ostler, R. (2025). “This whole journey was sacred”: Latter-day Saint parents’ process in coming to accept a transgender child. *Family Process*, *64*(1), e13038.

Birns, B. (1999). Attachment theory revisited: Challenging conceptual and methodological sacred cows. *Feminism & Psychology*, *9*, 10–21.

Bliwise, N. G. (1999). Securing attachment theory’s potential. *Feminism & Psychology*, *9*, 43–52.

Bowlby, J. (1988). *A secure base*. Basic Books.

Bowlby, J. (1952). *Maternal care and mental health*. World Health Organization.

Bracho, A., Lee, G., Giraldo, G., & Prado, R. (2016). *Recruiting the heart, training the brain: The work of Latino health access*. Hesperian Health Guides.

Cassidy, J. (2008). The nature of the child’s ties. In J. Cassidy & P. R. Shaver (Eds.). *Handbook of attachment: Theory, research, and clinical applications* (pp. 3–22). Guilford.

ChenFeng, J. L. & Galick, A. (2015). How gender discourses hijack couple therapy—and how to avoid it. In C. Knudson-Martin, M. A. Wells, & S. K. Samman (Eds.). *Socio-emotional relationship therapy: Bridging emotion, societal discourse, and couple interaction* (pp. 41–52). AFTA Springerbriefs in Family Therapy, Springer.

ChenFeng, J., Kim, L., Knudson-Martin, C., & Wu, Y. (2016). Application of socio-emotional relationship therapy with couples of Asian heritage: Addressing issues of culture, gender, and power. *Family Process*, *56*, 558–573.

Collins, P. H. (2000). *Black feminist thought: Knowledge, consciousness, and the politics of empowerment*. Routledge.

Cozolino, L. (2016). *Why therapy works: Using our minds to change our brains*. Norton.

Diamond, G. M., Boruchovitz-Zamir, R., Nir-Gotlieb, O., Gat, I., Bar-Kalifa, E., Fitoussi, P. Y., & Katz, S. (2022). Attachment-based family therapy for sexual and gender minority young adults and their nonaccepting parents. *Family process*, *61*(2), 530–548.

Diamond, S., Diamond, M., & Levy, S. A. (2014). *Attachment-based family therapy for depressed adolescents*. American Psychological Association.

Doherty, W. J. (2020). The evolution and current status of systemic family therapy. In K. S. Wampler, R. B. Miller, & R. B. Seedall (Eds.). *The handbook of systemic family therapy* (Vol. 1, pp. 33–49). Wiley.

Drain, C. & Han, M. (2023). Innovations in parent education: Attachment interventions and the family map inventories, *National Council on Family Relations Report*, *68*(4), F4–F5.

Edelman, M. W. (1987). *Families in peril: An agenda for social change*. Harvard University Press.

Edelman, M. W. (1980). *Portrait of inequality: Black and white children in America*. Children’s Defense Fund.

Edwards, C., Allan, R., & Wittenborn, A. (2026). Queer contextualized emotionally focused therapy. In E. E. Hartwell & L. L. Edwards (Eds.) *Queer-contextualized family therapy: Toward radically inclusive theory and practice* (pp. 95–117). Routledge.

Edwards, C., Wittenborn, A. K., Morgan, P., Pratt, F., & Heiden-Rootes, K. (2025). The transition to teletherapy: Experiences of emotionally focused therapists. *Family Process*, *64*(1), e13068.

Esmiol Wilson, E. (2015). Relational spirituality, gender, and power: Application to couple therapy. In C. Knudson-Martin, M. A. Wells, & S. K. Samman, (Eds.). *Socio-emotional relationship therapy: Bridging emotion, societal context, and couple interaction* (pp. 133–144). AFTA SpringerBriefs in Family Therapy. Springer.

Esmiol Wilson, E., Knudson-Martin, C., & Wilson, C. (2014). Gendered power, spirituality, and relational processes: Experiences of Christian physician couples. *Journal of Couple and Relationship Therapy*, *13*, 312–338.

Fishbane, M. D. (2013). *Loving with the brain in mind: Neurobiology & couple therapy*. Norton.

Franzblau, S. H. (1999). Historicizing attachment theory: Binding the ties that bind. *Feminism & Psychology*, *9*, 22–31.

Fricker, M. (2007). *Epistemic injustice: Power and the ethics of knowing*. Oxford University Press.

Fuller, B. & Coll, C. G. (2010). Learning from Latinos: Contexts, families, and child development in motion. *Developmental Psychology*, *46*, 559–565.

Furrow, J. & Palmer, G. (2024). Emotionally focused family therapy (EFFT): Stepping into EFT with Families. In *Stepping into Emotionally Focused Therapy* (pp. 305–320). Routledge.

Garcia, M., Košutic, I., & McDowell, T. (2015). Peace on earth/war at home: The role of emotion regulation in social justice work. *Journal of Feminist Family Therapy*, *27*, 1–20.

Gordon M. (2018). Empathy as strategy for reconnecting to our common humanity. In N. Way, A. Ali, C. Gilligan, & P. Noguera (Eds.). *The crisis of connection: Roots, consequences, and solutions* (pp. 250–273). New York University Press.

Greenberg, L. S. & Goldman, R. N. (2008). *Emotion-focused couples therapy: The dynamics of emotion, love, and power*. American Psychological Association.

Hardy, K. V. (2016). Mastering context talk: Practical skills for effective engagement. In K. V. Hardy & T. Bobes (Eds.). *Culturally sensitive supervision and training: Diverse perspectives and practical applications* (pp. 136–145). Routledge.

Hughes, D. A. (2011). *Attachment-focused family therapy workbook*. Norton.

Hughes, D. A. (2009). Communication of emotions. In D. Fosha, D. J. Siegel, and M. F. Solomon (Eds.). *The healing power of emotion: Affective neuroscience, development, and clinical practice* (pp. 280–303). Norton.

Jenks, A., Adams, G., Young, B., & Seedall, R. (2024). Addressing power in couples therapy: Integrating socio-emotional relationship therapy and emotionally focused therapy. *Family Process*, *63*(1), 48–63.

Johnson, S. (2019). *Attachment theory in practice: Emotionally focused therapy (EFT) with individuals, couples, and families*. Guilford.

Johnson, S. (2008). *Hold me tight: Seven conversations for a lifetime of love*. Little, Brown, & Company.

Johnson, S. M. (2004). *The practice of emotionally focused couple therapy* (2nd ed.). Brunner-Routledge.

Johnson, S. M. (2002). *Emotionally focused couple therapy with trauma survivors: Strengthening attachment bonds*. Guilford.

Johnson, S. M. & Lee, A. (2000). Emotionally focused family therapy: Restructuring attachment. In C. E. Bailey (ed.). *Children in therapy: Using the family as a resource* (pp. 112–136). Norton.

Knudson-Martin, C. (2025). *The socio-emotional relationship workbook: Closing the gap between the relationship you want and the relationship you have*. Routledge.

Knudson-Martin, C. (2024). *A Step-by-step guide to socio-emotional relationship therapy: A socially responsible approach to clinical practice*. Routledge.

Knudson-Martin, C. (2013). Why power matters: Creating a foundation for mutual support in couple therapy. *Family Process*, *52*, 5–18.

Knudson-Martin, C. (2012). Attachment in adult relationships: A feminist perspective. *Journal of Family Theory and Review*, *4*, 299–305.

Knudson-Martin, C. & Huenergardt, D. (2010). A socio-emotional approach to couple therapy: Linking social context and couple interaction. *Family Process*, *49*, 369–386.

Knudson-Martin, C. & Kim, L. (2023). Socioculturally attuned couple therapy. In J. Lebow and D. Snyder (Eds.) *Clinical handbook of couple therapy*, (6th ed., pp. 267–291). Guilford.

Knudson-Martin, C. & Silverstein, R. (2009). Suffering in silence: A qualitative meta-analysis of post-partum depression. *Journal of Marital and Family Therapy*, *35*, 145–158.

Lareau, A. (2003). *Unequal childhoods: Class, race, and family life*. University of California Press.

Levy, S., Mason, S., Russon, J., & Diamond, G. (2021). Attachment-based family therapy in the age of telehealth and COVID-19. *Journal of marital and family therapy*, *47*(2), 440–454.

Loscocco, K. & Walzer, S. (2013). Gender and the culture of heterosexual marriage in the United States. *Journal of Family Theory & Review*, *5*, 1–14.

Mauthner, N. S. (1999). "Feeling low and feeling really bad about feeling low": Women's experiences of motherhood and postpartum depression. *Canadian Psychology*, *40*, 143–161.

McDowell, T. (2015). *Applying critical social theories to family therapy practice*. AFTA Springerbriefs in Family Therapy, Springer.

Medina, J. (2013). *The epistemology of resistance: Gender and racial oppression, epistemic injustice, and resistant imaginations*. Oxford University Press.

Mikulincer, M. & Shaver, P. R. (2012). Adult attachment orientations and relationship processes. *Journal of Family Theory and Review*, *4*, 259–274.

Minuchin, P. (2002). Cross-cultural perspectives: Implication for attachment theory and family therapy. *Family Process*, *41*, 546–550.

Pandit, M., Kang, Y. J., ChenFeng J., Knudson-Martin, C., & Huenergardt D. (2014). Practicing socio-cultural attunement: A study of couple therapists. *Journal of Contemporary Family Therapy*, *36*, 518–528.

Piercy, F. P. (2020). The future of systemic family therapy: What needs nurturing and what does not. In K. S. Wampler, R. B. Miller, & R. B. Seedall (Eds.). *The Handbook of Systemic Family Therapy* (Vol. 1, pp. 753–770). Wiley.

Porges, S. W. (2009). Reciprocal influences between body and brain in the perception and expression of affect: A polyvagal perspective. In D. Fosha, D. J. Siegel, & M. F. Solomon (Eds.). *The healing power of emotion: Affective neuroscience, development, and clinical practice* (pp. 27–54). Norton.
Reichert, M. C. & Nelson, D. (2018). I want to learn from you: Relational strategies to engage boys in school. In N. Way, A. Ali, C. Gilligan, & P. Noguera (Eds.). *The crisis of connection: Roots, consequences, and solutions* (pp. 344–360). New York University Press.
Rothbaum, F., Rosen, K., Ujiie, T., & Uchida, N. (2002). Family systems theory, attachment theory, and culture. *Family Process*, *41*, 328–350.
Sabey, A. K., Lafrance, A., Furrow, J., Diamond, G., & Hughes, D. (2024). A family reunion of "clinical cousins": Attachment and emotion in four family-oriented therapy models. *Family Process*, *63*, 1119–1144.
Seedall, R. B. & Sandberg, J. G. (2020). Attachment and other emotion-based systemic approaches. In K. S. Wampler, R. B. Miller, & R. B. Seedall (Eds.). *The handbook of systemic family therapy* (Vol. 1, pp. 391–415). Wiley.
Siegel, D. J. (2023). *IntraConnected: MWe (Me + we) as the integration of self, identity, and belonging*. Norton.
Siegel, D., J. (2020). *The developing mind: How relationships and the brain interact to shape who we are* (3rd ed.). Guilford.
Siegel, D. J. & Hartzell, M. (2014). *Parenting from the inside out: How a deeper self-understanding can help you raise children who thrive* (10th anniversary ed). Jeremy P. Tarcher/Penguin.
Smoliak, O., Rice, C., Rudder, D., Tseliou, E., LaMarre, A., LeCouteur, A., Gaete, J., Davies, A., & Henshaw, S. (2024). Emotion regulation as affective neoliberal governmentality. *Family Process*, 00, 1–18.
Taylor, S. E. (2002). *The tending instinct: How nurturing is essential to who we are and how we love*. New York Times Books.
Trevarthen, C. (2009). The functions of emotion in infancy: The regulation and communication of rhythm, sympathy, and meaning in human development. In D. Fosha, D. J. Siegel, & M. F. Solomon (Eds.). *The healing power of emotion: Affective neuroscience, development, and clinical practice* (pp. 55–85). Norton.
Tronick, E. (2009). Multilevel meaning making and dyadic expansion of consciousness theory. In D. Fosha, D. J. Siegel, & M. F. Solomon (Eds.). *The healing power of emotion: Affective neuroscience, development, and clinical practice* (pp. 86–111). Norton.
Tuttle, A. R., Knudson-Martin, C., & Kimi, L. (2012). Parenting as relationship: A framework for assessment and practice. *Family Process*, *51*, 73–89.
Van der Kolk, B. (2014). *The body keeps the score: Brain, mind, and body in the healing of trauma*. Penguin.
van der Spek, N., Dekker, W., Peen, J., Santens, T., Cuijpers, P., Bosmans, G., & Dekker, J. (2023). Attachment-based family therapy for adolescents and young adults with suicide ideation and depression: An open trial. *Crisis: The Journal of Crisis Intervention and Suicide Prevention*.
van Ijzendoorn, M. H. & Sagi-Schwartz, A. (2008). Cross-cultural patterns of attachment: Universal and contextual dimensions. In J. Cassidy & P. R. Shaver (Eds.). *Handbook of attachment: Theory, research, and clinical applications* (pp. 880–905). Guilford.
Vatcher, C. A. & Bongo, M. (2001). The feminist/emotionally focused therapy practice model: An integrated approach for couple therapy. *Journal of Marital and Family Therapy*, *27*, 69–83.
Walsh, F. (2009). Human–animal bonds I: The relational significance of companion animals. *Family Process*, *48*, 462–480.
Wells, M. A., Lobo, E., Galick, A., Knudson-Martin, C., Huenergardt, D., & Schaepper, J. (2017). Fostering trust through relational safety: Applying SERT's focus on gender and power with adult-survivor couples. *Journal of Couple & Relationship Therapy*, *16*, 122–145.
Wetherell, M. (2012). *Affect and emotion: A new social science understanding*. Sage Publications.
Willis, A. B., Haslam, D. R., & Bermúdez, J. M. (2016). Harnessing the power of play in emotionally focused family therapy with preschool children. *Journal of Marital and Family Therapy*, *42*, 673–687.

9 Socioculturally Attuned Bowenian Family Therapy

In the 1950s, Murray Bowen made the groundbreaking proposition that symptoms such as depression, alcoholism, or physical illness need to be understood as a dynamic process involving the family as a unit, rather than the individual. He described human behavior as part of interlocking emotional systems through which people receive information from the environment, adapt, and respond (Bowen, 1978; Kerr & Bowen, 1988). Beginning in response to Freudian theory, Bowen argued that the principles governing emotional connectedness are "written in nature" and common to all natural systems (Kerr & Bowen, 1988, p. 26). Two natural life forces are involved: those that promote self-interest and those that promote the group. These innately affect functioning across all systemic levels from the cellular to the societal. Differentiation of self within these systems is considered key to more optimal functioning, with a balance of connectedness and autonomy (Bartle-Haring & Whiting, 2024).

In Bowen Family Systems theory (BFST), emotion is the energy that drives relationships (Bowen, 1978). When tension and conflict are high, like an "emotional magnet," family members or groups automatically react to each other (Titelman, 2014, p. 22). Symptoms and relational problems are a reflection of the underlying emotional system. While Bowen therapists typically help people observe themselves and the patterns in their relationships so they can respond reflectively rather than reactively (White, 2024), BFST is best understood as an integration of feeling and thinking (Brown & Errington, 2024). What appears to be rational thought is often more emotional (Kerr, 2019). Patterns of emotional reactivity are transmitted from generation to generation.

Applications of Bowen theory continue to inform the importance of family of origin work, however they have evolved to incorporate new findings from neuroscience and integrate more experiential approaches (Hargrave & Houltberg, 2020). While the family is the unit of analysis, Bowen therapists often work with individuals. Addressing the impacts of societal level inputs such as discrimination, government-level violence, the emotional effects of socio-economic status, environmental stress, and disconnection from nature is consistent with the emphasis on emotional connectedness across all systemic levels in BFST (Burke & Post, 2024; Collier & Mader, 2024; Lassiter, 2022).

•←→•

Third order change is facilitated from a Bowen perspective when clients see themselves and their concerns not only as part of multigenerational family systems but also as part of ongoing sociocultural systems.

•←→•

In this chapter, we first explore five key aspects of family therapy based on Bowen theory and then consider how to integrate principles of socioculturally attuned therapy with guidelines for practice and a case example.

DOI: 10.4324/9781003493426-9

Primary, Enduring Family Therapy Concepts

Differentiation of self is the core developmental process and is at the heart of Bowen therapy. It is described as the ability to "maintain emotional objectivity while in the midst of an emotional system… yet at the same time actively relate to key people in the system" (Bowen, 1978, p. 485). We view the following five components of Bowen family therapy as central to increased differentiation and relationship functioning: 1) differentiation of self, 2) transgenerational patterns and transmission, 3) the flow of anxiety, 4) maintaining emotional engagement, and 5) therapist's family of origin work.

Differentiation of Self

A child is born. Her parents named her Arielle. Arielle is born into a web of emotional connections that predate her and extend across generations. According to Bowen theory, from the moment of birth—or even prior to birth—Arielle will experience an automatic pull toward this togetherness (Bowen, 1978; Titelman, 2014). She will also experience a natural pull toward individuality. Differentiation of self is how the tension between these two forces is managed. Arielle's development of self will move along a continuum from low to (potentially) high differentiation. On the low end is *emotional fusion* in which individual responses are highly reactive to others. On the high end, is a *solid self* that enables reflective and differentiated responses. Arielle's capacity to move from emotional fusion inherent at birth to differentiation depends on the level of emotional fusion in her family of origin. It is an individual *and* family-level process.

Arielle's African American family values tightly knit family bonds. In a nearby neighborhood, Eric is born. His European American family prefers more personal space and emphasizes individual achievement. According to Bowen theory their process of differentiation is the same. It begins with functioning based on automatic responses similar to emotional reactions among other life forms. For example, Carmen's horse demonstrated emotional reactivity when he would sense danger, tense up, and step around the shadow of a mailbox every time he passed one. He did not have the capacity to reflect on the current meaning of a shadow. He reacted not only on his experience but from instinctual "horse" experience across generations. At this level of differentiation, there is no ability to observe oneself separate from the group or context. Differentiation increases when intellectual functioning or awareness enables one to distinguish a sense of self and respond in a less reactive or automatic way.

Transgenerational Patterns and Transmission

Arielle and Eric's basic levels of differentiation depend primarily on how their families handle the intrinsic melding of family members' emotional states, that is, their degree of fusion. It is important not to confuse emotional fusion with preferences for physical closeness and deep caring about one another. Arielle's African American family enacts family-centered values within a relatively well-differentiated family system. People in her family like each other's company and participate in many shared activities. They enjoy spirited disagreement and have lively family conversations on many topics. When faced with a crisis, such as the great-grandmother's recent diagnosis of Alzheimer's disease, the extended family discussed many options for how to share her care. Individual family members felt respected and freely reflected on what they could and could not do to help. Even though the emotional demands on the family are high, they are able to lovingly and non-reactively respond to Arielle's needs as a newborn while also helping care for their great-grandmother. Growing up in this well-differentiated family environment promotes Arielle's individual differentiation.

In contrast, Eric is growing up in a much less differentiated emotional context. Family members have never been able to tolerate differences among them. People attend family gatherings as expected and are careful not to upset each other. Eric's aunt refuses to participate. When Eric was born, she brought a gift at a time when no other family members would be present. The conflict between this aunt and the rest of the family causes Eric's mother, Jamie, considerable distress, and she expends significant energy trying to keep the peace. She is similarly cautious about upsetting her husband (Eric's father) and often feels lonely and unappreciated. Though Eric's parents and extended family genuinely love him, the low level of differentiation in this family system is accompanied by intense intergenerational anxiety. The high level of emotional reactivity will make it difficult for Eric to differentiate within this system.

By the time Arielle and Eric are born, the emotional functioning of their family systems has been evolving for many generations. Arielle's family has historically been able to respond to important nodal and socio-contextual issues—including the civil rights movement, job loss, and the death of Arielle's grandfather in the Vietnam War—with considerable self-awareness on the part of individual family members and the ability to support each other without sacrificing autonomy. Arielle is therefore likely to develop a well-regulated emotional system and approach adult relationships from a non-reactive, reflective position. This will help her sustain a network of supportive relationships and enable authentic emotional expression (Brown & Errington, 2024; Kerr & Bowen, 1988).

Eric will probably experience more difficulty forming healthy and satisfying adult relationships (Thomas et al., 2021; Ogan et al., 2024). His historical legacy includes multiple generations in which family members responded to immigration to the US with high anxiety about economic success and fitting into societal expectations of the dominant culture by which they judged themselves. No deviations from rigid roles and expectations were allowed. When Eric's grandparents lost a child to cancer, they were never able to speak of it. Since she was a child, Eric's mother, Jamie, responded to familial distress by trying to make her parents happy. This pattern is repeated in her relationship with her husband, Robert, who is frequently angry and not attentive to her. This fused emotional context will inhibit Eric's movements toward differentiation of self.

Flow of Anxiety

According to Bowen theory, anxiety in response to interpersonal differences or life's challenges is a natural response to low levels of differentiation (Papero, 2024; Willis et al., 2021). An important part of assessment in Bowen therapy is to track the flow of anxiety within the shared emotional system. Not everyone is equally affected. Some constantly seek relationships and try to please; others deny their need for relationships and keep their distance. Substance use, eating disorders, physical symptoms, and traits such as obsessiveness, grandiosity, perfectionism, aggressiveness, paranoia, and hopelessness can all be ways anxiety is bound in a system, as are polarizing beliefs (Kerr & Bowen, 1988). "In general, the more anxious people become, the less constructive their responses to others tend to be" (p. 124).

When tension is high between two people, they will often diffuse their anxiety by directing attention to another person or activity. This is called *triangulation.* Triangulation happens quite naturally and may not be intentional. For example, when upset with Robert, Jamie directs her attention to her newborn son Eric. This calms her. The connection she experiences with her son makes it possible for her to avoid addressing her unhappiness in the marriage. Eric absorbs the tension. If this pattern continues, Eric is likely to become a symptom-bearer. This is an example of what Bowen theory terms the *family projection process*, that is, the anxiety of one generation is passed to another through a series of interlocking emotional triangles.

Maintaining Emotional Engagement

The ability to maintain genuine relationships in the face of stress or turmoil is the outcome of differentiation. The Bowen clinical approach emphasizes learning to make "inner-directed" decisions from within the self, rather than "coercion or persuasion from others" (Kerr & Bowen, 1988, p. 105). The goal is to respond less on the basis of emotional reactivity and more from a *solid self* that can tolerate intense feelings and reflectively respond. Turning to her infant son when there is stress between Jamie and her husband may be a sign of emotional fusion. Others may respond to emotional fusion by neglecting or abusing others or by cutting off from them in order to maintain emotional distance (Papero, 2024). For example, Robert reactively responds with anger when his wife disagrees with him. When his son Eric cries for long periods of time, Robert has little ability to tolerate the intensity. He disengages and puts his focus elsewhere. He might react to emotion in the system by physically or emotionally abusing Eric or his wife, having a sexual affair outside the marriage, or directing all his energy and attention to work or some other activity rather than engaging with his wife and child. Low differentiation perpetuates this pattern, making it increasingly hard for him to engage.

People can increase basic differentiation by developing awareness of the emotional patterns in their lives, the social and family contexts that invite these responses, and how their own emotional reactivity contributes to sustaining the patterns. This enables more choice about how one responds, reduces the anxiety in the family system, and has an impact on the emotional transmission process for future generations (Bowen, 1978). It is important to remember that in Bowen theory differentiation and connectedness work together. In Text Box 9.1 Monica McGoldrick extends the idea to include the larger community and world.

Text Box 9.1 Monica McGoldrick, MSW, PhD

Monica McGoldrick is co-founder and director of the Multicultural Family Institute in Highland Park, NJ, and adjunct faculty at Robert Wood Johnson Medical School. She is among those who continue to evolve the practice of Bowen theory and is a well-known author and editor of books related to gender, culture, diversity, lifecycle, and family therapy. Her words below are from *The Genogram Casebook* (McGoldrick, 2016):

In order to make the best choices, we human beings need to appreciate that we are all connected to each other and to the earth, to the past and to the future of each other and of our planet. So making the best choices means aiming toward positive connectedness with family, friends, community, coworkers, and nature that surround us... Before people can make the best possible choices for their lives, they must first be centered and able to think clearly where they are and what their connections mean to them... Assisting clients to view themselves in the context of their genograms is aimed at helping them figure out how to live in respectful relationship with others and with nature, to care for and be cared for by others as appropriate, and without exploitation or disregard for our world or for future generations (McGoldrick, 2016, pp. 2–3).

All systems are interconnected. Thus when a client begins to see his or her own behavior as related to that of others, [they have] *a choice how to participate in each relationship moving forward. This helps people take back their power to relate to others according to their own values for relating rather than letting themselves be defined by other family members or cultural rules they do not accept... Helping clients work on their genograms means helping them get past focusing only on the behavior of others, and learning to focus on their own part in the system, so they can make decisions to take responsibility for how they conduct their lives, no matter what others do. Recognizing their connections to others can often give them the courage to do what is required to resolve their issues* (McGoldrick, p. 5–6).

Therapist's Family of Origin Work

Bowen theory suggests that therapists must work from a differentiated sense of self. This enables them to avoid emotional fusion with clients' anxiety. It requires developing a clear sense of self, knowing our place in the world, and what matters to us (McGoldrick, 2016). Like a coach, Bowen therapists are then able to stay outside of the system, asking the kinds of questions and making observations that help clients in their own process of self-discovery. The therapist is a "witness on the sidelines…inspiring clients to undertake their own work" (McGoldrick, 2016, p. 111). Containing anxiety requires a calm presence that makes it safe for people to engage in the therapeutic process.

Integrating Principles of Sociocultural Attunement

Human systems are both natural (e.g., biological) and sociocultural. Bowen focused on human behavior as part of natural systems in common with all life forms and biological evolution. He did not draw on knowledge from social sciences, such as how key processes like differentiation intersect with societal power dynamics (Innes, 1996). However, Bowen theory emphasizes the reciprocal flow of anxiety between individuals, families, institutions, and society at large (Kerr & MacKay, 2024). Attention to the impact of sociocultural, political, and economic systems can enhance the model and increase the potential to transcend destructive patterns invited by societal isolation and inequities (Lassiter, 2022) and environmental crises and disconnection from nature (Collier & Mader, 2024)

In this section, we examine differentiation in societal context, why power processes are important, and how awareness of one's sociopolitical, cultural, and historical contexts can be the foundation for empowerment and third order change. We also show how neuroscience supports this expanded application of Bowen theory (Damasio, 1999; Kerr 2019; Lassiter, 2022; van der Kolk, 2014).

Differentiation in Societal Context

Therapists must be cautious regarding judging differentiation. What looks like low differentiation may sometimes more appropriately be understood as the effects of discrimination and/or limited power.

Anxiety in the Macrosystem

Bowen postulated similar emotional processes at the societal level as in organizations and families. When anxiety is high, groups within the system are isolated from each other (Bowen, 1978; Kerr & Mackay, 2024). People tend to take sides on issues without hearing each other (Friedman, 2007). In times like today when people are socially polarized, we are "constantly bombarded" by other people's reactivity (Friedman, 2007, p. 62). Bowen noted that people or groups respond to the anxiety by scapegoating persons in subordinate positions, such as People of Color, low-income people, sexual or gender minorities, immigrants, and those with mental illness. Unfortunately, the theory also sometimes seemed to reflect a scapegoating of disenfranchised populations, suggesting that their acts of resistance (i.e., protests or divorce) are a sign of emotional immaturity and that "over-lenient" public officials keep low-income people "one-down" (Bowen, 1978, p. 445). An approach more informed by critical theories (McDowell, 2015) would focus on resilience and motivation to claim a self embedded in "acting out" behavior (McGoldrick, 2016; Unger, 2015). This approach would challenge those with more power to be open to hearing from those with less power, making it safe for them to speak, even when what they have to say makes us uncomfortable.

↔

Societal projection processes such as discrimination, scapegoating, and entrenched power hierarchies are likely to disproportionately affect targeted or marginalized groups.

↔

Living on a day-to-day basis at lower levels of the societal power hierarchy increases stress hormones, inflammation, reduced immune function, and poorer health outcomes, even when controlling for access to health care (Lantz et al., 2005; Lassiter, 2022). Societal stressors become embodied in neuroendocrine and immune systems (Sternberg, 2001). For example, people raised with fewer economic resources are more likely to get sick when exposed to a cold virus than people raised with more affluence, even when economic circumstances have improved later in life (Cohen et al., 2010). From a Bowen perspective, these are examples of the inequitable effects of embodied societal anxiety, in which the well-being of one group comes at the expense of another. While living with the effects of discrimination and inequities can affect the differentiation process, persons in more privileged positions are not necessarily more differentiated. Their apparent health may be a facade held in place by their dependence on others to automatically meet their needs or accommodate to their positions of power (McGoldrick, 2016). It is important to consider all the intersecting factors.

For example, Julia, a lab technologist who had been working at the same hospital for over 20 years sought therapy because she was so depressed she could barely get out of bed. Going to work produced considerable anxiety. She felt ashamed that she could not cope better and took people's teasing personally. The intense, emotional way she spoke, the questioning of her own competence, and the judgmental statements she made about others all lined up to easily think of her as "poorly differentiated." But as the therapist expanded the lens to ask about the changes happening in the hospital as a result of the pandemic, and in medical services more broadly, a series of interlocking triangles became evident. Anxiety in the larger health care system moved to multiple levels of managers in this hospital, which increased the pressure on her team to perform an extraordinary amount of work, with no mistakes, in a very short amount of time. This chain of events led to others scapegoating Julia for being different in age and ethnicity.

Julia was probably no less differentiated than the others in her workplace. She was targeted because anxiety in the larger system made it difficult for the workgroup to tolerate differences. But she was the one showing the symptoms and being most affected. As Julia reflected on the anxiety in the system and how various people responded to it, she was able to consider her options and develop a strategy for how to deal with it. Since her managers seemed unable to respond in ways that changed the work environment, the burden fell on Julia to change her own response, including the ramifications of possibly deciding not to work in this setting. Naming the inherent unfairness in the situation was important.

Intersection of Differentiation and Culture

The concept of differentiation of self applies across cultures (Gallego et al., 2024; Neophytou et al., 2021), with culture as emotional context (Brown & Errington, 2024; Chan, 2024). As we saw in the cases of Arielle and Eric, cultural patterns intersect with emotional differentiation processes.

Eric's less well-differentiated family enacted ideals of autonomy and achievement in ways that limit positive connection and adaptation. Arielle's better-differentiated family enacted the cultural ideal of sticking together to face adversity (Cowdery et al., 2009).

•←→•

When differentiation is high, people are able to apply cultural values in relatively functional ways. When differentiation is low or in times of distress, cultural values can become exaggerated.

•←→•

Takeshi Tamura (2016), a family therapist in Japan, called this exaggeration "cultural overdose." For example, Japanese culture tells adolescents that they should achieve for the sake of family honor. According to Tamura, when anxiety is high, Japanese youth are likely to isolate themselves and avoid social situations, increasing the risk of suicide, depression, and self-harm. In the US, cultural pulls toward independence are often reflected in acting out and externalizing behaviors.

In a video presentation to the International Family Therapy Association, Tamura (2016) cited the example of a family in Korea. When the video opens, two adolescent daughters are arguing about using the computer. The mother—with some tension in her voice—tells the older daughter that she needs to shut down the computer and go to bed in a few minutes, reminding her that she has school tomorrow. When the daughter does not do this and the two girls begin to scream at each other, the mother also begins to scream and threaten the older daughter. Tamura explained that the anxiety in this household reflects societal performance expectations that make going to school highly anxious for the daughter. The resulting family conflict is triangulated with societal projection processes in a way that holds the mother responsible for the daughter's performance.

Societal Transmission of Collective Trauma

Just as past family emotional processes are passed on from generation to generation and affect current relationship functioning even when people are not aware of these histories, collective historical traumas continue to perpetuate heightened anxiety and reactivity. Watson (2013) described the collective nervousness that many African American people experience regarding how they appear to others. For example, she told of her experience as a Black woman in a restaurant with a White friend. When Black people at a nearby table were loud and noisy and rude to the waiter, she felt ashamed and embarrassed. It is unlikely that her White friend would have felt similarly shamed had the rude diners been White. Watson attributed this emotional response to the legacy of slavery, where "if one slave got out of line, all slaves might feel the lash, or worse." Internalized Black inferiority leaves people "on the edge…obsessed with how we and other blacks look, talk, and act because we were enslaved and then discriminated against for having black skin" (p. 50). The feeling of shame says more about the societal power context of the situation than Dr. Watson's level of differentiation.

•←→•

It is important to recognize, acknowledge, and name realities of collective trauma and unsafe contexts. The problem may be a history of collective trauma lived out and repeated in individual lives.

•←→•

When a Black mother was referred to therapy because she demonstrated angry and disruptive behavior at her daughter's school, she was quickly described by supervision group members as "paranoid." Under that label, no one asked about her experience with schools, especially schools like this one where the teachers, principal, and most of the students were White. They did not seek to understand her expectation and fear that her daughter would be treated unfairly. They could only see that her reaction to the school appeared "out of proportion" to the issue at hand, individualized and medicalized the problem, and did not recognize the historical context of systemic racism.

Value of Belonging

In Bowen theory the self can never be defined separately from significant relationships and contexts (Kerr, 2019). The goal is to define a "self" while staying in relationship (Brown & Errington, 2024). However, dominant Western discourses tend to value individuality and autonomy over more connected ways of relating. Despite the emphasis on maintaining emotional connection in Bowen theory, this bias can be seen in how Bowen theory is often presented and applied (Knudson-Martin, 1994, 1996).

Socioculturally attuned therapists resist the temptation to view individual autonomy as more important than relationships.

For example, therapists may be more likely to support a decision for a wife to move to advance her husband's career (an individualistic goal) than for a wife to not move in order to stay close to her sisters—a relational goal (McGoldrick, 2016). Socioculturally attuned Bowen therapists will counteract this tendency to prioritize individual goals over relational ones. They will emphasize that people need community to sustain their well-being and to have the strength to resist oppressive forces of society. In fact, sources of healing are embedded in clients' cultural communities. A clear cultural or racial connection has been associated with high levels of differentiation (Skowron, 2004).

As another example of the importance of relational connection to the process of differentiation, consider Marie, a 35-year-old European American woman who strongly identified with her conservative Christian denomination. Marie felt depressed and powerless in her marriage and told the therapist she wanted a more equal marriage, but also believed in the principles of her religion, including that the husband was the leader of the family. The feeling that she needed to choose between equality or her religion distressed and isolated her. With the therapist's encouragement, Marie sought a woman in the church she thought would understand. Marie returned to therapy the next week, saying, "All the women in the church feel the same way I do!" (Silverstein et al., 2006, p. 401). As Marie explored her Christian identity, she was also better able to connect to her religion in a personal way and more genuinely engage in her church community. Marie did not need to differentiate *from* her faith; she needed to differentiate *within* it.

Value of Intuition and Feeling

Bowen Family Systems Theory has been criticized for valuing objectivity over intuition, subjectivity, and emotional expression (Knudson-Martin, 1994, 1996; Luepnitz, 1988). Bowen emphasized using the intellectual system to mediate responses to the emotional system and advocated clinical strategies that stressed cognitive awareness and distinguished thinking from feeling.

Such approaches fail to acknowledge or value self-knowledge that comes through feeling and affective awareness and discount the experience of many women and cultures. Nouvelle, an African American nurse in her mid-thirties described her subjective, "gut knowing:"

> I think that growing up as a person of color in this society, you develop something more instinctual and survival-like. It's a different kind of smart and a different kind of sense… It's much more visceral, it's much more down here [points to stomach].
>
> (Goldberger, 1996, p. 352)

When people experience a disconnect between what their bodies or experience tell them and what is expected or known in the dominant culture, they are likely to discount or silence their own knowing (Jack & Ali, 2010). Their bodies may register the diminishment with a stress response even if unaware or only dimly aware of the social rejection (Lassiter, 2022). Rather than a unitary self, people in subjugated positions may develop a shifting consciousness in which they simultaneously perceive multiple realities (Hurtado, 1996). The ability to apprehend multiple consciousnesses enables them to make sense of the complexities in their lives and negotiate multiple and stigmatized social identities as they move from context to context. For example, Hurtado spoke of the need for Women of Color to navigate danger and anger to successfully manage marginality:

> There develops an intuitive sense of danger that is primarily kept at bay through anger. Putting a "bit" on anger is of primary importance for survival… The challenge is to "know what you know" *and* be able to circumvent the consequences of that knowledge while being true to yourself. (p. 378)

•←→•

A socioculturally attuned application of Bowen theory appreciates and draws from many forms of knowing.

•←→•

Differentiation and Societal Power Processes

The ways of relating associated with high differentiation such as direct communication, "I" statements, and the ability to respect differences and deal with conflict presume relatively equal power positions. But power imbalances are built into social structures and norms (Mahoney & Knudson-Martin, 2009; Komter, 1989), and have an impact on differentiation processes.

Power Structures, Fear, and Anxiety

Societal inequities based on race, class, gender, sexuality, or other differences require emotional fusion, whereby the dominant group's interests are supported at the expense of subordinate groups (McGoldrick, 2016). Norms of the dominant culture will be privileged.

•←→•

Members of more powerful groups are largely unaware that members of less powerful groups accommodate them.

•←→•

Survival for the Women of Color quoted above required them to be attentive to the potential emotional responses of the powerful. They needed to manage their emotions in relation to the power situation (e.g., put a "bit" on their anger). Without taking power into consideration this could seem "overly" focused on others (less differentiated). Instead, this attention to context is important to their well-being.

•←→•

Until those in powerful positions develop an awareness of their dependence on being accommodated by others, they remain emotionally fused with societal power processes.

•←→•

Inequities inspire anxieties (Lassiter, 2022). A well-differentiated system would recognize and address fairness issues openly and directly. In contrast, autocratic/totalitarian leadership styles seek to contain anxiety (Friedman, 2007). Those in positions of power maintain power by inciting fear among the less powerful. This may be unintentional through unquestioned expectations, such as when a boss expects an employee to be available for shifts at any time of the day. They may also intentionally incite fear through threats, intimidation, or force. The boss may threaten employees with losing their jobs if they don't comply.

In less differentiated systems, responsibility for managing anxiety often falls on the less powerful. For example, Bryan Stevenson (2014), a Black civil rights attorney, described the anxiety he experienced early in his career when he was sitting in his car listening to music on the radio after parking near his apartment. He looked up and saw a White policeman pointing a gun at him,

> My first instinct was to run. I quickly decided that wouldn't be smart… "Move and I'll blow your head off!" The officer shouted the words, but I couldn't make any sense of what he meant. I tried to stay calm… I put my hand up and noticed that he seemed nervous… I don't remember deciding to speak, I just remember the words coming out: "It's all right. It's okay… I live here." I hated how afraid I sounded and the way my voice was shaking. (p. 40)

Stevenson's relatively high level of contextual awareness helped him defuse the situation, but the unacknowledged injustice and assault to his dignity continued to impact him. When he got into his apartment, Stevenson kept saying over and over again, "They never even apologized" (p. 42). Stevenson attributed his ability to think through the situation—a differentiated response—to his years of study and legal training (which his instincts told him not to disclose), but the fear and humiliation he experienced were related to his subordinate position and vulnerability because of what the color of his skin represents on a societal level.

Situated Emotion and Power

Emotion occurs at the intersection of sociopolitical life and daily interactions (Knudson-Martin, 2024; Smoliak et al., 2024). It is situated in a complex material and relational field never separate from a person's power position in the setting (Wetherell, 2012). The feeling of humiliation experienced by Stevenson is an example of his body reading and recording the meaning of the racial hierarchy surrounding the event (Lassiter, 2022). Had the same event happened to a White attorney (which in itself seems unlikely), the emotional experience of the participants would have been different, with the attorney likely experiencing indignation rather than humiliation.

•←→•

Socioculturally attuned therapists must listen for, and seek to understand, the societal contexts in which family histories are embedded in order to identify and name issues of fairness and injustice.

•←→•

Relational Justice and Differentiation

Inequitable power processes at the societal level create power imbalances within couples and families. Relationships with a high level of differentiation are characterized by equality (Gilbert, 2006). One person does not function at the expense of another. Each is open to hearing and understanding the other. There is direct, mutual conversation in which partners freely communicate their own thinking, and each is actively engaged in listening. Power imbalances inhibit this kind of direct, mutually engaged communication and tend to be connected to societal-based power differences such as gender, race, and socio-economic status (Knudson-Martin, 2024; Mahoney & Knudson-Martin, 2009). On the other hand, relational equity facilitates increased differentiation.

It is important to consider how power dynamics in a family or relationship affect differentiation. Power imbalances create an unsafe environment in which those with less societal power (often women and children) must constantly be vigilant and on guard. The lines between emotional fusion and survival become blurred. It is difficult to move toward differentiation when one's social and/or relational contexts are not safe. Importantly, as discussed above, at first glance, those in powerful positions may appear more differentiated, especially if their reactive responses appear rational rather than emotional, though they are not. Whether they are overtly dominating and abusive or maintain power through more subtle dominance and intimidation, enacting power by disinterest in and lack of empathy for the experiences and perspectives of others is a sign of low differentiation.

↔

Socioculturally attuned therapists must attend to the relational power context, and not confuse power with differentiation.

↔

Empowerment and Third Order Change

In a socioculturally attuned approach to Bowen, increasing one's level of differentiation provides a foundation for empowerment and third order change. This approach takes very seriously Bowen's proposition that we cannot understand emotion out of context (Burke & Post, 2024). Doing so requires intentionally weaving the connections between interpersonal neurobiology, relational dynamics, and societal power processes (Fishbane & Wells, 2015; see also Chapter 15, SERT).

The Sociocultural Brain

Bowen emphasized distinguishing thought and feeling as part of the differentiation process. More recent work shows that these two cannot be separated. No parts of the brain are specifically cognitive or specifically emotional (Damasio, 1999). There is no such thing as a "non-affective thought" (Duncan & Barrett, 2007). This new information actually reinforces Bowen's ideas that the individual does not biologically exist and that social processes become embodied as we interact (Burkitt, 2014; Gilbert et al., 2012; Lassiter, 2022). Without awareness of our context, we are thus likely to remain emotionally fused with social forces, which are often invisible to us and limit personal choice.

↔

Larger societal processes are part of the nearly instantaneous neurological sequence in which the contextual and situational nature of relationships register in the body and are felt.

↔

In an effort to apply Bowen theory to women and less individualistic cultures, Knudson-Martin (1994, 1996) advocated for the use of visceral feeling-based knowledge and movements toward healthy togetherness. From this perspective, rather than primarily using the "higher" brain to overcome the more primitive brain, differentiation would also include developing awareness of one's sensory experience and activating social connection. For example, Julia, the lab technologist described above, was very agitated as she described what was happening at work. The therapist recognized that the part of her vagus nerve that impeded social engagement in response to stress/fear was activated (Porges, 2009). Before trying to expand systemic understanding of the situation or strategize a response to her hostile work environment, she stayed engaged with Julia, gently reflecting resonance with her contextually inspired emotion, "It so unfair. You know you're competent, but you feel so humiliated... You just want to do your job." This empathic engagement calmed Julia's anxiety and enabled her to move into a more reflective position. The therapist then invited Julia to take some deep breaths and feel the anxiety in her body. Julia found that allowing herself to recognize and feel these physical sensations was important to her empowerment process.

Critical Awareness

As suggested by Paolo Freire (1971/2000), consciousness and critical self-reflection are the first steps toward liberation and playing an active role in the direction of one's life. Awareness of the system and one's role in it makes this possible. Though neglected by Freire, awareness of one's emotions and being able to intentionally respond to them is important to developing critical consciousness (Garcia et al., 2015).

↞↠

A socioculturally attuned understanding of Bowen theory encourages critically examining how personal biographies are interwoven with societal relationships in the experience of feeling.

↞↠

Reflective consciousness always involves attuning to and engaging the bodily sensations; without them, words and the images associated with feelings and emotion are empty and meaningless (Burkitt, 2014).

Differentiation from Dominant Cultural Values

Therapists need to be well differentiated and able to invite reflections that go beyond societal emphasis on autonomy, competition, materialization, goal-directedness, and objectivity (Knudson-Martin, 2024). Because the language used in Bowen theory can obscure values more commonly associated with women and less individualistic cultures, clinicians need to be aware of the social context of their own values and experiences (Stone & ChenFeng, 2020).

↞↠

Socioculturally attuned therapists consider what values they want to represent in their work, asking questions that help expose taken-for-granted societal expectations. They do this while standing aside to enable clients to reflect on the values *they* prefer and make informed choices from positions of self and contextual awareness.

↞↠

This is an active, not a passive role. Therapists take a clinical stance that greater equity leads to differentiation and, as McGoldrick (2016), one of the first family therapists to apply Bowen theory from a socioculturally attuned perspective described, "come back again and again…to help clients expand their perspectives on their values" (p. 63).

Practice Guidelines

The goal of socioculturally attuned Bowenian therapy is to increase individual empowerment so that clients are able to make choices about how to respond to the circumstances of their lives and create equity-based relationships that, in turn, create a context in which differentiation is possible. The steps involved are not discrete, and therapy is likely to move back and forth between them. The following guidelines promote critical awareness of the systems within which one is embedded and differentiation that enables equity, flexibility, and options.

1. Expand Presenting Problem to Larger Contexts

When people initially seek therapy, they are likely to be in an emotionally reactive state. The therapist's questions, comments, and observations help to deescalate the anxiety. The therapist builds trust and demonstrates respect through careful **attunement** that demonstrates thoughtful interest in the sociocultural and relationship contexts surrounding their concerns. In doing so, the presenting issues begin to feel more manageable. The therapist expands the conversation to include clients' social identities and locations, paying special attention to how these inform emotions and meaning. In Text Box 9.2 Monica McGoldrick points to the importance of addressing sociocultural issues from the outset, even though it may feel uncomfortable.

It is important to recognize and **name** the power processes in the immediate situation and validate emotional experiences related to injustices. Therapists promote optimism and hope by providing information about the process of change, emphasizing that through their work together, clients will come to understand and gain perspective on their lives and the patterns and contexts that influence them; that this will enable them to expand options and determine the direction they want to take.

Text Box 9.2 Monica McGoldrick, MSW, PhD

I ask clients about their cultural backgrounds right up front… I try to help clients identify cultural patterns that were part of their family's history—values about education, money, work, religion, family rituals, communication and so forth… Where there is disparity [between therapist and clients] *in race, sexual orientation, gender, socioeconomic class, or social location…we should assume there* ***will*** *be a certain level of discomfort… The key is the therapist's willingness to help clients explore their cultural background and become comfortable with such conversation, since it is not generally part of social discourse… It is always relevant to take account of your own experiences, genogram history, culture, life cycle stage, and current stresses in thinking about what issues to watch out for in working with a particular client* (McGoldrick, 2016, pp. 28–29).

2. Stabilize Immediate Situation

The process of thoughtfully discussing the client's situation and beginning to expand the context around it calms anxiety. Clients may also need to make decisions about the current stressors. Anxiety around these issues can easily pressure a therapist to solve the problem for clients and invite judgments that pathologize clients and undermine equity. Therapists need to have developed a critical contextual consciousness to help them be aware and respond justly (Stone & ChenFeng, 2020). Emotions stimulated by clients' situations—such as anger, sadness, helplessness, or shame—provide useful information, particularly regarding the power contexts underlying the presenting issues. Being aware of one's own emotional response can help therapists mindfully determine the most appropriate and helpful action (Garcia et al., 2015).

3. Assess Differentiation Through a Relational Lens

As discussed earlier, thinking and feeling are connected. The ability to be empathic and connected to others is essential to well-being. In the process of self-discovery and differentiation, clients need to draw on and develop all of these. Because Western society privileges values such as individualism, rationality, and competition, therapists need to actively **value** feeling, intuition, empathy, and connectedness. They should encourage clients to be aware of their emotions, accept them, and use them to help clarify what is important to them (Garcia et al., 2015). They should also help clients identify and connect with people and communities that enhance their sense of belonging and support. According to McGoldrick (2016),

> Clinicians and policy makers who do not consider clients' deep-seated need for continuity and belonging…are likely to increase the trauma of the original experience by ignoring the importance of their clients' connectedness. (p. 12)

4. Develop and Support Critical Consciousness

Bowen therapists often use genograms to map the people, places, contexts, and communities that are important in clients' lives (see McGoldrick, 2016; McGoldrick et al., 2008 for detailed guides). Questions suggested by McGoldrick, et al. begin with the immediate household and life cycle changes: Who lives there? What do they know about the problem? How do they view it? Where do other family members live? What has been happening recently? Questions expand to the current community, workplace, school settings, and to wider intergenerational, cultural, and societal contexts: What ethnic, religious, racial, trade, or professional groups do you feel part of? How was your family perceived in the community? What experiences have been most stressful for your family in the US? This work may be done relatively quickly or expanded upon in depth over many sessions. As therapists help clients track family patterns over time and space, they raise questions that call automatic cultural assumptions into question and that help clients recognize and resist societal patterns that reinforce inequity.

For example, in this exchange between Monica McGoldrick (2016, p. 63) and a male client, she persisted in raising questions about his resistance to needing help:

MM: What do you think about what I am saying, that the strongest man is a collaborator, not a do-it-yourself guy who never needs anything? Do you believe that?

Client: … I still believe it's like my father was. You're the man of the house and take care of the family. That's it.

MM: And how did that work for him?

Client: I don't know. He did his best…

MM: … And you've always had the sense, maybe because of the "man thing," your father didn't let himself connect as much as maybe you needed… But my thoughts are that the rules for men have been very unfair and not worked well…

Socioculturally attuned therapists can also consider using cultural and critical genograms to acknowledge aspects of clients' histories that have been influenced by injustice and marginalization as well as sources of resilience (Hardy & Laszloffy, 1995; Košutić et al., 2009). What sources of pride and shame are related to your culture of origin? What beliefs and dreams did your ancestors have? How have you been wounded by wrongs done to your people? How have you been complicit in wrongs done by your ancestors? What values are important now? Questions like these evolve as clients tell their stories. As the therapist listens through a sociocultural lens, new questions emerge, new stories are told, and clients develop a contextual understanding of themselves and their life choices. They may do research to learn more about the sociopolitical context of their family history.

5. Help Client Observe Their Own Part in the System

In this phase of therapy, clients hone in on the most troubling or persistent patterns in their lives. They become observers of themselves in the present, connect current behavior to sociocultural patterns and family histories, and learn to recognize their own emotional triggers. Clients need support to tolerate the pain they may feel as they confront their sociocultural contexts and patterns that have been shaping their lives. Attention to emotions such as fear, anger, or shame arising from contextual experiences may catalyze reflective action (Garcia et al., 2015). Clients in power positions need to become aware of the consequences of their actions on others (Samman & Knudson-Martin, 2015).

As clients reflect on themselves and realistically assess their contexts, they acknowledge what they predictably do when anxiety gets high and begin to identify empowering actions they can take. People in all power positions may also experience "felt resistance" (Garcia et al., 2015, p. 5) as they consider changes that resist or disrupt established power systems and the status quo. Being aware of anxiety and reflecting on it enables clients to shift toward action and balance responsibility for self with responsibility toward others. They can **envision** change and develop a plan for how they will respond differently to familiar patterns.

6. Increase Equity and Flexibility in the System

Clients are now ready to do the work of making choices, trying new responses, and developing more authentic and genuinely connected ways of relating. Instead of automatically reacting according to prior family patterns and societal stereotypes or on the basis of one's power position, clients use knowledge of their own experiences and situations to respond more intentionally. Therapists **intervene** by serving as a coach and mirror, asking questions about what happens and challenging clients to break through societal patterns that encourage withdrawing, triangulating, or other forms of reactivity. Therapists serve as an advocate for equity and flexibility, supporting all participants to expand beyond their comfort level to resist taken-for-granted pulls back to the status quo. As clients move toward increasing differentiation, they become more flexible, less bound by fusion with sociocultural stereotypes and expectations. **Transformation** occurs as they are able to relate to each other from more equitable positions and join together to effectively resist discriminatory and marginalizing larger systems.

7. Plan Meetings with Family and Community

Bowen therapy may be conducted with individuals, couples, or families or applied in community settings such as workplaces and churches (e.g., Friedman, 2007; Gilbert, 2006). Regardless of who is involved in the sessions, the differentiation process involves thoughtfully planning and preparing for meetings with family members and other significant relationships and settings. Meetings may be part of researching information about one's family, history, and culture or steps to engaging with significant people and contexts in new ways. Ultimately, the goal is to be able to connect with one's own family history and sociocultural contexts and to build and maintain these continuing relationships from a differentiated sense of self.

Case Example

At the suggestion of their attorney, Cloé (aged 23) first visited Judy, a White 56-year-old cishet female licensed marriage and family therapist, just several weeks after discovering that their boss had installed cameras that enabled him to secretly view Cloé from under their desk. They reported that apart from a visit to their attorney, this was the first time they had left their apartment since the discovery. Judy's intake form asked several questions that helped her begin to orient to her clients' sociocultural contexts. She learned that Cloé identified as "gender queer" and preferred pronouns "they," "them," and "theirs." They had been married to James (age 23) for three years, held a BA in English literature, cited Swedish cultural background, and said religion was not important to them.

Since Judy had a daughter about Cloé's age and positioned her clinical work to counteract societal inequities, she was aware that the case raised feelings of both anger and protectiveness for her. As a socioculturally attuned Bowen therapist, she drew on awareness of these feelings to take a differentiated stance in relation to Cloé that was clear about the values that guided her work while allowing Cloé the space to define themselves.

Expand Presenting Problem to Larger Contexts

Judy began by asking Cloé about what happened at work and their relationships with the people who worked there. She learned that it was a small accounting office consisting only of her employer, a White male in his 50s who appeared to be widely liked in the community and had long-standing relationships with the clients he served, a Black female office manager who had worked with him for over 20 years, and a young single mother who assisted with the accounting on a part-time basis. In exploring the incident, Judy assessed how the job fit into Cloé's sociocultural identity.

Cloé had felt lucky to have a full-time job as an office assistant because it provided benefits and seemed more personal and flexible than larger places. They said that working for a large corporation would not fit with their values; that they and their partner James wanted a lifestyle connected to nature and the local community. Learning that their employer had violated them in this way was not only a betrayal by someone they trusted, but put into question their own judgment. They had thought of this man and the women she worked with almost as family. Their fear about leaving the apartment now was in reaction to the loss of their identity as a confident person who could make their own way in the world.

Judy named the violation Cloé had experienced; making it clear that it made sense that it would call into question everything they believed about themselves. She shared her experience that when people are violated in this way, they often feel shame even though they had done nothing to deserve the assault. Cloé agreed that they were not at fault—that was why they had hired an attorney. Yet they were paralyzed, not able to trust themselves, while he [perpetrator] went about his business. Judy reiterated the unfairness and her genuine sadness and anger that this had happened to Cloé,

"You did nothing to deserve this. I am so sorry this happened to you. I get angry when I hear stories like yours." This differentiated expression of the therapist's own beliefs and response to the injustice helped to set the tone for the critical self-reflection and action that their work together would inspire.

Focusing on the meaning and context of the violation started to expand the presenting issues within just a few minutes. Judy then further expanded the context by asking how their husband James reacted to the assault and about their history together. Cloé described James as "completely supportive," "angry on their behalf," and "a good listener." Cloé and James had married as young undergraduates at a small liberal arts college. James represented values different from Cloé's family of origin, who "were good, loving people who did not understand them." Cloé and James had traveled and lived in several different places, looking for communities that were "more open and accepting" than the small town in Minnesota where Cloé had grown up. James fully supported Cloé's queer identity, which they embraced more fully in recent years. However, Cloé was still cautious about their gender identity and had "passed" as cisgender at work.

Judy sketched a brief genogram in her notes and used it to raise additional questions regarding relationships with family of origin and other significant community connections.

Judy: You said your parents are "good people." What does that mean to you?
Cloé: My dad's a deacon at church. My mom and dad would do anything for anyone. Dad's a teacher; mom's a nurse. They care about people.
Judy: How was that for you growing up? Would they do anything for you, too?
Cloé: I always knew they loved me. I still talk with them every week. They're just so different from me. They can't understand. They know I don't go to church, but we don't talk about it.
Judy: Have you told them about what happened?
Cloé: Not really. I told them I quit my job. When I call I ask them about their lives. It makes me feel better to talk with them, but I don't want to upset them and they'd want me to come home. Or mom would come out here.
Judy: So you still keep a connection with your parents, even though you feel you have to keep this big piece of your life to yourself… Are there other people? Friends? Community here?

As the initial conversation continued, Judy picked up on key sociocultural themes and invited Cloé to expand on them. For example, Judy noted that Cloé described their parents as religious and that their intake form said religion was not important to them. She asked Cloé to say more about that. She also asked about their experience of living outside the gender binary. By the end of the first session, Judy and Cloé had developed a picture of the trauma as an assault to Cloé's identity as a queer person and a demonstration of patriarchal societal patterns that they worked hard to resist.

Stabilize Immediate Situation

Judy was concerned that Cloé had not left the house in almost three weeks and had mostly been sleeping. She was aware of her impulse to make decisions for Cloé. Instead, she engaged directly with them about the seriousness of the situation, inviting Cloé to think through how best to address these concerns,

Judy: I'm wondering what you think about not leaving the house for almost three weeks?
Cloé: I just couldn't. James is worried about me. He tries to get me to go places with him.
Judy: Are you worried?
Cloé: Not so much worried… I know this isn't me. I just need some time.

Judy continued the conversation with questions that contrasted Cloé's current isolation with their pattern of taking on challenges. Together they used anger at the injustice as a motivator for planning some steps to break out of the isolation:

Judy: From what you've been telling me, I get the sense that it's not like you to hole up by yourself. Is that right?
Cloé: I've always been so free, so bold. I think maybe I've been naive.
Judy: It seems to me more about the injustice—it's not fair that you're not able to be you… How do you respond to that?
Cloé: It makes me mad! I want my life back. I don't want to be a victim.
Judy: What do you think would be a first step that you could do to take your life back?

Cloé decided that it was too soon to go out on their own, but that they would arrange to go on a hike with James on the weekend. Judy also suggested that James join them for the next session.

Assess Differentiation Through a Relational Lens

Given the family of origin history and early marriage that Cloé described, some therapists might have approached the couple with an assumption that the two were emotionally fused and needed to individuate. Judy began the couple session with a conversation about how they supported each other. She reinforced the value of James's focus on Cloé, his ability to empathize with them and to temporarily give up some of his needs to help them through this hard time:

Cloé: [to James] I worry that I'm being unfair to you. You're so willing to be there for me. And it just seems like all I can do to focus on me right now.
James: You don't need to worry about me. I just want you to get better.
Judy: Cloé, you said James is such a good listener, a real support to you. Has this been a pattern throughout your relationship?
Cloé: I think we've always been there for each other, but maybe sometimes I've needed James more than he's needed me. I think I struggle more than he does.
Judy: James, are you aware of that capacity they say you have to listen and empathize with them?
James: Well I care about them. And, yeah, [smiles] I think I might be better at empathy than a lot of guys.
Judy: I know the give and take is a little out of balance right now. But it seems like your ability to be there for each other when you need it is a real strength.

At this point in the therapy, Judy wanted to focus on the strengths in their relationship, to see their connectedness as a foundation for healing and further differentiation. Judy also encouraged Cloé to be aware of their feelings. Rather than continuing to resist the feelings of helplessness and unfairness, Cloé decided to journal about them and make drawings based on them. They and James began to take daily walks together, while Cloé continued with therapy sessions individually. The more comfortable Cloé was accepting James's care, the more able they were to engage in the work of self-discovery.

Develop and Support Critical Consciousness

Cloé had developed considerable critical consciousness related to oppressive societal norms and structures in their college classes. Together with James, they had taken active steps to avoid falling into taken-for-granted societal norms and create a life more consistent with their values. These were moves toward increased awareness, differentiation, and choice. Yet, as might be expected given their stage of life, these changes also involved some cut-off from connection to Cloé's sociocultural roots and family. In the next sessions, Judy guided Cloé in continuing to explore how their response to the violation inflicted upon them related to key themes and patterns in their family of origin, culture, religion, and sociopolitical context. Through questions that challenged assumptions, expanded the focus outward, and invited reflection and integration, Judy maintained a curious and supportive partnership with Cloé.

"Men are violent and unsafe," was identified as a family and sociopolitical theme brought to the surface by Cloé's assault:

Judy: So now you think that all men are unsafe? How has that been for the women in your family?
Cloé: My mother is always telling us to be careful. Not to trust men. To be careful where you go. In her work as a nurse, she has seen so many women who were raped or beaten.
Judy: How do you think this message that men are unsafe has affected your mother?
Cloé: My mother is very cautious. She doesn't go to many places by herself. My sister is just like her.

As the conversation continued, Cloé realized that they didn't actually know much about their mother's experiences with men or the experience of women in previous generations. Their father and spouse were described as "exceptions," warm, loving, and nonviolent. Judy expanded the topic of male dominance from the family to the larger society,

Judy: You said your father is very kind. How does power work between your mother and father?
Cloé: No one really questions my father… They're very traditional really.
Judy: But you question male dominance—a lot, it seems to me.
Cloé: Yeah. But it's everywhere, everywhere I look. That's why [explicative] like [employer] gets away with it. Because they can!
Judy: Yeah. That's how power works, isn't it? But you're not letting him get away with it. You're taking him to court. You're holding him accountable. What else do you think is important to counter the male dominance in our society?

Framing their assault as an example of a larger system of male dominance was an important step in Cloé's ability to develop a thoughtful response to it. Several other key themes evolved as Judy continued to expand their genogram work. For example, "doing good" by following a religious code was a major moral theme across multiple generations. Independence and stoicism were connected to survival and success for their immigrant great-grandparents from Sweden and continued to be valued family traits. Holding back from full engagement was a common "solution" to potentially disruptive disagreements.

Help Client Observe Own Part in the System

Cloé became better able to name the marginalization they experienced as a queer person living in a world still organized around a gender binary, heteronormativity, and male dominance. It began to make sense that they hid this identity much of the time, both because of very real societal discrimination and because family patterns encouraged only partial engagement of the self. Cloé also recognized that their sense that they should cope with the trauma of the assault primarily on their own was also part of family and cultural patterns that they had unconsciously continued. Through conversations with Judy, they began to track how their response to injustice maintained isolation.

Judy: How has the journaling about your feelings been going? What have you noticed?
Cloé: I've noticed that I am very lonely. I want to share my feelings, but I can't.
Judy: What do you think stops you?
Cloé: It just feels wrong.
Judy: Like you're breaking a rule?
Cloé: Yes! It might seem silly, but it's scary to think about telling someone what I'm feeling—even James.
Judy: How do you think people would respond? I'm guessing maybe some people would be more able to hear you than others?
Cloé: Yeah. Probably. I think I just don't want to bother people. To upset them. To be a burden.

Increase Equity and Flexibility in the System

Judy began to coach Cloé in initiating a plan of action with four goals, all related to living out the family legacy of "doing good" in a differentiated way: 1) to become engaged in collective action to combat male dominance, 2) to expand safe spaces for authentically expressing their voice and identity, 3) to develop their own spiritual practices, and 4) to update and deepen their bonds with James and their family. One week Cloé came in with an announcement that they had told their parents about the assault:

Cloé: I told my parents what happened!
Judy: Wow. That was a big step. Did it go as you expected?
Cloé: They were great! I told them that I had not told them before because I didn't want to worry or upset them. They seemed to understand that. They listened really well.
Judy: How do you think you were different in the way you talked to them?
Cloé: I had decided that I didn't care how they reacted. I just needed to be honest with them.
Judy: So you wanted them to know what was really going on with you. You wanted to be you. Were you prepared that they might not be able to handle it well?
Cloé: I thought through all that. I decided that I could handle it. I knew they loved me.

Cloé made similar changes in how they related to James, not only accepting his care, but also being more able to focus on what he needed. This change promoted more genuine equality between them:

Judy: It's interesting that you are more able to focus on James's needs now. Do you think this is because the effect of the violation at work is letting up, or do you think something else is going on?
Cloé: It's both. I always followed James's lead. I liked that he wanted to travel and live in different places. I liked that he accepted me for who I am. But I didn't feel like I could disagree with him. I didn't even let myself have those kinds of thoughts. So I think I also kept my distance a little bit. If I let his needs be too important, I would have felt dominated.

Plan Meetings with Family and Community

Much of Judy's work with Cloé involved expanding their interpersonal connections and strategizing how to do this. This included being able to connect with the women they had worked with to tell them what happened and preparing to tell their story in court. Judy was always careful to recognize and validate the real dangers and stresses involved, and to support Cloé in working through what responses were right for them. Another important step was volunteering in two community groups for young people. One provided support for children and adolescents questioning their gender identity; the other provided education to teenage girls regarding sexual violence. Cloé invited James to several therapy sessions to help them work through the changes in their relationship as Cloé took a more differentiated position. In these sessions, Judy also helped James become aware of the hidden power he held in their relationship and to be able to receive disagreement from Cloé.

Cloé and James took a trip to visit their family in Minnesota. One of the issues Cloé decided they wanted to share with their parents was their newly evolving spirituality. After the visit, Cloé returned for a final therapy session. They said they were surprised at how better able they were to be themselves with their family. They realized how much they had missed being more connected to them. As a result, Cloé and James were discussing using the settlement Cloé received from [perpetrator] to start a small farm-to-table restaurant in Minnesota, a few hours away from their family. Cloé had initiated the idea and felt confident that they could thoughtfully work through this decision on equal par with James. Whether or not they started this business, Cloé wanted more connection with their family and was better able to engage with them even though their parents could not fully understand their identity and lifestyle.

Summary: Third Order Change

Bowen theory promotes systemic thinking. Understanding symptoms or patterns always requires going larger (McGoldrick, 2016) so that clients can see themselves, their concerns, and their multigenerational family systems as part of ongoing sociocultural systems. Third order change involves being able to critically reflect on how societal context and power processes are part of one's situation and making choices regarding how to resist these dominant societal discourses and contexts from a less reactive, more reflective position.

Cloé and James had begun this process. They recognized systems of systems and elected to live outside the dominant social structure as much as possible. Yet, at their stage of differentiation, their responses demonstrated the tenacity of emotional fusion within both larger societal and family systems. Much of their resistance to dominant societal values had been reactive in nature, cut off from bonds that connected them to family and sociopolitical contexts. Cloé's differentiation work in response to the sexual assault enabled third order change; that is, greater ability to recognize and navigate complex social forces while staying genuinely engaged in their social worlds.

The clarity and sense of self that comes with third order differentiation involves awareness and respect for one's interconnectedness with the larger group (e.g., Lassiter, 2022; Wiseman & Papero, 2011). It may be compared to Freire's (1970/2000) idea of liberation through grassroots consciousness-raising and action. Through critical thinking and awareness of self-in-context, people discover their situatedness and how their own internalized images have been emotionally fused with dominant social systems, leaving them trapped inside a socioemotional web rather than able to make freely informed choices about their lives. Reflection on the self and the systems within which one is embedded enables transformative action. This reflection enables awareness of community, which in turn supports increased empowerment.

Reflexive Questions

- If societal projection processes such as discrimination, scapegoating, and entrenched power hierarchies are likely to disproportionately affect targeted or marginalized groups, which groups do you think are most affected in your community?
- In less differentiated systems, responsibility for managing anxiety often falls on the less powerful. What thoughts or reactions do you have to this statement?
- If inequitable power processes at the societal level create power imbalances within couples and families, and relationships with a high level of differentiation are characterized by equality, then what would this mean for your intimate partner relationship, past or present?
- What would this understanding mean for the couples you work with as a Bowen-informed couples therapist?
- Has there been a time when you have mistakenly confused someone's power with differentiation? How did you know?

References

Bartle-Haring, S. & Whiting, R. (2024). Perceived overlap and therapy outcomes among couple clients. *Journal of Marital and Family Therapy*, *50*(4), 821–839.

Bowen, M. (1978). *Family therapy in clinical practice*. Jason Aronson.

Brown, J. & Errington, L. (2024). Bowen family systems theory and practice: Illustration and critique revisited. *Australian and New Zealand Journal of Family Therapy*, *45*, 135–155.

Burke, K. & Post, A. (2024). Intimate partner violence and Bowen family systems theory: promoting safety and expanding capacity of families. *Australian and New Zealand Journal of Family Therapy*, *45*, 190–208.

Burkitt, I. (2014). *Emotions and social relations*. Sage.

Chan, P. (2024) Bowen theory, culture and therapeutic applications to Asian families. *Australian and New Zealand Journal of Family Therapy*, *45*, 244–256.

Cohen, S., Janicki-Deverts, D., Chen, E., & Matthews, K. A. (2010). Childhood socioeconomic status and adult health. *Annals of the New York Academy of Sciences*, *1186*(1), 37–55.

Collier, C.E. & Mader, A. (2024) The language of nature in Murray Bowen's writings: how connection to nature informs Bowen theory and is essential to human survival. *Australian and New Zealand Journal of Family Therapy*, *45*, 218–234.

Cowdery, R., Scarborough, N., Knudson-Martin, C., Lewis, M., Seshadri, G., & Mahoney, A. (2009). Gendered power in cultural contexts part II: Middle class African American heterosexual couples with young children. *Family Process*, *48*, 25–39.

Damasio, A. (1999). *The feeling of what happens: Body and emotion in the making of consciousness*. Harper Collins.

Duncan, S. & Barrett, L. F. (2007). Affect is a form of cognition: A neurobiological analysis. *Cognition and Emotion*, *21*(6), 1184–1211.

Fishbane, M. D. & Wells, M. A., (2015). Toward relational empowerment: Interpersonal neurobiology, couples, and the societal context. In C. Knudson-Martin, M. A. Wells, & S. K. Samman (Eds.). *Socio-emotional relationship therapy: Bridging emotion, societal discourse, and couple interaction* (pp. 27–40). AFTA Springerbriefs in Family Therapy: Springer.

Freire, P. (2000). *Pedagogy of hope*. Continuum. (Original work published 1970).

Friedman, E. H. (2007). *A failure of nerve: Leadership in the age of the quick fix*. Seabury Books.

Gallego, A., Schweer-Collins, M. L., Osorio, A., & Rodríguez-González, M. (2024). Differentiation of self in adolescents: Measurement invariance analysis across six Spanish-speaking countries. *Current Psychology*, *43*(16), 14581–14589.

Garcia, M., Košutić, I., & McDowell, T. (2015). Peace on earth/war at home: The role of emotion regulation in social justice work. *Journal of Feminist Family Therapy*, *27*, 1–20.

Gilbert, R. M. (2006). *Extraordinary leadership: Thinking systems, making a difference*. Leading Systems Press.

Gilbert, S. F., Sapp, J., & Tauber, A. I. (2012). A symbiotic view of life: We have never been individuals. *Quarterly Review of Biology*, *87*, 325–341.

Goldberger, H. (1996). Cultural imperatives and diversity in ways of knowing. In N. Goldberger, J. Tarule, B. Clinchy, & M. Belenky (Eds.). *Knowledge, difference and power: Essays inspired by women's ways of knowing* (pp. 335–371). Basic Books.
Hardy, K. V. & Laszloffy, T. A. (1995). The cultural genogram: Key to training culturally competent family therapists. *Journal of Marital and Family Therapy*, *21*, 227–237.
Hargrave, T. D. & Houltberg, B. J. (2020). Transgenerational theories and how they evolved into current research and practice. In K. S. Wampler, R. B. Miller, & R. B. Seedall (Eds.). *The Handbook of Systemic Family Therapy* (Vol. 1, pp. 317–338). Wiley.
Hurtado, A. (1996). Strategic suspensions: Feminists of color theorize the production of knowledge. In N. Goldberger, J. Tarule, B. Clinchy, & M. Belenky (Eds.). *Knowledge, difference and power: Essays inspired by women's ways of knowing* (pp. 372–392). Basic Books.
Innes, M. (1996). Connecting Bowen theory with its human origins. *Family Process*, *35*, 487–500.
Jack, D. C. & Ali, A. (2010). *Silencing the self across cultures: Depression and gender in the social world.* Oxford University Press.
Kerr, M. E. (2019). *Bowen theory's secrets: Revealing the hidden life of families*. WW Norton & Company.
Kerr, M. E. & Bowen, M. (1988). *Family evaluation: An approach based on Bowen theory*. Norton.
Kerr, M. & MacKay, L. (2024). A personal reflection on Bowen family systems theory by Dr Michael Kerr. *Australian and New Zealand Journal of Family Therapy*, *45*(2), 266–273.
Knudson-Martin, C. (2024). *A step-by-step guide to socio-emotional relationship therapy: A socially responsible approach to clinical practice*. Routledge.
Knudson-Martin, C. (1996). Differentiation and self-development in the relationship context. *The Family Journal*, *4*, 188–198.
Knudson-Martin, C. (1994). The female voice: Applications to Bowen's family systems theory. *Journal of Marital and Family Therapy*, *20*, 35–46.
Komter, A. (1989). Hidden power in marriage. *Gender and Society*, *3*, 187–216.
Košutić, I., Garcia, M., Graves, T., Barnett, F., Hall, J., Haley, E., Rock, J., Bathon, A., & Kaiser, B. (2009). The critical genogram: A tool for promoting critical consciousness. *Journal of Feminist Family Therapy*, *21*, 151–76.
Lantz, P. M., House, J. S., Mero, R. P., & Williams, D. R. (2005). Stress, life events, and socioeconomic disparities in health: results from the Americans' changing lives study. *Journal of Health and Social Behavior*, *46*(3), 274–288.
Lassiter, L. (2022). The emotional side of socioeconomic status. *Family Systems: A Journal of Natural Systems Thinking in Psychiatry & the Sciences*, *17*(1), 9–29.
Luepnitz, D. A. (1988). *The family interpreted: Feminist theory in clinical practice*. Basic Books.
Mahoney, A. R. & Knudson-Martin, C. (2009). The social context of gendered power. In C. Knudson-Martin & A. R. Mahoney. *Couples, gender, and power: Creating change in intimate relationships* (pp. 17–29). Springer Publishing Co.
McDowell, T. (2015) *Applying critical social theories to family therapy practice*. AFTA Springerbriefs in Family Therapy, Springer.
McGoldrick, M. (2016). *The genogram casebook*. Norton.
McGoldrick, M., Gerson, R., & Petry, S. (2008). *Genograms: Assessment and intervention* (3rd ed.). Norton.
Neophytou, K., Schweer-Collins, M. L., Rodríguez-González, M., Jódar, R., & Skowron, E. A. (2021). The differentiation of self inventory–Revised: A validation study in the Greek cultural context. *The American Journal of Family Therapy*, *49*(2), 185–203.
Ogan, M. A., Monk, J. K., Thibodeau-Nielsen, R. B., Vennum, A., & Soloski, K. (2024). The role of emotional dysregulation in the association between family-of-origin conflict and romantic relationship maintenance. *Journal of Marital and Family Therapy*, *50*(1), 28–44.
Papero, D. V. (2024) The family emotional system. *Australian and New Zealand Journal of Family Therapy*, 45, 156–167.
Porges, S. W. (2009). Reciprocal influences between the body and the brain in the perception and expression of affect. In D. Fosha, D. S. Siewgel, & M F. Solomon (Eds.). *The healing power of emotion: Affective neuroscience, development & clinical practice* (pp. 27–54). Norton.
Samman, S. K. & Knudson-Martin, C. (2015). Relational engagement in heterosexual couple therapy: Helping men move from "I" to "we." In C. Knudson-Martin, M. A. Wells, & S. K. Samman (Eds.). *Socio-emotional relationship therapy: Bridging emotion, societal discourse, and couple interaction* (pp. 79–92). AFTA Springerbriefs in Family Therapy, Springer.

Silverstein, R., Bass, L., Tuttle, A., Knudson-Martin, C., & Huenergardt, D. (2006). What does it mean to be relational? A framework for assessment and practice. *Family Process*, *45*, 39–405.
Skowron, E. A. (2004). Differentiation of self, personal adjustment, problem solving, and ethnic group belonging among persons of color. *Journal of Counseling and Development*, *82*, 447–456.
Smoliak, O., Rice, C., Rudder, D., Tseliou, E., LaMarre, A., LeCouteur, A., … & Henshaw, S. (2024). Emotion regulation as affective neoliberal governmentality. *Family Process*. Advanced on-line publication. DOI: 10.1111/famp.13064
Sternberg, E. (2001). *The balance within: The science connecting health and emotions*. H. W. Freeman.
Stevenson, B. (2014). *Just Mercy: A story of justice and redemption*. Random House.
Stone, D. J. & ChenFeng, J. L. (2020). *Finding your voice as a beginning marriage and family therapist*. Routledge.
Tamura, T. (2016). *Family therapy: East meets West. Plenary presentation at the 2016 International World Family Therapy Congress*, Waikoloa, HI.
Thomas, R., Shelley-Tremblay, J., & Joanning, H. (2021). Anxiety explains self-differentiation: Implications for Bowenian approaches to marriage and family therapy. *The American Journal of Family Therapy*, *49*(5), 534–549.
Titelman, P. (2014). The concept of differentiation of self in Bowen theory. In P. Titelman (Ed.). *Differentiation of self: Bowen family systems theory perspectives* (pp. 3–64). Routledge.
Unger, M. (2015). Varied patterns of family resilience in challenging contexts. *Journal of Marital and Family Therapy*, *42*, 19–31.
van der Kolk, B. (2014). *The body keeps the score: Brain, mind, and body in the healing of trauma*. Penguin Books.
Watson, M. F. (2013). *Facing the black shadow*. BookBaby.
Wiseman, K. & Papero, D. V. (2011). How Bowen theory can be useful to people in the workplace: A conversation between Kathy Wiseman and Daniel V. Pepero. In *Bringing systems thinking to life: Expanding the horizons for Bowen family systems theory* (pp. 209–217). Routledge.
Wetherell, M. (2012). *Affect and emotion: A new social science understanding*. Sage.
White, K. L. (2024). Moving around the system: a way of working clinically using Bowen family systems theory. *Australian and New Zealand Journal of Family Therapy*, *45*, 235–243.
Willis, K., Miller, R. B., Yorgason, J., & Dyer, J. (2021). Was Bowen correct? The relationship between differentiation and triangulation. *Contemporary Family Therapy*, *43*, 1–11.

10 Socioculturally Attuned Contextual Family Therapy

Contextual family therapists take the view that humans are fundamentally connected and responsible to each other. Ivan Boszormenyi-Nagy devised contextual therapy as a socioethical umbrella under which other approaches may be leveraged (Boszormenyi-Nagy, 1987). Its emphasis on our ethical responsibility to care for one another (Boszormenyi-Nagy & Krasner, 1986; van der Meiden et al., 2019) is unique and counters dominant Western ideas of utilitarian self-interest. When developed, contextual therapy represented a shift from an emphasis on intrapsychic change to facilitating change in the ethical contracts between people. Like postmodern therapies, this approach views the "self" as a relational process rather than an individual construct (Ducommun-Nagy, 2025).

Contextual therapy encompasses five levels: 1) facts regarding the circumstances that impact life experience including where one is born, key life events such as traumas, losses, and transitions; 2) individual psychology, or the meaning that individuals make of their experience and how that is internalized; 3) transactional patterns involving family communication, structures, and interactions; 4) relational ethics—fairness in what we give to each other—as the overarching contextual framework; and 5) the fundamental ontic need to relate to others that serves as a healing resource when people "recognize the uniqueness and full humanity of the other and treat each other fairly" (Ducommun-Nagy, 2025, p. 9).

The contextual approach to family therapy continues to evolve and is especially helpful in identifying and addressing the relational impact of unjust social systems and contexts (Daneshpour, 2025; Gangamma & Le, 2026; Rootes, 2013; Sude & Gambrel, 2017; van der Meiden, 2020). Its integrative framework invites many styles of practice and focuses on resources rather than pathology (Dankoski & Deacon, 2000; Glebova et al., 2025; Hargrave & Pfitzer, 2003).

•←→•

Socioculturally attuned contextual therapists inspire third order change by addressing how larger social contexts and societal power inequities affect relationality and the balance of fairness in people's lives.

•←→•

In this chapter, we first highlight five enduring family therapy concepts that guide contextual therapy: 1) interpersonal consequences, 2) the balance of fairness, 3) entitlement, 4) intergenerational loyalty, and 5) multidirected partiality. We then show how to apply them from a socioculturally attuned perspective and illustrate with a case.

Primary Enduring Concepts

In Nagy's framework, context refers to the ethical connections within which individual development and interpersonal dynamics occur (van Heusden & van den Eerenbeemt, 1987). Whether we

DOI: 10.4324/9781003493426-10

work with an individual or a family, these ethical considerations are always present. A look at the case of Barbara, a 25-year-old Anishinabe (sometimes referred to as Chippewa or Ojibwe) woman with a five-year-old daughter, will help us understand the concepts in contextual family therapy. Barbara sought therapy because she was in a new relationship with Karl, aged 32, whom she described as a "good" man and did not want to "lose." Both the men in her previous relationships were in prison. She said she could afford one session a month from her job as a waitress and would not accept a reduction in the fee. From a contextual perspective, this therapy is about what Barbara has a right to expect in the relational give and take between herself and others (Boszormenyi-Nagy & Krasner, 1986), with an emphasis on giving care as a source of healing absent in most other clinical approaches (Daneshpour, 2025; Ducommun-Nagy, 2025; Fishbane, 2023).

Interpersonal Consequences

Nagy was strongly influenced by Martin Buber's (1958) view that personhood is founded on relationship rather than self-interest, living *with* the world rather than *in* it (Boszormenyi-Nagy & Spark, 1973; Fishbane, 1998). He viewed relationships as a dialogical I–thou process of "receiving through giving, through caring about the other," and approached therapy with "responsibility for all those who will be affected by his or her work" (van Heusden & van den Eerenbeemt, 1987, pp. 4–6). In Barbara's case, this included her relationships with her daughter Cora and partner Karl, but also her mother, step-father, former foster care parents, former partners, people in her community and at work, and future grandchildren.

Contextual therapists believe that what we do inevitably has consequences for others. Symptoms occur when there are violations of this foundational ethical contract (Hargrave & Pfitzer, 2003). Like many clients, Barbara had a long history of interpersonal wounds and betrayals. She "inherited" a mother who was addicted to drugs and engaged in survival sex work and a stepfather who sexually abused her. She suffered physical abuse from her first partner and left him when she learned she was pregnant. These relational injustices were rooted within legacies of historical injustice and trauma suffered by the Anishinabeg (which means first people) as Euro-Americans systematically took their land and culture from them. As we will see, the consequences of the trauma inflicted upon her people continued forward through multiple generations.

Contextual therapy emphasizes that Barbara was entitled to care and respect *and* helps her be responsible for the consequences of her responses to these prior injustices. Her therapist is empathic and stresses that Barbara is not responsible for the abuse she endured. She also asks about how these previous experiences affect the way Barbara parents Cora and her ability to be a trustworthy partner with Karl. Rather than considering only pathology in her family history, contextual therapy helps her find resources that she can carry forward (Boszormenyi-Nagy & Spark, 1973; Glebova et al., 2025). The work is intergenerational and seeks to rebalance fairness in these relationships, with attention to the consequences for all family members.

Balance of Fairness

Justice is a synthesis of the reciprocity balance among family members (Boszormenyi-Nagy & Spark, 1973). This means that people must openly acknowledge the positive contributions that they have made to others and that others have made to them (Goldenthal, 1996). Nagy called this *due crediting.* This is not just a behavioral action. It includes the capacity to be sensitive to others, to see from their perspective, and "above all give care to others" (p. 19). When the giving and taking of care is out of balance, the relationship is not just. Persons with marginalized identities or limited power are less able to feel seen and heard; therapists must be able to name and acknowledge the unfairness and play an active role in facilitating a more equitable and ethical balance of care (Gangamma & Le, 2026). Helping family members balance the ledger of fairness—who owes what to whom—is a core goal in contextual therapy and is important for the giver as well as the receiver (Ducommun-Nagy, 2025).

Justice is not simply a 50–50 exchange; "I do this for you, and you do this for me." It is based on genuine care and giving what is needed in the circumstances. It means providing care when someone is sick or disabled, but also acknowledges ways those receiving may also be giving all in the context of valuing the relationship itself (Fishbane, 2023). Justice involves commitment to the well-being of one another over the long term. In the case of a parent such as Barbara, reciprocity is not "tit for tat;" as an adult Barbara is responsible to create a safe and nurturing environment for her daughter. In her relationship with Karl, Barbara is entitled to mutual support (Knudson-Martin & Huenergardt, 2010).

Entitlement

All persons are entitled to care and nurturance from others. This is especially true of children from adult caregivers. Boszormenyi-Nagy used the notion of *constructive entitlement* to describe the outcome of receiving positive and responsive care. Having received care as children, we have the capacity to give care to others as adults and to pass it along. When entitlement to care during childhood is not met, the person approaches adult relationships from a position of *destructive entitlement*. According to Boszormenyi-Nagy and Krasner (1986), "destructive entitlement is one end result of the parental failure to honor the inherent entitlement with which each infant is born" (p. 110). Because they feel as though they are owed a debt, they may lack or deny sensitivity to others and cause pain or harm. As stated by Boszormenyi-Nagy and Krasner (1986), "credit earned by victimization predisposes people to repetitive, substitutive claims for restitution…and are disinclined to feel pangs of remorse or guilt." (p.111). As in Barbara's case, destructive entitlement may also skew a person's perceptions of justice so that they do not feel entitled to care and do not expect to receive it from others. They may always do for others without receiving care in return. Either way, the balance of care in current relationships is unfair.

Sometimes destructive entitlement weakens parental boundaries such that the child must assume the role of a *parentified child*. Barbara had been expecting five-year-old Cora to show care and respect for her feelings, something she was entitled to and did not receive as a child or in prior relationships with men. While a five-year-old can and should learn to respond sensitively to others (Siegel & Hartzell, 2003), Barbara had been expecting a level of validation from Cora that a child could not provide. When she understood this, Barbara was able to respond to Cora from a position of care rather than anger.

On the other hand, Barbara had been uncertain whether she was entitled to the care and sensitivity Karl demonstrated to her. She began to feel emotionally indebted, fearful that he would leave her if she asked or expected too much. The therapist facilitated several couple sessions that helped Karl explicitly credit Barbara with all that she gave to him, reinforced her entitlement to care, and clarified what mutual care and support would look like for them.

Intergenerational Loyalty

In contextual therapy, Barbara's current relationships cannot be understood apart from her loyalty to her family of origin. Loyalty is defined differently than we may usually think of it. Here, it is an existential bond that connects us to our origins, but may be invisible to us. According to Boszormenyi-Nagy and Krasner (1986), "it is almost synonymous with the essential irrefutability of family ties" (p. 15). We may consciously disavow or disconnect from family members but remain drawn to our indebtedness to them. This can include invisible or split loyalty to larger social contexts and connections (Gangamma & Le, 2026).

Barbara left home at the age of sixteen and had not seen her mother since. The doubt, uncertainty, and inability to trust Barbara experienced when Karl demonstrated caring and treated her well are examples of *invisible loyalty*. She did not want to be obliged to the therapist by not paying the full fee but was unaware of the ways she unconsciously maintained loyalty/obligation to her mother and prior generations. From a contextual perspective, finding ways to express healthy filial loyalty to her parents was an important developmental task (Fishbane, 2005). It would free her to new possibilities in her own life and help her engage responsibly with Cora and Karl. It meant learning to see her mother in the broader context and giving her credit for her positive contributions to Barbara's life. In contextual therapy, this process is called *exoneration*, or "lifting the load of culpability of a person who has previously been blamed for a violation" (Hargrave & Pfitzer, 2003, p. 139). Ideally, but not necessarily, it is also linked to processes of forgiveness in which love and trust are reestablished (Hargrave & Pfitzer, 2003).

Multidirected Partiality

Multidirected partiality is at the heart of what contextual family therapists do (Goldenthal, 1996; Roberto, 1992; van der Meiden et al., 2020). Therapists demonstrate empathy to everyone while highlighting issues of *relational ethics* (Sibley et al., 2015). They take into consideration the relational claims of each person, whether or not they are in the room. Through the technique of *due crediting*, therapists highlight relational injustices that each person has experienced and acknowledge their efforts and contributions. For example, Barbara's therapist recognized and empathized with the pain and injustice she suffered as a child and in her prior relationships. However, she also brought the interests and contributions of her birth and foster parents into the room.

Contextual therapists explore the past but emphasize due crediting as a current process. The therapist asked Barbara what she learned about relationships from her foster family. Though Barbara had not previously focused on the resources this family had provided to her, it was easy for her to identify the stability and love they had offered. The value of these important contributions had been lost to Barbara due to *split loyalty*; the invisible pull of loyalty to her birth family kept her focused on what they owed her, rather than what she had actually received from the foster family. As a result, she had not maintained a connection with them. When she contacted her foster parents and thanked them, they were overjoyed and still available to her.

Rebalancing trust and fairness when there are legacies of injustice such as trauma and abuse can require many sessions (Wells et al., 2017); but not always (Goldenthal, 1996). Barbara did not know much of her mother's story but knew how to find her. The therapist and Barbara discussed what it would mean to invite her to a therapy session, and the uncertainty of not knowing what to expect. Barbara was motivated to transform her life and ready to take this important step. In the intervening time, her mother had done a lot of her own transformative work and was active in a twelve-step program. She welcomed the opportunity to revisit her relationship with Barbara. The therapist began the one two-hour session with an assumption that there were relational resources that could be accessed. She invited the mother to tell her story, helping them look not only at what Barbara was entitled to as a child, but to hear and credit the mother's anguish at willingly giving up her child because she did not believe she could care for her. The mother recounted how her desire to get her child back had motivated her to get clean and marry an older man (now deceased) who could provide economic stability.

The role of the therapist is not neutral (Goldenthal, 1996). Therapists align with different persons at different times and use their power to help balance relational ledgers or *ledgers of merits*. This is an active role based on multidirected caring and empathy (Glebova et al., 2025; Sibley et al., 2015). Barbara's therapist moved back and forth between caring and empathy for Barbara and for her mother. The therapist used her role to facilitate a conversation about what Barbara and her mother needed from each other now. She addressed their shared sadness at never knowing Barbara's birth father and Barbara's experience of sexual abuse, which the mother had not known. Barbara recounted how she had purposely protected her mother from knowing this because she did not want to hurt her (an example of invisible loyalty).

Exoneration of past injustice occurred as Barbara began to understand why she was not given her due and began to see her parents as real people (Fishbane, 1998). Barbara and her mother developed a plan for maintaining limited contact with each other and for Cora to know her grandmother. This was facilitated by their shared interest in reconnecting with generational legacies of injustice, community, and pride as members of the Anishinabeg nation. Following this session, Barbara reported a fundamental transformation in her sense of self. She felt more comfortable with, and entitled to, a mutually supportive relationship with Karl and more confident in herself as a loving parent, while also gradually building a relationship with her mother and claiming her identity as an Anishinaabe woman. The therapist's active use of multidirected partiality enabled the family to rebalance the generational ledger and intentionally redirect their responses to old wounds.

Integrating Principles of Socioculturally Attuned Family Therapy

Though applications and study of contextual therapy are growing (e.g., Daneshpour, 2025; Gangamma et al., 2015; Gangamma & Le, 2026; Sibley et al., 2015; van der Meiden et al., 2019), the approach has been underutilized and understudied. This could be in part because notions such as sensitivity, integrity, and relational responsibility and justice do not resonate with individualistic Western patriarchal culture (Dankoski & Deacon, 2000). The relational justice focus of contextual therapy can be expanded to clarify the impact of broader societal systems and power to enable third order change.

•←→•

Justice within a family system can never be separate from justice within the larger societal context.

•←→•

Societal Systems

How family members experience care, what they owe each other and what they are entitled to is shaped by cultural norms and values, structural inequities, and legacies of sociopolitical injustices and traumas. In fact, as noted by Gangamma & Le (2026), the concept of family often assumed in this model may further decenter and colonize diverse family forms, including LGBTQ+ families. Socioculturally attuned contextual family therapy demands expansion of the concept of family to include families of choice and broader systems of care.

Justice, Privilege, and Entitlement

Nagy emphasized the need to look beyond the immediate give and take to place relationship patterns in context of the ledger of indebtedness across generations and the group's history. Entitlement is earned through caring about others and goes hand in hand with reciprocal indebtedness

(Boszormenyi-Nagy, 1987; Ducommun-Nagy, 2025). It is both a human right and a human obligation. This ethical commitment transcends transactional patterns and carries important consequences for the future.

Privilege, as we use it in this text, refers to unearned benefits (care) that one gains simply because of their social locations, for being White, for being male, for being straight, etc. It is a societal-level process that contributes to interpersonal processes. From the lens of relational ethics, unacknowledged social privilege results in "exploitative oppression" (Boszormenyi-Nagy, 1987, p. 317), which engenders destructive entitlement. When people acknowledge and are accountable for their privilege, they are more able to be responsive to the needs of others and earn constructive entitlement. On the other hand, when processes of privilege result in discrimination and injustice, destructive entitlement may accrue, damaging personal and relational health and potentially be expressed in a variety of harmful behaviors or symptoms.

•←→•

A socioculturally attuned approach links person-to-person exploitation to structural exploitation that may be oppressing all participants, including the therapist.

•←→•

Values

Unlike dominant economic systems, contextual therapy values the work of caring and equity. It challenges the myth of the rugged individual (Fishbane, 1998) and views justice as collaborative rather than competitive. It can be easy for persons raised in Western cultures to think of ledgers or give and take from a more individualistic exchange perspective. Instead of helping people negotiate, "I'll do this for you and you do this for me," socioculturally attuned therapists help people approach each other with empathy rather than blame, and encourage them to attune to each other and the relationship overall. Through this approach, addressing conflict is an opportunity for relational trust and individual growth (Daneshpour, 2025).

•←→•

When persons genuinely take on the experience of another, they also begin to demonstrate more responsibility for the effect of their actions on them.

•←→•

Knudson-Martin and Huenergardt (2010) described therapy with Damon, a European American university student who considered himself a "geek" and not people oriented, and his female partner Ellie. The couple described an incident in which Damon got angry with his aunt (with whom they lived) and walked out of the room, leaving Ellie to deal with the aunt. The therapists did not automatically accept the cultural idea that men, especially computer nerds, are not relational. Instead, they encouraged Damon to imagine what it was like for Ellie when he walked out. They stayed with Damon until he could take in her experience. When he did, he began to see the unfairness and was motivated to engage more equitably with Ellie, which increased trust in the relationship for both of them.

Helping clients identify their relational needs and commitments enables more choice regarding what cultural values mean to them, which they want to enact, and how they perform them. In addition to thinking that geeks could not be people persons, Damon also believed in fairness and genuinely valued and loved Ellie. He needed help enacting caring values that male dominant culture discouraged. In this way, contextual therapy aligns with feminist therapies and ethics of care (Daneshpour, 2025; Fishbane, 2023; Smoliak et al., 2022).

Historical Injustices and Trauma

Millions of people suffer from intergenerational effects of historical injustices such as slavery, religious oppression, genocide, and colonization that systematically destroy their culture, land ownership, spiritual practices, and humans themselves (Brown, 2008). This kind of historical trauma weakens traditional cultural coping strategies and creates stress and trauma that affects present-day circumstances. Because it was not safe for disenfranchised survivors to express hostility toward oppressors, they often internalized anger, grief, sadness, loss, shame, and inferiority that is passed on and affects the next generation (Brave Heart & DeBruyn, 1998). Groups with these historical injustices endure high rates of depression, violence, substance abuse, and suicide (Brown, 2008). From a contextual therapy point of view, when the reality of these injustices is acknowledged, it is possible to transform what they mean going forward (Glebova et al., 2025).

Consider the effect of the cultural genocide of Indigenous people on Barbara. European colonization of the Anishinabeg homeland forced social changes that disrupted her ancestors' balance of life, leaving them facing death, disease, and starvation and increasingly reliant on foreign commodities (Brave Heart & DeBruyn, 1998; Brownlie, 2008). In the 19th century, her people were removed from their traditional lands. Those who survived were consigned to small tracts, reservations with few resources. Women, who had held high status prior to European encroachment, found their roles and value diminished (Brownlie, 2008).

Barbara's grandparents grew up in the economically devastated conditions of one of these reservations. Her grandfather was sent to a boarding school designed to solve the "Indian problem" by teaching native children dominant cultural values (Brave Heart & DeBruyn, 1998, p. 63). He was beaten for speaking his native language, not allowed to see his family all year, and labeled as a failure. As a young man, he was sent to an urban relocation center where he was not prepared to succeed, developed problems with alcohol, and drifted back and forth between the reservation and the city. Barbara's mother grew up in this environment, with a father who was frequently absent and violent when he was present. She did not see jobs or opportunities for herself and felt ashamed of her heritage. At the age of sixteen, she left the reservation with an older man. Soon she was alone and drug-addicted, with no way to support herself.

The effects of sociohistorical and continued injustice upon Indigenous people had been experienced and passed forward in Barbara's family and community for many generations. Barbara had grown up unaware of the strength of women and spiritual resources within her Anishinabeg roots and with limited awareness of what her ancestors suffered. Naming the injustice was very important. This freed Barbara and her mother to embrace their Anishinabe identity, overcome internalized shame, and develop new life patterns that honor their shared history. For the colonized, refugees, immigrants, and other marginalized people, being viewed as "thou" rather than dehumanized as "it" is a necessary relational resource to facilitate in therapy and in larger communities (Glebova et al., 2025).

Environmental Justice

The balance of justice extends beyond the family to communities, nations, and social systems (Boszormenyi-Nagy, 1987). Nagy argued that family therapists have an ethical responsibility to contribute to the survival of the planet; that this is "therapy's ultimate mandate for humanity" (p. 321). Many people today are disconnected from the earth and unaware of their ethical relationships to it (Hernandez-Wolfe, 2019; Laszloffy, 2019). Dialogue about environmental issues can help families and communities consider their ethical relationships to the planet, each other, and future generations (Fraenkel & Cho, 2020; Nesmith et al., 2021).

Mental health is highly correlated to where we live and our access, not only to services but to a safe and life-sustaining environment (Hudson, 2012; Magistro, 2014). What is the quality of the air our clients breathe? Do they have access to greenspace? How crowded are their living conditions? Many families have limited choices about where they live, the number of hours they work, or the availability of safe and affordable green places (McDowell, 2015). Engagement in collective action can help transform the balance of fairness. For example, when Sarah Delgado (as described in Esmiol et al., 2012) encouraged a group of houseless immigrant Latina women to reflect on how environmental factors impacted their relational functioning, they began to share their needs [entitlement] and develop their own form of activism. Rather than turn injustice inward in the form of depression and hopelessness, they "grieved…their 'invisible' status here in America" (Esmiol et al., 2012, p. 583) and developed strategies for hope and survival based on trustworthy relationships with each other.

↞→

The contributions that people from parts of the world with fewer economic resources make to the lives of those in more affluent parts of the world is often overlooked.

↞→

Justice across Cultures and Contexts

Many people leave their families and homelands to provide services such as child care and farm labor that promote the well-being of other people's families. Relational justice requires crediting these contributions and accountability to those who make them. For example, Rena's (a heterosexual coparent living in an upper-class neighborhood) therapy focused on her depression and the effects of trauma in her life. When the therapist inquired about how she attended to her middle-school-aged daughters when she was feeling low and self-focused, Rena said that Josephina, her housekeeper from the Philippines, was "around." The therapist wondered how Josephina's contributions to the family were recognized. He asked Rena about the relationship with Josephina, her circumstances, and their agreement about her services. As a result, Rena acknowledged Josephina and developed a more equitable contract that included compensation for child care. This was important because Josephina had been doing extra hours and shopping to make sure Rena's daughters were cared for. Her uncompensated work perpetuated societal and relational injustices. And, like many who care for children of the affluent, she had to leave her own two young children in the care of a neighbor.

Power

Societal power inequities affect whose needs and interests are noticed and attended to. This occurs in the larger society and in interpersonal communication processes. Preemptive silencing happens when people are never asked about what they think and their interests are not included in discussions (Medina, 2013). Decisions are made to develop a neighborhood, but residents themselves are not included in the discussion. Similarly, a family debates whether to go to the beach (which the children want) or hiking in the mountains (which the father wants). No one asks what the mother wants. In another family or community the experience of a gay or gender non-conforming child may be overlooked, misinterpreted, or made hypervisible (Gangamma & Le, 2026).

Recognizing Power Imbalances

Sometimes people participate in communication exchanges, but their credibility and perspectives are minimized. This would happen if in the family above the mother says she has a lot of things to do and, whatever they do, wants to get an earlier start, but her concern is overlooked by the father and dropped from the conversation. Latent power (Komter, 1989) happens when participants automatically focus on the needs of the dominant person, primarily because societal norms and expectations limit the options. For example, the owner of a home has a right to sell it. Unless regulations protect renters, they have no legitimated voice. Or, a family moves for the husband's job without fully considering the impact on the wife and children. They may relate to children and their activities with heteropatriarchal assumptions, making it difficult for other experiences to be recognized or heard (Gangamma & Le, 2026).

↔

In order to facilitate relational justice, therapists need to assess the power context of communication patterns.

↔

There are differences in how people see fairness, depending on their power location. Those in higher power positions tend not to notice that others attune to them and accommodate their needs. Worldwide, women are likely to feel more gratitude for the contributions of male partners than men do for women's contributions (Coltrane, 1996; Matta & Knudson-Martin, 2006). Promoting relational ethics requires that therapists' observations and questions make these subtle power dynamics and their relational effects visible. For example, Kirstee Williams (2011) described her work with a female couple in which one, Michelle, had an affair. Michelle's partner, Nicole was older, made substantially more money, and judged Michelle's "emotional" communication style as "immature" (Williams, 2011, p. 524). Michelle's affair was an indirect response to the power imbalance. "Naming the power difference enabled them to come face to face with the ways their differing societal power positions interfered with attaining their egalitarian ideals" (p. 524).

Therapist Power

Multidirected partiality does not mean neutrality (Dankoski & Deacon, 2000; Glebova et al., 2025). Contextual therapists care equally about all participants, but are prepared to use their power to temporarily "side with one person" in order to help create more balanced relationships (Goldenthal, 1996, p. 11).

↔

From a socioculturally attuned perspective, therapists need to be accountable for which values they promote and how their actions affect relational justice.

↔

Third Order Change

Like other family therapy models, contextual therapy draws on systemic understandings and interventions that include second order change in transactional patterns, e.g., change in the rules by which the relationship operates. Contextual therapy places this work within a larger ethical context—how individuals are responsive and accountable to relational connections beyond themselves (Boszormenyi-Nagy & Krasner, 1986).

↔

Socioculturally attuned contextual therapy seeks third order change in which family members see themselves not only as connected and ethically responsible to each other, but also see their relationships and loyalties in context of their societal position and are accountable to the wider community.

↔

A third-order shift in consciousness provides family members perspective on their social situations and ethical responsibilities and increases their ability to make intentional choices about how their actions contribute to posterity and the systemic balance of fairness. For Barbara, this meant she saw her own life in the larger scheme of history and actively engaged with her mother, Karl, and their community in ways that help restore gender and cultural justice. They were able to intentionally promote the kind of future they want for Cora and society by balancing care and fairness within their own relationship, in parenting, and in their relationships with the wider society.

Therapists are also accountable for the impact of their interventions and the values they reinforce (Melito, 2003). They are answerable for how their clinical actions help undo societal inequities or reinforce them. In Text Box 10.1 Stephanie Brooks describes her contextual approach to third order change.

Text Box 10.1 Stephanie Brooks, PhD, LCSW, LMFT

Stephanie Brooks is the inaugural Dean of the College of Health at Cleveland State University. She describes herself as an African American cisgender woman, parent of two daughters, and educationally privileged with a productive career in academia and private practice. Her interests include MFT education and training, supervision, ADHD in Black couples, trauma, depression and addiction, and leadership. Nagy's contextual therapy provides an overall ethical framework for her socioculturally attuned integrated approach to practice.

I center how the dominant culture informs clients' experiences/relationships, presenting problems, and coping. This approach allows me to explore how power, privilege and oppressive systems reinforce and shape interactions and understand how our (therapists and clients) identities and experiences will influence the therapeutic journey with the larger goal of inviting options and possibilities for change.

I was privileged to be trained in the mid 80s in the Intersystem Approach developed by Gerald Weeks. This approach then and now enabled me to honor the client's entire self by assessing across individual, interactional, and intergenerational parts embedded in layers of larger systems and to construct appropriate interventions that consider and fit the client's worldview. This meta framework explores the inner dialectics (individual, biological, psychological) and outer dialectics (systems—sociological/cultural/historical). Therefore, I intentionally weave in and out of modern, postmodern and social construction family therapy constructs with a critical eye on freedom and liberation. As a therapist, I engage in self-interrogation and inquiry (self of the therapist) while keeping an eye on what Nagy referred to as the "between" —what happens in the between therapist–client relationship.

I try to attune to the client's sociocultural experience by noting what is said, seen, and known and by being curious about what is not said, unseen (hidden), and unknown. I believe systems of power, oppression, and submission are always present, and as a therapist I need to understand how they translate to the client experience as well as serve as a disrupter. I identify and name these issues through maintaining a curious stance and questioning. I use focused genograms, ecomaps, and storytelling as tools for amplifying what has been silenced and marginalized.

Creating space for clients' agency and value is important. I use Hardy's Validation, Challenge, and Request (VCR) intervention to interrupt unjust relationships and systems. I also use my own power and role to facilitate structural and systemic change. One method is to engage clients to be curious and question how they became who they are, which includes exploring family origin dynamics, geographical, economic, gender scripts etc. This exploration and questioning creates openings to connect the influence on the presenting problem and typically highlights their perspective and limitations for change. It also opens conversations about how they respond to power/powerlessness, who defines power, how they are expected and want to be treated in relationships. My work encourages transformative, third order change by elevating clients' voices and experiences and naming what is considered taboo, which facilitates valuing their own experience and creates space to imagine what their change would look like if they were seen and heard.

Practice Guidelines

Socioculturally attuned contextual therapy expands the relational ethics lens to include the sociopolitical context of intergenerational family processes. Goals go beyond symptom relief or behavioral change to love and trust grounded in a balance of fairness. As noted earlier, therapists are not neutral; they actively position their interventions to catalyze justice. They are likely to engage as many family members as possible, including extended family and family of choice. The seven guidelines below are interconnected and inform clinical decisions and therapist actions throughout the course of therapy; 1) practice multidirected sociocultural attunement, 2) discuss socio-historical context/background, 3) identify and acknowledge unfairness, 4) assume people want to give, 5) encourage due crediting, 6) encourage accountability, and 7) focus forward.

1. Practice Multidirected Sociocultural Attunement

As therapists seek to understand and **attune** to each person's sociocultural experience and empathize with it, clients feel felt (Pandit et al., 2014; Sibley et al., 2015). This sets the stage for family members to also experience empathy for one another, to acknowledge the hurts and injustices each has experienced, and to begin envisioning potential pathways to healing (Sibley et al., 2015; van der Meiden et al., 2020). Identifying the societal contexts that give rise to expectations and feelings helps reduce blame and opens family members to each other's experiences, even for those who are not in the room and/or have deceased. They become more willing to be accountable for the effect of their actions on others.

2. Discuss Socio-historical Context/Background

Socioculturally attuned contextual family therapy focuses on justice as the bridge between the past and the future (e.g., Hargrave & Pfitzer, 2003; van der Meiden et al., 2020). Therapists help clients explore and **name** the sociopolitical context of their family legacies. They want to know about the effect of historical events such as war, immigration, and economic conditions, as well as the family's ethnic background and position relative to others in the community. How was the family treated and regarded by others? What messages did prior generations receive about their value and worth? How might these have been related to social identities such as gender, sexuality, religion, race, ethnicity, or ability? As therapists and clients collaboratively create a sense of these sociocultural contexts, it becomes possible to develop empathy and/or understanding of parents and prior generations. People begin to see themselves as a transformative link in the evolving family and sociocultural history.

3. Identify and Acknowledge Unfairness

Socioculturally attuned contextual therapists assess the balance of fairness within relationships and social experience. Through observation and questioning, they track the giving and receiving of care across generations and within intimate relationships. When people have suffered injustice in their families and/or as part of societal processes of power, privilege, and oppression, having the unfairness recognized, **valued,** and witnessed is empowering (Glebova et al., 2025; Weingarten, 2003). **Naming** the ethical violation is an important aspect of healing (Gangamma & Le, 2026). Socioculturally attuned contextual therapists look for and explore experiences of relational and societal-level violence to the self and to one's group. We use violence broadly here to refer to direct physical attack and witnessing death, etc. to the insidious effects of continued disparagement, invisibility, or limited access to economic and other valued resources.

4. Assume People Want to Give

Societal discourses around autonomy and competitiveness can mask or pathologize people's desire to give to and support others. People who have been hurt by injustice and are owed care sometimes find it difficult to give to others, and people in power positions may not notice what others need. Contextual therapists know that at our core, people want and need to give to others and **intervene** accordingly. They approach each family member with these expectations and, without minimizing hurts they may have caused, also ask about ways that each has been, or would like to be, helpful. Conversely, it is a great gift to know how to receive, and not just give. By graciously receiving a gift, we are giving a gift in return. Identified patients/persons, e.g., those who have been defined as the problem, are invited to give as well as take. If the therapist is attuned to this process between give and take, as Nagy and Krasner (1986) suggested, then clients will be able to recognize relational goals and name interest in another's well-being. These shifts focus away from pathology toward resources each can provide others. Importantly, the giving of care is validated and honored rather than overlooked or framed as a problem. This shift toward a relational perspective actively counters models of human nature based primarily on self-interest.

5. Encourage Due Crediting

Once naming and validation of harm and injustice have been clearly acknowledged, therapists encourage due crediting; e.g., giving the other credit for positive contributions to one's life and to the relationship. This must never seem to positively connote abusive or harmful behavior, but it does involve seeking to find genuine contributions (Goldenthal, 1996, p. 68). For example, Ruben had a history of relationships that ended because he was not able to make a long-term commitment such as marriage. He, his current partner, and their therapist all agreed that his ongoing experience since childhood of needing to care for and protect his mother due to the effects of living with bipolar disorder made it hard to commit to taking emotional risks. The therapist credited his entitlement to care from his mother, especially as a child:

Therapist: (after Ruben described his childhood anxiety about his mother's needs) You were just a child. You needed her to be there for you. All children do.

Ruben: I know. It's not her fault. She did her best.

Therapist: She did her best, but she wasn't able to mother you the way I imagine she wanted to, the way you had a right to be parented.

Ruben: She tells me she's sorry. But it's still a one-way street you know. It's still about what she needs from me.

After more dialogue that explored and validated Ruben's right as a child to have an adult he could count on to look after his needs and that recognized the abandonment from his father, the therapist moved the conversation to ways his mother had given to him:

Therapist: We know your mother wasn't able to parent you the way she would have wanted to… I'm curious, though; I'm guessing there are also things she *has* given to you. Do you have any ideas about what those might be?
Ruben: She loved me! I always knew that! I still know that. She tells me all the time.
Partner: You're so loving. That's what I love about you. You got that from your mother. I see that.

Both aspects of due crediting are key to rebalancing Ruben's relationships going forward: crediting what he deserved or was entitled to that he didn't receive, but also acknowledging what he *did* get. Since mothers tend not to be credited and are frequently blamed for their children's problems (i.e., mother-blaming), helping Ruben acknowledge and credit what his mother did give him was an important social justice intervention.

6. Encourage Accountability

Contextual family therapists raise issues of responsibility and accountability regarding the consequences of what clients say and do on others. For example,

Therapist: It makes sense that you would hold yourself back a bit from commitment. How do you think your holding back affects [partner]?
Ruben: She doesn't like it. But I tell her I just need time.
Therapist: (persists with effect on partner). What do you think it is like for her?

Socioculturally attuned therapists are also attentive to how relational accountability intersects with societal power dynamics. Ruben's sense of destructive entitlement from his family of origin combined with societal gender entitlement (Wells, et al., 2017). The therapist helped him explore the gendered nature of injustice in his relationship:

Therapist: A lot of men I work with have a hard time staying present when their partners are upset. They have a hard time really wanting to hear her. Is that something you're aware of?
Ruben: ummmm. Yeah!
Therapist: What do you think society teaches men that gets in the way of being there for a partner?

7. Focus Forward

As clients develop a fuller understanding of the sociopolitical and interpersonal contexts of their parents and communities, they are freed from invisible loyalty to the past and past injustices. Socioculturally attuned contextual therapists help people be intentional about how they want to interrupt the impact of family and societal injustice, what they **envision** going forward for themselves, their children, and posterity. This opens space for **transformation.**

Case Illustration

Let's return to Rena, the mother with the housekeeper from the Philippines. About a year prior, Rena (45), a cishet (cisgender heterosexual) woman of Jewish descent, moved to the Midwest from the East coast when her husband Gideon (age 53) was relocated by the airline for which he was a pilot. Daughters Anah (age 12) and Ellen (age 11) went to a small private school. Rena sought therapy with Peter, stating that she battled depression due to a trauma history and that before the move she had seen a therapist twice a week for seven years. She had tried several other therapists in the new community but was not satisfied with any of them. Peter, a 55-year-old European American who earned his LMFT after an earlier career in pharmaceutical sales, was the single parent of three teenagers following his wife's death two years earlier.

Peter approached Rena's case with the conviction that she would be better able to manage depression and the effects of trauma if therapy focused on these as part of a larger set of ethical relationships. He was aware that his wife's death and his earlier career change highlighted for him the importance of being accountable to one's relationships and deepened his commitment to, and hope for future generations. Though Peter was careful to distinguish his personal history from Rena's, as a socioculturally attuned contextual family therapist, he actively directed his clinical actions to advance relational and societal justice.

Multidirected Sociocultural Attunement

Although Peter typically invited all involved family members to attend the first session, in this case, he first met individually with Rena because she was so clear that she was looking for a therapist that would support her. He wanted to begin to know her and demonstrate multidirected partiality toward the well-being, interests, and perspectives of other family members as well. His questions focused on what family members needed from each other and what they were able to give. He also clarified what Rena needed from him and what each was willing to give to the therapeutic process. Peter began by letting Rena know that what she suffered was wrong, that she was entitled to better:

Peter: (after Rena described an overview of the history that brought her to therapy) You have endured so much! People have hurt you and treated you unjustly. A teacher who was supposed to support your dignity and growth sexually harassed you. Young men you thought were friends brutally assaulted you, and your first husband raped and assaulted you too. And no one seemed to care or notice. No one should be treated like you have been! You were entitled to teachers and friends who supported you and a husband that cherished you. You had a right to expect others—your parents, your friends, the school—to stand up for you. And you didn't receive that.

Rena: (softly). No one has ever said that to me before.

Peter: You have suffered unfairly. I work from the idea that everyone needs loving and supportive relationships—in their families and also in their schools and communities. I see many people who live with the effects of the trauma and injustice they suffered. I see them turn the impact of these legacies around to create a better future for themselves and those they love and to make the world a better place. Does this fit with what you're looking for?

Rena: Absolutely! You seem to understand how hard it is. I think I could work with you.

In this statement, Rena conveyed that the therapist offered her what she felt she was owed: understanding and safety. Peter then introduced the idea that Rena also owes others, especially her children.

Peter: I would like to work with you. I'm wondering also how your girls are doing? How will the work we are doing here affect them?

Rena: They're doing OK. The move has been hard for them. Their new school is kind of hard to break into. You know how kids are.

Peter: I imagine that you want to be there for them, make their transition easier. What do you think they need from you?

With this line of questioning, Peter established from the very beginning that he sees Rena's therapy connected to the give and take between her and others, to what she is entitled to as well as what she owes others. He also laid the foundation for exploring inequity in her marriage and extended family relationships:

Peter: How about your relationship with Gideon? How does he attend to what you need?
Rena: (tears) Gideon is gone so much. And he's under a lot of stress. Pilots in their 50s have to prove they're healthy enough to fly. When he gets home, he needs to relax.
Peter: It sounds like you try to be aware of Gideon's stress and what he needs. Is he aware of yours?
Rena: I don't know. Maybe sometimes. I try to be careful not to upset him.

Peter also learned that Rena had limited connections with her parents, her two brothers, and their families. She perceived that they did not care about her, except in the most perfunctory of ways, such as attending family events and observations. Peter's response also showed multidirected partiality to them and to the family's ethical commitments to each other:

Peter: What do you think your family is missing out on by not knowing you better?
Rena: They don't know me at all really. They never did!
Peter: I imagine there is a lot of you that you wish they could know. I wonder what has gotten in the way?
Rena: (shrugs). Who knows? They always seemed more concerned about what others would think than about me.
Peter: That must have been very hard, especially for a child… As an adult now, do you have any idea what would have made them so concerned about making a good impression on others?

Discuss Socio-historical Context/Background

In the next session, Peter began a discussion of the socio-historical context of Rena's relational experience and the traumas she suffered.

Peter: What was it like for you growing up in [East coast city]?
Rena: I was always kind of lonely. Kids teased me about my curly hair. I tried to stay in the background.
Peter: You said on the intake that you are ethnically Jewish. Were there other Jewish kids? Do you think they teased you because you were Jewish?
Rena: There were only a couple of other Jewish kids in my school. I know there were other neighborhoods with lots of Jewish people, but not where I lived. I was embarrassed that I looked different and we didn't celebrate Christmas like the other kids.
Peter: How was your family connected to the Jewish community?

As this line of conversation continued, Peter learned that Rena had always felt isolated. Though her working-class family had lived in the same house all her life and were considered "respectable" by the neighbors, they seldom engaged socially with them. Her family did not practice Judaism or participate in the large Jewish Center in a nearby community. Peter also asked about gender:

Peter: What messages about being a girl did you receive from your family and school?
Rena: That I was supposed to be pretty…but I wasn't. I had a funny nose and unruly hair. I was skinny. Most people in my school didn't have expensive clothes, but the girls dressed cute, you know? I was always plain. My parents didn't allow short skirts or makeup.

Peter began to see that Rena found herself alone and in a one-down position at school. He explored more about this experience and asked where she found support:

Rena: I had a friend, Erin. She didn't have friends either. Nobody liked her. My parents didn't like her; they didn't like her values and Erin's mom didn't care where she went.
Peter: What did you value about your relationship with Erin?
Rena: I could just be me. She listened to me…sometimes. She made me laugh.

Peter asked about the sexual harassment from a teacher, placing this in context of her social location:

Peter: Being with Erin must have been a relief. You didn't have to be on guard. She accepted you. I can see why Erin was important to you. School was a pretty unsafe place for you. You were teased. You felt like an outsider and didn't fit what it seemed girls were supposed to be like.
Rena: (tears). If it wasn't for my friend Erin, I don't know what I would have done.
Peter: You said a teacher sexually harassed you. What happened?

Rena had been surprised when the male music teacher asked if she would like to help him with the music and instruments. She had never been singled out in a way that felt special before. When he started making comments about her body and sexual innuendos, she didn't know what to do. Erin told her it was nothing to be worried about; it was what men did. Rena felt uncomfortable but did not dare stop working for him. Her parents had seemed so pleased that she had been selected for this honor; she never told them how hard it was being with him. Several years later, when assaulted by multiple teenage boys at a party, she didn't tell anyone, not even Erin.

Peter also began to explore what Rena knew about her parents' history. She knew both came from families that immigrated to the United States from Poland shortly before World War II, when it became apparent that it was increasingly dangerous for Jewish people. Since her family seldom talked about the past, she did not know much about their experience growing up at this time in history, only that both families scraped by with very limited economic resources and were grateful to be alive. Peter wondered aloud what it must have been like for them and how their experiences may continue to affect them:

Peter: I wonder what it was like to grow up in families who left everything they knew and loved? I wonder how people treated your grandparents when they got here and what it was like to raise young children in a place where they were considered foreigners? This must have affected your mother and father and how they parented you.
Rena: I don't know. I never really thought about it (reflective pause) maybe that's why my parents were always so worried about what other people thought, why my dad just seemed to keep his head down and keep going.
Peter: You're probably right. I think it might be helpful to know more about this history.

Identify and Acknowledge Unfairness

Rena entered relationships from a position of destructive entitlement. In other words, she brought a ledger of unfairness from the past with her. The trauma and injustice she experienced as a result of bullying, harassment, and rape were not separate from, and were intensified by her marginalized female, economic, and Jewish identities. Her family had responded to the historical trauma of the Jewish Holocaust by keeping quiet and trying not to call attention to themselves in their new homeland. Stripped of their economic wealth, living in a neighborhood with few Jewish people, and not knowing what to expect, they avoided close affiliation with their neighbors and kept their Jewish identities quiet. As Rena learned more about her personal and family histories and shared it with Peter, he took care to name the injustice:

Peter: The injustice done to your family can never be repaid. Your grandparents ran for their lives and for the lives of their children. They faced threats of death, discrimination, and poverty—not of their making.

Peter helped Rena recognize how these past injustices contributed to inequity in her relationships with men, including messages she received about her worth:

Peter: All those ideas about how girls are "supposed" to look, how do you think they have disadvantaged you or put you at risk?
Rena: They made me think I was ugly, that I wasn't worth much. So I didn't expect much.
Peter: Do you think this is still true with Gideon? That you don't expect much?

Peter suggested Gideon join some of their sessions. This enabled both Rena and Gideon to recognize and name the inequity in their marriage, an inequity perpetuated by differences in social class and economic and resources, as well as gender. The disparity was present from the beginning of their relationship:

Gideon: I was attracted to Rena because she seemed so pretty and so vulnerable. Just being with her made me feel good!
Peter: How did she make you feel good?
Gideon: She was there for me. She liked to be with me and do the things I like to do. She was a great listener! She still is.

Rena said that she was attracted to Gideon because he was stable; he knew what he liked and was "mature." She said she was surprised he would be interested in her. He came from a higher SES family, had economic security, and (in her mind) could have his pick of women. Recognizing a likely disparity, Peter began to explore their balance of give and take:

Peter: Gideon, you said you were attracted to Rena because she was a good listener and liked to do things with you. How does this work in your relationship now? Are you a good listener for her?
Gideon: (pauses). hmm. I'm tired when I get home. She usually asks me what I'd like, how my trip went.
Rena: I try to focus on him. He deserves it. It would be nice if he listened to me, but my life isn't very interesting.

After more fully exploring this imbalance and Rena's need and right for care and attention, Peter named the inequity and asked Gideon if he'd be interested in knowing more about Rena's life.

Peter: Gideon, you really appreciate the care and attention Rena gives you. It seems like a pattern has developed where she focuses on you. When you come home, she stops what she was doing and tries to be there for you. She doesn't have the sense that you're also interested in her. You've gotten used to her tending to you. Is this a pattern that you'd be interested in changing, that you could be there for her as well?

Gideon: Of course. I love Rena. She just never seems to have anything to say.
Peter: I think Rena has a long history of learning that people, especially men, aren't very interested in what she has to say. How do you think you could make it safer for her, how could you show her that you're interested?

Note that in this example, accountability for change was directed first toward Gideon, since he was the beneficiary of the imbalance. Giving care would also be beneficial to him.

Assume People Want to Give

Peter began with the assumption that Gideon cared about his wife and would want to help create a fairer balance of give and take. Rather than primarily seeing Rena individually, Peter encouraged couple sessions. This act of commitment to Rena and their marriage on Gideon's part was an important step in rebalancing the ethical ledger. In the past, frequent individual therapy sessions helped to fill the void in her life, but could not correct the imbalance of relational fairness that sustained Rena's depressive symptoms. Both partners began to look forward to the couple sessions, in large part because Peter recognized and highlighted their love and concern for the other, even when the going was tough. For example, one day the couple came in very distressed. Gideon was visibly angry; Rena was pale and silent. She seemed almost invisible in the room and surely her past injustices had been triggered. Peter joined with Gideon around his desire to be there for Rena:

Peter: (to Gideon). I don't know if I've ever seen Rena look so scared. I know you're angry. I can see that. I also know how much you love Rena, that you don't want to hurt her, that you want to be there for her… What do you think happened that made her so scared right now?

Acknowledging Gideon's relational resources helped him feel calm and engage in the process of working through the situation. It helped reassure Rena that she had not lost his love.

Peter also assumed that Rena and Gideon loved their daughters and wanted to provide a safe and loving environment for them. He regularly asked about their well-being and included their concerns in their sessions. He also suggested several family sessions and one with Rena and the girls. These sessions included the premise that the girls had something to give:

Peter: (to Anah and Ellen) We've been talking a lot about what you need from your parents. That's important. And I'm guessing you also want to give to them. What do you think you have to give that might make it easier for your mother?

When asked, the girls showed considerable insight into their mother and seemed energized to think that they could help her:

Ellen: Mom really loves flowers! I could pick them from the garden and bring them to her. That would make her feel cared about.
Anah: I think mothers don't get cared about very often. Mom feels better when I tell her about my day and I ask her about hers. But I forget to do that. I should do that more often.

Peter also assumed that Rena's parents, who were in the late 70s, also wanted to give and that Rena would want to give to them.

Encourage Due Crediting

Rena had spent most of her life focusing on what she had missed. Crediting her parents for what they had already given to her was an important part of her healing. Rena was grateful that both her parents were still alive and that she could tell them in person. She experienced an important internal shift when she understood that her parents had always cared deeply about her and tried to protect her in the ways they knew. She looked forward to visiting them and her brothers and called them more frequently. Rena acknowledged the courage and sound judgment her grandparents demonstrated in leaving Europe before it was too late and how their immigrant experience was an act of love. She was surprised by how willing her parents were to talk to her about their lives when she asked.

Encourage Accountability

In addition to providing support and validation for what Rena was owed, Peter encouraged her accountability and responsibility to others from the very first session. He helped Rena develop strategies to stay engaged with her daughters, even on down days. Rena discovered that this outward focus often helped her feel better. She learned to be accountable for what she expected from Gideon, her children, and her parents. As Rena became clearer that she was entitled to receive love and care, that she was worthy, Peter also encouraged her to be intentional in how she wanted to relate to others and what she wanted to contribute, not only to her own family, but to the future.

Focus Forward

Understanding the effect of past injustices in her life and rebalancing the give and take in her marriage and with her children helped Rena move from hopelessness to optimism for the future. She made conscious choices about how to respond to her Jewish legacy and the isolation her family experienced as a result of the Holocaust and immigration. She became involved in Bend the Arc, which is a Jewish Partnership for Justice, where she learned how to advocate for the values she cared about. She also joined a knitting group at the Jewish Community Center that provided friendship and conversation in her new community and she volunteered for a committee at her daughters' school. She and Gideon took advantage of the many beautiful parks in their area, hiking as often as they could. Though still on antidepressant medication, Rena was working with her physician to lower the dosage with the expectation that she may not need to continue them over the long term.

Summary: Third Order Change

Rena's case illustrates how contextual therapy can catalyze third order change that transforms historical injustice and indebtedness to create an ethical balance in current and future relationships. The therapist positioned his work to be accountable to values of fairness and responsibility to others, actively engaging with clients in ways that moved away from dominant culture ideals of self-interest, to our responsibilities toward others. This intentional shift on the part of the therapist was the result of third order thinking in how he viewed his professional role and responsibilities, with a focus on how the effects of his work ultimately affect the next generation and which societal values are transmitted. He recognized choices in how systems operate and that his actions were not neutral. This reflective stance served as an overarching lens through which Rena and her family could see themselves as a transformative link between the past and the future.

The therapy moved from a focus on individual pathology to the underlying relational and societal injustice and uncovered family members' desire to give. As they began to see their connections to social structures and sociohistorical events, they recognized how these had limited their responses to each other in ways that perpetuated isolation, loss, and trauma. Naming the injustice and unfairness while also crediting what family members had given each other enabled "exoneration," or starting fresh, so that they could envision an ethical balance of fairness and transform their ways of relating to each other and the wider community based on awareness of systemic choices. They moved from isolation to love, connectedness, and social action.

Reflexive Questions

- How would you describe the sociopolitical context of your family legacies?
- How would you describe the ways in which the giving and receiving of care across generations are culturally informed and reinforced?
- Did you experience destructive entitlement due to needs and care not being given to you in childhood? If so, how does that affect your familial relationships and work with others professionally?
- Do you need to be freed from an invisible loyalty from the past and past injustices? If so, can you name it and envision a more just and equitable future for yourself?
- "If reciprocity of commitment and earned entitlement are so fundamental to a viable and balanced life context, why has the ethical dimension in family life basically remained unaddressed?" (Boszormenyi-Nagy & Krasner, 1986, p. 211)

References

Boszormenyi-Nagy, I. (1987). *Foundation of contextual therapy: Collected papers of Ivan Boszormenyi-Nagy, M.D.* Brunner/Mazel.

Boszormenyi-Nagy, I., & Krasner, B. R. (1986). *Between give and take: A clinical guide to contextual therapy*. Brunner/Mazel.

Boszormenyi-Nagy, I. & Spark, G. M. (1973). *Invisible loyalties: Reciprocity in intergenerational family therapy*. Harper & Row (reprinted by Brunner/Mazel, 1984).

Brave Heart, M. Y. H. & DeBruyn, L. M. (1998). The American Indian holocaust: Healing historical unresolved grief. *American Indian and Alaska Native Mental Health Research*, *8*(2), 56.

Brown, L. S. (2008). *Cultural competence in trauma therapy: Beyond the flashback*. American Psychological Association.

Brownlie, R. J. (2008). "Living the same as the White people": Mohawk and Anishinabe women's labour in southern Ontario, 1920–1940. *Labour/Le Travail*, 41–68.

Buber, M. (1958). *I and thou* (R. G. Smith, Trans). Charles Scribner's Sons.

Coltrane, S. (1996). *The family man: Fatherhood, housework, and gender equity*. Oxford University Press.

Daneshpour, M. (2025). Couples therapy and the challenges of building trust, fairness, and justice. *Family Process*, *64*, p.e13072.

Dankoski, M. E. & Deacon, S. A., (2000). Using a feminist lens in contextual therapy. *Family Process*, *39*, 51–66.

Ducommun-Nagy, C. (2025). The essence of contextual therapy, its place in the field of family therapy, and its role in the future. *Family Process*, *64*, p.e13070.

Esmiol, E., Knudson-Martin, C., & Delgado, S. (2012). How MFT students develop a critical contextual consciousness: A participatory action research project *Journal of Marital and Family Therapy*, *38*, 573–588.

Fishbane, M. D. (2023). Couple relational ethics: From theory to lived practice. *Family process*, *62*(2), 446–468.

Fishbane, M. D. (2005). Differentiation and dialogue in intergenerational relationships. In J. Lebow (Ed.). *Handbook of clinical family therapy* (pp. 543–568). Wiley & Sons.
Fishbane, M. D. (1998). I, thou, and we: A dialogical approach to couples therapy. *Journal of Marital and Family Therapy*, *24*, 41–58.
Fraenkel, P. & Cho, W. (2020). Reaching up, down, in, and around: Couple and family coping during the coronavirus pandemic. *Family Process*, *59*, 825–831.
Gangamma, R., Bartle-Haring, S., Holowacz, E., Hartwell, E. E., & Glebova, T. (2015). Relational ethics, depressive symptoms, and relationship satisfaction in couples. *Journal of Marital and Family Therapy*, 41, 354–366.
Gangamma, R. & Le, A. (2026). Queer contextualized contextual family therapy. In E. E. Hartwell & L. L. Edwards (Eds.) *Queer-contextualized family therapy: Toward radically inclusive theory and practice*. (pp. 141–159). Routledge.
Goldenthal, P. (1996). *An integrated model for working with individuals, couples, and families*. Norton.
Glebova, T., Lal, A., & Gangamma, R. (2025). Relational ethics in immigrant families: The contextual therapy five-dimensional framework. *Family Process*, 64, p.e13071.
Hargrave, T. D. & Pfitzer, F. (2003). *The new contextual therapy: Guiding the power of give and take*. Brunner-Routledge.
Hernandez-Wolfe, P. (2019). Eco-informed couple and family therapy: Systems thinking and social justice. In T. A. Laszloffy & M. L. C. Twist (Eds.). *Eco-informed practice: Family therapy in an age of ecological peril* (pp. 33–44). AFTA SpringerBriefs in Family Therapy, Springer.
Hudson, C. G. (2012). Disparities in the geography of mental health: Implications for social work. *Social Work*, 57(2), 107–119.
Knudson-Martin, C. & Huenergardt, D. (2010). A socio-emotional approach to couple therapy: Linking social context and couple interaction. *Family Process*, *49*, 369–386.
Komter, A. (1989). Hidden power in marriage. *Gender and Society*, *3*, 187–216.
Laszloffy, T. A. (2019). What is an eco-informed approach to family therapy? In T. A. Laszloffy & M. L. C. Twist (Eds.). *Eco-informed practice: Family therapy in an age of ecological peril* (pp. 7–19). AFTA SpringerBriefs in Family Therapy, Springer.
Magistro, C. A. (2014). Relational dimensions of environmental crisis: Insights from Boszormenyi-Nagy's contextual therapy. *Journal of Systemic Therapy*, *33*(3), 17–28.
Matta, D. & Knudson-Martin, C. (2006). Couple processes in the co-construction of fatherhood. *Family Process*, *45*, 19–37.
McDowell, T. (2015). *Applying critical theories to family therapy practice*. AFTA Springerbriefs in Family Therapy, Springer.
Medina, J. (2013). *The epistemology of resistance: Gender and racial oppression, epistemic injustice, and resistant imaginations*. Oxford University Press.
Melito, R. (2003). Values in the role of the family therapist: Self determination and justice. *Journal of Marital and Family Therapy*, *29*, 3–11.
Nesmith, A. A., Schmitz, C. L., Machado-Escudero, Y., Billiot, S., Forbes, R. A., Powers, M. C., … & Sloan, L. M. (2021). *The intersection of environmental justice, climate change, community, and the ecology of life*. Berlin: Springer.
Pandit, M., Kang, Y. J., ChenFeng J., Knudson-Martin, C., & Huenergardt D. (2014). Practicing socio-cultural attunement: A study of couple therapists. *Journal of Contemporary Family Therapy*, *36*, 518–528.
Roberto, L. G. (1992). *Transgenerational family therapies*. Guilford.
Rootes, K. M. H. (2013), Wanted fathers: Understanding gay father families through contextual family therapy. *Journal of GLBT Family Studies*, *9*, 43–64.
Sibley, D. S., Schmidt, A. E., & Kimmes, J. G. (2015). Applying a contextual therapy framework to treat panic disorder: A case study. *Journal of Family Psychotherapy*, *26*, 299–317.
Siegel, D. J. & Hartzell, M. (2003). *Parenting from the inside-out: How a deeper understanding can help you raise children who thrive*. Penguin Putnam, Inc.
Smoliak, O., Rice, C., LaMarre, A., Tseliou, E., LeCouteur, A., & Davies, A. (2022). Gendering of care and care inequalities in couple therapy. *Family Process*, *61*(4), 1386–1402.
Sude, M. E. & Gambrel, L. E. (2017). A contextual therapy framework for MFT educators: Facilitating trustworthy asymmetrical training relationships. *Journal of Marital and Family Therapy*, *43*, 617–630.
van der Meiden, J., Noordegraaf, M., & van Ewijk, H. (2019). How is contextual therapy applied today? An analysis of the practice of current contextual therapists *Contemporary Family Therapy*, *41*, 12–23.

van der Meiden J., Verduijn, Noordegraff, M., & van Ewijk, H. (2020). Strengthening connectedness in close relationships: A model for applying contextual therapy. *Family Process*, *59*, 346–360.
van Heusden, A. & van den Eerenbeemt, E. (1987). *Balance in motion: Ivan Boszormenyi-Nagy and his vision of individual and family therapy*. Brunner/Mazel.
Weingarten, K. (2003). *Common shock: Witnessing violence every day–How we are harmed and how we can heal*. Dutton/Penguin Books.
Wells, M. A., Lobo, E., Galick, A., Knudson-Martin, C., Huenergardt, D., & Schaepper, J. (2017). Fostering trust through relational safety: Applying SERT's focus on gender and power with adult-survivor couples. *Journal of Couple & Relationship Therapy*, *16*, 122–145.
Williams, K. (2011). A socio-emotional relationship approach to infidelity: The relational justice approach. *Family Process*, *50*, 516–528.

11 Socioculturally Attuned Cognitive Behavioral Family Therapy

Cognitive behavioral therapy refers to a range of problem-focused approaches that address the reciprocal influences between thoughts, feelings, and observable behavior. With roots in behavioral psychology, early models emphasized stimulus–response patterns, goal setting, and behavior modification strategies. The addition of the cognitive component in the 1970s emphasized how people's thoughts or ideas about a situation impacted their responses. In what has been called "the third wave" of behavior-based therapies (Hayes et al., 2006), a variety of new, more contextually focused approaches, such as dialectical behavior therapy and acceptance and commitment therapy, have emerged. Recent applications are also more attentive to emotion in both the evolution of problems and in creating change (Epstein & Falconier, 2024; Fischer et al., 2016).

Though most CBT approaches still tend to focus primarily on individual experience (Craske, 2010; Dattilio et al., 2023), cognitive behavioral family therapy (CBFT) (e.g., Dattilio, 2010; Epstein & Baucom, 2002) and CBT in couples therapy (e.g., Epstein & Baucom, 2002; Epstein & Falconier, 2024) were developed to deal with the more complex, systemic ways couples and family members' underlying belief systems, emotional responses, and behaviors influence each other. Proponents assert that CBFT integrates well with other models and can also take larger societal contexts into account (Epstein & Dattilio, 2020; Parker & McDowell, 2017). For example, Epstein and Falconier (2024) encourage cognitive behavioral therapists to take an active role in identifying the impact of sociocultural contexts in people's lives and promoting equity. Others call on behavioral analysts to use their skills to promote caring beyond self and address injustices at larger systemic levels (Sadavoy & Zube, 2022).

Yet, even as cognitive-behavioral approaches are increasingly used across the globe to address a wide variety of clinical issues and support family members in creative ways through group settings or the use of apps, these new applications seldom help clients see their concerns through a socioculturally attuned lens (e.g., Bäckström et al., 2024; Dover & McGuire, 2023; Golboni et al., 2023; Petrinec et al., 2021).

↞→

In contrast, socioculturally attuned cognitive behavioral couple and family therapists create third order change by attuning to systems of systems that maintain problematic societal patterns and inequities within relationships and shared ways of thinking.

↞→

Primary Enduring Family Therapy Concepts

CBT begins with the premise that troublesome behaviors, emotions, and thoughts are acquired, at least in part, through learning and experience and thus can be changed (Craske, 2010; Epstein & Dattilio, 2020). The goal is to help people identify problematic emotional, behavioral, and cognitive

DOI: 10.4324/9781003493426-11

sequences and replace them with more adaptive ones. When applying this process within a systemic framework, five concepts are particularly foundational: 1) mutual behavioral reinforcement, 2) schemas, 3) cognitive distortion/incongruent thinking, 4) relational patterns of thought, emotion, and behavior, and 5) therapist as coach.

Mutual Behavioral Reinforcement

According to learning theory, the consequences of an individual's behavioral response have an effect on its future occurrence (Craske, 2010). So, if a child cries when a mother leaves and the mother responds by giving the child attention and delaying her leaving, the child may be more likely to cry the next time the mother leaves. Cognitive behavioral family therapists focus on these kinds of observable patterns of interaction and the ways in which family members serve as *both* stimulus and response for each other (Epstein & Dattilio, 2020). Integrating Bandura's (1973) ideas of continual social reinforcement with the systemic notion of circular causality, one person's behavior becomes the prompt for another's. CBF therapists would not only focus on the mother's impact on the child's behavior; they would be interested in how the child's behavior impacts the mother.

CBF therapists are interested in how mutual behavioral reinforcement cycles influence family communication and problem-solving patterns. Historically, they have not usually attended to how interlocking patterns within relationships are connected to larger sociocultural processes. For example, they might not ask how the mother's response is related to sociocultural expectations about mothering or gender inequalities in family life and the workplace. However, a recent guide calls on the field to expand beyond CBCT stereotypes of behavioral contracts and challenging irrational beliefs to address the "complex interplay among cognitions, behaviors, emotions, and contextual factors" and help people address the impact of dominant discourses and oppression in their lives (Epstein & Falconier, 2024, p. *x*). Cultural and larger context considerations are relevant at each domain of CBT (Baucom et al., 2023; Dattilio & Schoenly, 2023).

Schemas

The notion of schemas is central to how cognition is linked to behavior (Beck, 1967; Dattilio, 2001). Schemas are "deeply rooted cognitive structures and beliefs that help define a person's identity in relation to others" (McKay et al., 2012, p. 9). They are experienced as taken-for-granted "truths" about the world and our role in it. Schemas are acquired from repeated messages about the self as we engage in social situations. They organize the huge quantity of information in the environment into meaningful patterns that help us predict the future. Schemas are tied to emotion and thus serve as triggers for behavior. Maladaptive schemas such as the belief that others are unreliable, will harm you, or won't meet your needs, are often connected to early childhood experience (McKay et al., 2012). From a CBFT perspective, attachment working models (see Chapter 8) are an example of a schema (Epstein & Dattilio, 2020).

Schemas such as beliefs that one is inferior, unlovable, different, inadequate, or superior and deserving are examples of how core beliefs about the self affect how one approaches relationships and responds to others. If your internal truth is that you need to put the needs of others over your own, then when someone is upset, you will likely feel guilty. But if your internal truth is that you are entitled to having your needs met, you may respond with anger if someone seems to ignore you. These fundamental orientations to others arise within a person's web of relationships and societal contexts such as gender, culture, race, ethnicity, socioeconomic status, sexual orientation, and other relevant social locations that inform our position relative to others (Parker & McDowell, 2017; Silverstein et al., 2006).

Though schemas are considered relatively stable over time, they evolve as we travel through life, go to school, engage in the workforce, move across cultures, and utilize technology (e.g., video games, television, movies, the internet). For example, children in the same family may have very different schemas based on their experiences at school. One child may develop a sense of herself as competent and the world as supportive and responsive; another may see himself as picked on and view the world as a hostile place where he has to fight for recognition or respect.

Cognitive Distortion/Incongruent Thinking

An important idea in CBFT is that family members perceive and interpret each other based on relatively stable internalized schemas that provide roadmaps for how to respond (Dattilio, 2005). The problem is that schemas can be inflexible and create distortions in thinking and attributions that create distress and conflict. For example, conclusions may be drawn about a family member's behavior without knowing all the facts or circumstances. Information about another may be taken out of context, for example, if a man makes a decision without consulting his female partner, she may believe he does not care about her. The behavior of a family member may be overgeneralized, magnified, or minimized, as in when a woman raises a concern and her female partner responds, "I can never do anything right!" Or "I am worthless." How family members perceive each other affects their interaction. As they interact, they not only create perceptions but also see what they expect to see, filtering out information that does not fit.

For example, Frank's schema suggests that Jenny should be available when he wants her attention. He does not notice Jenny's schedule or what her needs are, and acts upset or disappointed when she is not available. In turn, Jenny starts to see Frank as demanding and self-centered. Given that her schema tells her she must satisfy him and keep the peace, she accommodates him quickly in order to avoid conflict and keeps her resentment to herself. Frank sees their relationship as comfortable and is not aware that she experiences him as selfish.

After interacting together over many years, couples and families develop shared beliefs, or family schemas (Dattilio, 2005), e.g., "we can't upset Dad" or "it's best to keep our thoughts to ourselves." Entrenched ideas about how each member behaves and how a family functions and solves problems are foundational to the way a family operates. Oftentimes, these are helpful, such as when children learn that sharing their feelings is expected and welcomed or when partners expect each other to share their concerns and are responsive to them. Schema can also become rigid, restricting the interpretation of events and limiting choices and flexibility (Dattilio, 2005). CBF therapists focus on how schemas can create distortions and omissions in thinking that affect family communication processes (Baucom et al., 1989).

Relational Patterns of Thought, Emotion, and Behavior

Systemic therapists do not believe it is possible to separate one person's patterns of thought, emotion, and behavior from the relational systems within which they are embedded. They are likely to be interested in breaking down or deconstructing the patterns of beliefs, attributions, and experiences that create and perpetuate destructive relationship patterns. In the case of Frank and Jenny, the CBF therapist would help the couple identify how each person's schema connects to their core beliefs about coupling and family life and how these guide their assumptions about how to behave and what they can expect from the other. Each will have brought their own schemas about relationships from their families of origin, and these will have been impacted by their life experiences (Dattilio, 2001).

For example, even though Frank's mother had a full-time job, she organized her schedule so that she was always home before her husband. Jenny observed more mutuality between her parents and had learned to put relationships first. When Frank did not seem to notice her needs, her schema of self and others was challenged, leaving her hurt and surprised. When Frank got angry, her idea that she should preserve relationships influenced her to respond in ways that would calm him and, in the process, silence her concerns.

When people form adult relationships, they also create a union of their beliefs as they interact and respond to each other. This combination of ideas and life experiences becomes the family of origin schema passed on to their children (Dattilio, 2005). The family schema includes the beliefs, experiences, and perceptions of all the family members and evolves over time as circumstances and experiences change and new family members enter (e.g., birth or marriage) or leave (e.g., death or divorce). Individual cognitions thus reflect shared experience across multiple systemic levels. Jenny and Frank (and their children) are now part of each other's cognitive, behavioral, and emotional systems. They have unwittingly enacted a model of male dominance that is now part of their own and their children's relational schema. Societal level male privilege influenced their relational patterns and meaning-making.

Shared schemas guide how we derive meaning from interpersonal experience and serve as important underlying organizational mechanisms for communication and relational/family interaction. Because societies and cultures are constantly changing, our shared schemas also continuously evolve. Just the other day Carmen overheard a six-year-old say to his brother, "When you grow up, do you want to marry a boy or a girl?" This statement reflected societal-informed schema about himself and others and what he can expect in life that had clearly been passed on to him by the people around him and legal changes in the US that made this option possible.

Therapist as Coach

Cognitive behavioral family therapy is described as collaborative (Craske, 2010; Dattilio, 2010; Dattilio et al., 2023). The image of a coach is a good metaphor for the CBF therapist role. CBF therapists are likely to begin by educating clients about the approach and some of the key concepts, such as automatic thoughts, core beliefs, etc. They engage clients in the process of observing repetitive patterns of thought, behavior, and emotion. For example, they might ask Frank and Jenny to identify and record their automatic thoughts about each other and to note how each thought influenced their responses to each other. The therapist might then engage with them in a functional analysis of their interaction, pinpointing problematic schema formations that are leading to cognitive distortions.

Like a coach, therapists work with clients to identify clear goals with specific objectives for change. They then work to develop homework assignments and/or communication and problem-solving exercises that will help clients attain their goals. The therapist is a facilitator and educator that helps couples and families take new perspectives and try new approaches to familiar situations. Because CBFT focuses on the complex relationships between thoughts, emotions, behaviors, and context, treatment plans are flexible, with therapists sometimes drawing on interventions from other models to help clients reach their targets (Fischer et al., 2016).

One common CBFT intervention is to highlight and challenge thinking errors. Though these thinking errors can differ among family members, cognitive distortions are often shared. Both Jenny and Frank may assume that the burden for regulating emotion in the family falls on Jenny; that it is her job to keep Frank calm. Or perhaps Frank's masculinity-informed schema leads to the idea that if someone loves him, they will always do what he wants and not question him.

Years of shared interaction have confirmed this perception, and he and Jenny may now share aspects of this idea. The therapist may help the couple challenge this belief, consider alternative cognitions that might produce different responses, and help them develop a plan to change this interaction.

The CBFT process requires active participation and motivation for change on each participant's part. CBF therapists keep therapy focused on defined goals, help clients create an agenda for each session, and provide useful information. The therapist may help family members practice good expressive and listening skills, facilitate conversation about their interlocking communication patterns, and/or develop contracts with each other. Because CBF therapists play active educational and structuring roles in the process of therapy, their actions and input to therapy have a major impact on whether or not clients learn to see their problems as manifestations of individual deficits or as connected to sociocultural systems and the associated power processes.

•←→•

Therapists help determine whether or not new relational alternatives generated in therapy replicate and maintain societal inequities or promote equity and justice.

•←→•

Integrating Principles of Sociocultural Attunement

Practicing socioculturally attuned cognitive behavioral family therapy begins by recognizing the subjective and influential nature of the therapist's role, taking stock of one's own conceptual frameworks about reality (Epstein & Falconier, 2024).

> Therapists need to be aware of the values and traditions associated with their social location and background. These influence what therapists notice about clients and what they are unaware of or tend to ignore. This is especially the case when the therapist's social locations and cultural background involve belonging to dominant groups in society. (p. 43)

Therapists must make sense of the vast and often conflicting ideas, experiences, values, and beliefs that inform how we understand and work with individuals, couples, and families, i.e., our schema of schemas (Parker & McDowell, 2017), and acknowledge that these organizing frameworks are not neutral.

•←→•

Socioculturally attuned therapists begin with the view that social schemas are inseparable from personal and family schemas; they organize therapy in ways that attend to power dynamics inherent in creating and maintaining these schemas, including within the therapy process itself.

•←→•

Contextual Nature of Schema

Ideas integral to CBFT, such as the value of having goals or that people can and should take active steps to shape the direction of their lives, tend to be linked to Western social schema prizing individual autonomy and an orientation to the future. If we apply these measures of clinical outcome non-reflexively, we may neglect cultural practices and resources inherent to client solutions (Charlés & Bava, 2020). Learning to recognize how our own social schemas implicitly organize what we see is an ongoing process, with some social schemas easier to recognize than others. Changing them requires intentional action (Williams et al., 2022).

↞→

Shared social schemas are deeply embedded into every level of society and tend to be almost invisible to us; they are so taken for granted that we often don't see how they shape and organize us.

↞→

Societal schemas shape the experience of self and relationships from a very young age. A major error in thinking typically occurs at birth when children are assigned a gender category based on the appearance of their genitals (Welch-Ross & Schmidt, 1996). This creates and reinforces the idea that there are two distinct gender groups and that people must fit into one or the other. This gender schema limits the allowable options for everyone and disregards or renders invisible a much wider range of experiences. Parents, caregivers, and other children believe in these binary differences and relate to children in ways that anticipate and reinforce them, even though the biological differences between male-identified and female-identified babies are minimal (Eliot, 2009). For example, when parents expect a male child to be more active, they are likely to encourage and reinforce energetic behavior while being more apt to calm a female child. Societal gender schemas also typically presume heterosexuality as seen in a t-shirt for a male infant that reads "chick magnet." The slogan not only implies heterosexuality, but carries power differences in the construction of gender by characterizing females as diminutive. When children do not fit this message, they learn that they are different, inferior, or incompetent.

Heteronormativity and patriarchal gender systems tend to reinforce each other. Thus, parents of a young boy whose behavior seems "feminine" (i.e., sensitive, submissive, emotional) might worry that he will "grow up to be gay" and experience the negative effects of homophobia. Though the parents would be confusing sexual orientation with gender, this is a societal-level error, not just a personal one. Conflating sex and gender is another societal-level cognitive error, assuming that biological sex and gender identities are the same when they are not. In order to optimally support their child, the parents may need help distinguishing the real effects of not conforming to these societal gender schemas and how to advocate for their child from their own unhelpful fears and beliefs (Malpas, 2011).

The impact of social schemas on families and family therapy involves the broadest levels of social, economic, and political arrangements. When therapists **attune** to core beliefs within clients' schema, there is nearly always an opportunity to examine how these connect to societal norms and values that reflect and maintain larger social systems. For example, Tony, a cishet (cisgender heterosexual) working-class father of three, sought therapy to address impulsive behavior that he described as "sabotaging his relationship." As he and the therapist detailed the sequence of thinking and feeling surrounding this behavior; his acting out was connected to core beliefs that "family men had to give up their creativity to keep a job." Rather than see this as simply a reflection of Tony's individual distorted thinking, the therapist engaged him in examining and **naming** the values and structure of the workplace, societal expectations for men around work and family, and how these affected his personal schema and relational well-being.

The effects of patriarchy, capitalism, and democracy came together in Tony's schema in ways that were inherently contradictory. The idea that men have to give up their creativity to keep a job reflects Tony's low-status role in the workplace hierarchy. Yet the cultural measures by which Tony judged himself also included values such as free choice and entitlement to respect that reflect and maintain the privilege of the dominant group (i.e., White, upper class, able-bodied, heterosexual, cisgender privileged adult males). Patriarchy also requires males to develop characteristics that will allow them to take power-over gendered positions congruent with traits valued in capitalism (McDowell, 2015). Men are thus trained to respond to others within a hierarchical schema of how relationships work (Tannen, 1994). In Tony's case, this meant he was supposed to comply with orders and policies delivered in a top-down fashion while at work and then take a leadership role in his family. These hierarchical relationship schemas left him feeling disconnected both at home and at work. As he learned to recognize how these societal schemas impacted him, he was able to give more **value** to the relational role he wanted with his children and better understand his frustrations at work and develop strategies for how to respond.

Conflicting societal messages also place women and girls in a cognitive bind. They are socialized to develop relational schema (Jordan, 2009; Tannen, 1994). They are expected to be emotionally attuned to others, yet also learn that thoughts and logic are valued over emotions and intuition. Even though relational skills are institutionally and historically devalued, if women do not demonstrate them, they are likely to be viewed as shrill, cold, uncaring, or self-centered. Holding a stereotypical female schema inherently requires accepting a less valued societal position in order to be desired or accepted.

Power and Social Schemas

Therapists need to **name** whose interests are reflected in the social schemas embedded in their clients' schemas. For example, African American family therapist and scholar, Marlene Watson (2013) tells the story of her grandmother who said, "I was never pretty like my sister Brazolia. She was the pretty one. I was black and ugly" (p. 1). Though a Black woman, her schema of self and others reflected the societal framework that people with darker skin are inferior (i.e., colorism). Social schemas generally promote the cultural capital (Bourdieu, 1986) of the dominant group by privileging how *they* think and what *they* do, while marginalizing the cultural capital and schemas of other groups. Like Dr. Watson's grandmother, people will unintentionally adhere to schemas that reflect and support unjust social arrangements in their communities, living conditions, work settings, and intimate relationships.

•←→•

Power processes in the broader society tend to be reflected in the power dynamics within intimate and family relationships.

•←→•

CBF therapists should not assume that each family member contributes equally to creating the family schema or that each feels equally free or entitled to express their thoughts. For example, in the case of Frank and Jenny above, the entire family operated according to schemas that privileged Frank's experience and caused everyone else to avoid saying or doing things that might upset him. Jenny's relationally oriented schema from her family of origin, her experience as a woman, and more egalitarian models of marriage were subsumed over time by Frank's schema of male power and entitlement, even though he was largely unaware of his expectations or how Jenny and the children accommodated him. Expecting Jenny to challenge her schema-driven thoughts before Frank adjusted his would be difficult, given Frank's inherent power in the family system (Knudson-Martin, 2015). In some relationships, encouraging a less powerful voice to express herself could be dangerous.

Prejudice and Discrimination as Cognitive Distortion

Prejudice is a form of cognitive distortion (Parker & McDowell, 2017). As discussed in Chapter 1, economic and political systems play a large, and often contradictory, part in determining which qualities and characteristics are socially valued and which groups are privileged. Societal messages about the deficits and inadequacies of non-dominant groups are integrated into our schemas, along with those promoting the superiority of other groups. Those in marginalized groups are described in negative or less valued terms while positive attributes are associated with members of the most privileged groups; as when some people are thought to be smarter, more athletic, and better looking than others.

Though based on inaccurate thinking, processes surrounding prejudice maintain existing systems of power and privilege and support the idea that exceptions to our social schemas (e.g., the "poor" kid who becomes wealthy) are primarily dependent on individual motivation and hard work (Unger, 2019). CBF therapists can easily become inducted into promoting these prejudicial systems (Williams et al., 2022).

•←→•

If therapists are not intentional about expanding their lenses beyond individual and family schemas, they will likely label problematic symptoms as individual deficits or flaws in thinking.

•←→•

For example, imagine a therapist is working with a teen from a low socioeconomic group who has been identified as "a behavior problem." If they help the youth recognize his belief that "I will fail no matter what I do," as distorted thinking, without exploring the societal messages that tell him he is a failure, then the youth will see only himself as the problem—or he will resist therapy—and the systemic nature of prejudice remains unchallenged.

Prejudices are collectively enacted and maintain systematic discrimination throughout society. Social norms, laws, policies, and precedents result in unequal access to social influence and material resources (Jones, 1997).

•←→•

Those in dominant groups tend to internalize positive messages about themselves such that their schema of self and others includes little or no awareness of their privilege due to their group membership.

•←→•

In the US, this enables middle-class White males to view their economic successes and achievements as the outcome of individual hard work (i.e., the myth of meritocracy). This is a cognitive distortion based on a partial truth; while hard work is important, the contribution of other social supports and access to relevant knowledge and resources is overlooked (Parker & McDowell, 2017; Unger 2019).

Like the African American grandmother we discussed earlier, people in marginalized groups frequently internalize negative messages about their group. These destructive ideas adversely shape beliefs about personal worth and abilities. For example, a woman may view herself (and be viewed by others) as too emotional to make good decisions. Three social schemas are involved here: one says that men are more capable leaders than women, another that men are less emotional than women, and the other privileges intellect over emotion. Moreover, this kind of systematic distortion (i.e., prejudice and internalized oppression) results in discrimination that maintains the dominant social structure. That is, leaders of an organization are more likely to be male and, regardless of who fills the position, expected to disavow empathy in order to put the success of the institution over the needs and well-being of workers. These social schemas also tend to denigrate those who receive welfare as unfairly "living off others," while viewing upper-class wealth made from the work of those in the middle and lower classes as fair.

Social schemas that support established larger systems are reflected in the attitudes, values, and behavior of individuals and families. For example, in the US the economic system depends on the willingness of people in the middle and lower classes to work hard, which is reflected in how values play out within families. Family members may be in conflict over what work counts, whose work is more important, and so on. The tendency to value paid work over family work is directly linked to societal schema connected to capitalism (Folbre, 2001). These schemas likely contribute to the power Frank holds in his family and Jenny's tendency to accommodate his work schedule.

Impact on Equity and Well-being

Socioculturally attuned CBF therapists should be alert to and **intervene** in the impact of societal schemas that suggest who is worth more—who deserves what and why. These schemas contribute to health and well-being in multiple ways, from viewing environmental and structural inequities as "fair" or "normal," to the stress of living daily with discrimination, to treatment protocols that do not fit the reality of one's experience or cultural values. This helps explain why the quality of people's health in the US depends on their race, socioeconomic class, gender, sexual orientation, age, and ability (Watson et al., 2020; Chapter 1, this volume).

↔

Client symptoms should always be examined in relation to their location in larger systems of stratification, power, privilege, and oppression, as well as the patterns of thinking and doing that perpetuate prejudice and discrimination.

↔

For example, Deidre, a White, single parent mother of four, was referred to a community clinic for depressive symptoms. At first, Deidre appeared difficult to engage and somewhat hostile. When the therapist expanded the assessment of the presenting issues to include the sociocultural context, Deidre became more engaged. The therapist learned that the family was living in a homeless shelter, the children needed to get to three different schools, and no school buses served the shelter. Deidre feared that she was at risk of losing her children if they were late for school again.

Deidre's automatic thoughts were that it was hopeless to deal with the school system and that she was a failure as a mother. Even so, she did not give up. She made an appointment to see the school official monitoring her case but returned feeling defeated and even more fearful. Applying third order thinking, the therapist and Diedre could **envision** more equitable possibilities by visiting the school together. The therapist's role was to work with the school official to identify the patterns of thinking (i.e., prejudices and oppression) within the larger system that made it difficult for the official and Diedre to find a more adaptive solution. This enabled a **transformative** systemic shift in thinking and the school to help develop a more workable plan. Though Deidre continued to address her role as a mother, her depressive symptoms improved almost immediately. If the therapist had focused the therapy primarily on developing more positive thoughts about herself and ways to be more organized in preparing the children for school, Deidre would have continued to internalize ideas that she alone was responsible for her children's success or failure and the school system would continue to see her as a problem parent.

Third Order Change

The possibility of third order change depends on seeing the systems we are embedded in and envisioning alternative options and choices. It helps to realize most cultures are complex and people enact cultural models in many different ways. For example, a study of heterosexual couples in Iran found that they drew on multiple societal schemas when describing their relationships and there appeared to be considerable diversity in how Iranian couples integrated and responded to potentially contradictory societal schema (Moghadam & Knudson-Martin, 2009). Though the powerful impact of male dominant social norms was evident as women reported ways husbands could use the law to limit where they went, others spoke of values inherent in Islam that promoted expectations of mutuality and respect for women, and described these values manifested in their marriages. The authors concluded that couple and family therapists should help clients explore religious, cultural, and legal values and ask what their faiths or cultural norms teach about justice and respect, rather than assume that these social schemas are not open to reflection or able to be enacted differently.

↔

Conflicts inherent in social schemas are common and create openings for third order change.

↔

For example, a couple's power dynamics might be influenced by the deeply embedded expectations one or both hold about who has the right or is more qualified to make major decisions (patriarchy), alongside the expectation that each should have equal voice (democracy). While these contradictions can be the source of cognitive distortion, they are also potential fertile ground for developing more adaptive relationship patterns. People are usually not aware of the impact of contradictory societal schemas in their lives. When these are made visible, they have more choice. If Frank is asked whether he thinks Jenny's needs should be important, he is likely to draw on beliefs regarding equality and say they are.

The ability to transform destructive patterns is enhanced when people are aware of the multiple values inherent in their social schema, the consequences of each, and whose interests these represent and maintain. In Text Box 11.1 Elizabeth Parker describes how to help couples break societal gender schemas into the nitty gritty of how they show up in the division of labor, and how doing so helps couples address conflict and be more intentional about how they divide family labor.

Text Box 11.1 Elizabeth Parker, PhD

Elizabeth Oshrin Parker (she/her) is a family therapist and researcher. She has done research on a variety of topics including complex trauma, effects of discrimination on mental health, and quantitative research methodologies.

Many couples come to therapy citing "communication" as a primary issue in their relationship. People say if they could communicate better and be "nicer" to each other, then their relationship would function better. However, after clinical assessment, we find an imbalance in the relationship, where one person—most often the woman, in male/female relationships—is carrying more responsibility. This can include tangible duties such as care tasks and childrearing, and also intangible requirements of a functioning relationship, such as tending to the emotional health of the relationship or carrying the mental load (for example, remembering what and when things need to be done).

What this often looks like is both partners working paid jobs outside of the home, but with the woman in charge of all the tasks that make a family run smoothly. Sometimes, this manifests as the female partner doing all the care tasks (cleaning dishes, washing floors, changing sheets, buying soap, etc.), and sometimes it looks like both partners are doing care tasks at home, but with the female partner in charge of carrying the mental load of these tasks. Carrying the mental load means that the female partner is remembering when the sheets need to be changed, knowing the preferred soap of each family member, or doing the logistical work of setting up interviews for a nanny. She might ask her partner to help, and he might do so willingly, but she is still in charge of remembering each task and knowing the when, what, and where of these tasks.

The concept of schema can be helpful in examining the greater societal expectations of husband and wife roles that have been inherited and absorbed in the relationship, and can also help in breaking down the more concrete and day-to-day workings of family life. Take meal preparation: Say the woman does the majority of the cooking, but one night she asks her husband to cook dinner because she is feeling tired. He agrees and cooks the dinner that she was planning on cooking. Now, while this might look like sharing the responsibility of dinner, the cooking of the actual meal is only one part of meal production. The woman had already decided what to make, learned the ingredients that go into the meal, gone shopping for those ingredients, and put away the food from the store. If the man has the schema that "making dinner" is the physical act of preparing the meal and the wife has the schema that "making dinner" includes all of the preparation previously mentioned, this mismatch can cause inequity and conflict within the couple. The man may have in his mind that he has taken a task off of his partner and could be frustrated that "she's still not satisfied," while the female partner still feels run-down and exhausted by all of the other components that go into meal preparation.

Schemas are useful for helping couples take unconscious expectations of what relationships and tasks should look like and turning them into conscious choices between partners. It is important to spend time with the couple to look closely at how their relationship functions and then break down all of the components of their family life. Many have schemas inherited from their families or modeled by society that the woman is in charge of family life and the man contributes partially to tasks. You can see this when the couple describes the man as "helping" with laundry or babysitting his kids. Recall the example of meal preparation and the different understandings of what the task entails. Helping the couple come together on a mutually agreed definition of what a task is and who is responsible for it can help them restructure their expectations of each other in order to have a more equitable distribution of family life and ultimately take the strain off the couple's relationship.

•←→•

Though it is not easy to step outside dominant social schema, practicing from a socioculturally attuned perspective can lead to more options and third order change.

•←→•

Practice Guidelines

The following five practice guidelines help family members recognize commonly held societal schema, track their effects on their relationships, and develop alternative relationship models that work better for them (Parker & McDowell, 2017). It is helpful to note that they are not always implemented sequentially and may move fluidly back and forth over the course of the therapy.

These five practice guidelines include: 1) identify problematic schemas, 2) track patterns at multiple levels, 3) connect individual, family, and societal schemas, 4) commit to alternative relationship models, and 5) create behavioral change based on new schemas.

1. Identify Problematic Schemas

Socioculturally attuned CBF therapists systematically gather information about how client families function, identifying the schemas and cognitive distortions that contribute to concerns that brought the family or couple to therapy.

Socioculturally attuned cognitive behavioral family therapists look to the larger context to help pinpoint societal schemas that underlie problematic behavior, provide contextual meaning to family interaction, and affect the way family members perceive and impact each other.

Table 11.1 provides questions that can help guide therapists' initial assessment of potential sources of societal schemas that contribute to the problematic schemas affecting each client.

2. Track Patterns at Multiple Levels

CBF therapists help family members track how their thoughts, feelings, and behaviors are part of circular interactional patterns that include multiple family members. In this process, they make explicit how problematic schemas underlie the targeted emotions and behaviors. Tracking patterns provides an opportunity to begin to discuss the beliefs and ways of making meaning that guide family members' expectations of each other and makes the thinking behind the behaviors visible. Socioculturally attuned therapists approach this task with interest in how the patterns they are identifying are part of cultural, historical, and sociopolitical processes and seek to expand and contextualize them (Pandit et al., 2014). As the therapist develops questions and hypotheses that

Table 11.1 Sources of societal schemas and influence

Source of Societal Schemas	*Therapist Listens for the Following:*
Place	In what kinds of contexts is the client embedded? How have they changed over time? How much mobility is possible?
Gender	What societal messages about gender has the client internalized?
Socioeconomic status	How do socioeconomic status and economic situation impact schema of self and other?
Sexual Orientation	How have societal messages about sexual orientation influenced client's internalized identity and expectations about life cycle?
Sociocultural Location	How do clients' culture, religion, age, race, ethnicity, and disabilities impact schema of self and relationships?
Larger Systems	How do client relationships with legal structures (immigration, justice system, and so on) impact their schema of self worth and agency?
Social Power	How much personal, interpersonal, and institutional power do clients experience as a result of their societal position?
Societal Position	What overall messages about self in relation to others are perpetuated by client's position in societal context?

Adapted from Silverstein, Bass, Tuttle, Knudson-Martin, & Huenergardt (2006) p. 399.

clarify the repetitive patterns and cognitive distortions, family members begin to see themselves responding to each other and develop an interest in the source of the schemas influencing their relationships. Therapists use a variety of techniques to visualize these patterns of influence, such as the downward arrow technique (Beck, 1995) (see Figure 11.1 in case example, p. 249).

3. Connect Individual, Family, and Societal Schemas

Therapists must be intentional in helping families become aware of the ways they are enacting commonly held societal schemas. When family members see themselves caught in patterns larger than themselves rather than as simply something wrong with them, their experience is less pathologized (Pandit et al., 2014). Once thoughts, feelings, and behaviors are identified, there are many ways therapists can help people explore the underlying assumptions or values that societal schemas impose on them and how these impact their behavior. Video clips from movies or psychoeducation groups can be helpful sources of consciousness-raising conversation. Therapists can recognize societal schemas embedded in clients' automatic thoughts and directly identify them and track their consequences in the relationship. For example, when a woman says that her thought was that she didn't want to upset her male partner, the societal idea that "women should protect men's emotions" could be named as a societal expectation and its consequences on her and the relationship identified. A column for messages from society can be added to a thought record (See Table 11.4). Opportunities to critically reflect on the connection between personal, family, and societal schemas from a meta-perspective are empowering (Hernández et al., 2005). Table 11.2 provides examples of questions that can help make this link.

Table 11.2 Questions to link personal, family, and societal schemas

1 The idea that [insert distorted individual thought] is interesting.

- Where do you think you learned [insert parallel societal stereotype or expectation]? How did/does [your family] enact this pattern?

2 I noticed that when [interpersonal trigger] you responded by [insert societally stereotyped or inequitable behavior].

- What thought was going on for you right then? Is the idea that [client answer] common among other [relevant social group] that you know?

3 The idea that [cognitive distortion] is that causing you to [problematic behavior]?

- How do you suppose this kind of idea has affected other people [or men, women, etc] in our society?
- How do you think this idea has emerged in history?
- How does the thought that [distorted societal idea] affect others in your family?

4 When you feel [troubling emotion] what thoughts about yourself as a [relevant social group/role] pop up for you?

- What messages in society encourage this thought?
- What expectations about [social role] do you take in?
- What parts of yourself do you have to keep hidden?
- How does this impact others?

5 How do others in your community view [problematic behavior]?

- What moral codes or societal expectations are tied to your [distorted thought]?
- Who in society benefits when you think this way?
- How did you learn to think this way?
- How has this kind of thinking affected your family/relationship?

4. Commit to Alternative Relationship Models

As consequences of destructive societal schemas are linked to the sequence of thoughts, emotions, and relational patterns, family members become interested in other options. Values associated with alternative ways of relating can be explored, which enables family members to take more ownership of the values that they want to guide their life (McKay et al., 2012; Williams et al., 2022). Recognizing how their reactions to each other have been connected to restrictive and/or inequitable societal models decreases self-blame and makes it more possible to label barriers, observe impulses to act with old schema coping behaviors, and develop values-based strategies to move beyond them. To help overcome the power of dominant societal schemas, therapists provide leadership in engaging family members in examining and experimenting with relationship models that support the well-being of all. They support couples and families in envisioning an agreed-upon plan for change.

5. Create Behavioral Change Based on New Schemas

Core schemas of self and others are very persistent. Clients are now ready to actively engage in an intentional process of responding to each other based on the new schemas to which they have committed. This requires activities that help each of them recognize when problematic emotions and thoughts arise and to do something different. The therapist may provide education about practices that help enable this kind of behavioral change. For example, they may teach mindfulness skills to facilitate emotional regulation (McKay et al., 2007) or strategies to face emotions rather than avoiding them. The therapist helps family members and partners track their new responses to each other and identify how they overcame the old emotional cues and thoughts, as well as the pieces involved in enacting something new. They provide support and guidance that enables people to persist even when powerful emotions and old thoughts arise. Part of the coaching role is to remind people of the values and goals they identified and help families develop homework activities that keep the new relational schemas visible, such as a communications checklist or values intentions worksheet. Table 11.3 is an example. Other good examples of exercises that help people see and transform the impact of societal and power influences in their lives may be found in Knudson-Martin's (2025) *Socio-Emotional Relationship Workbook.*

Case Example

Jared (35) and Pamela (29), a European American cishet working class couple married for eight years, sat straight, their bodies stiff as they described the concerns that brought them to the CFT training clinic. They said that about the only time they talked was when they were "fighting about the boys." Aaron (aged 13) did not want to go to school, Jason (aged 12) got into fights, and they feared that Dillon (aged 9) worried too much about all of them. Pamela reported feeling "depressed" and "exhausted all the time." Their therapist, Claudia, a Latina family therapy graduate student, aged 35, was also a married cishet woman and mother of a toddler. As the session began, Claudia noted that the couple seemed nervous and approached her as an authority. Jared said that he "wanted to learn what he was doing wrong."

Claudia was aware that the couple's subservient orientation to her was very different from how she had learned to approach authorities in her relatively affluent home. She was mindful that her context for parenting was likely to be very different from this family's. She checked her own feelings about Pamela having become a mother at such a young age. While mostly experiencing awe for how anyone could manage this, she was also conscious of some beneath the surface judgment that Pamela "should have planned her life better" and recognized this as part of what she had learned was important in order to be successful. When she did not plan, Claudia felt inferior, less than. She had been especially careful to avoid the stereotype that Latinas get pregnant at a young age. This self-reflection helped Claudia orient herself to the couple with respectful curiosity about how they made meaning of their responses to each other and an interest in how the world around them influenced their schemas.

Table 11.3 Relational practices checklist

Rate yourself and your significant other (usually, sometimes, seldom).
Discuss. Where there is a discrepancy in your perceptions, discuss how your internalized social schemas may contribute to your differing perceptions.
Identify areas for discussion and practice in our therapy sessions.

Relational Practices	Perception of Self	Perception of Other
Attunement to others ✓ How interested are you in knowing and understanding the other's experience and perspective? ✓ Do you listen to your partner? Your children? About what? In what circumstances? ✓ To what extent do you notice and respond to the other's feelings and needs?		
Openness to vulnerability ✓ How willing are you to show weakness, uncertainty, or mistakes in your partner's presence? ✓ How safe and willing do you feel to share innermost thoughts and feelings with your partner? ✓ How likely are you to seek relationship repair by expressing a feeling or concern?		
Accepting influence ✓ How able are you to engage the other in addressing issues that concern you? ✓ How free do you feel to directly express your opinions or make requests? ✓ How readily do you accommodate your interests/schedule to fit your partners'/the family's needs and schedule?		
Relational responsibility ✓ To what extent do you focus on what is needed to maintain or improve your relationship? ✓ To what extent do you keep track of what needs to be done in the house? For the children? For the relationship? ✓ How responsible are you for doing the emotional work in the relationship?		

Adapted from the Circle of Care. Knudson-Martin & Huenergardt, 2015; Knudson-Martin & Kim 2023 (see Chapter 15, this volume)

Identifying Problematic Schemas

Claudia wanted to get background information about the family's context and the factors that might influence their personal and family schemas. She also wanted to engage the couple in an exploration of their interaction patterns and begin to develop hypotheses about the sequence of thoughts, emotions, and behaviors causing distress. After she gave the couple hope and a vision of how change could occur by describing the process of therapy, she explained that problems were often related to living in environments that created toxic and distorted ideas about ourselves and how we relate to others. She invited the couple to describe the problem that brought them to therapy.

When Jared said he was frustrated and didn't know what to do, she asked questions that helped to detail his view of the problem, "What happens? Who does what? What thoughts go through your mind? She was especially interested in understanding the context in which he felt so helpless. Jared described fights between Pamela and the boys. He would raise his voice and tell the boys to stop arguing with their mother, but this did not help and seemed to make Pamela even more upset. When Claudia asked him what he did when his efforts didn't help, Jared replied that he felt "useless" and usually "gave up." Using the questions in Table 11.1 as a guide, Claudia recognized his feelings as connected to societal schemas that create the distorted expectation that men must always be competent and in charge.

Turning to Pamela, Claudia was aware that not all voices in a relationship come from equal positions and made sure to not automatically follow Jared's definition of the problem and to instead invite another perspective, "Jared says that it's upsetting to see you and the boys fighting and to feel useless in making the fighting stop. That's his point of view. What do you see as the problem?" Pamela described being worried about the boys and needing to protect them. She was quick to praise Jared, who was not the birth father, for being there for them. Claudia asked questions to detail what happened from Pamela's point of view and began to establish a picture of how her responses connected to Jared's. For example, Pamela repeatedly spoke of how indebted she and the boys were to Jared. When Jared would yell at the boys, it triggered thoughts that she had no right to expect much of him. They began to pinpoint Pamela's underlying schemas about self and others—that it was not safe to trust anyone and that she was unworthy if she upset a man. Claudia wondered how these personal schemas connected to larger sociopolitical systems and how these impacted what happens within this family.

Claudia immediately began to widen the lens to learn more about the societal contexts surrounding their problems and expanded upon this in the next session. She asked about the neighborhood they lived in and their experiences with school, economic, and legal systems. She asked about how others had viewed their families growing up and what they learned about things like gender, social class, and sexual orientation. She encouraged reflection about how these affected their expectations and responses. Together, using questions like those illustrated in Table 11.2, the therapist and couple began to pinpoint a troublesome sequence in which the emotions and automatic thoughts generated around parenting resulted in responses that distanced them from each other and increased arguments with their children.

Tracking Patterns

The boys were invited to several sessions to further track interactional patterns. Claudia helped the family observe their responses to each other, systematically detailing how each served as triggers for the others. For example, when Pamela said that 12-year-old Jason was getting in fights at school and needed to change his behavior, Jason told her to back off. Nine-year-old Dillon came to Jason's defense, and 13-year-old Aaron rolled his eyes. When Pamela raised her voice and repeated her concern, telling Jason that fighting was dangerous and would get him in trouble, Jason directed an angry curse toward her. Jared told him to respect his mother.

The therapist guided the family in identifying each person's automatic thoughts and reactions, making visible a behavioral sequence they could all recognize and bringing new awareness regarding their situation. Underneath Jason's reaction was the idea that if he did not fight, he would never be respected at school; that he would not survive. Aaron anticipated increased distress between his parents that he could do nothing about and squelched his fear that Jared would leave the family by telling himself he didn't care. Nine-year-old Dillon broke into tears, saying that Mom should leave Jason alone; that she was making everyone unhappy. Pamela became visibly depressed, a reaction supported by the idea that she was worthless because she failed to keep all members of the family safe and was upsetting them. Jared physically pushed his chair back, saying, "I give up." The therapist helped clarify the desire for family members to be able to express disagreements and still love each other. All agreed that helping mom and dad stay connected to each other during times of stress was a primary goal.

Pamela: Women's Worth and Children	Jared: Men's Leadership and Children
Women's worth is defined by men.	Men must be in charge.
Men's opinions matter more than women's.	To be in charge I must know what to do.
When a man treats me badly I am worthless.	People expect me to be competent.
It's my job to learn how to please a man.	If others see me as incompetent I am a failure.
It hard to know what will please a man.	It is not acceptable to be a failure.
I must be very careful not to upset a man.	When I cannot handle the boys I am a failure.
When Jared yells at me I am worthless.	Men are not allowed to be a failure.
Without Jared my children and I are nothing.	For me to be a man, the boys must behave properly.
My children must not upset Jared.	For me to be a man Pamela must keep the boys in line.
I am worthless if my children upset Jared.	

Figure 11.1 Downward arrow illustration

In their couple sessions, Claudia helped Pamela and Jared create a downward arrow diagram to visualize the connection between their contexts, core schema, and responses to parenting. As illustrated (Figure 11.1), parenting was connected to core schemas about self-worth and gender for both parents. When the boys acted out or were distressed, Pamela experienced an almost automatic cascade of thoughts connected to the societal idea that "women's worth is defined by men." This led to the irrational thought that "she is worthless if the children upset Jared." Jared reacted to underlying societal schema regarding male leadership that in the end translated to the distorted idea "that for him to be a man, Pamela had to keep the boys in line and doing well." The couple readily recognized these thoughts as errors that did not really represent how they viewed parenting or their relationship with each other, but escalated in times of stress.

Connecting Individual, Family, and Social Schemas

Claudia helped the couple develop strategies to observe their own behaviors, recognize when they were being triggered, and identify their underlying automatic thoughts. They discussed situations that happened and what they noticed. As they talked in session, they created "thought logs" that included the triggering event, feeling, thought, response, and associated societal expectation. An example is illustrated in Table 11.4. Expanding the pattern to detail how their environment contributed to the family pattern helped Jared and Pamela feel understood and validated, and more able to approach their problems without blaming themselves or each other.

For example, the high cost of housing in their urban area meant that they could not afford to own a home near Jared's work, even though he had to drive three to four hours every day. Claudia asked questions that helped the couple examine taken-for-granted assumptions about owning a home and how this society-driven need was related to social schemas about class and economics that made owning a home a measure of personal worth and success, especially for Jared.

They discussed how the schools in their neighborhood suffered from limited resources and Pamela's fears about violence on the school grounds. When she saw Jason fighting, she feared that he was taking on male models of violence that triggered her own experience with men. They also examined the racial composition of schools and how, as parents of White children, their fears might be related

Table 11.4 Thought log with societal schemas

Triggering Event	*Thought*	*Feeling*	*Societal Schema*	*Response*
Pamela: School calls because Aaron is not in school.	School is unsafe. I'm a bad mother.	Guilt Worthlessness	Stereotype that Black kids are violent and hate gay kids. Schools judge parents.	Call Jared to ask him to talk to the school.
Jared: Pamela calls me at work.	The guys think I'm a "wus". My boss might see.	Embarrassment Anxiety	Men shouldn't let women "hang on them." Work and family should be separate.	Anger at Pamela. Refusal to call the school.
Pamela: Asks Jason to turn down the music and do his homework.	Jared's worked hard; the noise will upset him. I can't even get Jason to do his homework.	Guilt Worthlessness	Women need to calm men. Mothers are responsible.	Yells at Jason that he won't be able to go to the party unless he does his homework.
Jared: Jason calls Pamela "bitch," slams his door, & turns up the music.	Pamela is too controlling. I'm entitled to some peace and quiet.	Anger Anger	Boys should not be over-protected. Work is a man's priority; he should be able to relax at home.	Yells at Pamela, "why are you always over-reacting?" and goes out.

to racial stereotypes and biases regarding Children of Color. They began to consider how to talk about racial issues with their sons without perpetuating discrimination and irrational racist fears.

Pamela was especially concerned for Aaron's safety, as he had recently told his parents that he thought he might be gay. They examined each parent's responses to these safety concerns in light of internalized societal ideas about masculinity, sexual orientation, and appropriate behavior for boys. Though both parents said they accepted Aaron's sexual orientation, they needed help examining how internalized homophobia limited their ability to engage with Aaron and support him. Jared, who already felt unsure and disengaged from his role as a father, was especially at a loss regarding how to develop a relationship with a gay son.

Pamela, who became a mother at sixteen and had lived in a world dominated by poverty and male violence before meeting Jared, felt extraordinarily grateful for his financial support. They examined how her ideas about herself were influenced by societal schema that valued people based on their income and limited what people with little money felt entitled to. Jared, who was brought up in a middle-class family with a physically violent father, adamantly resisted using physical force. With no positive model for how to engage with the family, he focused most of his personal identity on work. Jared began to recognize how his anxiety at work was linked to underlying societal schemas that valued his performance at work more than his relationships and caused him to resist missing work for family matters but take time from family to "go out with the guys" after work. Pamela came to see that part of her depression was internalized anger at the unfairness in their relationship and gendered and classist ideas that, though she desired more emotional closeness with Jared, said she was not entitled to it.

Commit to Alternative Schemas

Jared and Pamela began to have a sense of the systems of schemas influencing them. They saw how the schemas into which they had been socialized, together with their prior life experiences, generated automatic thoughts and emotions that triggered behaviors that added to their stress, increased conflict, and created emotional distance. To achieve their goal of staying connected even in the face of conflict, they not only needed to change the way they communicated, but they also needed to identify and commit to a new relational schema. Because societal schemas limit the options people are able to envision, the therapist gave them a handout illustrating a model of relationship based on equality and mutual support that she integrated from socio-emotional relationship therapy (see Chapter 15, Figure 15.1) and used it as a guide to help them examine and identify values that were important to them. She also engaged them in conversations about ideals they wanted to model and support for their boys as they form relationships and participate in social systems outside the family.

With Claudia's encouragement and support, Pamela and Jared made a list of the values to which they wanted to commit. For example, they decided they liked the idea of shared relationship responsibility. This meant they had to resist societal schemas that said women needed men but men didn't need women, that women were responsible for raising children, and that men always had to have the answers and be competent. They wanted to know Aaron as a person and not just accept him as "gay." This meant they had to relate outside gender and sexual binaries and stereotypes. Jared wanted to learn to have a father–son relationship with him and their other sons. Overall, they wanted to organize their family more around relationships and less around economic measures of success and to equally support the well-being of every family member.

Creating Behavioral Change Based on New Schemas

Though Pamela and Jared did not have the time or comfort with writing to keep regular thought records at home, they created a special place to keep copies of those made in session easily accessible. They also found it helpful to tape a copy of the model of mutual support (see Chapter 15,

Figure 15.1) where they could see it. Pamela and Jared showed the diagram to the boys and told them they were trying to model a new way to respond to each other. The therapist also helped the couple practice letting themselves sit briefly with their stressful emotions, recognize them, and name the family and societal messages underlying them. This made it easier to respond differently. When the couple reported triggering events that resulted in the old cycle, Claudia coached them in identifying new responses that would help them attain their goal of staying connected during times of stress.

One of the most transformative sessions included the boys. Claudia guided a conversation about masculinity between Jared and them. Jared spoke of what he had learned about the destructiveness of needing to be "in charge" and how he had not really learned how to focus on others in the family. He told Aaron that he wanted to not let his fears about homosexuality limit their relationship. With Claudia's encouragement, Aaron was able to risk sharing his ideas about what he'd like from his father. And, following Aaron's lead, Jason and Dillion described how they'd like to engage more fully with Jared. Witnessing this event between her husband and sons helped Pamela solidify a new schema about men, women, parenthood, and her worth. Claudia asked her to share these ideas with her family. The family examined the list of values they had previously made in terms of both the progress they had made and the new challenges they gave themselves. They had learned to take a meta-perspective on societal schemas and were moving into third order change, intentionally developing a new shared family schema less constrained by inequitable and limiting societal messages and structures.

Third Order Change: Summary

Socioculturally attuned cognitive behavioral family therapy is well suited to the process of third order change. The approach encourages people to raise consciousness about societal influences on their thoughts and how these are connected to their emotions and interactions. Couples and families can recognize the impact of societal inequities in their lives and decide to create more just relationships and challenge discriminatory social distortions that maintain them.

In the case of Pamela and Jared, first order change occurred when Pamela learned to pause and be aware. She was able to recognize that the extent to which she worried about upsetting Jared was problematic. She began to respond in ways that helped her feel better about herself and the marriage. Second order change occurred when Pamela and Jared redefined their shared family schema to include more options for who does what. Family members no longer held Pamela responsible for everyone else's behavior. Third order change occurred as they began to develop social awareness, to consider the systems of systems that influenced them, and began to see how their life was organized around prescribed roles.

Pamela and Jared no longer automatically followed societal norms and expectations. They still experienced times of conflict and confusion, but their response to the conflict was different and brought them together as they reminded themselves of the societal schemas they were resisting. If automatic thoughts from earlier schemas were triggered, they recognized their oppressive nature and were able to draw on a different view of the world. The ability to see multiple sets of societal schemas and make choices in relation to them was transformative.

Reflexive Questions

- If you could make a list of five societal schemas (schemas that reflect dominant societal values and beliefs) that have shaped your experience of self and relationships, what would they be?
- How do you think these societal schemas affect your thoughts, feelings, actions, and interactions in personal and professional relationships?

- If prejudice is a form of cognitive distortion, what makes it sustain over time? How can it be disrupted by cognitive behavioral couple and family therapy?
- What are your reactions to this statement? "If therapists are not intentional about expanding their lenses beyond individual and family schemas, they will likely label problematic symptoms as individual deficits or flaws in thinking."
- How can you help families disrupt disempowering societal schemas and transform them to schemas that reflect their needs, interests, and vision?
- What are the tools, interventions, or means by which you have helped others recognize the impact of societal inequities in their lives? How did these processes lead to more just relationships and challenge discriminatory social distortions that maintain them?

References

Bäckström, B., Rask, O., & Knutsson, J. (2024). Adolescent and family-focused cognitive-behavioral therapy for pediatric bipolar disorders: An open trial and individual trajectories study in routine psychiatric care. *Child Psychiatry & Human Development*, *55*(6), 1502–1513.

Bandura, A. (1973). *Aggression: A social learning analysis*. Prentice Hall.

Baucom, D. H., Epstein, N. B., Fischer, M. S., Kirby, J. S., & LaTillade, J. J. (2023). Cognitive-behavioral couple therapy. In J. L. Lebow & D. K. Snyder (Eds.). *Clinical handbook of couple therapy* (6th ed., pp. 533–578). Guilford.

Baucom, D. H., Epstein, N., Sayers, S. L., & Sher, T. G. (1989). The role of cognition in marital relationships: Definitional, methodological, and conceptual issues. *Journal of Counseling and Clinical Psychology*, *57*(1), 31–38.

Beck, J. S. (1995). *Cognitive therapy: Basics and beyond* (1st ed.). Guilford.

Beck, A. T. (1967). *Depression: Clinical, experimental, and theoretical aspects*. University of Pennsylvania Press.

Bourdieu, P. (1986). The forms of capital (R. Nice, trans). In J. Richardson (Ed.), *Handbook of theory and research for the sociology of education* (pp. 46–58). Greenwood.

Charlés, L. & Bava, S. (2020). Systemic family therapy and global mental health: reflections on professional development and training. In Wampler, K. S., Rastogi, M., & Singh, R. (Eds.). *The Handbook of Systemic Family Therapy* (Vol. 4, pp. 549–567). Wiley.

Craske, M. G. (2010). *Cognitive-behavioral therapy*. Theories of psychotherapy series, American Psychological Association.

Dattilio, F. M. (2010). *Cognitive-behavioral therapy with couples and families: A comprehensive guide for clinicians*. Guilford.

Dattilio, F. M. (2005). The restructuring of family schemas: A cognitive-behavior perspective. *Journal of Marital and Family Therapy*, *31*, 15–30.

Dattilio, F. M. (2001). Cognitive-behavior family therapy: Contemporary myths and misconceptions. *Contemporary Family Therapy*, *23*(1), 3–18.

Dattilio, F. M. & Schoenly, A. (2023). Families in crisis. In F. M. Dattilio, D. I. Shapiro, & D. S. Greenaway (Eds.). *Cognitive-behavioral strategies in crisis intervention* (4th ed., pp. 225–243). Guilford.

Dattilio, F. M., Shapiro, D. I., & Greenaway, D. S. (2023). Crisis intervention: An overview. In F. M. Dattilio, D. I. Shapiro, & D. S. Greenaway (Eds.). *Cognitive-behavioral strategies in crisis intervention* (4th ed., pp. 3–23). Guilford.

Dover, N. & McGuire, J. F. (2023). Family-based cognitive behavioral therapy for youth with Misophonia: A case report. *Cognitive and behavioral practice*, *30*(1), 169–176.

Eliot, L. (2009). *Pink brain blue brain: How small differences grow into troublesome Gaps*. Mariner Books.

Epstein, N. B. & Baucom, D. H. (2002). *Enhanced cognitive-behavioral therapy for couples: A contextual approach*. Washington, DC: American Psychological Association.

Epstein N. B. & Dattilio, F. M. (2020). Behavioral and cognitive-behavioral approaches to systemic family therapy. In K. S. Wampler, R. B. Miller, & R. B. Seedall (Eds.). *The Handbook of Systemic Family Therapy* (Vol. 1, pp. 365–389). Wiley.

Epstein, N. B., & Falconier, M. KI. (2024). *Treatment plans and interventions in couple therapy: A cognitive-behavioral approach*. Guilford.

Fischer, M. S., Baucom, D. H., & Cohen, M. J. (2016). Cognitive-behavioral couple therapies: Review of the evidence for the treatment of relationship distress, psychopathology, and chronic health conditions. *Family Process*, *55*, 423–442.

Folbre, N. (2001). *The invisible heart: Economics and family values*. The Free Press.

Golboni, F., Alimoradi, Z., Potenza, M. N., & Pakpour, A. H. (2023). The efficacy of an online family-based cognitive behavioral therapy on psychological distress, family cohesion, and adaptability of divorced head-of-household women in Iran: A randomized controlled trial. *Asian Journal of Social Health and Behavior*, *6*(3), 133–140.

Hayes, S. C., Luoma, J., Bond, F., Masuda, A., & Lillis, J. (2006). Acceptance and commitment therapy: Model, processes, and outcomes. *Behaviour Research and Therapy*, *44*, 1–25.

Hernández, P., Almeida, R., & Dolan-del Vechhio, K. (2005). Critical consciousness, accountability, and empowerment: Key processes for helping families heal. *Family Process*, *44*, 105–119.

Jones, J. M. (1997). *Prejudice and racism* (2nd ed.). McGraw-Hill.

Jordan, J. (2009). *Relational-cultural therapy*. American Psychological Association.

Knudson-Martin, C. (2025). *The socio-emotional relationship workbook for couples: Closing the gap between the relationship you want and the relationship you have*. Routledge.

Knudson-Martin, C. (2015). When therapy challenges patriarchy: Undoing gendered power in heterosexual couple relationships. In C. Knudson-Martin, S. K. Samman, & M. A. Wells (Eds.). *Socio-emotional relationship therapy: Bridging emotion, societal context, and couple interaction* (pp. 15–26). AFTA SpringerBriefs in Family Therapy, Springer.

Knudson-Martin, C. & Huenergardt, D. (2015). Bridging emotion, societal discourse, and couple interaction in clinical practice. In C. Knudson-Martin, M. A. Wells, & S. K. Samman (Eds.). *Socio-emotional relationship therapy: Bridging emotion, societal context, and couple interaction* (pp. 1–13). AFTA SpringerBriefs in Family Therapy. Springer.

Knudson-Martin, C. & Kim, L. (2023). Socioculturally attuned couple therapy: Socio-emotional relationship therapy. In J. L. Lebow and D. K. Snyder (Eds.). *Clinical handbook of couple therapy*, (6th ed., pp. 267–291). Guilford.

Malpas, J. (2011). Between pink and blue: A multi-dimensional family approach to gender nonconforming children and their families. *Family Process*, *50*, 453–470.

McDowell, T. (2015). *Applying critical social theories to family therapy practice*. Springer.

McKay, M., Lev, A., & Skeen, M. (2012). *Acceptance and commitment therapy for interpersonal problems*. New Harbinger Publications.

McKay, M., Wood, J. C., & Brantley, J. (2007). *The dialectical behavior therapy skills workbook*. New Harbinger Publications.

Moghadam, S. & Knudson-Martin, C. (2009). Keeping the peace: Couple relationships in Iran. In C. Knudson-Martin & A. Mahoney (Eds.). *Couples, gender, and power: Creating change in intimate relationships* (pp. 255–274). Springer Publishing Co.

Pandit, M., Kang, Y. J., Chen, J., Knudson-Martin, C., & Huenergardt D. (2014). Practicing socio-cultural attunement: A study of couple therapists. *Journal of Contemporary Family Therapy*, *36*, 518–528.

Parker, E. O. & McDowell, T. (2017). Integrating social justice into the practice of CBFT: A critical look at family schemas. *Journal of Marital and Family Therapy*, 43, 502–513.

Petrinec, A., Wilk, C., Hughes, J. W., Zullo, M. D., Chen, Y. J., & Palmieri, P. A. (2021). Delivering cognitive behavioral therapy for post-intensive care syndrome family via a mobile health app. *American Journal of Critical Care*, *30*(6), 451–458.

Sadavoy, J. A. & Zube, M. L. (2022). *A scientific framework for compassion and social justice*. Routledge.

Silverstein, R., Bass, L. B., Tuttle, A., Knudson-Martin, C., & Huenergardt, D. (2006). What does it mean to be relational? A framework for assessment and practice. *Family Process*, *45*, 391–405.

Tannen, D. (1994). *Gender and discourse*. Oxford University Press.

Unger, M. (2019). *Change your world: The science of resilience and the true path to success*. Sutherland House.

Watson, M. F. (2013). *Facing the black shadow*. BookBaby.

Watson, M., Bacigalupe, G., Daneshpour, M., Han, W., & Parra-Cardona, R. (2020). Covid-19 interconnectedness: Health inequality, the climate crisis, and collective trauma. *Family Process*, *59*, 832–846.

Welch-Ross, M. K. & Schmidt, C. R. (1996). Gender-schema development and children's constructive story memory: Evidence for a developmental model. *Child Development*, *67*, 820–835.

Williams, M. T., Faber, S., Nepton, A., & Ching, T. H. W. (2022). Racial justice allyship requires civil courage: A behavioral prescription for moral growth and change. *American Psychologist*, *77*(1), 55–67.

12 Socioculturally Attuned Solution-Focused Family Therapy

Solution-focused family therapy (SFFT) evolved from the work of Steve de Shazer, Insoo Kim Berg, and their colleagues during the early 1980s in the United States (US) at the Brief Family Therapy Center (BFTC) in Milwaukee, Wisconsin. Those at BFTC developed a collaborative, eco-systemic approach that assumes families have the solutions they need to solve problems (Dolan, 2024; Lipchik, 2002; 2017; McKergow, 2021). The Mental Research Institute played a vital role in the development of strategic family therapy and solution focused therapy. According to De Jong (2019) in his interview with Steve deShazer and Kim Insoo Berg,

> The story begins in the 1970s at the Mental Research Institute (MRI) in Palo Alto, California. There, the likes of Don Jackson, Jay Haley, and John Weakland had been developing a form of brief therapy since the inception of MRI in 1958. Steve and Insoo, both from Milwaukee but unknown to each other at the time, came to Palo Alto wanting to learn more about the ideas and practices of MRI. They learned, among other things, that MRI's practice was, in part, inspired by the work of the psychiatrist Milton Erickson. Some of MRI's therapists, including Haley, would visit Erickson in Arizona and talk to him about his cases. Haley, especially, has written about Erickson's work describing many of his cases (Haley, 1986). Erickson's practice with clients was short term, sometimes included hypnosis, and always involved Erickson doing something to bring about change. Steve became fascinated by Erickson's work. While Erickson did not develop and write about a detailed model of doing therapy, he did describe many cases and what he did with them. (pp. 9–10)

This work continues to be influential today. SFFT shares several tenets with other brief systemic models, such as solution-oriented family therapy (O'Hanlon & Weiner-Davis (1989/2003). While conceptualizing from relational and interactional perspectives, SFFT is based on the assumption that change can happen quickly. Therapists focus on the here and now, with the idea that small change can lead to more significant change. SFFT is grounded in a social constructionist, post-structural framework that aligns with other postmodern models such as collaborative and narrative family therapy (Chenail, et al., 2020). The approach can be integrated into a variety of other family therapy models (Dolan, 2024; Nelson, 2019).

Solution-focused family therapy is more about creating change than understanding problems. In fact, understanding the problem is not viewed as necessary to begin finding solutions, which may not even be directly related to the problem (Dolan, 2024). Consider parents who enter therapy with their four-year-old child who is having angry outbursts. The therapist acknowledges the problem but assumes the child does not always have outbursts. They ask parents about places in which outbursts do not occur, question the family about times when outbursts are less severe, and search for times when the child starts to have an outburst but quits. As a solution-focused brief therapist,

DOI: 10.4324/9781003493426-12

they put their energy into what works. The family is seen as the ultimate experts on their own lives, while the therapist is seen as an expert on the clinical process and in asking the right questions to create and sustain preferred solutions (Dolan, 2024). They help the family determine what is different about their thoughts, feelings, behaviors, and interactions during times when the problem is not occurring (i.e., when the family is engaging in preferred behaviors and interactions). The therapist works together with the family to identify and amplify solutions that have been overlooked, while avoiding hypothesizing about the cause of the problem (i.e., that the parents don't have enough control, the child is expressing pent up feelings, or the child is caught in marital conflict). Solution-focused family therapy relies on the idea that change is always happening and there are always times when presenting problems don't occur or at least are not as severe (Dolan, 2024; Nelson, 2019; McKergrow, 2021).

•←→•

Socioculturally attuned solution-focused family therapists encourage third order change when they help families choose and amplify solutions that support equitable and just relationships.

•←→•

As is true with most family therapy models, the practice of SFFT has developed over time, adding new concepts and practices for the "next generation" (p. 73) of clinicians (McKergow, 2021). In this chapter, we describe enduring and evolving family therapy concepts and practices related to SFFT and offer a set of guidelines for socioculturally attuned practice. We share a case illustration to demonstrate how to create third order change by integrating societal systems and attention to power into solution-focused practice.

Primary Enduring Family Therapy Concepts

While no family therapy model is without theoretical underpinnings, SFFT is more about language than theory; about asking the right questions at the right time (De Jong & Berg (1998). That said, SFFT is often misinterpreted as simply a set of techniques that are often used with other models. Therapists who too rigidly and quickly move from one solution-focused question to the next often overlook relevant information, (e.g., undisclosed problems and experience, feelings, meaning-making, and relational dynamics). Therapists who avoid problem stories can leave clients feeling like they have not been heard, putting at risk a meaningful collaborative therapeutic relationship (Lipchik, 2017). It is essential for solution-focused therapists to demonstrate genuine curiosity and compassion. According to Dolan (2024) solution-focused therapists "use a tone and manner that clearly communicates serious interest in hearing what the other person says in answer to questions" (p. 9). This authentic curiosity helps therapists and clients find strengths and solutions within the rich tapestry of life that extends from the most intimate thought and feeling to the broadest and most complex societal systems. As McKergow (2021) noted, it is important for solution-focused therapists to engage clients in "stretching the world" (p. 86) to expand affordances and opportunities.

There are many guidelines for working from a solution-focused stance that are beyond the scope of this chapter and published elsewhere (e.g., de Shazer & Dolan, 2007/2021; Dolan, 2024; McKergow, 2021; Nelson, 2019; Nelson & Thomas, 2007). Following, we share the hallmarks of SFFT, including: 1) resolute attention to the use of language, 2) a collaborative stance in which therapists rely on clients' strengths and expertise, 3) careful construction of therapeutic goals, 4) finding and amplifying exceptions, and 5) the role of hope in change processes.

Use of Poststructural, Social Constructionist Language

In SFFT, therapists and clients work together to construct meaning in ways that help solve problems. All therapies rely on language, but SFFT pays particular attention to the use of language from social constructionist and poststructural perspectives. de Shazer and Berg relied heavily on Austrian-British philosopher Ludwig Wittgenstein's understanding of language games to create change through therapeutic conversations (Bidwell, 2007; de Shazer & Berg, 1992; de Shazer, 1997; McKergow, 2021). From this perspective, words without specific referents are fluid, and boundaries around them can become easily blurred. This is helpful in SFFT because it allows therapists to participate in the co-construction of meaning in ways that can make problems more solvable. This is particularly important to the process of moving away from being defined by problems. Initially asking about clients' best hopes for working together, rather than delving into the problem, helps set the stage for change, challenging the assumption that the future is determined by the past (McKergow, 2021).

Take as an example a White middle-class father, Daniel, who entered therapy after his wife has been incarcerated. His only child, Maya, is 8 years old. They entered therapy after the school called Daniel to tell him that Maya had been getting into fights. Their therapist, Aziza, was an upper middle class, Arab American Muslim, who identified as a cishet (cisgender heterosexual) woman.

Aziza: So tell me about your best hopes for our work together.
Daniel: I am hoping we can help Maya get along with the other kids at school. She has been getting into fights. She never used to be aggressive but since her mom went to prison, she hasn't been herself.
Aziza: I see, so your mom is in prison now?
Maya: Yes, and I hate it! I want her to come home.
Daniel: So do I, but it doesn't help for you to be aggressive! (Turns to therapist) I know she is depressed, but she can't take it out that way.

Aziza recognized Daniel's description of his daughter as aggressive and depressed as contributing to the stuckness of the problem. She responded to Daniel's statement in a way that began to shift meaning from Maya being defined by characteristics or qualities of aggression and depression to Maya experiencing those states. She encouraged Daniel to describe specific observations that lead him to conclusions about his daughter.

Aziza: What tells you Maya is feeling depressed?
Daniel: She is irritable and spends most of her time alone in her room. She also cries a lot.
Aziza: So Maya, your dad has seen you crying a lot and spending a lot of time in your room. You are feeling sad?
Maya: Of course I am. My mom is in prison and everyone knows it!
Aziza: The kids at school know?
Daniel: Her best friend told a few of the kids and now they all know.
Aziza: That must be difficult and upsetting, Maya.

Aziza began to move away from the father's description of his daughter as being aggressive and depressed in favor of moving toward a co-construction of the problem as Maya being upset and sad because she is going through a difficult situation. Aggressive and depressed are terms with fluid boundaries that give way to the equally fluid, but more solvable and transient problems, of upset and sad. Changing the description of the problem affects meaning and alters future interactions.

It is important not to immediately accept problems as clients understand and present them. Doing so often contributes to therapists getting stuck where clients are stuck. The therapist in this situation worked with the family to contextualize the problem. SFFT has been critiqued for failing to place problems in social context (Dermer, et al., 1998), however, contextualizing language, meaning, experience, relationships, and roles is a basic premise of this model (Sundman, et al., 2020). As we argue later in this chapter, there is room to expand the context further without abandoning the core of how language can be used to co-create solvable problems and well-designed goals.

All questions shape meaning, including what therapists expect by asking them. SFF therapists carefully use questions to inspire the expectation for change. Questions are open-ended, often using words like "when" and "will." A SFF therapist is likely to say "tell me about a time when…" rather than "has there ever been a time when…?" and "what will it look like when" rather than "what would it look like if…?" Let's jump ahead in the therapeutic conversation with Daniel and Maya.

Aziza: Tell me about times when you feel sad or upset about your mom when you are at school but you don't get into a fight?

Maya: I don't know. I guess when the teacher is looking at me.

Aziza: So when the teacher is looking at you, you decide to do something different? What do you do?

Maya: I just think "don't get in trouble" and keep my head down.

Aziza: Really? You are able to keep your head down and remind yourself not to get into trouble?

Maya: Yeah, I guess.

Aziza: How about other times when you feel sad or upset about your mom at school but you don't get into a fight?

Maya: When I am with my friend or I see my dad is there to pick me up.

Aziza: So when you are with your friend or getting ready to be with your dad you don't start a fight? I am curious about that. What is it like for you to be with your friend or your dad? How does that help?

Maya: I don't know. I guess I know they care about me.

These questions demonstrated Aziza's belief that change is possible and exceptions are already occurring. Maya's strengths began to emerge. In time, Aziza and the family discovered that Maya is someone who cares deeply about others, appreciates close caring relationships, and has the ability to resist acting out her feelings. This questioning continued until Maya, her father, and the therapist had a clear plan for how and when to amplify the exceptions they identified.

The types of questions most frequently used in SFFT include *miracle questions*, *scaling questions*, and *coping questions*. There are volumes written about why and how to ask these and other types of questions (e.g., de Shazer & Dolan, 2007/2021; Dolan, 2024; Lipchik, 2002; McKergow, 2021; O'Hanlon & Rowan, 2003; Selekman, 1997; Walter & Peller, 1992). What follows here are some comments about the foundational role these questions play as interventions in the practice of SFFT.

According to de Shazer & Dolan (2007/2021) the miracle question serves several important functions. First, it is useful in setting goals. If the therapist asks something like "If you wake up tomorrow to a miracle, and the problem is solved…?" or "How will we know when the problem is solved and we are done with therapy?" they are inviting clients to imagine solutions. Asking questions like "What will each of you be doing differently?" "If we had a movie of your family when this problem is resolved…?" or "What will each of you notice…?" help the therapist and family understand the current impact of the problem and descriptions of solutions. Second, the miracle question provides an emotional experience. Through imagining, clients can experience some of what it will be like after they make the desired change. Imagining is a powerful tool that motivates us and gives us hope in everyday life. Third, the miracle question sets the stage for finding exceptions. Clients' descriptions of what will be different provide them and the therapist with clues—specific feelings, behaviors, thoughts, interactions—that are likely already occurring to some degree at least in some contexts (de Shazer, 1988). Finally, miracle questions help clients move from digressive stories (i.e., what has or is getting worse) to progressive stories (i.e., what has or is getting better).

Once the therapist and clients establish goals, scaling questions may be used to assess progress toward goals and focus on exceptions (de Shazer & Dolan, 2007/2021). Scaling questions send the message that the problem is not static; that there are times when the problem is less present and/or solutions are more accessible. For example, a therapist might ask a couple questions like, "On a scale of 1–10, with one being not giving each other the benefit of doubt at all and ten being really giving the other the benefit of doubt (one of the clients' goals), where were each of you on the scale when the fight broke out? How about times when you were getting along? Or when during the week did you notice you gave the other or they gave you a little more benefit of the doubt (e.g., going from a 5 to a 6)?" These types of questions imply that clients have control over giving each other the benefit of doubt and that at times they do just that. They help explore the connection between giving each other the benefit of the doubt and getting along. Scaling questions can also be used to help clients describe their inner world of emotions (de Shazer & Dolan, 2007/2021; Lipchik, 2002), which can then be connected to what is happening relationally.

Typically, therapists use scaling questions around exceptions that reflect positive goals (i.e., what is happening rather than what is not happening). The following example demonstrates a slightly different use—using scaling questions to identify and deal with emotions. The example also explores one of many ways to scale without the use of a numeric measure, to which children may have more difficulty relating. While SFFT relies heavily on moving toward positive goals (i.e., what is rather than what isn't), it can be helpful at times to make space for unwanted emotions. Let's go back to Daniel and Maya:

Aziza: So Maya, if I had a big thermometer that went from the floor to the ceiling, and the bottom is not sad at all and the top is as sad as you can ever imagine (uses hand gestures to describe the thermometer), how sad are you right now?

Maya: About here (holds her hand up to about the middle of the imaginary thermometer).

Aziza: What do you notice when you are about this sad (uses hand gesture to show the point in the thermometer Maya indicated)? What do you usually do?

Maya: I just maybe read a book or watch tv.

Aziza: How does your dad know when you are this much (hand gesture to the same spot) sad?

Daniel: She gets quiet and won't talk to me.

Aziza: What helps you go from here (on the imaginary thermometer) to here (a little lower on the thermometer)?

Maya: Maybe when dad and I play a game or grandma comes over.

Aziza: So when you and dad play a game or grandma comes over, you feel a little better. What do you do differently when you are a little less sad? When you are playing a game or spending time with grandma?

Aziza was able to assess Maya's current level of sadness. She would likely want to compare that to the previous week and carefully investigate what was better when the sadness lessened. The series of questions helped the family and the therapist identify a solution they are already using, such as talking to each other and having some fun. In the future, once the family has had enough time to talk about sadness, Aziza might want to change the scale to one indicating a positive outcome like happiness rather than sadness.

Finally, coping questions (Dolan, 2024; Lipchik, 2002) are used when clients cannot identify exceptions to a problem. There are times when problems are so overwhelming that it is hard to even imagine life without them. For example, a client who is devastated over the loss of a child is likely to feel hopeless about ever feeling anything but sadness and loss. In these situations, SFF therapists ask coping questions such as "How have you been able to keep breathing?" "How have you managed to just get from one day to the next?" or "What keeps you going?" This often reveals rich and meaningful information about strength and resilience that can be built on over time (Bolton et al., 2017). Answers such as "I have to keep going for my other children," "I turn to God every minute of every day," or "I know my child would want me to" point to strengths such as a sense of duty, parental integrity, fierce determination, and unwavering faith that can be further explored. At other times when no exceptions can be identified, the therapist might simply ask the family to "do something different" (de Shazer & Dolan, 2007/2021; O'Hanlon, 1999).

Collaborative Therapeutic Relationships

The therapist may be the expert in the process of therapy, but clients are experts of their own lives (Anderson & Goolishan, 1992; Dolan, 2024). SFF therapists recognize that each client is unique and avoid assuming they know what clients need based on theory or clinical experience. Therapists take a "not knowing" (Anderson & Goolishan, 1992), unassuming, tentative stance so they are always in the position of learning from clients (Thomas & Nelson, 2007; Nelson, 2019). Past clinical experience is used as a last resort when clients are stuck and unable to imagine solutions. At these times, SFF therapists may tentatively contribute something like "I don't know if this is helpful, but a lot of people I work with who are in your situation tell me…" (Lipchik, 2002). Clients take on an active role in discovering exceptions through examining thoughts, feelings, behaviors, and interactions along with the therapist. When clients say "I don't know" the therapist believes them and helps them discover what was previously out of their awareness.

Successful SFFT depends on therapists genuinely believing clients have what they need to solve problems. Therapists need to be authentically hopeful, curious, respectful, and positive (Nelson, 2019; Thomas & Nelson, 2007). According to Sundman et al. (2020), "the practitioner builds on hope, positive emotions, virtues, caring, love, compassion, gratitude, and sympathy for the clients and their environment" (pp. 35–36). SFF therapists are deeply committed to believing in and finding strengths, which helps them persevere when clients doubt their own abilities to overcome problems. Therapists who successfully use this model not only ask poignant questions but listen deeply to clients. They allow clients time and space to share problematic stories so that they are truly heard. Problem stories also offer therapists opportunities to explore strengths, including how clients got through hard times.

While there is a clear focus on solutions, exceptions are embedded in both problem and solution patterns (Choi, 2019). SFF therapists can track problem patterns in order to notice exceptions in and out of sessions. For example, a common problem pattern for a couple might be to immediately distance when they start to have conflict. In this case, the therapist would want to notice times when a couple stayed engaged, regardless if they were aware of these exceptions. The therapist might say to a couple, "I noticed just now that you stayed in the room and in the conversation, even though you both became angry. How were you able to do that?" The couple might respond with, "It is because you are here," which only speaks to motivation. The therapist would press further, "I understand you are motivated to do something different when you are in therapy and I am sitting with you, but I am still really interested in *how* you were both able to stay in the conversation." This is not a simple question and would most likely take the couple and therapist some time to unravel.

Therapists must enter clients' worlds—the way clients make meaning—to cooperate with them on solutions. What other models see as resistance is viewed as therapists not cooperating the way clients expect or need. The therapist gently leads from behind. While most SFF therapists consider customers for change to be those who share a goal for change and are willing to do something about it, many invite all family members to treatment to recruit as many customers as possible to help resolve problems.

SFF therapists, having faith in clients' strengths, connect deeply and authentically with all members of a family and inspire expectation for change through their own unwavering optimism (Lipchik, 2002). Therapists join with clients in part through compliments and seeing the best in clients, however, compliments are genuine rather than paternalistic. For example, a therapist would be taking a one-up patronizing stance by saying something like, "That is so amazing, good for you for not giving up!" but would be taking an authentic stance when saying something like, "I notice that you don't give up easily on what is important to you and your family; that you are tenacious and determined."

Focusing on Client Goals

Goals must be important to clients (Nelson, 2019); however, it is not accurate to assume the therapist simply accepts the goal as first delivered by clients. The therapist attends to clients' best hopes while playing an instrumental role in facilitating the process of helping clients develop workable goals that meet a variety of criteria. This requires exploring clients' experiences, the meanings they make of their situation, their opinions of each other, their sometimes conflicting hopes and dreams, their past struggles, and as we will introduce further along in this chapter, their sociocultural context.

Well-defined (Walter & Peller, 1992), or well-formed (Nelson, 2019) solution-focused goals are stated in several ways: in positive form (e.g., what will be vs. what won't be); refer to process (e.g., backing each other up as parents vs. each making decisions on how to parent on our own;); in the here and now (e.g., get along better vs. get married someday); address the right level of specificity (e.g., I want to be more efficient vs. I want to get my filing done on time); are within the client's control (e.g., We want to follow through on rules and consequence vs. We want our son to do his chores); and use the client's language (e.g., you want to get along as a family vs. you want to function better as a family unit). The goals are designed to be achievable and include a role for all family members who are in therapy (Nelson, 2019).

To clarify, the therapist attends to clients' language throughout therapy while actively engaging in co-constructing new language and meaning. In the example of Daniel and Maya, Aziza would not accept as a goal the first explanation of what the client wanted to achieve. Aziza would have made a mistake if she had said:

Aziza: So tell me about why you came in today.
Daniel: Maya has been having fights at school. She never used to be aggressive but since her mom has been gone, she hasn't been herself.
Aziza: So fighting at school is a problem? Do you agree with your dad, Maya?
Maya: Yes.
Aziza: What do you want Maya to do instead of fighting, dad?
Daniel: I just want her to get along with the other kids.
Maya: Duh dad. Like I don't want the other kids to like me.
Aziza: So both of you want Maya to get along better with the kids at school? Tell me about times when you do get along, Maya.

In this scenario, the therapist accepted the definition of the problem too quickly, without exploring what was going on in the family or hearing Maya's story about her mother being incarcerated. This type of goal could be instrumental in finding exceptions to fighting as the therapist pursues what getting along looks like, what each person is doing, and so on. The problem with this goal, however, is that it is not at the right level of specificity. It too narrowly defines the problem. It also includes only one member of the family, inadvertently implying the child is the problem and missing opportunities for more significant systemic change. Notice the difference in the type of goal that can be set after exploring the problem more fully:

Aziza: O.K. So when you are talking to dad or grandma and having some fun you are not quite so sad. Dad, what are you doing differently at these times Maya is talking about?
Daniel: Well, I guess I am talking more too, having some fun. It is nice when my mom comes over. It gives me someone to talk to.
Aziza: Helps you feel better too?
Daniel: Yeah. It has been hard on me, too and on my mom. Well of course, on Maya's mom especially. We all worry about her.
Aziza: Sure, it has been hard on everyone—everyone worries. It sounds like it helps though when you talk to each other and stop every once in a while, and remember to have fun?
Daniel: Yeah, I guess so.
Aziza: Maya, how about at school, what helps you get along with everybody as often as you do?
Maya: Sometimes I don't think about it. Maybe I am having fun with my friends or doing schoolwork.
Aziza: I will be interested in knowing more about times you start to think about it or start to worry but decide not to and times when you are thinking about it but manage not to get into fights… but right now I am wondering if you are both saying that it is important to take a break from thinking and worrying about mom sometimes.

Here the therapist builds on exceptions that include having some fun and not worrying to ask the family to consider the idea that they can take a break from the problem. This implies that the problem is not always occurring and points toward further exceptions.

Daniel: I suppose it doesn't help any of us to just dwell on it. I know Maya's mom wouldn't want that. We need to start getting back to normal.
Aziza: Maya what does your dad mean when he says "getting back to normal?"

Aziza picks up and repeats Daniel's statement about getting back to normal. This metaphor (Zatloukal et al., 2019) uses the client's words to capture a way of being and has the potential to meet the criteria required to co-construct a well-defined, solution-focused goal.

Maya: I don't know…maybe doing things we used to do, wrestling, watching tv together, eating dinner at the table…just normal stuff.
Aziza: So as a family you would like to get back to normal? As normal as you can be given what's going on? Maybe at school too?
Maya: Yeah. Everywhere. I just want to get back to normal.
Daniel: I know her mom wants that too.

Aziza didn't force a goal or accept the first idea that came along. She kept talking with the family until the right type of goal emerged. This goal is at the right level of specificity. It may seem broad at first glance, but "back to normal" serves as an umbrella goal under which many more specific interactional solutions can be identified. This is a goal that has a solution embedded in it because it refers to a time when the problem did not exist while still taking into account the family's difficult situation. This goal is also helpful to everyone and includes all of the family in the solution. Finally, the goal makes sense as the family is identifying what many families report, such as maintaining family routines during a time of crisis enhances resilience.

Discovering and Amplifying Exceptions

Exceptions to any problem can be found, created, or imagined. Focusing on the positive helps nudge clients in the direction of the desired change. SFF therapists are continuously operationalizing goals and identifying anything that clients do that moves them toward desired outcomes. They encourage doing more of what is working and examine how clients are able to do things differently when change is spontaneous. Let's continue with our example of Daniel and Maya. Aziza would want to identify what is included in "back to normal," trusting that the family knows what this will take, even if they can't immediately describe it. She would believe that the family has the strength and resilience to accomplish this goal.

Aziza: So Dad and Maya, let's imagine that we are meeting for the last time because we all agree that you are as back to as normal as you can be until mom gets home. What will we notice? What will each of you be saying? Better yet, let's say you bring in a movie to show me how things are back to normal. What will we see you doing in the movie?

Maya: We will be talking and laughing. Dad would be tickling me.

Daniel: Maya would be coming home, saying she had a good day at school.

Aziza follows these more global statements like a good day at school with specific, observable behaviors.

Aziza: The two of you will be talking and laughing more. You will be wrestling and tickling and Maya will have good days at school? [therapist repeats replacing the word "would" with the word "will" moving from hypothetical to expected change]

Daniel: Yes. And Maya won't be so sad all of the time.

Aziza: And you, dad?

Daniel: Well, I suppose I wouldn't be so sad either.

Aziza: So what will you both be feeling instead of so sad? [looking for the positive vs. absence of negative].

Daniel: Maybe less worried about Maya's mom being O.K.

Aziza: So less worried and sad. Tell me about times now when you are a little less worried and sad. [continues to use this language because it still seems most meaningful and useful to the client]

Daniel: I think when I remind myself that Maya's mom will be alright. That we will get through this.

Aziza: You have been through other difficult things in your life? [looking to transfer solutions from one context to another]

Daniel: Yes. My father died a couple of years ago. Maya was really sick when she was a baby.

Aziza: (lowers voice, speaking more slowly) How did you remind yourself that you could get through those hard times—that things would be alright?

Daniel: (tears up) I just told myself that I could do it. That I wasn't alone and that eventually, things would get better.

Aziza: How are you teaching your daughter to have that kind of courage and deep optimism as she is going through her first really hard time?

Daniel: I think I could do better. [turns softly to daughter] Sweetie, things are going to be alright. Your mom is safe and will be home by next summer. We can make it. She wants our lives to be as normal as we can make them while she is gone.

Maya: (quietly) I know Dad. I'll be alright.

Toward the end of session:

Aziza: So I am wondering if you would be willing to do an experiment this week? It seems like you both want things to be as normal as possible and that you agree you can get through this. Would you be willing to do something every day that will reassure the other that things are going to be OK? You know, something normal! [all laugh]

Now we have some exceptions that are related to the goal, can be used across contexts, are relational, and are within the client's control. The therapist knows enough about the problem to notice exceptions when they may be out of the family's awareness. Aziza would also be keen to watch for exceptions that occur in session. For example, if Maya, Daniel, and Daniel's mother are in a session and the therapist notices them teasing each other, she might say, "Is teasing each other one of those things that you normally do?"

Hope

Hope and expectancy play an essential role in change processes in general, but these are particularly highlighted in solution focused therapy (Singer, 2024). Helping clients identify their "best hopes" clarifies goals and ensures goals can be put in positive terms. Questions that identify strengths and movement toward goals encourage hope that pathways to desired outcomes are possible and doable (Courtnage, 2025; Reiter, 2010). Courtnage (2025) identified three phases related to hope in solution focused therapy: hope identification, hope activation, and hope empowerment. Hope identification helps clients determine desired outcomes and amplifies the desire to change. Hope activation promotes agency, including clients' beliefs that they have the capacity to change. Hope empowerment involves clients discovering pathways to their goals. The therapist's role centers on believing clients are capable and supporting the change processes. This process is the antithesis of therapists identifying problems and providing solutions.

Throughout their conversation, Aziza is relying on her belief that change is possible; that Daniel and Maya have the strengths they need to move forward; that solutions are already available. Aziza repeatedly invites hope into the conversation by asking questions that assume there are exceptions and point to strengths, as well as presupposing that change is both possible and likely.

Integrating Principles of Sociocultural Attunement

SFF therapists support social equity by challenging power dynamics between clients and therapists, seeing clients as experts of their own lives, and taking a collaborative, power-sharing stance. SFF therapists also serve as activists when they avoid pathologizing clients, refusing to focus on problem-saturated descriptions and labels. Socioculturally attuned SFF therapists go beyond the family, however, to include the impact of, and potential solutions within, the broader societal context.

↞→

Socioculturally attuned solution-focused family therapists help clients access personal and contextual strengths and resilience by integrating critical awareness of societal context and power dynamics.

↞→

Solutions in Societal and Cultural Context

SFFT is based on social constructionist and post-structural thought, which centers the relationship between culture, societal context, and meaning. Solutions to problems emerge from cultural and social frameworks that both expand and limit possibilities. Cultural groups within societies collectively generate solutions over time. This long list includes things like rituals that help mark change or deal with loss, acts of resistance through the use of language and song, and rules that support caring family relationships. Cultural and societal norms are not apolitical, however; they advantage some over others, and those with greater influence in societies have greater impact on meaning-making. According to Bidwell (2007), "social constructionist theory does not necessarily reject an underlying 'reality'" (p. 73). Uneven influence over meaning-making has real material consequences, including access to adequate employment, health care, and housing, level of food security, safety, influence in the legal system, and so on. While SFFT is well suited for practice across cultures and societies (Neipp & Beyebach, 2024), due to social constructionist underpinnings, therapists and clients will be limited in imagining and discovering solutions if they fail to realize the potentially restricting aspect of unexamined cultural frameworks and societal systems. The question is how we do this without imposing a theoretical framework on clients.

A number of scholars and practitioners have advocated integrating Paulo Freire's (1970/2000) approach to raising critical consciousness using dialogue, reflection, and action into the practice of family therapy (Korin, 1994). There are several points of convergence between Freirean ideas and SFFT. Chief among these is the belief that people are the experts on their own lives. Like SFF therapists, Freire viewed emancipatory education as helping people become aware of what they already know. SFF therapists focus primarily on clients' expertise of themselves and each other and what they know works to eliminate their problems. Freire focused on encouraging people to recognize their expertise on their environment and societal context. The main difference is that SFFT aims to help people *discover* what is helpful on a personal and interpersonal level. Emancipatory education aims to help people *uncover* societal realities so they are in a better position to take necessary action to improve their lives. What they know about themselves and the world is transformed by an understanding of the reality of broader cultural and societal dynamics.

↞→

Inviting clients to explore societal forces that affect their lives can increase potential solutions and encourage discovering and amplifying a broader set of exceptions.

↞→

SFF therapists are pragmatic—willing to explore what works. They rely on asking nuanced questions and avoid getting caught in theoretical word games. It is not so difficult to imagine integrating social and cultural awareness into SFFT practice. Take for example, Janise, an African

American single parent living on low income, who is balancing the demands of motherhood while pursuing a college education. A SFF therapist is likely to ask Janise questions about where she lives, who is in her life, what social support systems she has (e.g., church, peers at college), interactions between family members, and so on. The therapist would work to co-create a goal that is in positive form, for example, "being the mother I want to be" despite her challenging situation. The therapist would then help Janise operationalize what this means and explore times when she is able to do so; complete her school work while parenting, act according to her values and beliefs, and enjoy being with her child.

A socioculturally attuned SFF therapist would extend the context and word questions in ways that would help Janise and the therapist become more aware of the effect of her societal context. Questions might include, "You mentioned that most of your peers at school are single, middle class, White students. What is your experience in that context? How do you make sense of the racial and social class dynamics?" As Janise and the therapist uncover the impact of oppressive sexist, racist, and classist educational and other societal systems, Janise would be able to make new meaning of her situation. This would not alleviate her financial stress or the "isms" she is faced with on a daily basis, but would expand potential solutions and better acknowledge existing strengths. Solution-focused questions that follow might include things like "How do you think Black women have historically been able to survive and thrive when there has been so much working against them?" and "How have you been able to do this for so many years? How are you able to be successful in school and still be a caring mother, despite the racism and sexism you experience and with so few financial resources?" These questions would help Janise move from the broader context, including the strengths Black women in her situation have historically shared, to her own strengths and solutions.

↞↠

Clients and therapists can move from seeing the client as having unique solutions to a private problem, to being part of a collective with both common and unique solutions to a shared public problem.

↞↠

Language, Meaning, and Power

The relationship between language, meaning, and power in socioculturally attuned SFFT takes us back to the beginning—to de Shazer's (1997) reading of Wittgenstein, who postulated that meaning associated with words emerges only when used and heard in context (Pitkin, 1972; Sundman, et al., 2020).

↞↠

Socioculturally attuned solution-focused family therapists critically analyze discourse as it unfolds in therapeutic conversations, attending to words, tone, body language, and emotion to understand how power shapes meaning.

↞↠

This includes attention to the role of power and meaning and context in how problems are understood and goals are identified. We might think of socioculturally attuned SFF therapists as routinely searching for meaning while engaging in a type of informal critical discourse analysis to understand how group power dynamics are part of the context in which meaning is made and social arrangements are reinforced. According to van Dijk (2015), critical discourse analysis "studies the way social-power abuse and inequality are enacted, reproduced, legitimated, and resisted by text and talk in the social and political context" (p. 466). Let's explore how societal context and power dynamics impact the meaning embedded in even the most seemingly simple questions and solutions. Suppose a therapist echoes a remark by a family that the mother "is a strong woman." This won't evoke the same image or description for all of us, but for many it means something like "she can endure a lot" or "she can stand up for herself and won't take being put down." The meaning of the statement is inseparable from gendered power dynamics.

SFF therapists must attend closely to meaning to ensure questions and solutions support social equity. The therapist might follow with questions like, "You mention that you see your partner as a strong (woman/man/person). Can you describe what you mean? What do you and others notice that leads you to describe them in this way?" These questions open space for discussing gender and other power dynamics using specific, here-and-now examples. If being a strong woman includes enduring a lot or not taking being put down, questions that follow would include identifying how a client is able to stand up to others as well as what is happening relationally that requires standing up to others.

Third Order Change

Third order change can occur when the experience of all family members is fully explored within their sociocultural context. Slowing the process of imagining values, solutions—expanding what is both possible and preferable to include equitable relationships—mirrors the model's expectation of collaboration between therapist and clients. When offered space to do so, families and therapists can envision, identify, and amplify *just* solutions. This requires extra steps to ensure what has been silenced can be named and voiced; that therapists intervene to encourage families to develop the willingness to respond to each other; and exceptions are noticed and amplified that encourage transformation toward *just* relationships within and beyond the family. In Text Box 12.1, Toni Schindler Zimmerman describes practicing SFFT from an equity-based framework.

Text Box 12.1 Toni Schindler Zimmerman, PhD, LMFT

Toni Schindler Zimmerman (she/her/hers) is a Professor in the Human Development and Family Studies Department at Colorado State University. She identifies as White, female, cisgender, upper-middle class, heterosexual, unaffiliated religion, able bodied, Euro-American.

Clients, therapists, and supervisors are embedded in systems of privilege and/or oppression based on their social location (e.g., race, sexual orientation, ethnicity, gender and gender expression, socioeconomic status) in their personal and professional lives. As therapists and supervisors, it is essential that we understand how these systems were set up, how they continue today, and the real and significant harm that is caused as a result. The mental health system has participated and contributed to oppression and discrimination, and worse.

In order to dismantle systems of oppression in mental health, we must be fully committed to examining and changing our policies, practices, and the way we interact with clients and others in our work. This commitment involves gaining significant knowledge about the history and current realities and the disparities and barriers imposed upon those with marginalized identities by those who hold power. In addition to a commitment to learning and unlearning, we must also be in a continuous state of self-examination. Systems of oppression and discrimination are so foundational to everyday life that if we are not vigilant to our implicit bias, stereotypes, microaggressions, and deficit assumptions that can show up in the therapy and supervision process, we can do real harm. Systems of oppression in relationships can show up in the therapy room where power is unjustly distributed (e.g., couples, parent–child, therapist–client) and in the workplace itself (e.g., supervisee–supervisor, a caste system among employees, harassment). In all areas, we must actively work to create an environment and provide services that are socially just. This is the foundational value that I strive to work from.

My work is guided by a systems perspective, including attunement to systems of oppression at all levels. I utilize a variety of models, including solution focused, which I will talk about here. From a solution focused model, I focus on strengths and the remarkable ability to cope that so many clients and supervisees exhibit. The lived experience of so many persons with marginalized social location identities is that of being underestimated, overlooked, single storied, and attended to from a deficit lens. Connecting some of these experiences in their personal lives to the way in which this is also happening at the societal level is useful to provide context for the pain and suffering they are experiencing.

The message can sound like "our societal structures value and reward people who make more money, and even see them as more important, and often give them more of a say. So, it is no wonder that in your relationship you have this dynamic. It is surprising that you have so many areas of your relationship where you are functioning as equals, without who makes more money having influence in decision-making. How can you do more of that?" "Given the unjust (e.g., homophobic, transphobic, misogynistic, racist, etc.) society in which we live, how have you coped in your work, in your relationships?"

Highlighting exceptions in the therapy room can be a way of identifying and naming power inequities. For example, a therapist might say something like "the way you spoke to your partner was not from a place of power over her and shutting her down; instead you accepted her concerns and listened and validated her. I wonder if that is why she was able to find the courage to speak up even though she was worried about your response."

I might say something like "The way you listened and didn't interrupt just now gave your partner the opportunity to feel valued and heard, how were you able to do that when you have been taught to win in conflicts?" An example of what interrupting unjust relationships might look in therapy could be, "I have to stop you there. It is no wonder given the "father knows best" society we live in that you want to be in charge. Earlier you were able to listen to your son without judgment and with an open heart and mind and that is when I saw you being the best father."

I sometimes use the concept of envisioning a future without the problem. For example, "when you both approach decisions with equality—valuing both of your ideas equally—what impact do you think that will have on your feelings of closeness with each other?" I would add that I believe in providing ongoing opportunities for all voices to be heard in organizations, anonymously or not. Listening to clients, staff, students, etc. and valuing all voices is essential for transformation. No voice is too "small" to be heard. No voice is so "big" to drown others out.

Practice Guidelines

Following are four guidelines for practicing socioculturally attuned SFFT. These include 1) inviting clients to explore the societal context in which they live, 2) considering equity when setting goals, 3) broadening the search for solutions to the wider societal and historical context, and 4) discovering and amplifying just solutions.

1. Invite Clients to Explore Societal Context

Socioculturally attuned SFF therapists invite clients to examine the relationship between societal context and presenting problems in order to expand possibilities for solutions and support equitable relationships. Therapists need to have the social awareness to know where to look and what to ask, but not assume they know the social reality of clients' lives. Therapists and clients explore social dynamics together, engaging in mutual consciousness raising. It is assumed that each family has a unique relationship to its societal context, and therapists must **attune** to their specific situation. In other words, societal context plays out differently across families, and the therapist must take a stance of inquiry to help families explore context as integral to the meaning they make of the world, including how they relate to each other.

2. Consider Equity in Co-constructing Client Goals

Socioculturally attuned SFF therapists work with families to ensure goals include as many members as possible and support relational equity. Imagine asking a few well-placed questions in addition to the typical miracle question, such as: "So you have described that when this problem is gone all of you will be communicating more. I am curious about how you **envision** each of you being heard by the others. Whose voice will carry the most influence and be heard the loudest? Who is likely not to be heard or have as much influence in conversations?" and/or "What will it look like when you all have the influence you need to feel heard and get your needs met?" As clients answer these questions, they are likely to negotiate goals that include attention to power dynamics. The therapist might **name** the impact of the family's societal context by asking questions like, "What will be the difference between how males and females are heard in your family?" "How will this be the same or different from your experience in the rest of your lives?" Socioculturally attuned SFF therapists continue to check with clients about the impact of goals relative to their relational power throughout the course of therapy.

3. Broaden Search for Solutions to Wider Context

SFF therapists listen carefully to clients' values that may not be directly expressed but are implicit in conversation (Sundman, et al., 2020). Socioculturally attuned SFF therapists also broaden the search for solutions by **valuing** the wider social and historical context. This includes working with clients to identify collective resistance and resilience. Clients are encouraged to consider the exceptions of their ancestors, those in their social identity groups, and those whom they admire. Having ancestors who maintained their humanity even when enslaved, practicing religion in spite of discrimination, or being part of a group that continues to practice cultural traditions in spite of colonization and attempted genocide are examples of the power of the collective. Individuals within these collectives are also important sources of strength, resilience, and exceptions (e.g., a grandmother who left an abusive relationship to raise children on her own, a sibling who came out in spite of family disapproval, a leader in the Civil Rights movement, a parent who went to college later in life). Exploring these resources often exposes shared characteristics or solutions that can be amplified. Questions might include: "In what ways are you like your grandmother?" "How have the many generations of your religion been able to stay faithful in spite of discrimination?" and "How have you been active in keeping cultural traditions going?"

4. Identify and Amplify Just Solutions

Therapists and clients work collaboratively to identify and amplify exceptions. They expand available solutions and then choose from possibilities. Each member of the family is asked to identify exceptions and prompted to do more of what works. Socioculturally attuned SFF therapists add a step to this process by **intervening** to ensure that what works is just; that exceptions which are amplified are those that all members of the therapeutic system agree to support, or at least don't interfere with relational equity, and that equity is supported in all relationships, such as relationships in the workplace, social groups, and religious communities. Socioculturally attuned SFF therapists pay constant attention to societal stereotypes and systems of discrimination and oppression. Consider a male client answering a question such as "What seems to help the two of you get along better?" with "When she listens to me!" Of course listening to each other helps most of us get along, yet few therapists would proceed with "So do you agree that listening to your husband helps the two of you get along better?" It would not be uncommon, however, for a therapist to say something like "So do you both agree that you get along better when you listen to each other?"

A socioculturally attuned SFF therapist again takes a few extra steps toward **transformation,** resisting the temptation to gloss over the power imbalance indicated in the original statement. The therapist might ask the husband "So you would like your wife to listen to you. What does that mean for you? How do you know when she is listening to you? How does she know when you listen to her?" and then ask the wife "What do you think he means when he says he wants you to listen to him? How do you know when he is listening to you?" and so on.

Socioculturally attuned solution-focused family therapists ensure that family members do not act in ways that oppress or limit each other's strengths and solutions. Rather, the therapist works with the family to ensure equitable relationships that support the well-being of all members.

Case Illustration

Tina, age 40, immigrated from Taiwan to the US when she was 25 and married a European American man, David, age 39. Most of her family still lives in Taiwan, including her parents and two siblings, and their children. Her nephew, Eric, did not do as well as the family hoped on the Taiwanese national Form III exam at the end of junior high and was placed in a less than desirable high school. The likelihood of Eric not passing college entrance exams in Taiwan loomed over the family. Eric's parents also wanted Eric to become more fluent in English than was possible in compulsory English language courses and costly after school programs. Simply put, like most parents, they wanted their child to have opportunities for a better life. The extended family collectively decided Eric would live with Tina and David to attend high school and college in the US.

Within months of arriving, Eric had become isolated, spending most of his time in his room. Try as they might, Tina and David were not successful in drawing Eric out to be an active member of their family. David had become irritated with Eric's seeming unwillingness to contribute to basic family chores. David complained to Tina about Eric leaving his plate on the table or having to be asked to gather his dirty laundry week after week. Eric had also become increasingly unhappy with his aunt, whom he expected would be there to help him more than she was. Tina was caught in the middle, feeling burdened by her brother's expectation that she would take on the responsibility of raising her nephew and worrying she was burdening David with her family problems.

Eric felt lost in the US, unable to speak the language fluently or understand the culture. He was not making friends at school, relying on communicating mainly with his aunt, and playing video games with kids back home whenever he got the chance. Tina and her sister-in-law talked daily about Eric and how Tina and David might help him adjust. Things did not improve, however, despite their efforts. Eventually, Tina asked Eric's parents for permission to take him to therapy. Tina was referred by one of her friends to a Taiwanese American family therapist, Alice, who worked from a solution-focused framework.

Invite Clients to Explore Societal Context

The therapist explored the relationships between David, Tina, and Eric, including how they saw the problem within their societal and cultural context. Eric described his Aunt Tina as "not having Chinese thinking." He expected his aunt to offer him more guidance, help him more with daily decisions, monitor his homework, and instruct him in what she expected him to do around the house. Eric respected his aunt as his elder, but there had been little connection between them before he arrived in the US. David wanted Eric to be more independent and thought that by now he should be able to see what needed to be done and take responsibility for his own schoolwork. David and Eric agreed that they expected Tina to be the bridge between them. Following is an excerpt from their therapy conversation:

Alice: So Tina, you mentioned that you are sort of a bridge between Eric and David. Also, between your family here and your family in Taiwan?

Tina: Yes, I guess I am. I want to support my brother and nephew but also want to make sure David doesn't have to take on my whole family.

Alice: So trying to bridge what everybody needs?

David: She is the one everybody goes to. She is the bridge for Eric too.

Alice: Eric, you go to your aunt when you need something, or don't understand something about being here?

Eric: Yes. My aunt helps me the most.

Alice: So Tina is the bridge because she knows both countries—knows how to think Chinese and to think US. How do each of you think gender expectations might play into this on both ends of the bridge? To Tina's role in helping everyone understand each other?

Alice continued to help the family explore the transnational contexts, which were impacting their daily lives and each of their contributions to helping the family adjust, before moving on to co-construct goals. It was evident that Tina was expected to take on the most responsibility for cultural translation. As a Taiwanese American woman living with a European American man, she had been the one to culturally accommodate. David did not put equal effort into bridging the cultures, assuming Tina would take on this burden. Gender dynamics were also at play as Tina's husband, brother, and nephew all expected her to solve family problems.

Consider Equity in Co-constructing Client Goals

After exploring cultural and societal context, Alice was in a better position to co-construct equitable goals. The family went on to talk about what it will look like when they no longer need a bridge or a cultural translator. They agreed that one of their goals was everyone learning to live in two cultures at once.

Alice: When you have all adjusted to living together in two cultures, what will we notice? What will you see each other and yourselves doing differently?

David: Eric will be talking to us more, spending more time trying to make friends...contributing to the household without always being asked...

Alice: And what will you be doing differently, David?

David: Maybe not going to Tina every time I don't understand Eric or don't like what he is doing? Taking more on myself.

Alice: Tina, what will you be doing differently when you are no longer carrying most of the burden of being the bridge in the family?

In the excerpt above, David begins answering the miracle question with what he wants from Eric. Alice continues to ask questions that will co-construct a goal that encourages equal participation and holds everyone equally accountable for change. The conversation continued in this way until all members of the family and the therapist co-created the goal of everyone working together to learn how to live in two cultures at the same time. The goal was then carefully defined and described. This might include recognizing when cultural norms and values are at odds, making room for multiple traditions, and learning key words in both languages. This goal challenged the inequity of those in the most marginalized cultural positions (i.e., outsiders from the less globally powerful Taiwan) needing to be the ones to adjust to those in the most centered and dominant cultural positions (those in the most privileged group in the more powerful host country). Likewise, contributions were expected to be equal among all genders.

Broaden Search for Solutions to Wider Context

Alice searched for exceptions by identifying ways David and Tina were already able to live together and adjust to living in two cultures at once. Exceptions included each of them explaining cultural differences to their families, negotiating different values, beliefs, and cultural practices, and thinking about cultural differences rather than assuming the worst when differences arose between them. Alice also asked about Eric's willingness to come to a new country, his ability to navigate school, and times when he was aware of cultural differences. Alice helped the family draw from collective successes. These included drawing from the rich history of Chinese and Taiwanese people in the US, including how they coped with discrimination and cultural differences and stories of those like Tina who found ways to successfully live in the US without losing connection to core cultural values or family in her home country.

Identify and Amplify Just Solutions

The therapist in this case was careful not to promote or amplify solutions that worked for some but were not just solutions for others. For example, asking Tina to continue to work harder than the rest of the family to bridge the two cultures may have worked and in fact, had been working to some extent, but was not a just solution. Alice could reasonably assume that amplifying unjust solutions would lead to further problems later on. Identifying and amplifying just exceptions and solutions included times when David and Tina talked together with Eric to help him interpret differences in US and Taiwanese culture. It also included times when David worked to understand and support Taiwanese cultural beliefs, values, and practices in ways that matched Tina's work to learn about and fit into European American culture. Alice helped the family amplify times when David and Eric spent time together, and when Eric went to David for help and David advised him.

Summary: Third Order Change

Third order change occurred in this family when there were major shifts in how they saw the world and the problems they were having within this expanded view (Ecker & Hulley, 1996). The family was able to consider more possibilities for how to organize their relationships when they were able to take a metaview of culture and transnational power dynamics, as well as gender across two societies. This helped them realize the impact of these broad social arrangements on their most intimate relationships and to make more conscious choices about how they wanted to live. The therapist invited the family into third order change by asking questions that placed their lives within cultural and societal context.

The family continued to work on bridging two very different cultures in a single household, but now did so from a perspective that broadened options. They could more consciously share the burden of living in two cultures rather than Tina having to do all of the cultural accommodating. They developed a more critical view of the relationships between countries and the tendency for one partner's culture and gender to dominate the other. Third order change made it impossible to automatically assume the prescribed and stereotypical roles of a female cultural outsider who must learn to live in the US and a White US male who married an accommodating Asian female. This arrangement was now one of many possibilities that Tina and David could choose for their lives together and with Eric.

Reflexive Questions

- Solution-focused family therapy is more about amplifying strengths and creating change than about understanding or treating problems. How is this stance countercultural within psychotherapy/mental health fields? What values does it represent?
- When considering your work as a solution-focused family therapist, how do you see yourself supporting social equity? What factors enable you to do this?
- If you were to write a list of societal forces that increase solutions, what would they be? What broader set of exceptions could be amplified?
- How do you challenge power dynamics between yourself and your clients? What values, beliefs, and knowledge enable you to see your clients as experts of their own lives and to work in collaborative and power-sharing ways?
- How is it that choosing to amplify strengths and refusing to focus on problem-saturated descriptions and labels are forms of activism? What sociocultural forces are being resisted or challenged?
- How do you determine if the solutions or exceptions to the problem you are asking each member of the family to identify are just and equitable?

References

Anderson, H. & Goolishan, H. (1992). The client is the expert: A not-knowing approach to therapy. In S. McNamee & K. J. Gergen, (Eds.). *Therapy as a social construction* (pp. 25–39). Sage.

Bidwell, D. R. (2007). Miraculous knowing: Epistemology and solution-focused therapy. In T. S. Nelson, & F. N. Thomas (Eds.). *Handbook of solution-focused brief therapy* (pp. 65–88). Haworth Press.

Bolton, K., Hall, J., Blundo, R. & Lehmann, P. (2017). The role of resilience and resilience theory in solution-focused practice. *Journal of Systemic Therapies*, *36*(3), 1–15.

Chenail, R., Reiter, M., Torres-Gregory, M. & Ilic, D. (2020). Postmodern family therapy. In K. Wampler, R. Miller, & R. Seedall (Eds.), *Handbook of systemic family therapy* (Vol. 1, pp. 417–442). Wiley & Sons.

Choi, J. (2019). A microanalytic case study of the utilization of "solution-focused problem talk" in solution-focused brief therapy. *The American Journal of Family Therapy*, *47*(4), 244–260.

Courtnage, A. (2025). Solution focused single session therapy: Small conversations for big social change. In A. Wulf and J. Von Cziffra-Bergs (Eds.). *Women's perspectives on the solution-focused approach: International applications and interventions* (pp. 55–74). Routledge.

De Jong, P. (2019). A brief, informal history of SFBT as told by Steve de Shazer and Insoo Kim Berg. *Journal of Solution-focused Practices*, *3*(1), pp. 9–16.
De Jong, P. & Berg, I. K. (1998). *Interviewing for solutions*. Thomson Brooks/Cole Publishing Co.
Dermer, S. B., Hemesath, C. W., & Russell, C. S. (1998). A feminist critique of solution-focused therapy. *The American Journal of Family Therapy*, *26*(3), 239–250.
de Shazer, S. (1997). Some thoughts on language use in therapy. *Contemporary Family Therapy, 19*(1), 133–141.
de Shazer, S. (1988). *Clues: Investigating solutions in brief therapy*. WW Norton & Co.
de Shazer, S. & Berg, I. K. (1992). Doing therapy: A post-structural re-vision. *Journal of Marital and Family Therapy*, *18*(1), 71–81.
de Shazer, S. & Dolan, Y. (2007/2021). *More than miracles: The state of the art of solution-focused brief therapy*. Routledge. (Original work published in 2007, Hawthorn Press.)
de Shazer, S., Dolan, Y., Korman, H., Trepper, T., McCollum, E., & Berg, I. K. (2021). *More than miracles: The state of the art of solution-focused brief therapy* (2nd ed.). Routledge.
Dolan, Y. (2024). *Solution-focused therapy: The basics*. Routledge.
Ecker, B. & L. Hulley. (1996). *Depth oriented brief therapy: How to be brief when you were trained deep and vice versa*. Jossey Bass.
Freire, P. (1970/2000). *Pedagogy of the oppressed*. Bloomsbury. (Original work published in 1970).
Korin, E. C. (1994). Social inequalities and therapeutic relationships: Applying Freire's ideas to clinical practice. *Journal of Feminist Family Therapy*, *5*(3–4), 75–98.
Lipchik, E. (2017). My story about solution-focused brief therapist/client relationships. *Journal of Systemic Therapies*, *36*(4), 76–89.
Lipchik, E. (2002). *Beyond technique in solution-focused therapy: Working with emotions and the therapeutic relationship*. Guilford Press.
McKergow, M. (2021). *The next generation of solution-focused practice: Stretching the world for new opportunities and progress*. Routledge.
Neipp, M. C. & Beyebach, M. (2024). The global outcomes of solution-focused brief therapy: A revision. *The American Journal of Family Therapy*, *52*(1), 110–127.
Nelson, T. (2019). *Solution-focused brief therapy with families*. Routledge.
Nelson, T. & Thomas, N. (Eds.). (2007). *Handbook of solution-focused brief therapy*. Haworth Press.
O'Hanlon, B. (1999). *Do one thing different: And other uncommonly sensible solutions to life's persistent problems*. William Morrow & Company.
O'Hanlon, B. & Rowan, T. (2003). *Solution-Oriented Therapy*. Norton.
O'Hanlon, B., & Weiner-Davis, M. (1989/2003). *In search of solutions: A new direction in psychotherapy*. Norton. (Original work published 1989.)
Pitkin, H. (1972). *Wittgenstein and Justice*. University of California Press.
Reiter, M. (2010). Hope and expectancy in solution-focused brief therapy. *Journal of Family Psychotherapy*, *21*, 132–148.
Selekman, M. D. (1997). *Solution-focused therapy with children: Harnessing family strengths for systemic change*. Guilford Press.
Singer, S. (2024). *Brief therapy for clients with challenging or unique issues*. Routledge.
Sundman, P., Schwab, M., Wolf, F., Wheeler, J., Cabie, M-C., van der Hoorn, S., Pakrosmis, R., Dierolf, K., & Hejerth, M. (2020). *Theory of solution-focused practice*. European Brief Therapy Association, Books on Demand.
Thomas, F. N. & Nelson, T. (2007). Assumptions and practices within the solution-focused brief therapy tradition. In T. S. Nelson & F. N. Thomas (Eds.). *Handbook of solution-focused brief therapy* (pp. 3–24). Haworth Press.
Walter, J. & Peller, J. (1992). *Becoming solution-focused in brief therapy*. Brunner/Mazel.
van Dijk, T. A. (2015). Critical discourse analysis. In D. Tannen, H. Hamilton, & D. Schiffrin (Eds.). *The handbook of discourse analysis* (2nd ed., pp. 466–485). Wiley.
Zatloukal, L., Žákovský, D. & Bezdíčková, E. (2019). Utilizing metaphors in solution-focused therapy. *Contemporary Family Therapy 41*, 24–36.

13 Socioculturally Attuned Collaborative-Dialogic Family Therapy

Collaborative practice (Anderson, 1997), also known as the collaborative language systems approach (Anderson, 1993, 1995; Anderson & Goolishian, 1988), collaborative-dialogic practice (Anderson 2023), and the postmodern collaborative approach (2012a), attends to the relationship between client and therapist, listening and responding to client's narratives through a dialogic process that generates new thought and action (Anderson, 2023). Originally, Anderson and Goolishian (1988) conceptualized this new theoretical perspective as therapists working within "a linguistics system" distinguished by those who are "in language about a problem" instead of people organized by social organizations, such as families, parents, couples, etc. They contended that the role of the therapist is that of a "master of conversation, an architect of dialogue, whose expertise creates the space for and facilitates dialogical conversation" (p. 372). Leaders in the field of family therapy such as Harlene Anderson, Harry Goolishian, Lynn Hoffman, Tom Anderson, and Peggy Penn were instrumental in developing these practices; however, they are now applied across many disciplines (Anderson & Gehart, 2023).

Collaborative-dialogic family therapists are known for taking a humble, unassuming "not-knowing stance" and examining multiple narratives and perspectives in order to create new meanings and possibilities. Anderson asserted that working from this collaborative stance is a philosophy of life in action; "a way of thinking with, experiencing with, relating with, and responding with the people we meet in therapy (Anderson, 2007, p. 43)." It is a political and ethical value position that counters dominance inherent in the therapist role through practices that engage clients as equals (Anderson, 2023; Bava, 2023). This way of working is not considered a model, theory, or framework. Instead, Anderson described it as a way of *being* with others that demonstrates that they are seen, listened to, respected and appreciated as unique and important people. This *withness*, first proposed by Lynn Hoffman in 2007, refers to a relationship that shares space in a communal, collective, and intimate manner. These relationships and conversations invite and encourage others to participate in ways that are equitable (Anderson, 2012a).

↞→

Collaborative-dialogical practices encourage third order change through generative dialogue that expands possibilities for more equitable relationships in families and society.

↞→

In this chapter, we identify core enduring concepts of collaborative-dialogic practices and then integrate the tenets of socioculturally attuned family therapy into the practice of collaborative therapy. We illustrate these ideas by sharing a case example of a Latino family in crisis due to the deportation of their son.

DOI: 10.4324/9781003493426-13

Enduring and Foundational Concepts

Below, we describe what we believe are enduring concepts of collaborative-dialogic practices, including 1) social construction of meaning, 2) therapy as a dialogic process between conversational partners, 3) a therapist's not-knowing stance, and 4) therapy as a mutual endeavor toward possibilities.

Social Construction of Meaning

Social constructionists assume that knowledge and meaning evolve through interactions between people. It is impossible to know outside of context (Rosen, 1996). Words do not have meaning in and of themselves. They derive their meaning from the contexts in which they are created and change from one context to another (Bava, 2019a). Language is more than just the words and gestures that are expressed or performed. Meaning emerges from the cultural practices that define and shape our interaction, and the boundaries between self and society become blurred (Chenail et al., 2020). Through language, we construct the manner by which thoughts, feelings, and behaviors are produced, which is historically and culturally located (McNamee & Gergen, 1992; Monk & Gehart, 2003). Collaborative-dialogic therapists exude the belief that those with whom they meet are important and have something worthy to say and worthy of being heard.

Therapists also need to be aware of what they bring to the conversation. "Similar to mindfulness, it takes practice to learn how to quiet one's inner meaning-making narrator" (Gehart, 2023, p. 57). It is important to meet clients without judgment of past, present, or future. Therapists are aware of their biases, preferences, and meaning-making, but do not have a hidden agenda. As described by Gehart, collaborative-dialogic practitioners learn to balance their focus on what is being said—the outer dialogue—with their own inner dialogue, so that over time, a natural rhythm will emerge.

The practice of *withness* (Hoffman, 2007, 2012; Hoffman, 2018) is a participatory process that is mutual rather than hierarchical and dualistic (Anderson, 2007; Anderson, 2012b). According to Anderson (2023, p. 25), "withness challenges an expert–no-expert dichotomy by respecting the expertise, knowledge, and resources that each person brings." Therapists honor their own education, knowledge, lived experience, and awareness of cultural discourses, but shift their relationship to what they think they know so as to be open and curious about other perspectives and emergent possibilities (Bull & D'Arrigo, 2026). It is within this space of mutual dialogic exploration that unpredictable newness can emerge. The therapist must set the stage for collaboration and generativity, focusing on how relationships and conversations mutually influence each other. The dialogue requires a commitment to the relationship and vice versa.

Conversational Partners

Before meeting or knowing anything about the clients, therapists assume clients will be collaborators or co-investigators (Guilfoyle, 2006). At the most basic level, the primary aim of the therapist is to facilitate a generative conversation in which all persons are engaged and heard by each other (Mills & Sprenkle, 1995). This dialogic process is the primary "intervention." The pacing of the conversation is often slower than other conversations in order to allow space and time for inner dialogues to shape and take new forms. Through the subtle shifts of inner and outer dialogue, each person's perspective and experience of the problem shifts (Monk & Gehart, 2003). It is not possible to predict how the story will unfold or how it will end. The dialogical process is an *intentional, generative, dynamic mutual activity* that feels distinct from other forms of language, such as a discussion, debate, or simply chatting (Anderson, 2007). This philosophical stance is a way of being and becoming with others (Anderson & Gehart, 2023).

Therapists facilitate a process that keeps all voices in motion and contributing to the conversation. They model honesty and sincerity, being receptive to hearing and being engaged in each other's story. Each client should feel as though they are equally important and that their version of the narrative is as important as that of others. Therapists are intentional about not siding with any one particular person, but being "for" all persons simultaneously. However, as we'll discuss later in the chapter, therapists must also be aware that societal power processes create imbalances that complicate this practice and can leave some important views unsaid (Bull & D'Arrigo, 2026).

Humility and Uncertainty

Taking a not-knowing stance is one of the most important, and also potentially misunderstood, aspects of collaborative practices (Anderson, 2005). Collaborative therapists walk a tightrope between understanding and not understanding, knowing and not-knowing. The not-knowing stance does not mean that the therapist does not know. That would be impossible. It means that therapists bracket or suspend what they believe they know so that assumptions can be avoided and new understandings can emerge (Anderson, 2012b). Remaining curious and attending to clients' local knowledge and their lived experience is at the core. Not knowing also involves keeping an open and receptive mind to whatever the client is saying so as to remain alert for openings for newness and possibilities (Gehart, 2023).

From this stance, participants continuously challenge their assumptions and are receptive to alternatives and untapped potential. This means welcoming multiple and sometimes contradictory narratives. Although a therapist is always informed, prepared, educated, well-trained, and knowledgeable, the stance of not-knowing is about having the willingness and humility to remain in a respectful, unassuming, learner position. It also means being willing to experience the discomfort that arises when venturing into new, often previously marginalized, space (Bava, 2019b). According to Malinen et al., (2012), "the therapist is not burdened with being 'right' but with being present and responsive" (p. xiii). Certainty has the potential of limiting and shutting down possibilities and blocking our abilities to be experience near (Gertz, 1974) and relationally responsive in our work with clients.

Expanding Possibilities

Possibilities unfold when both clients and therapists are in the moment and open to being influenced. The dialogic process invites participants to influence and be influenced, to shape and be shaped by the interaction, and to mutually co-create meaning. Through this rich process, the *not-yet* said or heard meanings can emerge (Guilfoyle, 2003). Being open to possibilities, instead of dogmatically holding on to predetermined scripts and "shoulds," enables participants to explore paths that are better suited for their lives, contexts, and preferred ways of living and being. Doors can open in ways that were previously limited by social constraints. Clients might say things like, "I have never thought of that before," "I could not have imagined doing something like this before now," or "No one has ever mentioned this to me in this way." These types of comments reflect ways in which clients experience the opening of spaces for new realities and possibilities to emerge.

Integrating Principles of Sociocultural Attunement

Hare-Mustin (1994) said a therapy room can be like a mirrored room in which a therapist and client can only openly discuss what is reflected in the dialogue between them. If the therapist or clients feel unable to address larger social issues (i.e., racism, classism, xenophobia, homophobia, transphobia, ableism, sexism, etc.) because the client has not brought these discourses into the room, then third order change is not likely (Ellis & Bermúdez, 2021). Hare-Mustin suggested that it is the responsibility of the therapist to develop consciousness about larger systemic issues and invite these topics into the room so that these social forces do not remain silent. In the words of Bull & D'Arrigo (2026): "What is radically revised in queer-contextualized collaborative therapy is the silence inherent in the theory, the lack of guidance to talk about how social positions materially impact peoples' lives. There is a whiteness to that silence, one that makes too much room for status quo replication" (p. 211). Socioculturally attuned collaborative therapists open these dialogues, knowing that while language can marginalize and constrain, it can also empower and liberate (Chenail et al., 2020).

Societal Context

Collaborative-dialogic therapists view language as not just the way we talk, but as a way we create and are created by the world. As such, justice is manifested in the ways we relate to one another and in the interplay between larger structural and systemic forces and discursive processes (Bava & McNamee, 2019; Bava, 2022). Saliha Bava (2022) described the interplay between these forces as a relational loop (2022), and posited collaborative-dialogic practices as an "antidote to the dominance-based approaches" (p. 37). In Text Box 13.1 Bava explains the relational discursive loop and how she works with it in therapy.

Text Box 13.1 Saliha Bava, PhD, LMFT

Saliha Bava (she, hers, hers, they) is a Professor and MFT Program Director at Mercy University in New York and does private practice and organizational consultation. She orients to collaborative-dialogic practices and draws on Anderson, Gergen, McNamee and Shotter's social constructionism, critical theory, communicative action, Bakhtin's dialogism, Bateson, Wittgenstein, Boal's theater of the oppressed, performance theory, and Milton Erickson's offerings, among others.

I view all practices, and by extension, my work, as political. Political is "what people…do together and what their doing ***makes****" in the world (McNamee, 2009, p. 62). I see my "work" as being relationally responsive to how we are shaping this world even as it shapes our everyday encounters. Such relational responsiveness, which is a political activity, positions us to see how our somatic experiences, local knowledge, language, and participation are deeply intertwined discursive processes in creating the structural and the systemic processes, which in turn shapes and is shaped by our storied realities as illustrated in the figure below.*

"My work"
It's a process of living in search for meaning
It's a play of liberation
It's a play of imagination
It's a play of dialectics

Sociocultural context is at the heart of it all; it is the water we swim in and what we produce from within our everyday engagements. Rather than view social locations and structures as static entities, my curiosity leans towards how the systemic structural processes are constructed from within the interactional and discursive, which in turn are shaped by the systemic structural—what I call the relational discursive loop (Bava, 2022).

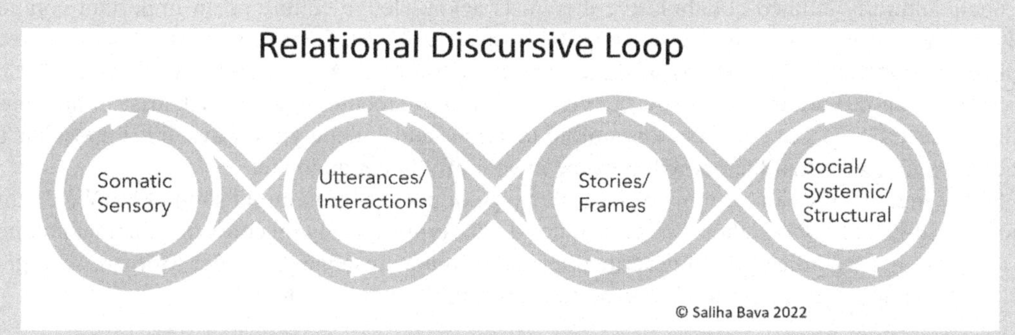

Figure 13.1 Relational discursive loop

I engage in what I call hyperlinked conversations (interviewing) (Bava, 2019a, 2019b), where we are listening to what matters to the person and how they are connecting the dots between the various spaces within the loop. My process includes attending to our presence, listening with curiosity to what is emerging, how context is shaping and being shaped, while noticing the power of withness talk. I call this relational play (Bava, 2020) an improvised contextually responsive, emergent play. It is a way of weaving back and forth with the other in the process of sensemaking between the broader and local contexts of people's storied lives. It is a frame from which to engage our differences, to listen for and respond from where someone is speaking, listening, or participating. It offers us a way to value each person's unique ways of participating while also inviting them to notice what their participation is creating in the world around them.

Working in NYC, where I encounter people from all over the world, it is hard to say that I will know what is silencing or marginalizing for each couple or family I meet. I follow the client's lead. I assume that each culture, as experienced and engaged by the client, has its own way in which the process of domination, subjugation, and liberation operates. And, it is by adopting a stance of cultural curiosity while leaning into uncertainty that I encounter the unspoken or even the unspeakable, but often with a felt presence that touches us. The felt presence can be a gaze, a gesture, a rush of words, tension, a sensation, sudden laughter, discomfort, etc. Thus, orienting towards the embodied, a felt presence with cultural curiosity and permission, I seek to engage that which might be silenced or marginalized while attempting to make sense of what is emerging with our engagement.

As is clearly illustrated by the present day social and racial equity movements, as social systems act on us, we act back on these systems. In recognizing this discursive flow of organizing life forces between the personal and the social, we can reclaim our agency and voice as participants within the socio-relational political processes. The transformative quality lies in not only noticing the discursive process but to see the choice points in our everyday participation—from orienting to our embodied sensations to the use of language, to the construction of stories/meanings, to the reconstructions of institutional systems. Such a perspective offers us a range of possibilities, as participants, to not only be consumers but also to be producers of preferred social organizing.

•←→•

Socioculturally attuned collaborative therapists engage in conversations with a heightened awareness of sociopolitical and contextual issues and how they affect our lives.

•←→•

Socioculturally attuned collaborative therapists acknowledge culture as an important component of local meaning-making (Anderson, 2023; Bava, 2023; St. George & Wulff, 2014) and recognize the material consequences of these contexts (Bull & D'Arrigo, 2026; McDowell, 2015). They do not know until they are in the conversation what sociocultural issues will arise or how they will manifest. Given that conversations unfold in unique and collaborative ways, it is impossible to predict which contextual factors will become meaningful in the dialogue.

Following, we offer an example of what this type of conversation might sound like. We do this understanding that our collaborative colleagues do not typically rely on conversational techniques or offer examples of dialogue to describe their philosophical stance. Consider Morgan, who presented to therapy with an expressed desire to transition from male to female.

Morgan: I always felt different.

Therapist: What do you mean? Would you be willing to tell me more about feeling different?

Morgan: I guess I just felt different… I was always teased and mocked at school for the types of clothes I wore, especially my old shoes.

Therapist: (curious about the societal context around the notion of "old shoes") Old shoes?

Morgan: It was humiliating, especially in middle school. We would mostly shop at the thrift store and garage sales…(long pause)… I hated going with my mom—I was embarrassed. I didn't fit in at school and my parents were struggling too hard to help me.

Therapist: I am curious about what you said about your parents struggling too hard to help you. Would it be ok to talk more about that?

Morgan: Sure. Maybe I sometimes resent them, but I get it. They grew up with nothing and they tried really hard. They never had enough money. They both had crappy jobs. I wanted nice things but then I also felt bad when they had to work so hard to get them. Sometimes I kind of felt guilty.

Therapist: Yeah, that seems really hard…growing up without enough money…with your parents working so hard.

Morgan was struggling financially and felt at risk of being evicted from their apartment. The therapist may have initially thought that the conversation would focus on Morgan's feelings around the desire to transition; however, the therapist realized as the conversation progressed that Morgan was concerned about their financial situation and struggled with resentment toward their parents.

The larger social constraints of poverty and classism were influencing Morgan's current struggles. As Anderson (2012a) suggested, we are born, live, and are educated within mostly invisible grand knowledge narratives, universal truths, and dominant discourses in societal contexts that we take for granted. The grand narratives of meritocracy and the intersection of gender and poverty affected Morgan's sense of self and relationship with their parents. It was essential that the therapist was able to remain experience near (D'Arrigo-Patrick et al., 2016; Newman, 2024) and engage as a conversational partner, gently examining the larger forces that impacted Morgan's life.

Therapist: How do you think those "old shoes" and all the struggle you have been through about not having enough affect you now?

Morgan: Well, I hate to say this, but I feel like I got ripped off somehow. I wasn't given a lot to build from like my friends and the kids in college. And I always work so hard and still feel like I'm broke all the time. I can never seem to just make it. And I know that people discriminate against me because I'm queer, especially at work. It just sucks all the way around.

Therapist: Sucks all the way around…hmm… Would it be ok to help me try to understand what that means for you? Can you say more about that?

The therapist continues to stay with Morgan, walking with them closely through their experience, through the effects of societal context.

•←→•

Given that grand narratives have so much power and authority in society, they seduce us into practices that can distance others and create dissonance for ourselves and our preferred ways of being.

•←→•

In addition to the grand narratives clients hold about their lives, as therapists, we also have grand narratives about ourselves, our work, and our profession. The names we use to describe the profession of family therapy, as well as the politics and economics of diagnoses, are also important grand narratives. For example, our field is often referred to as "mental health," "behavioral health," "behavioral medicine," among others. These names were constructed by larger social systems and have been used to define the practice of "psychotherapy." Socioculturally attuned collaborative family therapists remain vigilant about how these dominant narratives define us and our work, often constraining possibilities and putting therapists in positions of imposing these ideas through diagnostic categories. In the example with Morgan, the therapist was also in the position of serving as a gatekeeper in Morgan's ability to proceed with the transition process.

Grand societal narratives affect how people know themselves, construct their problems and solutions, and participate in therapy. For example, a therapist might diagnose Morgan with gender dysphoria to get approval for hormone treatment and insurance coverage. However, Morgan might be anxious about that, not knowing who would see the diagnosis and how this could impact their living situation (e.g., housing, insurance coverage, and employment). A socioculturally attuned collaborative therapist would name injustices embedded in the medical context and engage Morgan in conversations to ensure they have the opportunity to carefully navigate difficult decisions.

As socioculturally attuned therapists, we must remain vigilant about how and why we support or reject grand narratives. These narratives have a direct effect on how we engage as conversational partners. We must remain aware of how factors such as racism, classism, sexism, and homophobia affect the ways clients engage as conversational partners (Ashbourne et al., 2016) and what narratives may be voiced or heard (Bull & D'Arrigo, 2026), and make the connections between their experiences, ideas, and the larger sociocultural context transparent.

•←→•

Socioculturally attuned collaborative therapists do not remain neutral about the ways clients are affected by social inequality; they invite these perspectives into the dialogue.

•←→•

It is important to understand that, as conversational partners, therapists have a responsibility to bring a voice to the dialogue (Cheon & Murphy, 2007). In fact, clients may misinterpret silence as collusion with larger dominant discourses. Let's consider a therapist who listens intentionally, respectfully, and quietly for a long period of time as a client speaks of his religious beliefs. The client becomes notably anxious as the therapist continues to affirm minimally, with an "uh huh" and slightly nodding his head. The client is left unsettled because he feels vulnerable in sharing his experience and feelings and the therapist's level of engagement does not match that of the client, exaggerating the therapist's position of power by remaining silent and invulnerable. His silence is disconcerting and confusing to the client because he does not know where the therapist stands in response to what has been disclosed. The process needs engaged equitable conversational partners, each contributing to the dialogue in proportionate, transparent, and appropriate ways.

Socioculturally attuned collaborative therapists are transparent with their concerns about the impact of societal structures on dialogical processes and how these realities may limit possibilities generated in the clinical dialogue. D'Arrigo-Patrick and colleagues (2016) examined how therapists handle possible tensions between collaborative practices and addressing social justice. They found that therapists brought issues of fairness and larger context to the clinical conversation by asking questions that bring social justice to the forefront and staying close to the client experience. For example, a therapist might ask, "Could it be that racism plays a role in what you are experiencing?" Findings showed that the distinction between activism and collaboration was a false dichotomy. In varying ways, therapists balance raising these issues and maintaining relationships with clients. This balance can be strengthened when the therapist has a clear picture of the sociocultural context in which their therapeutic relationship is situated. In Text Box 13.2, Justine D'Arrigo describes how they attend to social justice issues in a collaborative manner, and how this varies depending on the power context of their various professional roles.

Text Box 13.2 Justine D'Arrigo, PhD, LMFT

Justine D'Arrigo (they/them) is a White queer Counseling and Therapy Associate Professor at California State University, San Bernardino. They are interested in the intersections of relational activism and therapy, navigating critical theory and poststructuralism, post-oppositional approaches to relationships and change, and exploring compositionism (Bruno Latour) and curiosity in therapy (moving beyond critique). Their work illustrates the careful attention to use of power when aligning with collaborative practices and other postmodern approaches.

As a White therapist and educator, I feel a tremendous responsibility to cultivate a deep awareness of sociocultural context. Some of what has made me so sensitized to this is my own queer identity. In many ways, I'm not able to see through any other lens but a sociocultural/sociopolitical one. I am always wondering **how**—*not if—various intersecting identities and social, cultural, and political contexts are shaping and informing story, experience, and meaning in some way.*

I name and identify these issues differently based on the contextual factors at play. Where there is high risk of harm, I might speak more explicitly about how I am attuning to issues arising from sociopolitical and sociocultural contexts. Most other times, I see curiosity as my greatest ally in attending to these issues in a way that exposes them without imposing them on clients. This might look like asking "How did you learn that this was expected of you in your marriage?" rather than asking "What messages have you received as a woman about how you should respond as a wife?" The first question might open space to expose some of the taken for granted ways gender structures relationship; whereas the second might impose gender as a way of making meaning.

My way of amplifying what's been silenced or marginalized happens differently in my faculty role than in a therapeutic context. As a faculty member who is White, I am intentional to explicitly name and speak to the practices that have a silencing and marginalizing effect. For instance, when a Colleague of Color is dismissed or spoken over, or when an older White cis male is taking up space to define for others, I will name this and call attention to it. In a therapeutic capacity, I rely on my curiosity. I make sure my curiosity is attentive and intentional in moving close to the places where people or experiences have been invisibilized.

I feel called to use my power to intentionally interrupt unjust practices at both the relational and systems level. In the university system over time, I have felt more compelled to use my power to challenge and hold myself accountable. With students, I feel compelled to use my power to both challenge and trouble things, while also creating a safe relational context that takes time to learn their experiences too. In a clinical capacity, I feel compelled to use my power to intentionally be tentative and curious.

I encourage third order change by always posing questions that work to expose whatever it is that is operating on our lives in a taken for granted and unquestioned way. I ask the questions that power wants to divert us from, for instance, Who benefits? Who might be harmed? What perspective is being privileged here? What perspective is possibly being overlooked or silenced? I think these questions allow folks to consider the many contexts within which our decisions, actions, and meaning-making processes are embedded. They often create a pause long enough for some self-reflexivity and cultural reflexivity to take root, which I see as supporting more just and equitable relationships. It is important to me, as someone who is White, to be thoughtful and careful with how I do this. I don't want to colonize others in a counter cultural way, particularly colleagues, students, and clients with minoritized identities, but I do want to be active in raising questions that might create even the smallest opening for change or difference in perspective.

Culture is created through the ways we create language, narratives, and social discourses (Laird, 2000). These narratives are both private (e.g., internal thoughts and processes) and public (e.g., as when we are talking to another person). We put our cultures into action through interactive processes that define ourselves and others.

•←→•

Socioculturally attuned collaborative therapists must attend to the relationship between the nuance of words, meanings, intonation, utterances, pauses, silences, and dominance.

•←→•

Cultural categories and language can justify stereotypes, power-over acts of violence (e.g., gay-bashing, victim-blaming), and cultural atrocities (e.g., ethnic cleansing, femicide, slavery). Conversely, compassionate words and the act of *listening* are important ways to enter people's lives by creating space for them to be heard. Language gains meaning from how we use it in our relationships, not just what we think our words represent (Strong, 2002).

•←→•

It is important to be mindful of the ways in which our social locations and intersecting identities affect the nuances as conversational partners within a collaborative relationship.

•←→•

How people communicate and participate as conversational partners depends in part on their cultural values and social locations. Laird (2000) asked, for example, "How is *this* person performing culture?" (p. 106). We add, how is this person or am I performing the intersections of gender, heteronormativity, middle-class, whiteness, etc.? Dominant discourses ascribe certain performances based on cultural norms (e.g., masculinity and femininity), which limit the possibilities generated. Socioculturally attuned therapists bring multiple possible perspectives or stories into the conversation.

Let's consider Don, a white Jewish man in his late 60s, known in the community for his collaborative practices with queer couples. He agreed to work with Tony and Gabriel, a gay Latino couple in their late 20s seeking help for Gabriel's "low sex drive." Upon meeting the couple, Don asked questions not simply to get answers, but in ways that allowed him to participate in the conversation in a curious way, responding to multiple perspectives, and to stay close to what is being said.

Don: Thank you for being here. I am eager to learn about what you both hope to accomplish by the end of our conversation. What would be most helpful for you to leave with today?

Gabriel: I want to tell Tony something I just discovered about myself. I want him to understand me and be OK with what I have to say.

Don: Would that be alright with you Tony? Is there something specifically you would like to see happen today, in addition to what Gabriel is wanting for your first session?

Tony: No, I'm good. I just really want to focus on what Gabriel wanted to talk to me about. I know it has been weighing heavy on his mind.

As a consequence, Gabriel disclosed to Tony that he thought he was asexual. He told Tony that he did not know he was asexual until he began to read more about it. Everything he read matched his perception of himself.

Don: Thank you for sharing that with us Gabriel. I am curious about what meaning this new identity has had for you personally, as well as for your relationship?

Gabriel: I feel liberated from my "fake self." I have always felt like I was playing a part; like I was performing being a man, which meant being sexual. I want to be loving and giving with Tony and share my life with him, but I am tired of pretending to be a man in that way.

Don wanted to contribute to and expand the conversation to include the possibility of addressing the impact of societal context on the couple.

Don: Could it be that social pressures and notions of masculinity and culture affected your desire to conform to those expectations?

Gabriel: For sure! No one understands it. All my brothers, my dad, and uncles, and friends are tough macho guys. They are always gay bashing and saying shit about women and "faggots" and "*culeros*" (derogatory and vulgar term in Spanish for gay men). It's exhausting and infuriating. I know that Tony is the only one who truly understands me. That is why I love him so much. I love you enough to be honest with you, Tony. I want to be fair to you.

Gabriel and Tony were able to engage in a generative dialogue that helped them understand each other and how they needed to redefine their relationship. The societal context in which they and most of us live does not support asexuality as an acceptable orientation for an attractive, Latino man in his late 20s, who is in a monogamous, committed relationship.

Gabriel told Tony that he loved him and was attracted to him and wanted to continue to share their lives together, but that he did not want to hold him back sexually. His sense of self as a sexual person was a part of him that did not feel authentic. Don gently invited questions into the discussion, such as "could it be that…?" and "I am curious about how…? These types of questions help examine how the larger societal context influenced Gabriel's thoughts and feelings about his sexuality. Both partners identified and talked about their experiences within multiple societal contexts and grand narratives in ways that helped them navigate and language their evolving relationship.

Power

Socioculturally attuned collaborative family therapists are aware of the ways power is relational and contextual. A person's power within any given context heavily influences the ability to engage in specific discourses or have voice to say what they need and want to say or to make the changes they would like to see. When a client is silenced or harmed by dominant discourses or when one family member is oppressed more than another, it is important that therapists position their dialogue to intervene in the imbalance.

•←→•

Thoughtful consideration of any relationship must include how the greater societal context informs interactions and the power dynamics embedded in those contexts.

•←→•

Socioculturally attuned collaborative therapists position themselves in relation to societally based power processes in order to effectively work with clients from their understandings and culturally informed dynamics of power. They ask questions that elicit cultural values of mutual respect, reciprocity, and shared commitment to relationships (Knudson-Martin, 2013). Clients also enter therapy with perceptions of themselves that reflect their positionality based on systems of oppression and/or privilege.

Let's consider Nasheema, a woman who presented for therapy because her parents were worried about her increasingly alternative "hippie" lifestyle (i.e., had many tattoos, facial piercings, wore mismatched old clothes, dyed hair), and was not doing well in college. Nasheema admitted that she was frustrated with college and not knowing what she wanted to major in or what she wanted for her future. She enjoyed her job at a coffee bar and worked 20 hours a week. Her parents were both professionals, and her siblings were academically and professionally "successful." Nasheema was the youngest of three and had never felt as though she fit into her family. Although she had been afforded many privileges and felt loved, she did not understand why they pressured her to do well in college and have a career. She claimed not feeling depressed or concerned about any other area of her life except for school and her parents' troubled and concerned reaction to her current situation. Her therapist, Renee, who was in her fifties, *appeared* to reflect many of the same values and beliefs as Nasheema's parents. It would have been easy for both of them to maintain positions that held each other in a negative light—ones that confirmed societal notions of power and privilege. Instead, Renee created the space in which Nasheema could authentically express herself.

Renee: You mentioned that you feel as though you don't measure up to your family's expectations of you. What do you think they are worried about?

Nasheema: They worry that I won't be able to support myself financially. They worked hard to give us a certain lifestyle with lots of opportunities, and I think they see me as throwing it all away by not taking advantage of the life I have been given. I feel like they see me as a bum, even though they would never say it. I can feel it. And it makes it worse that my sister and brother are so perfect. They worry about me too. They have it all together and all they care about is their jobs, nice things and expensive vacations. I don't care if I don't become something big.

Renee: I see. So to become something big, you have to make a lot of money and live a certain way? Can you help me understand that better?

Nasheema: That's right. It is as if I don't meet their expectations, then I am a failure in their eyes.

As the dialogue unfolded, they began to disentangle how power is embedded in cultural and societal scripts. Renee asked if Nasheema would be interested in learning more about the ways they both embraced, rejected, or reinforced certain culturally supported discourses. They brought up many issues; specifically, those related to social status, education, work, success, image, alternative lifestyles, familial expectations, youth, and aging. As they did so, Renee was open about her perspectives and possible biases. For example:

Renee: I imagine I come across as a pretty conventional person to you. I've done a lot of the things "society" defines as "success" —a college degree and all that.

Nasheema: (smiles) Yeah. You do look pretty conventional. I wasn't sure about you at first. But you seem interested in me.

Renee: Please let me know when I may not be understanding what matters to you. Honestly, I've always had a hard time understanding why people want tattoos, but I am appreciating it a lot more now.

Nasheema told Renee that it felt reassuring to know where Renee stood on certain issues and that she was frank about her stereotypes about people with tattoos; a bias and prejudice Renee was not proud to admit. They discussed how Nasheema began to feel as though certain possibilities were being blocked due to her appearance and beliefs, and that she felt judged for reasons that did not fit her perception of herself. She perceived herself as a kind, caring, thoughtful, creative, and helpful person. She said others saw her as a bum, living aimlessly without purpose—worthless. Renee stayed "experience near," continued to be transparent about her own thoughts, and asked questions that helped Nasheema make meaning of her experiences within multiple contexts of power and disempowerment.

Socioculturally attuned collaborative family therapists are keenly aware that we are all influenced by social forces that directly affect our sense of agency and actual agency to advocate for ourselves or others, and/or the ability to imagine equitable relationships. Renee had to position herself in her understanding of power dynamics; that all of us, in varying degrees, experience possibilities that are blocked due to institutional, structural, systemic oppression, while others who are members of dominant cultural groups benefit from the ties they have with those with sociopolitical and economic power. Nasheema has ties with people with societal power, such as her family and friends growing up, but their disapproval of her "lifestyle" did not enable her to fully benefit from the cultural and societal capital due to her association with them. Examining these power dynamics also helped Nasheema navigate what she wanted for her life while remaining connected to her family.

Another point to consider is the therapist's position of power. Regardless of the therapist's aim to "flatten the hierarchy" or have a collaborative relationship, therapists *do* have power (Larner, 1995). Larner (1995) stated that power, knowledge, and influence are intricately intertwined in the very experience of therapy and in the client's expectations of change. He challenged therapists to consider the wider social context in which a "not-knowing" or "non-intervening" conversation takes place, that while power is socially constructed, it is also tangible and felt. Therapists may prefer to "flatten the hierarchy," however, this remains *their* decision in a social context in which the professional role of therapist holds power.

•←→•

In the end, therapists must hold themselves accountable for their own power and for promoting shared power and equitable relationships among family members.

•←→•

Power is part of all social relationships (Guilfoyle, 2003). The idea that participants in a therapeutic dialogue are equal and power-free can obscure our understanding of power dynamics in therapy. Not all perspectives are equally heard or have the same weight in shaping conversations and reality claims. Just because multiple people are in conversation, including in a family therapy session, being in the same space doesn't grant equal voice or satisfaction with the process and outcome. We agree with Guilfoyle (2003), who asserted that mutual construction does not occur in the absence of attention to power. In fact, it is the ethical obligation of socioculturally attuned collaborative family therapists to promote fairness among family members.

↔

A potential trap of the collaborative approach is the belief that we equally co-construct reality. This stance can be mediated with critical consciousness.

↔

The ability to manage power varies based on a person's social location and diverse intersections of their identities. For example, it can be especially difficult for women, the very young or the very old, ethnic, racial, or sexual minorities, and others from discriminated or marginalized groups to experience power in contexts in which they are not part of the dominant group. It takes being in a powerful position to choose to embrace a not-knowing, unassuming stance to "flatten the hierarchy," downplay, or share power. As a Latina professor who is an immigrant, mother of three, the youngest of six children, and the only one to graduate from college, Maria is keenly aware of how choosing to take a stance of cultural humility when teaching a doctoral level class often works against her. Although it is her preferred stance due to her cultural values of *personalismo* and collectivism, and her philosophy of teaching and being a scholar, her social location within her professional context does not support this approach. Students and faculty will mistake her resistance to masculinist, hegemonic, and colonizing stances as her actually not knowing, being a leader, or doing or being enough. Her collaborative stance as a co-learner sharing her knowledge and power and equally honoring the knowledge of others is rarely noticed, acknowledged, or valued in her work setting.

If persons in positions of power, such as therapists, supervisors, and educators, are not members of a dominant group, then they may not have the cultural capital or position of privilege to minimize or share their power with others. Many may feel as if they need to amplify their power in order to have similar influence or respect that people from the dominant group might take for granted. This aspect of power and privilege may be overlooked by some collaborative therapists. According to Tatum (1997), there is no equal influence. She asserted, "Dominant groups, by definition, set the parameters within which the subordinates operate. The dominant group holds the power and authority in society relative to subordinates and determines how that power and authority may be acceptably used" (Tatum, 1997, p. 23).

Third Order Change

↔

Without a consciousness raising, action oriented, socioculturally attuned perspective, collaborative therapists risk replicating larger sociopolitical systems and beliefs that support social inequity and injustice.

↔

In socioculturally attuned collaborative family therapy, dialogue generates third order transformational change, including being able to recognize and navigate the social forces in one's life in more empowered ways. For example, if we have benefited and continue to benefit from cumulative advantage, then we must acknowledge our privilege and situate our success and our ability to assert ourselves or take action with confidence. Conversely, it is also important to recognize the material consequences of social inequalities, cumulative disadvantage, and other barriers due to a person's social location, as well as institutional and structural systems of discrimination and oppression.

Third order change includes consciousness and action; a form of transformative praxis that increases our ability to challenge, navigate, and mitigate systems that impede our ability to overcome adversity. From a collaborative perspective, such change is created through a shift in how we relate to one another and involves reflexive critique of everyday interactions (Bava & McNamee, 2019). Transformative dialogues are not always harmonious. In fact, according to Anderson (2023), sometimes having differences and tensions can be a resource for deeper dialogue and shared exploration. They also require intentionality in how helping professionals structure and approach their work to create dialogical space that engages clients from beginning to end, as experts in knowing what they need, and in which resilience and justice are emergent through the collaborative relational process (Bava & McNamee, 2019; Fraenkel, 2006; 2020; Palit & Levin, 2016). Peter Fraenkel describes the application of this stance to program development in Text Box 13.3.

Text Box 13.3 Peter Fraenkel, PhD, Licensed Psychologist

Peter Fraenkel, PhD (him, his), is a White, third-generation Jewish American upper-middle-class cisgender heterosexual man who tries to use his racial and educational privileges and the positions these privileges have afforded him to serve as a "White ladder and a White stepping stone" for his mostly Students of Color and first-generation immigrant students, and for the marginalized families with whom he works. His reflections are drawn from 14 years of work with graduate students at City College in New York City in which they developed, implemented, and evaluated a program for families living in homeless shelters. His collaborative, grounded theory approach to research and program development is described in several publications (e.g., Fraenkel, 2006, 2020).

I was asked to develop a program to support families that were homeless and living in shelters. Most of the families were African American, Afro Caribbean, or Latinx. The majority were single-mother families. Since legislation limited the length of time persons could receive welfare, shelters and other agencies were scrambling to provide employment and work readiness programs. I was told that many of the parents were not attending, dropped out before completion, or did not follow through with efforts to help them secure employment. This was cast as a problem of "engagement."

Given my social location as a White, upper-middle-class educationally privileged, cisgender heterosexual male mental health professional and researcher, and as a person who had never struggled with homelessness or joblessness or any location-based oppression, I used an approach that viewed the "families as the experts" on their challenges and existing coping approaches. This approach reversed the usual hierarchy of knowledge creation and program development and evaluation, in which persons who inhabit positions of privilege typically decide what families' challenges are and what they need to support them, and then evaluate the success of the program based on processes that do not include the voices and opinions of the persons receiving the program.

In introducing the nature of the project to families, we noted both in the Informed Consent forms and in the initial interviews, that we were "turning to them to learn from them about their challenges, their coping approaches, and what they wanted in a program if they wanted a program at all." We noted that we were taking this approach because none of us had the experience of being homeless, and therefore had no basis for understanding the impact and means of coping with homelessness.

The program provided the opportunity to offer ideas and advice to one another in the multiple family discussion groups, rather than providing "expert" knowledge on best ways to parent and to cope with various aspects of adversity. Parents are in a much better position to advise each other about how to work best with the staff of the shelter that either assists or impedes their movement towards employment and housing. Kids and teens also advised one another on how to cope with the stigma of being in a shelter, how to keep having fun while there, and how to keep their spirits up. Conversations about how to negotiate their many challenges equipped families with a new sense of empowerment and specific strategies to get what they need as best they can within the reality of structural racism, classism, and other structural constraints. Their feelings of oppression and outrage about being treated unfairly and unsympathetically were validated.

Both families and staff had a lot of fun in these meetings. Many commented that it was the sense of fun and pleasure that made them feel not like "clients" and us staff members as "workers," but that, in the words of one parent during a six-month follow-up interview, "You treated us like we were friends, and that's what made the difference." In other words, although the challenges facing families were many and serious, we encouraged a sense of pleasure and enjoyment as part of the process of addressing these issues. I hold a strong belief that social justice work is most sustainable when also pleasurable, and not approached only with a sense of dire seriousness and outrage, which can lead to burnout and bitterness. I often feel that our work was mostly about helping to "rehumanize and re-spirit" people whose spirits and family relationships were nearly crushed under the weight of these challenges and the larger oppressive forces from which these challenges flowed.

Practice Guidelines

Below we share guidelines for practicing socioculturally attuned collaborative family therapy. The five guidelines are partially informed by D'Arrigo-Patrick and colleagues' (2016) study of how social justice based therapists navigate critical and postmodern theories in their practice. They are as follows: 1) assume a critically informed stance, 2) participate with transparency, 3) remain sociocultural experience near, 4) attend to culture and power differences in dialogical processes, and 5) use inquiry to promote equity.

1. Assume a Critically Informed Stance

A critically informed stance requires therapists to bring critical consciousness to their work. On the one hand, socioculturally attuned collaborative therapists must know about the larger systems and sociopolitical context. On the other, they must remain curious and **attuned** to how these larger systems affect each individual in each family. Perils of not critically examining broader social contexts leave families vulnerable to therapists inadvertently supporting the status quo, including unequal and damaging family power dynamics.

↞↠

The critical knowing stance is every bit as important as taking a not knowing stance. This allows socioculturally attuned collaborative therapists to engage in liberatory processes while maintaining deep humility.

↞↠

2. Participate with Transparency

Transparency in clinical work requires that socioculturally attuned collaborative therapists are willing to have an open stance regarding what informs lines of questioning and curiosity, intentional about situating interest in social issues based on our own experience, and forthcoming with clients about the lens that shapes our distinctive approach. Therapists **value** all client voices and experiences. Clients value this open stance in which socioculturally attuned collaborative therapists reveal what informs their questions and curiosities. A therapist might say things like, "I see you as the expert on your own life because you live it. I will often share my thoughts and reactions to what you say, but my hope is that our conversations will help you decide what is best for you and what you want for your lives." Socioculturally attuned collaborative therapists might also say things like, "I will often ask questions and share my thoughts and reactions to what you are saying. If I notice something that seems unfair or a statement about what you *should* do that may be coming from the outside or bigger society, I will ask you about it."

3. Remain Sociocultural Experience Near

As seen in the examples above, therapists are attuned to the way clients experience and give voice to the impact of social issues. Therapists remain intentional, ensuring that questions attend to social issues as they directly relate to clients' experiences in their daily lives. This practice is instrumental in **naming** what is unjust or has been overlooked. It intentionally shares space and voice as collaborative conversational partners.

↔

The greater our ability to be curious about what happens for each one of us at individual, interpersonal, social, economic, and political levels, the greater our ability will be to walk closely alongside others.

↔

Broadening our lens increases the possibility of sharing connection with others that is simultaneously personal and sociopolitical. A socioculturally attuned collaborative therapist's personal experience is expanded by awareness of the experience of others across diverse social contexts. For example, Don, the therapist who worked with Gabriel and Tony, reflected on his own performance of gender within his cultural framework and became curious about what an asexual identity and experience might be like in other cultural and religious contexts and from various economic backgrounds. Don also found himself able to be more flexible in his own sexuality as a White male.

4. Attend to Culture and Power Differences in Dialogical Processes

↔

Socioculturally attuned collaborative therapists are acutely aware of how power shapes dialogic conversations and ensure marginalized and subjugated voices are valued and responded to in ways that support equity.

↔

In each of the examples in this chapter, the therapists do not presume equality. They know that larger societal scripts inform power dynamics. Socioculturally attuned therapists take their own and each participant's relative power positions into account to maintain a collaborative stance. They are alert to how space and freedom to speak is more available to some than others based on their positions within discourses that are culturally and socially, not individually, constructed (Guilfoyle, 2003; Knudson-Martin, 2013). Creating a collaborative dialogue involves responses that create space for marginalized identities and risk addressing the disconcerting and uncomfortable (Bava, 2019b). Genuinely collaborative clinical actions cannot be pre-scripted. As described by Justine D'Arrigo in Text Box 13.2, they depend on attention to how power is at play in what we are creating and on asking ourselves, "What questions does power want us to divert from?"

5. Use Inquiry to Promote Equity

Inquiry as **intervention** involves *asking* instead of *telling* clients about the effects of social issues, and allowing oneself, and each other, to be led more by curiosity than by theory or a stance of assuming or knowing. Socioculturally attuned collaborative therapists bring attention and awareness to larger contextual issues through the questions they ask. For example, rather than telling clients, "This is a gender issue," they might ask, "How might gender be affecting your experience?" Or they may introduce voices from outside the therapeutic milieu, such as "A lot of women talk about this…" or "There is some research on gender socialization and equity you might be interested in. Would you like to hear about it?"

Therapists are free to draw on any and all discourses that are relevant and potentially helpful. A collaborative, not-knowing stance means being curious and asking questions, and making statements that support relational equity and, by the very nature of asking the questions, can begin to disrupt oppressive power dynamics embedded in larger sociocultural systems and social structures. Socioculturally attuned collaborative therapists recognize that questions are never neutral or without purpose. They are intentionally moving us toward equitable practices. Conversations are generative as well as agentive, enhancing the ability to **envision** new realities. This dialogic process can lead to **transformational** change in how people engage with each other within their families and communities.

Case Illustration

In a small community less than ten miles from a large university in the southern US, families were awakened early on a Sunday morning by law enforcement loudly yelling and banging at their doors. Startled and scared, families opened their doors to armed agents from the Immigration Customs Enforcement (ICE) and Enforcement and Removal Operations (ERO) team, many of whom had identified themselves as parole officers or police just minutes before. That morning, fourteen men were handcuffed and taken from their homes in front of their terrified children, spouses, other family members and friends. Three days after the raid, at least five others were detained locally as part of ICE's "Cross Check" operation that ultimately arrested 2,059 individuals across the US in five days (Department of Homeland Security, 2015). Most of those detained following the raid opted for "voluntary departure," leaving behind traumatized, disrupted families and communities. In the days that followed, members of the community responded by providing economic, legal, logistical, and emotional support to these already marginalized families. Sandra was one of the local bilingual, licensed family therapists who responded to the community crisis. She was a Latin American immigrant and a trusted member of the community.

During the months following the raid, Sandra met with several families, including the Garcia family. Sandra was given the Garcia's number by a community liaison who lived and worked in their community. When Sandra called, Mr. Garcia stated that he was requesting help for his family, especially for his wife, who was having an "*ataque de nervios*" (nervous breakdown). Ms. Garcia was especially in crisis, crying uncontrollably, unable to sleep or eat, and completely at a loss as to how to help her son (age 20), who had been deported. Her grief was immense, and her husband did not know how to help her. She was also the primary provider for their family due to her husband incurring a back injury at work, for which he could not receive medical attention. Their eldest child, who was 20, was taken from their home, held at a detention center for months, and eventually deported back to his country of origin.

Assume a Critically Informed Stance

In a both/and manner, Sandra was intentional about maintaining a not-knowing stance while simultaneously maintaining an acute awareness of the larger sociocultural issues affecting this family. First, and rightfully so, there was mistrust of strangers within this community. To be invited into a home was indeed an honor. Sandra was aware of the importance of entering the family's home with a stance of embracing uncertainty and humility. This stance would be true for any therapist working in someone's home, but especially in the case in which there was an obvious social class difference; with the family representing an oppressed group and the therapist holding many privileges. In this case, the home was in a mobile home community of mostly Latinx people with mixed-legal status.

Although Sandra grew up in a working class family, her current social status rendered a visible difference due to her education and assimilation in the US. In Spanish, the literal translation of someone who is from a lower socio-economic status is "*una persona humilde*" (a humble person) and their home is a "*un hogar humilde*" (a humble home). Sandra had critical awareness that she was perceived as someone who represented the dominant societal group (i.e., white skin, English as her dominant language, highly educated, US citizen). This self-awareness helped her be mindful of her position of power in relation to theirs.

Sandra's stance of humility embedded in critical consciousness helped her acknowledge and honor *their* positions of power. For example, she asked them to address her by her first name, not by doctor. For Latinx culture, this stance would represent awareness of the values of hierarchy, which are based on social status, age, and gender, among other things. It is also based on *respeto*/ respect, which is not based on material wealth, but instead, earning respect due to treating others in a personal and respectful manner (Bermúdez et al., 2010; Falicov, 1998; Garcia-Preto, 2005). Honoring a family in their home and accepting their hospitality was an important way in which Sandra remained socioculturally attuned to how social class and cultural norms intersect. She was also careful to note how their ways of expressing themselves reflected larger narratives that were stripping them of their power.

As their time together continued, it became apparent that Mr. Garcia was blaming himself, instead of larger forces, for what happened to his son. He expressed an intense sense of guilt because he opened the door for the ICE agents and was later told that he did not have to open the door. Because he respects authority, he did not know that he could resist the unlawful entry of the agents if the door was closed. He said, "*fue mi culpa; yo les abrir la puerta.*" (It was my fault; I opened the door.) Sandra asked questions that helped him consider the larger forces that led him to believe that he had to open the door. "Could it be that you did not feel like you had a choice? That you believed you were doing the right thing?" she asked in Spanish. Mr. Garcia said he was taught to obey authority, and when they said, "Open the door!" he did. Because he and his son had the same name, he also thought they were looking for him. He was confused, and then so upset that they took his son instead of him.

Sandra tried to remain experience near, especially as they discussed the larger contextual factors affecting the Garcia family. They lived in a southern state in which there is a history of institutionalized discrimination, racism, and oppression against People of Color. Latinos were the latest target, with White supremacy groups gaining momentum using anti-Latino propaganda. The therapist was able to recognize their pain and struggle and discuss how the larger sociocultural forces influenced their family disruption (i.e., immigration policy in the US, anti-immigrant sentiment in the South, hostility, and discrimination toward dark skinned, low income, and non-English speaking Latinos) (Terrazas et al., 2020; Walsdorf et., 2020). Although they were loving parents and provided a stable home for their children, the effects of poverty, Mr. Garcia's health problems, and gang culture surrounding their home negatively affected and limited their access to alternatives. Mr. Garcia told Sandra, "*Queríamos una mejor vida para nuestros hijos, y siento que si estamos mejor aquí, pero nos duele sentir que en el país que tanto queremos, nos rechazan constantemente. Es difícil vivir asi.*" (We wanted a better life for our children, and I feel like we are better here, but it hurts to feel that in a country that we love so much, that we feel rejected constantly. It is hard to live this way.)

Both parents were devout Catholics who had religious shrines and candles lit in their home and prayed for their son's safety. They struggled with feelings of regret and doubt. They blamed themselves, but also were angry at their son for actively going against the way in which he was raised, which was to be a good person and a Christian:

Ms. Garcia: [crying and shaking her head] He knew better than that. We raised him to do the right thing. He knew he couldn't put himself and others at risk, but he felt like he was helping his friends. They drank too much and felt like they couldn't drive. He was the one that drank the least. They are all so young and just weren't thinking! He should not have been with them. We told him to stay away from them. They just cause trouble. Now they are free and my son is gone and we can't help him!

Both parents were upset that he was near the end of his probation when he was detained. The mother was also angry at the authorities and felt as though her son was treated unjustly due to being Latino, unauthorized, and from a low socio-economic status. Before he was arrested for driving without a license, her son had no prior record or legal problems. The parents were loving, kind, responsible, and insightful. They were a cohesive family. Their frustration stemmed not only from their self-blame and doubt but from the injustice they experienced due to their marginalized social status.

Their youngest daughter, Evelyn, was also able to gain greater consciousness about how her family was affected by her brother's detention and deportation. Evelyn, who was 10 years old, was deeply grieving the separation from her brother and was traumatized by the way he was taken. Sandra had to carefully measure her words, especially since Evelyn was present for most of their time together. She wanted to help Evelyn contextualize what happened in a way she could understand. In Spanish, Sandra told her, while her parents listened:

> Evelyn, I'm so sorry this happened to your brother and your family. He didn't deserve to be handcuffed and treated like a criminal. He is not a criminal. It wasn't his fault that he didn't have the papers that he needed to be here lawfully. Does that make sense to you? [Evelyn nodded yes]. For those of us who are not born in the US, we have to have certain documents that say we can be here legally. Not having the legal papers does not make someone a bad person or a criminal.

Sandra then turned to the parents and said,

> The way I see it is that your son had rights, and like many of us, you didn't know what those rights were—like not opening the door to authorities without a warrant for an arrest. You were not aware of your rights. I can't see how it's your fault.

They were able to have a frank dialogue in which the Garcia family felt heard and validated, while also understanding how their problem was situated within the larger social context. This critical stance would not mean as much without participating in an authentic and transparent manner. For many Latinx people, being treated with respect and connecting in an authentic and transparent manner is a core cultural value that transcends social class and other forms of hierarchy.

Participate with Transparency

The therapist listened carefully in an open, affirming, collaborative manner as the Garcias described the impact of larger structural, societal, and institutional realities. Sandra was aware of her power in relation to the Garcias. She remained transparent and had an open stance in terms of what informed her questions and was intentional about situating her interest in social issues (i.e., her social justice and equity based family therapy approach, especially with Latinos). She also talked about how her work was situated in her own experience of being Latina and having undocumented family members.

Sandra: Like many Latinos in the US, I also have family members that are undocumented. I know it's hard for them, but life is good for them too; much better than it was for them back in our home country. They feel so fortunate to be in the US and are doing OK, but it is hard for them sometimes. They have to work so hard physically to make ends meet. I sometimes feel guilty for having privileges that they don't have, especially for my education and the opportunities it has given me.

Sandra was also open about the reason she was there helping them. She was a family therapist who has devoted much of her energy to helping Latino families. This was her way of giving back. It hurt her to see how Latinos are treated for just wanting to have a better life. She was living the "American dream" in ways they couldn't. Sandra worked to remain honest and transparent. This leveraged her position to work with them as conversational partners and to share her power.

Remain Socioculturally Experience Near

As the therapy progressed, Sandra remained socioculturally experience near by being attuned to each family member's emotions and the ways they were affected by what happened. She attended to the specific ways in which they described and felt the impact of the effects of their son/brother being taken away, held in a detention center for months, and deported to a country where he did not have a strong grasp of the language and felt like an Americanized outsider. Sandra was also mindful of being experience near when attending to the child's (Evelyn's) narrative and her description of what happened. She let Evelyn explain things in her own words and asked questions directly related to what she said and tried to remain near Evelyn's lived experience, not just her parents' or their experience in general. When asked what this was like for her, Evelyn responded in English,

Evelyn: I miss my brother. He was so funny and nice.

Sandra: I'm so sorry about what happened to your brother. I can tell that you love him very much. I believe you when you say he is funny and nice. Is there something that you have here at home that can help you feel close to him while he is away—something that can make you smile and remember the things he said and did to make you laugh?

Evelyn ran to her room and got a stuffed animal. Sandra asked if she thought it was a good idea to hug her stuffed animal when she wanted to feel him close. She smiled and said "yes" and hugged it tight with tears in her eyes.

Attend to Culture and Power Differences in Dialogical Processes

Throughout their time together, Sandra remained attentive to how the various intersections of culture and power affected their communication as dialogical partners. As with many Latinx families, the father held greater power, but he seemed somewhat unconventional in that he displayed equal responsibility for the emotion work in the home. He initiated seeking outside support, attended to his wife's needs, and was very active in seeking help and being resourceful for his family. Ms. Garcia was also very active, but less so, given her greater language barrier and the extent of emotional crisis she was experiencing. The parents spoke very little English and did not have the means to hire a lawyer to help them help their son. Sandra also assessed how their different positions of power affected their sense of agency to mobilize them out of their crisis state. This was especially true when their son was in the detention center and they did not know how to help him.

Sandra made every effort not to replicate oppressive practices and to treat the family as an equal partner, although, from a societal standpoint, she had more power and voice. She was mindful that this family felt as though their son had been forced to accept a new life; that their sense of personal agency was taken from them. They felt they had to accept the reality that their son, who had lived in the US since he was four years old, did not know another place called home other than the US. His use of Spanish was limited, and he hardly remembered his life in his country prior to immigrating to the US. His mother did not know how her son could survive living there, especially in the violent, crime-ridden neighborhood where his grandmother lived.

After a few meetings, they felt comfortable enough with Sandra to ask if she would be willing to talk to their son by phone. They were worried about his well-being and wanted Sandra to offer some comforting words of hope. They also wanted her to encourage him to see things in a more positive light. They knew it was hard for him, but he was also living with his grandmother, which had the potential to be positive for them both. He was trying to be a source of support to her in the midst of his own crisis, but Ms. Garcia said that her son seemed too depressed and angry to make it more positive. Although they called him daily, they were very concerned. He had been recently assaulted by young men wanting to steal his phone and shoes and to hurt him. He was able to escape, but he was injured and strongly shaken by the experience. He felt as though he had lost all his sense of power, was having a terrible time adjusting, and missed his life with his family.

Ms. Garcia handed Sandra the phone. Sandra explained who she was and why she was there. She tried to be encouraging and asked questions about his well-being, what he wanted to do while he was there, and how he thought his family could help him. His parents were surprised that he talked as much as he did. They said their son was usually closed off emotionally, and it was unusual for him to talk to others about himself. After talking with the son, Sandra encouraged his parents to help him see the unexpected possibilities and to consider his strengths that could help him optimize his experience there—he spoke English well, had a high school education, and a home with his grandmother. He had access to resources that others did not have. These resources gave him power in his new cultural context in ways he could not fully understand.

Sandra was mindful of how her own power could help them gain access to internal and external resources during this crisis, while also remaining vigilant about how her position as a "helper" could potentially replicate exploitative or oppressive practices for the family. The Garcias had asked Sandra to help them, but given that they were not paying for her services and they were meeting in their home, the potential for boundaries to be crossed and for vulnerable persons to feel exploited was an ongoing potential threat. By remaining self-aware and transparent about her role—including that their work would be short term until the immediate crisis had subsided—and following the family's lead about how she could be helpful, Sandra took steps to avoid unintended exploitation.

Use Inquiry to Promote Equity

As described above, inquiry involves asking questions that lead people to examine the effects of social issues, as well as engage in dialogues that promote relational and social equity. Sandra talked with each family member so as to draw on any and all discourses that were relevant and potentially helpful. She asked questions about their sources of empowerment—in which they said church, family, neighborhood, and friends—and disempowerment, such as the legal system, Mr. Garcia's poor health, gangs in their neighborhood, and lack of work due to health problems. Through this respectful questioning, the family was able to name the specific things that were added stressors, as well as the things that gave them peace. They repeatedly mentioned their faith, so Sandra asked them more about it.

Rather than "teaching" the Garcias how to cope with stress and loss, Sandra turned to the family as the source of knowledge. She noticed they had a large image on their wall of *La Virgen de Guadalupe,* the Virgin Mary, the patron saint of Mexico. Along with this large image, they had flowers and a burning prayer candle. They mentioned their church often and Sandra, who was also Catholic, used their faith-based language in her inquiry. For example, she asked in Spanish, "*Creen que, con el favor de Dios, que van a poder restablecer su equilibrio y sentirse fuerte de nuevo?*" ("Do you think that, with the grace of God, you will be able to regain your sense of equilibrium and feel strong again?") *Qué es lo que más urgentemente quieren pedirle a la Virgen para que puedan salir de esta situation y seguir adelante en paz?*" ("What is it that you most urgently feel like you need to ask the blessed Virgin Mary to help you get out of this situation and to move forward in peace?") Sandra's questions about the Virgin Mary helped the Garcia family rally their faith to disrupt the immense feeling of powerlessness that had overtaken them. The process helped them limit the extent to which the larger system and grand narratives and experience of deportation had power over them individually and as a family. They had resources, especially in each other and their faith.

Sandra met with the Garcia family six more times. In the larger culture, the Garcia family had very little social and cultural capital. Sandra intentionally engaged with them as equitable, collaborative partners. By being a guest in their home, she was able to be in a space with the family in which *they* held the most power. The volunteer, in-home family work was a unique opportunity for the therapist to be there in ways that neither Sandra nor the family could have predicted. Sandra was able to be *with* them and to be an important resource to regain their sense of agency in an oppressive system. She continued to volunteer her time, be a source of support and encouragement, and connect them to community resources related to health, finances, and legal aid. With a focus on activism through countering injustice, Sandra was able to engage with the family to disrupt and challenge dominant ideologies and practices that kept them immobilized with fear, grief, and despair and generate a greater sense of resilience and hope for change.

Summary: Third Order Change

From a socioculturally attuned collaborative perspective, third order change for the Garcia family meant that they were better able to recognize and navigate the social forces creating crisis in their lives. The therapist integrated a critically conscious approach with a humble, not-knowing stance, while simultaneously leveraging her power, responding to the family's crisis with knowledge and resources, and continually engaging *with* the Garcia family in critical inquiry. Through this dialogic process, the Garcias felt more empowered to address their unjust situation by acknowledging and challenging racism, discrimination, and vulnerability due to lower socio-economic and unauthorized legal status. The ability of the therapist to respond during a time of crisis and offer a strong dose of *withness* and genuine support helped them regain their sense of hope and courage to keep moving forward and imagine possibilities.

Reflexive Questions

- What would it mean for you as a therapist if you were to embrace a socioculturally attuned collaborative stance? Would your current place of practice support this way of working? Why or why not?
- Have you ever taken an unassuming, not-knowing stance and were mistaken for not being informed, capable, or in charge? How did this affect you and your work?
- When thinking about your work as a socioculturally attuned collaborative therapist, how do you resist the temptation to remain neutral about the ways clients are affected by social inequality? How do you invite these perspectives into the dialogue? What blocks you from doing so?
- Given your social location and particular professional context, what would it mean for you to be *transparent* and willing to have an *open stance* regarding what informs your lines of questioning and curiosity? Does it require permission, safety, and/or protection from others for you to work in this way? If so, how?
- How can you be intentional about *situating your interest in social issues* and be *forthcoming* with clients about the lens that shapes your distinctive approach?
- How do you welcome sometimes contradictory social messages and sustain the courage and humility to remain in a respectful, unassuming learner position?

References

Anderson, H. (2023). Conceptual framework: Emerging orienting sensitivities for relationships and conversations that invite transformation and possibility. In H. Anderson & D. Gehart (Eds.). *Collaborative-Dialogic Practice: Relationships and conversations that make a difference across contexts and cultures* (pp. 3–18). Routledge.

Anderson, H. (2012a). Collaborative relationships and dialogic conversations: Ideas for relationally responsive practice. *Family Process*, *51*(1), 8–24.

Anderson, H. (2012b). Collaborative practice: A way of being "with". *Psychotherapy and Politics International*, *10*(2), 130–145.

Anderson, H. (2007). The heart and spirit of collaborative therapy: The philosophical stance "a way of being" in relationship and conversation. In H. Anderson & D. Gehart (Eds.). *Collaborative therapy* (pp. 43–52). Routledge.

Anderson, H. (2005). Myths about "not-knowing." *Family Process*, *44*(4), 497–504.

Anderson, H. (1997). *Conversations, language, and possibilities: A postmodern approach to therapy*. Basic Books.

Anderson, H. (1995). Collaborative language systems: Toward a postmodern therapy. In R. Mikesell, D. O. Lusterman, & S. McDaniel (Eds.). *Integrating family therapy: Family psychology and systems therapy*. American Psychological Association.

Anderson, H. (1993). On a roller coaster: A collaborative language systems approach to therapy. In S. Friedman (Ed.). *The new language of change: Constructive collaboration in therapy* (pp. 323–344). Guilford Press.

Anderson, H. & Gehart, D. R. (Eds.). (2023). *Collaborative-dialogic practice: Relationships and conversations that make a difference across contexts and cultures*. Taylor & Francis.

Anderson, H. & Goolishian, H. A. (1988). Human systems as linguistic systems: Preliminary and evolving ideas about the implications for clinical theory. *Family Process*, *27*, 371–393.

Ashbourne, L. M., Fife, K., Ridley, M. & Gaylor, E. (2016). Supporting the development of novice therapists. In S. St. George and D. Wulff (Eds.), *Family therapy as socially transformative practice: Practical strategies* (p. 41–55). AFTA Springerbriefs in Family Therapy, Springer.
Bava, S. (2023). A Relationally responsive world: The politics of collaborative-dialogic practices. In H. Anderson & D. Gehart (Eds.). *Collaborative-dialogic practice: Relationships and conversations that make a difference across contexts and cultures* (pp. 37–54). Routledge.
Bava, S. (2022). *A guide for conversations: The relational discursive loop*. https://medium.com/@thinkplay/a-guide-for-conversations-relational-discursive-loop-6f5ad6a8e3a3
Bava, S. (2019a). Hyperlinked identity: A generative resource in a divisive world. In M. McGoldrick & K. V. Hardy (Eds.). *Re-visioning family therapy: Addressing diversity in clinical practice* (3rd ed., pp. 318–335). Guilford.
Bava, S. (2019b). Responsive supervision: Playing with risk-taking and hyperlinked identities. In L. L. Charlés & T. S. Nelson (Eds.). *Family therapy supervision in extraordinary settings* (pp. 53–62). Routledge.
Bava, S. & McNamee, S. (2019). Imagining relationally crafted justice: A pluralist stance. *Contemporary Justice Review*, *22*, 290–306.
Bermúdez, J. M., Kirkpatrick, D., Hecker, L., & Torres-Robles, C. (2010). Describing Latino families and their help-seeking experiences: Challenging the family therapy literature. *Contemporary Family Therapy*, *32*(2), 155–172.
Bull, B. & D'Arrigo, J. (2026). Queer-contextualized collaborative family therapy. In E. E. Hartwell & L. L. Edwards (Eds.). *Queer-contextualized family therapy: Toward radically inclusive theory and practice*. (pp. 196–213). Routledge.
Chenail, R. J., Reire, M. D., Torres-Gregory, M., & Ilic, D. (2020). Postmodern family therapy. In K. S. Wampler, R. B. Miller, & R. B. Seedall (Eds.). *The Handbook of systemic family therapy* (Vol. 1, pp. 417–440). Wiley.
Cheon, H. S. & Murphy, M. J. (2007). The self-of-the-therapist awakened. *Journal of Feminist Family Therapy*, *19*, 1–16.
D'Arrigo-Patrick, J., Hoff, C., Knudson-Martin, C., & Tuttle, A. (2016). Navigating critical theory and postmodernism: Social justice and therapist power in family therapy. *Family Process*, *56*, 574–588.
Department of Homeland Security. (2015). 2,059 criminals arrested in ICE nationwide operation [Press Release]. Retrieved from http://www.dhs.gov/news/2015/03/09/2059-criminals-arrested-icenationwide-operation.
Ellis, E. & Bermúdez, J. M. (2021). Funhouse mirror reflections: Resisting internalized sexism in family therapy and building a women-affirming practice. *Journal of Feminist Family Therapy*, *33*(3), 223–243.
Falicov, C. J. (1998). *Latino families in therapy: A guide to multicultural practice*. Guilford Press.
Fraenkel, P. (2020). Collaborative family program development: Research methods that investigate and foster resilience and engagement in marginalized communities. In M. Ochs, M. Borcsa, & J. Schweitzer (Eds.). *Systemic research in individual, couple, and family therapy and counseling* (pp. 75–96). European Family Therapy Association Series, Volume 4. Springer Nature Switzerland.
Fraenkel, P. (2006). Engaging families as experts: Collaborative family program development. *Family Process*, *45*, 237–257.
Garcia-Preto, N. (2005). Latino families: An overview. In McGoldrick, M., Giordano, J., & Garcia-Preto, N. (Eds.), *Ethnicity and family therapy* (3rd ed., pp. 153–165). Guilford Press.
Geertz, C. (1974). From the native's point of view: On the nature of anthropological understanding. *Bulletin of the American Academy of Arts and Sciences*, *28*(1), 26–45.
Gehart, D. (2023). Curiosity as mindfulness practice: Following the moment-to-moment unfolding of meaning construction. In H. Anderson & D. Gehart (Eds.). *Collaborative-dialogic practice: Generative relationships and conversations across contexts and cultures* (pp. 55–68). Routledge.
Gómez-Lamont, M. F. & Bermúdez, J. M. (2023). *La terapia familiar sistémica y el pensamiento de tercer orden: Teoría crítica con perspectivas de género, multiculturalidad e interseccionalidad* (Systemic family therapy and third order thinking: Critical theories from gender, multicultural, and intersectional perspectives). National Autonomous University of Mexico.
Guilfoyle, M. (2006). Using power to question the dialogic self and its therapeutic application. *Counseling Psychology Quarterly*, *19*(1), 89–104.
Guilfoyle, M. (2003). Dialogue and power: A critical analysis of power in dialogic therapy. *Family Process*, *42*(3), 331–343.
Hare-Mustin, R. (1994). Discourses in the mirrored room: A postmodern analysis of therapy. *Family Process*, *33*(1), 19–35.

Hoffman, L. (2018). *Exchanging voices: A collaborative approach to family therapy*. Routledge.
Hoffman, L. (2012). The art of "withness": A new bright edge. In *Collaborative therapy* (pp. 63–79). Routledge.
Hoffman, L. (2007). The art of "withness": A new bright edge. In H. Anderson & D. Gehart (Eds.). *Collaborative therapy: Relationships and conversations that make a difference* (pp. 63–79). Routledge/Taylor & Francis Group.
Knudson-Martin, C. (2013). Why power matters: Creating a foundation of mutual support in couple relationships. *Family Process*, *52*(1), 5–18.
Laird, J. (2000). Theorizing culture. *Journal of Feminist Family Therapy, 11*(4), 99–114.
Larner, G. (1995). The real as illusion: Deconstructing power in family therapy. *Journal of Family Therapy*, *17*, 191–217.
Malinen, T., Cooper, S. J., & Thomas, F. N. (Eds.) (2012). *Masters of narrative and collaborative therapies: The voices of Anderson, Anderson, and White*. Routledge.
McDowell, T. (2015). *Applying critical social theories to family therapy practice*. AFTA Springerbriefs in Family Therapy. Springer.
McNamee, S. & Gergen, K. J. (Eds.) (1992). *Therapy as social construction*. Sage.
Mills, S. D. & Sprenkle, D. H. (1995). Family therapy in the postmodern era. *Family Relations*, *44*(4), 368–376.
Monk, G. & Gehart, D. R. (2003). Sociopolitical activist or conversational partner? Distinguishing the position of the therapist in narrative and collaborative therapies. *Family Process*, *42*(1), 19–30.
Newman, D. (2024). The effort and intricacies of generating experience-near language. *International Journal of Narrative Therapy and Community Work*, (1), 70–83.
Palit, M. & Levin, S. B. (2016). Collaborative therapy with women and children refugees in Houston: Moving toward rehabilitation in the United States after enduring the atrocities of war. In L.L. Charlés & G. Samarasinghe (Eds.). *Family therapy in global humanitarian contexts* (pp. 39–49). AFTA Springerbriefs in Family Therapy. Springer.
Rosen, H. (1996). Meaning-making narratives: Foundations for constructivist and social constructionist psychotherapies. In H. Rosen & K. T. Kuehlwein (Eds.). *Constructing realities: Meaning-making perspectives for psychotherapists* (pp. 3–51). Jossey-Bass.
St. George, S. & Wulff, D. (2014). Braiding socio-cultural interpersonal patterns into therapy. In K. Tomm, S. St. George, D. Wulff, & T. Strong (Eds.). *Patterns in interpersonal interactions: Inviting relational understandings for therapeutic change*. Routledge.
Strong, T. (2002). Collaborative "expertise" after the discursive turn. *Journal of Psychotherapy Integration*, *12*(2), 2188–2232.
Tatum, B. (1997). *"Why are all the black kids sitting together in the cafeteria? And other conversations about race*. Basic Books.
Terrazas, J., Muruthi, B. A., Thompson Cañas, R. E., Jackson, J. B., & Bermúdez, J. M. (2020). Liminal legality among mixed-status Latinx families: Considerations for critically engaged clinical practice. *Contemporary Family Therapy*, *42*, 360–368.
Walsdorf, A. A., Machado, Y., & Bermúdez, J. M. (2020). Undocumented and mixed-status Latinx families: Sociopolitical considerations for systemic practice. *Journal of Family Psychotherapy*, *30*(4), 245–271.

14 Socioculturally Attuned Narrative Family Therapy

Narrative family therapy (NFT) is a poststructural approach that assumes meaning is not stable, universal, or inherent. Meaning is socially constructed and relational, created through language and social interactions. There is no correct or single story about who we are; our lives are multi-storied. In other words, our experiences and identities are shaped by numerous influences and multiple narratives rather than a fixed, sole truth. Problems are created, located, and maintained within larger societal discourses rather than the individual psyche (Chenail et al., 2020; Combs & Freedman, 2016; Madigan, 2019). The underlying premise is that people are not their problems but that we suffer from the effects of problems, which can at times feel greater than our abilities to manage them. Therapists help people name the effects and manage their relationships with the problem to decrease the problem's power and increase personal and relational agency. Therapists take a collaborative, hopeful approach to help clients discover previously unrecognized possibilities and re-author their lives in ways that allow them to overcome problems.

In their groundbreaking book, *Narrative Means to Therapeutic Ends* (1990), Michael White and David Epston drew from the work of Michel Foucault (1982) and other poststructural thinkers to outline tenets of NFT. They asserted that as human beings, we story our experiences and in doing so, ascribe significance to events in our lives. According to White (1995), we live by the stories we tell about ourselves and others tell about us. The metaphor of story helps us consider problems as thin descriptions of our lives that have been co-written by social, cultural, and political contexts (Chenail et al., 2020; Freedman & Combs, 1996; Morgan, 2000). Therapists who do not explore these dominant discourses with clients before developing preferred stories are readily co-opted by them (Dumaresque et al., 2018; Gaddis, 2016).

At the core of narrative practices are deconstructive listening and questioning, externalizing the problem, making oppressive discourses evident, and reconstructing preferred narratives that allow for well-being in the present as well as expanded possibilities in the future (Freedman & Combs, 1996; Madigan, 2019; Morgan, 2000). More recently, there has been an "affective turn" in narrative therapy that includes the embodied and relational nature of affect, emotions as integral to the storying of our lives, and the importance of deconstructing dominant discourses about emotions (Beaudoin & Monk, 2024; Beaudoin & MacClennan 2021; Ewing et al., 2017; Zimmerman 2018). Stories are embodied as felt experiences and our emotional landscapes change as we re-story our lives. Rather than viewing affect and intellect as separate, they are understood as interconnected and fundamental to meaning making, identity, and change.

Narrative therapists have a firm conviction that people are separate from, not defined by, their diagnosis, condition, or problem. Change is not focused on solving the problem, but on creating the space for thoughts, actions, and narratives that no longer support the problem. Therapists assume clients have the abilities, skills, desire, and competence to overcome the effects of the problem.

DOI: 10.4324/9781003493426-14

With the help of scaffolding conversations (White, 2007; 2012), the therapist is able to help people disentangle themselves from what is known and familiar about their lives and to imagine what is possible.

•←→•

Third order change in socioculturally attuned narrative family therapy bridges the gap between critical theories and postmodernism. It involves individuals, couples, and families understanding how societal forces serve to create and support narratives, impact intimate relationships, and affect material realities.

•←→•

In this chapter, we describe key features of NFT and illustrate how therapists can integrate principles of sociocultural attunement and offer practice guidelines. We then share a case illustration in which a young woman and her family bravely stood up to resist oppressive forces that fueled feelings of victimization, vulnerability, and inability to take action.

Primary Enduring Concepts

There have been many contributions to the theory and practice of narrative therapy since Michael White and David Epston first published their seminal work in 1990 (e.g., Beaudoin & Monk, 2024; Freedman & Combs, 1996; Madigan, 2019; Morgan, 2000, White, 2007). Primary enduring concepts of narrative practices include that: 1) reality and meaning are socially constructed and mediated through language, 2) therapy is generative and time-oriented, 3) people are not defined by problems, 4) the life of the problem can be deconstructed, and 5) preferred narratives can be co-created and amplified to positively affect the future.

Reality and Meaning are Socially Constructed

The foundational principle of NFT is that reality is socially constructed, constituted through language; organized and maintained through narratives (Combs & Freedman, 2004; Freedman & Combs, 1996; White & Epston, 1990). We make meaning based on reflections of our experiences in the contexts of our families, communities, and cultures (Berg, 2009; White, 2002). While we might individually or collectively believe that our reality (or someone else's) is most true, narrative therapists assert that the concept of truth is socially and mutually constructed. There are multiple truths and perspectives, as well as endless ways of organizing and creating meaning in our lives. Narrative therapists are acutely aware that a person's context serves to create, maintain, and strengthen the life of the problem, as well as provide a source for co-creating possibilities, alternatives, and preferred narratives. The way we story our lives is informed by countless social, personal, interpersonal, political, cultural, familial, financial, and other factors.

Narrative therapists contend that the ways in which therapists interpret people's lives, relationships, and problems are influenced by dominant cultural ideas and the meanings connected to them (Freedman & Combs, 1996; Madigan, 2019, Morgan, 2000, White & Epston, 1990). As a result, the lived experience and collective discourses of entire groups of people can be marginalized, silenced, or dismissed by dominant discourses. As Beverly Tatum asserted (2017), those from dominant groups have the privilege to define, name, and decide what is valued; what we attend to and deem important.

Consider Ava (age 24) and Rob (age 23), who entered therapy when Ava began to feel uncertain about their relationship. Ava grew up in a middle-class family with her White mother and stepfather. She was six years old when her mother married her stepfather and had two sons. Her Haitian father was unaware of her birth and not part of the family's life. Her extended family never talked about her race, but treated her with less deference than her two brothers. This angered her mother, who would continually tell Ava how beautiful she was and remind her that "we are all the same." Rob grew up in a White middle-class family that had almost no contact with People of Color. His parents assumed a "color blind" stance, teaching Rob and his brother to treat everyone with respect. Among many other narratives, the couple shared a White liberal story about race being meaningful (socially constructed as real) yet not consequential (discoursed in a way that obscures White privilege).

According to White (2007), "many of the people who seek therapy believe that the problems in their lives are a reflection of their own identity or the identity of others… a reflection of certain 'truths' about their nature and their character or about the nature and character of others" (p. 24–25). Dominant and constraining narratives impact how we see ourselves and each other and become further entrenched as social discourses that become part of one's story (e.g., internalized sexism, racism, classism, ageism, homophobia). Continuing our example, Ava and Rob's relationship was influenced by narratives of race and gender, of which they were largely unaware. Ava described Rob as good looking, athletic, and smart. Rob stated Ava was the most amazing woman he had ever known. When they shared the story of how they met, they beamed with hope and excitement. Rob described Ava as being carefree, kind, and loving. Ava described Rob as being responsible, generous, and protective. Rob's family told their friends they were delighted that he had found such a "lovely girl," and Ava's family jokingly commented that now maybe Ava would "settle down."

Narrative family therapists focus on understanding and responding to the lived experience of each family member within all societal contexts. They intentionally attune to clients' words, stances, and responses to the forces that maintain problematic discourses as well as those that give life to preferred narratives. White (1995) asserted that the meanings derived through this interpretative process are not neutral. They have real effects and consequences in our lives. In our example, Ava's racial and gendered experience had been silenced for a lifetime. As a child, she was left trying to make sense on her own to navigate her identity as a bi-racial female, uncertain and unable to speak about how this social location affected her daily life in school, church, home, and the community. Rob was unaware of his male privilege and how this, along with his identity as a "non-racist" White person, contributed to silencing Ava as an adult. In effect, problems occurred when narratives too narrowly defined Ava and Rob's identities and dominant societal narratives (e.g., race doesn't matter; nowadays men and women are equal) were at odds with their lived experience.

Narrative family therapists engage clients in the process of re-authoring their stories through deconstructive listening and questioning. They ask questions from multiple viewpoints rather than searching for facts. They open space for considering alternative, subjugated stories and experiences, acknowledging marginalized stories of survival, resistance, and solidarity (Carr, 1998; Sen, 2021). Narrative family therapists do not re-author clients' lives, but take a decentered posture that allows them to "be acquainted with many possible stories about life" (White, 2007, p. 82), to help clients re-author their own lives or relationships. Alternative stories are explored and expanded via scaffolding conversations.

Scaffolding refers to providing support for developing new, more empowering stories. As inferred by the term "scaffolding," the therapist provides initial structure for building new story lines that are filled in or "thickened" over time. They invite the construction of alternative and/or amplification of subjugated stories by using questions aimed at deconstructing problem stories, discovering unique outcomes, and asking clients to fill in the details of preferred narratives. Let's listen in on the conversation between Ava, Rob, and their therapist, Wanda.

Wanda: So Rob, you said your family is very open and accepting of differences. I am curious how you know that.
Rob: Well, like my parents never objected to our relationship (glancing at Ava). In fact, they love Ava!
Wanda: Ava, I am wondering what you think Rob means?
Ava: That I am not White.
Wanda: And your family? What do they think about you being "not White?"
Ava: I think my mom has been through a lot with my grandparents…but I know they love me. My mom has been my biggest cheerleader.

The story that was emerging between the lines was one of Ava being "not White," but their extended families "not minding." This is a powerfully dominant racist discourse that shaped their daily lives and relationships. Wanda's tasks as a narrative therapist included helping Ava and Rob unearth, examine, deconstruct, and re-author the meaning of race/racism (as well as gender and other stories) and challenge the effect on their relationship. Wanda recognized Ava and Rob's lives as multi-storied and engaged them to create scaffolding that shapes a context in which people can separate from what is known, form a foundation upon which they can envision what might be possible (Chenail et al., 2020). It is through more complex, detailed, and robust stories—in this case including stories about recognizing, navigating, challenging, and overcoming racism—that we can engage in a process of identity enhancement through which to be our best selves, generate new possibilities for relationships, and realize better futures (Blanton, 2005; Combs & Freedman, 2004).

Therapy is Time-oriented and Generative

Narrative family therapy is considered generative because it encourages clients to construct preferred narratives that decrease the influence and power of problems to create space for more positive futures. White (2007) used the concept of maps to help clients explore parts of their life stories that have not been previously acknowledged. According to NFT, temporal notions of past, present, and future can be carefully assessed and mapped to understand the terrain of one's life; where we have been and where we are going. Events in our lives are seen as linked across time by themes, creating plots. Those that are included in our life stories tend to fit within plotlines, while contradictory events are left out. Narrative family therapists listen to stories with an ear to preferred values and positive understandings about oneself that have been missed, not thickened, or detailed. They ask questions that therapeutically restructure the re-telling of one's life story (Gaddis, 2016; White, 2007).

White (2007) advocated for therapists taking a decentered, yet influential therapeutic stance. Similar to the collaborative dialogical approach, the therapist honors the client's expertise on their lives, and the therapist's position reflects a curious and respectful stance in which the therapist is consistently checking their assumptions and biases about what clients mean, need, value, and how they should live their lives. Narrative therapists scaffold therapeutic conversations by helping clients bridge what they can think, feel, say, and do on their own, with what they can think, feel, say, and do with the help of the therapist.

Clients tend to enter therapy when stories about themselves and/or others become problem-saturated. They hold discursive identities, which reflect repeated definitions of who they are over time, which can create "I am," "you are," or "we are" discourses that can be particularly resistant to change or possibilities. Going back to our example, Ava and Rob had very different stories about belonging in their families. Ava was constantly aware that her presence in her family of origin was from a chapter that would have otherwise been closed. Ava's mother and birth father had a brief affair that would have become an inconsequential footnote in the plotline of Ava's mother's life before marriage if the affair had not produced a child. Rob's nativity story was one of two birth parents waiting anxiously after trying to have a child for several years; his arrival signaled the start of a family.

Wanda will be interested in how these stories of belonging have taken on meaning for Rob and Ava and affected how they live. She will look for entry points to a preferred story by asking them about times in which they had influence over the problematic issue or pattern. The therapist will ask Ava and Rob about what they would rather have done, identifying implicit hopes and values, inviting them to envision what it would look like (White, 2007). For example, the therapist might ask Ava about a story she has heard her mother recount about her birth that brought smiles or laughter to her mother's eyes when she told it. They would want to know all about that [seldom told] story and why it was so special to her mother. The therapist would not only ask about the details and meaning of this story in the past; they would ask what it means to Ava to know that this aspect of her birth was special in this way, and what this might mean to her as she charts her future with Rob.

White (2007) embraced "experience-near definitions of the problem" (p. 40), which focus on the particulars of each client's local knowledge and lived experience. This helps the therapist and clients get to know the unique and intimate details of problems and their effects. By doing so, therapists are in a better position to point out what is absent but implicit, broadening the story beyond the problem to explore what is important and valuable that is being overlooked in problem saturated stories. Therapists listen deeply and carefully to narratives to identify words, expressions, and experiences that don't fit with pejorative, harmful, or destructive dominant discourses. Through deconstructive listening and attuning to dominant narratives, therapists notice what gives the problem power and search for unique outcomes that support alternative, preferred narratives. This space allows clients to notice times when the problem is not present and what or who helped them act or respond differently. Having an understanding of how to situate oneself within multiple contexts and in a temporal dimension (past, present, future) is essential to moving toward preferred narratives.

People Are Not Defined by Problems

Unique to NFT is the idea that the problem is the problem. Instead of viewing a person or a relationship as pathological, dysfunctional, or defective, narrative therapists contend that persons are separate from their problems. Although we may feel like problems such as depression, anxiety, addiction, stress, or worry live inside us, narrative therapists contend that it is the problem-saturated belief or narrative that has become dominant in our lives, giving the problem more power than our ability to manage it. For example, a person may struggle with depression, anxiety, cancer, diabetes, HIV, bulimia, alcohol or drug abuse, or schizophrenia, but a person is not those things. It's the effect or the influence of these things that are "the problem." The illness, condition, or problem does not and should not define the person or relationship. When clients see themselves as separate, they can see the life of the problem and their relationship with it from many angles, perspectives, and contexts. More importantly, this process helps create the space for possibilities and for new and preferred narratives to emerge (Freedman & Combs, 1996; Parry & Doan, 1994; White & Epston, 1990).

Externalizing erodes the problem's power, allowing clients to enact agency by facing and defeating or weakening the effects of the problem. For example, by personifying the problem, clients can see how the problem can bully, manipulate, coerce, seduce, or trick them. These acts of violence, power, manipulation, and control can be so gripping that they inhibit us from exercising our own power, free will, and agency. Externalizing enables clients to claim or reclaim power that has been lost or diminished due to the effects of the problem. Although not all narrative therapists name and externalize the problem, externalization as a way of thinking about persons and their relationship with the problem permeates all aspects of the clinical process, from beginning to end (Bermúdez et al., 2009). The process is nuanced and can happen in many ways. It can involve one person, several people within a family, and/or an entire community (White, 1988; White & Epston, 1990). The externalization process commonly happens by naming, objectifying, and personifying a problem through a metaphor.

Beginning clinicians often think of externalization as a technique or an intervention, however, it is more accurately understood as a way of thinking and talking that invites a therapeutic process, generative stance, or philosophy (McGuinty et al., 2012; Payne, 2006; Roth & Epston, 1996). Furthermore, a novice might be tempted to simply accept and externalize whatever clients identify as the problem when they enter therapy without fully exploring narratives. In our example, Ava's definition of the problem as "uncertainty about the relationship" could be adopted and externalized as the problem without taking time to fully explore the situation. This would have inadvertently contributed to Ava being viewed as the one with the problem without deconstructing the dominant social narratives in which this problem is embedded (Gaddis, 2016). On further inspection, Ava's uncertainty was guiding the way; shedding light on the problems the family was struggling with, including racism and sexism. In fact, Ava's willingness to question was one of her strengths that had been repeatedly overlooked. Questioning and uncertainty would go on to take a central role in the couple's re-authored preferred narrative. Let's listen in again.

Wanda: I am curious about this uncertainty and questioning...did you notice that when you were a kid?

Ava: Sure. I was always uncertain about whether or not I really belonged in the new family. I kept wondering if it was because I looked different, or my stepfather wished my mother hadn't been with my birth dad before him, or if it was because I was the only girl...

Wanda: So lots of exploring what might be going on...what wasn't being talked about.

Ava: Yeah. I am good at that, right? [glances with a smile at Rob]

Rob: (chuckles) You are. She questions everything! I guess I just always accept things at face value.

Wanda: So Ava is the one who takes on the job of figuring things out and finding ways to talk about them?

Ava: I guess so.

Wanda: Makes sense...particularly when you are faced with so many unspeakables.

Ava and Rob: That's a good way to put it.

Wanda now has an agreement about how to language the problem and can move on to externalize "unspeakables." Racism, White privilege, gendered power dynamics, and unwanted pregnancies are all among what is unspeakable. Externalizing questions might include things like, "What do these unspeakables look like?", "Where do they mostly live?", "Who else do they affect and who is affected the most?", "How do you know unspeakables are nearby?", "Who else notices them?", and "When did unspeakables begin to interfere with your relationship?"

Deconstruct the Life of the Problem

In essence, problems have power, and problem-saturated stories need to be understood well in order to diminish or dismantle a problem's power. Rather than supporting pathologizing, deficit-based, internalized descriptions of problems, narrative therapists separate people from problems with the firm belief that problems will be eliminated when stories about our lives and consequent actions no longer support problems. Tilsen (2021) discussed the importance of queering narrative therapy by dismantling and deconstructing how we think and work in order to imagine new realities. Tilsen stated that deconstruction is aligned with queer theory's skepticism toward essentialist ideas by asking questions that would not usually be asked because they are thoughts, ideas, or practices that we perceive to be normal, common, or correct. By decentering dominance, space is created for lived experiences and realities to come forth. Therapists assume a role or clinical posture as a witness or audience whose goal is to be drawn into the story in ways that lead to externalizing the problem, uncovering alternative stories, identifying unique outcomes, and re-authoring preferred life stories and/or relationships with the problem. Therapists actively engage clients in exploring the meaning of the new behavior and expanding the new storyline.

Consider how Wanda might engage with Rob and Ava to map the problem—the "unspeakables." Wanda might use a whiteboard to draw a diagram of the problem to better understand how it affects individuals and relationships (see Figure 14.1).

Wanda: How do these unspeakables affect your relationship with your family?
Ava: It just feels awkward sometimes, like we all know something but just can't talk about it. Makes me feel like there is something to be ashamed of.
Rob: I guess it is like if we don't talk, then it doesn't exist. If we ignore differences or stuff from the past, it will just go away.
Wanda: But it doesn't?
Rob: No. I think it makes us tense and worried sometimes.
Ava: Definitely uncertain of our relationship.
Wanda: Like if we can't even talk about these things, they must be big?
Ava: Yes. I feel silenced a lot…maybe even invisible sometimes.

Once the problem is mapped, Wanda can encourage Rob and Ava to fight against its effects, which in turn are keeping it alive. For example, what is unspeakable leaves Ava feeling silenced; therefore, breaking the silence challenges the problem. Talking about race, gender, White privilege,

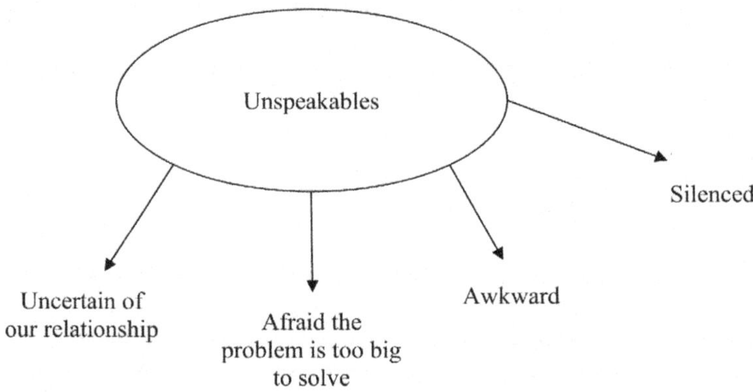

Figure 14.1 Diagram of externalized problem

and other unspeakable dynamics provides avenues for talking about difference, power, and negotiating their relationship within a social context. Not talking about these dynamics fuels Ava's uncertainty as she is not able to address "make it or break it" aspects of her relationship with Rob and their families. In turn, uncertainty fuels what is unspeakable as it increases anxiety over talking about real issues.

Co-create Preferred Narratives

Narrative family therapists listen deeply as they search for experiences, values, and meaning that counter problem-saturated stories and help co-create preferred narratives. These may be mere traces in the form of hopes, dreams, and intentions; moments when values and actions support subordinated stories of strength. Therapists remain committed to being curious, gathering support to thicken and more richly describe new or previously subjugated preferred narratives. This shift from the problematic to the preferred narrative happens by searching for examples of when people are stronger than the influence of the problem (e.g. unique outcomes, exceptions, or sparkling moments). White (2012) discussed these moments "of exception" as times of *initiative.* He stated that he preferred this term because it "evokes a sense of personal agency, that is, a sense that one has the capacity to play a part in the shaping of one's actions and the sense that, in some way, the world is responsive to the fact of one's existence" (p. 123).

White contended that (2012, p. 123), "scaffolding provides people with the support in the incremental and progressive distancing from the known and familiar toward what is possible for them to know and do without the assistance of the scaffolding." This gap is what Vygotsky referred to as the zone of proximal development. White (2007) applied this concept to therapeutic conversations as a way to understand the therapist's role in scaffolding dialogue and create the space for unique outcomes and preferred narratives. Madigan (2019, p. 173) added that "through the telling of a re-authored story, people can identify previously neglected but vital aspects of lived experiences—aspects that could not have been predicted from the dominant problem story."

In our case example, Wanda talked with Rob and Ava about how, as a couple, they had already begun to challenge the unspeakables of racism that can cause trouble in interracial relationships. This part of their story, the part that was challenging existing social norms, was thickened as an alternative plot. They agreed on the importance of race and gender equality but were uncertain about how these issues could be addressed. They struggled to talk about this in their relationship and succumbed to a White male-privileged stance of maintaining inequity by acting as if equality already existed between them. Furthermore, Rob's acceptance of things at "face value" may have been, at least in part, a function of his unspoken White, male privilege.

Understanding the *landscape of identity* and the *landscape of action* are important processes that lead clients toward preferred narratives and desired outcomes. The landscape of identity "emphasizes the irreducible fact that any renegotiation of the stories of people's lives is also a renegotiation of identity" (White, 2007, p. 82). For example, contrast the landscape of Ava's identity if she sees herself as a biracial woman from an unwanted relationship instead of a racially aware feminist. The landscape of action refers to concrete action that must be taken through intentional thoughts, actions, and interactions to bring preferred narratives to life in strong, tangible, and lasting ways. Following Ava, this might include her openly discussing race and gender equity and talking more openly about her birth father. That said, not all actions are possible in all contexts. People will still respond to her based on the color of her skin. There are societal and structural limits to action that can be taken on preferred narratives.

There are many ways to explore and amplify unique outcomes. For example, *remembering conversations* call on past relational knowings that contradict clients' dominant narratives that help elicit preferred, alternative stories. Those conversations thicken the preferred narrative and give it a stronger life in the future. According to White (2007),

> re-membering conversations provide an opportunity for people to revise the memberships of their association of life: to upgrade some memberships and to downgrade others; to honour some memberships and to revoke others; to grant authority to some voices in regard to matters of one's personal identity and to disqualify other voices. (p. 129)

A narrative therapist might ask, "Who in your life would not be surprised that you are now graduating from college?" This re-membering brings forth those individuals who team up with the client to thicken the plot of the preferred narrative. *Definitional ceremonies* (White, 2007), rituals, performances, art, creative expression, dance, letters, ceremonies, certificates, and the telling and retelling of the preferred narrative are also ways in which we can strengthen the life of the narrative that supports preferred ways of living, being, and relating to others. Bruner, as cited by White and Epston (1990), stated that "life experience is richer than discourse. Narrative structures organize and give meaning to experience, but there are always feelings and lived experience not fully encompassed by the dominant story (E. Bruner, 1986a, p. 143)." Narratives tend to be anchored in evocative moments; any experiential way of performing or telling the new narrative gives it more power, making it more likely that the developing narrative will translate into action (Zimmerman, 2018).

Integrating Principles of Sociocultural Attunement

The postmodern assumption that reality is socially constructed has been embraced by narrative therapists; however, several scholars have noted the limitations of this framework from a critical lens (Agger, 1991; McDowell, 2015; Miller, 2000; Slott, 2005). Many postmodern therapists, including narrative therapists, question critical social theory as relying on a modernist grand theory or singular truth claim. In turn, many critical social justice-oriented therapists argue that postmodernism relies too heavily on relativism. This can obscure injustice as a matter of pluralistic, equally valid perspectives, disregarding the real material consequences of social inequity. While narrative philosophy and practice are strongly situated in multicultural work (Laird, 1998), narrative therapists who neglect to attend to systems of power, privilege, and oppression risk maintaining the status quo by failing to address the impact of societal systems on their clients' lives and agency (Dumaresque et al., 2018).

Critical postmodernism and metamodernism attempt to reconcile tensions between theoretical perspectives. According to Boje (2001), "critical postmodern is definable as the nexus of critical theory, postcolonialism, critical pedagogy, and postmodern theory" (p. 433). Critical postmodernists join social constructionists in acknowledging that language does not reflect an objective reality and is not neutral. At the same time, they rely on analyses of societal structures to explain the inequitable distribution of influence and material resources. As noted in Chapter 2, we consider metamodernism to be an even broader framework that makes it possible to assume a superposition in relationship to competing epistemological and ontological paradigms. Taking a superposition allows socioculturally attuned narrative therapists to reflect on possibilities within, and relationships between, various systems of thought—including modernism, postmodernism, critical theory, Indigenous worldviews, local knowledge, and felt experiences. This expands and opens space for diverse ways of thinking, being, feeling, and doing.

In Text Box 14.1, narrative family therapist Laurel Salmon describes critically deconstructing how sociocultural contexts are part of each case she sees or supervises.

Text Box 14.1 Laurel Salmon, MS, LMFT

Laurel Salmon, MS, LMFT is the owner and operator of Ask Laurel, a mental health practice based in Nyack, NY, where she provides trauma-informed, socially just therapy and consulting services for youth, families, and adults. Laurel is also an adjunct professor in the Marriage and Family Therapy program at Mercy College. Formerly the Executive Director of CANDLE in New York, she has focused her career on community support, integrating strategies to interrupt oppression, and understanding the ways sexism, racism, heteronormativity, and religious oppression impact therapy. Laurel is dedicated to advancing equitable mental health care and empowering marginalized communities through clinical practice, training, and advocacy.

I tend to see all therapeutic clients through the lens of narrative therapy blended with elements of emotionally focused and attachment-based approaches. These models are about how clients experience relationships and the world through their lived experience. I always come from a place of stating what exists versus what we are told is true. I validate the internal resistance oppressed and marginalized people experience and highlight it. This practice helps people to identify how they want to be treated.

My work provides a framework for third order thinking around oppression and how it impacts the people we work with. I developed "Four Questions" to analyze how clients experience the world through the various systems they interact with and the social constructs the world applies to them. The Four Questions framework includes:

1. *What are the common stereotypes about each of the groups that [the client] falls into?*
2. *What is the dynamic between us because of oppression?*
3. *How can I expect to oppress [the client] inadvertently if I am not careful?*
4. *How are the current presenting problems related to oppression? (Salmon, 2017, p. 14)*

Once those factors are front and center, it pushes the clinician and or supervisor to identify how the therapeutic or supervisory relationship is impacted. I always name the unspoken context of unjust interactions. I err on the side of possibly overstating in order to balance how early we are conditioned to leave certain inequities unnamed. I routinely take the time to express who has the power to silence and marginalize by naming and highlighting the unspoken and unseen. I think it is our role to identify and examine these dynamics as part of our therapeutic work.

I spend a lot of time examining larger systems that we involuntarily interact with, like criminal justice, education, medical, social service, and mental health systems. I make an effort to externalize ideas that people have integrated into their sense of self, that come from the way they experience these systems. I also spend a lot of time talking about power dynamics and how they give all our relationships (with people and systems) a context that assigns meaning to all interactions. For example, if I have power over you—earned or unearned—it will impact how you feel about my interpretation of your behavior and how you will take guidance from me. If you feel like I value you as a person and respect your choices, it will adjust the context of how you experience me.

This perspective on power dynamics can be applied to any relationship, not just therapeutic relationships. It exists in courts, in schools, between doctors and patients, and in any other capacity where people interact. My hope is that by constantly giving voice to this, both marginalized and dominating groups will be slowly pushed toward more equitable relationships.

Societal Context and Discourses of Resistance

Socioculturally attuned narrative family therapists are keenly aware of how complex, interconnected social, structural, cultural, political, and economic realities contribute to unequal division of labor and resources, as well as uneven influence in decision-making and agency within and across all societies. Language plays a significant role in promoting and/or resisting societal systems; in how these systems are maintained, justified, challenged, and/or transformed. The aim of socioculturally attuned NFT includes helping clients deconstruct dominant discourses that maintain problems, co-create new narratives, and take action in support of preferred narratives. It also includes exploring with clients collective discourses of resistance to socially unjust dominant discourses.

•←→•

Socioculturally attuned narrative family therapists assume dominant discourses are among many competing and interrelated discourses for which there is greater or lesser social support.

•←→•

Support for discourses is garnered in several ways, including establishing and protecting truth claims (e.g., this is how it is) and/or appealing to one's interests, beliefs, and/or values (e.g., this is how it should be). When discourses are at odds, hybrids are formed. New stories emerge in the epistemological borderlands within and between global, societal, and familial contexts. For example, in the US, dominant discourses of democracy and capitalism are at times congruent and at times conflicting (McLaren & Farahmandpur, 2001). Contested interpretations of these value-based ideologies inform the broadest (e.g., Supreme Court decisions about same-sex marriage, laws banning hate crimes, banking deregulation) to the most intimate (e.g., our relationships with money, reproductive rights, who we listen to) public and personal decisions. Spin off discourses that have emerged as a result of the inherent incongruence of these and other dominant discourses include the myth of meritocracy, prosperity theology, heteronormativity, Christian nationalism, and colonial narratives of eugenics that associate skin color and phenotype with evolution (e.g., race).

The practice of NFT, with its emphasis on authoring one's preferred narrative, can inadvertently support the belief that anyone can "pull themselves [up] by their own bootstraps," hence supporting the myth of meritocracy (McNamee & Miller, 2004). Socioculturally attuned NFTs will recognize that the socially constructed discourse of an equal playing field (democratic ideal) in a system that requires some to be at the economic bottom (capitalism) draws attention away from the inherent conflict of these narratives by placing the problem squarely on those who have suffered lifetimes of cumulative disadvantage (Merton, 1988).

•←→•

Just as all discourses are acts of collective meaning-making, dominant discourses and discourses of resistance are also shared narratives.

•←→•

These various discourses are not seen simply as an array of personal choices, but as value-driven propositions which many of us cast our votes for or against. When dominant discourses go unnoticed as natural, inevitable, or assumed right by nature of their widespread support, we at best, inadvertently cast our vote in favor of, or fail to vote against, what may not align with our values, best interests, experience, or epistemology. Again, therapists must "be acquainted with many possible stories about life" (White, 2007, p. 82), and we argue this includes discourses of resistance to which clients can be introduced (Sen, 2020). Consider the impact discourses of resistance might have on our couple, Ava and Rob. Wanda might introduce them to websites for multiracial families (e.g., Project RACE), invite Rob into a men's group that actively challenges male privilege and patriarchy (e.g., National Organization of Men Against Sexism), and/or offer titles of books (e.g., bell hooks and Michael Kimmel). All of these resources are sites of collective resistance that challenge oppressive dominant discourses.

Dominant discourses may privilege some members of families over others, contributing to relational inequity. Socioculturally attuned NFT attends to conflicting narratives within families. This includes exploring who is supporting them and why, as well as how narratives may benefit some over others. Therapists carefully attend to ways in which certain family members are valued by each other, by society, or by other important people and contexts in their lives. Again, considering Ava and Rob, the narrative of Rob as being a non-racist White man inadvertently placed the burden of change on Ava by masking Rob's accountability for White male privilege.

Culture and (De)Colonization

As described in Chapter 2, colonialism refers to a process in which dominant group cultural practices, ideologies, and beliefs are centered as more right and true. The ideologies, beliefs, and cultural practices of non-dominant groups are subjugated and actively interrupted. This privileges dominant groups by centering their cultural capital (Bourdieu, 1986) to create and maintain the colonizers' advantage. Socioculturally attuned NFT is informed by decolonizing frameworks. As others have detailed, this requires reflexively considering the Western origins of narrative therapy and how it is conceptualized and practiced (polanco, 2016), as well as how narrative therapy is regularly co-opted by mental health delivery systems without considering how the treatment system itself upholds structural causes of oppression and problematizing world views (Dumaresque et al., 2018).

Like all models, narrative practices do not directly transfer or adapt to other cultures (polanco, 2016). An emphasis on space and linear time is, in itself, a colonizing act as the temporal epistemology of the West and Global North is privileged in most therapy. For example, therapists typically consider only one dimension of space over a single lifetime. This is in stark contrast to many Indigenous concepts of space, which exist simultaneously across multiple dimensions and time, in a nonlinear fashion. Stories are not always depicted in spoken or written words, as noted in our case illustration at the end of this chapter. Meaning is also co-constructed in ways that are non-verbal, expressive, visceral, and performative.

For example, marcella polanco (2016) described needing to develop a different way of practicing narrative therapy when working in her native Colombian Spanish, of having what she terms "un-reason-able conversations" (p. 73):

> I had to search for…the making of narrative therapy conversations which…make possible the made-up-ness of extraordinary, ordinary, unreal real realities not normally verifiable by the mind of Western reason, logic or sensory perception… I seek to turn reasonable conversations unreasonable, when displacing reason and logic as the only legitimate means for conversation—hence dethroning the brain as the only organ of our bodies that possess the capacity to become knowledged… I ask questions like these [regarding suicide]: What did your body know about you and your relationships that although your mind had decided to die, your body proceeded to live? At the moment in which your mind starts taking charge with its deadly plans, what part or parts of your body do you remember taking the lead in the

execution of such plans, and how was it like for them to engage in the plan?… I have learned that when given the opportunity, parts of our poetic, imaginative bodies, may have grown minds of their own. They are begging us to let them speak their minds, since they are often shrouded in secrecy. (pp. 74–75)

↔

It is difficult to make sense of one's experience when there is no language, no discourse through which it can be described. Not only are experiences outside of dominant cultural discourses marginalized by others, they are often marginalized within us—kept silent, secret and foreign to who we think we should be.

↔

Socioculturally attuned NFTs are attentive to hermeneutical injustice (Fricker, 2007), referring to inequities in whose experience is understood and given social credibility. They recognize how readily dominant cultural narratives are imposed or unchallenged in therapy if therapists do not externalize these normative judgements and invite counter-stories (Dumaresque et al., 2018; Sen, 2021). Shelja Sen (2021), a narrative therapist who works with young women in India dealing with gender-based trauma, uses therapeutic conversations to "develop solidarity against generations of patriarchy" (p. 61). Shawn Giammattei (Text Box 14.2) details a similarly decolonizing approach in his work with transgender, non-binary, gender expansive (TGE) clients and their families.

Text Box 14.2 Shawn V. Giammattei, PhD, Clinical Family Psychologist

Shawn Giammattei is a clinical psychologist with a group family therapy practice in California. He is the Associate Director of Mental Health for the Child and Adolescent Gender Center at UCSF, Benioff Children's Hospital, and founder of the Gender Health Training Institute and the TransFamily Alliance. He teaches at the California School of Professional Psychology, is a research consultant to Kaiser Permanente and Emory University, and a World Professional Association for Transgender Health (WPATH) certified gender specialist and mentor. While he draws on many clinical models, Shawn situates his work in a narrative paradigm.

The narrative paradigm keeps me attuned to the sociopolitical context. It requires me to deconstruct the heteronormative and cisnormative elements of the theories and techniques we use, and to do so in a culturally conscious way. I am a White, 2nd generation American, highly educated, and well resourced. I am also a gay man who was assigned female at birth and began the journey of authentic embodiment at the age of 36. I live with an invisible disability and have experienced the extreme impact of transphobia despite the privileges of the color of my skin and access to education. I am one personification of the resilience in this community. I am also keenly aware of how much easier my path has been compared to my trans siblings, particularly QTBIPOC, due to my levels of privilege.

Transgender people are often viewed in negative and pathologized ways by the world, their families, and themselves. Their difficulties are not appropriately seen as a medical issue, but as a cultural one. Parents are blamed for not properly gendering their children, and trans people are often treated like they don't have any family or that no one will ever love them or want to partner with them, so they aren't even considered in the context of a family or community other than as a throwaway human. My whole practice, whether working with clients directly, training clinicians, or acting as an advocate, is to disrupt these notions so we move to seeing trans people as humans with families, relationships, and something amazing to offer this world because of who they are, not in spite of it.

It would be very easy to exploit transgender, non-binary, gender diverse (TGD) clients and their families and become gatekeepers to their medically necessary care. We must understand not only the obvious issues impacting these families but also the more subtle cultural narratives around gender and sexuality. It is absolutely necessary for any therapist working with this community, regardless of their social location, to do the self of the therapist work, understand who they are in relation to their clients and how that impacts their work, the questions they ask, and what they think is possible for their clients.

The TGD population is incredibly marginalized. This is exponential when one holds more than one marginalized identity. On top of that is the impact of sociocultural narratives on family acceptance or lack thereof. Clinicians need to stay very close to our clients and understand these interactions and experiences, and not place our own lens and expectations on the families with whom we work. Sometimes, a simple question about whether they might be experiencing something opens up a whole story about what's happening culturally for them. I also use many tools, including genograms and cultural maps to get a better sense of their stories and experience. I pay very close attention to my own personal reactions to what I'm hearing. Once I recognize an issue is present or I'm aware that something is happening politically, socially, or culturally, I highlight it by asking questions about the impact of those things, or by exploring the history of behaviors that may be influenced by those factors or power dynamics. This is especially true at this time in history.

When I sense a power imbalance of some sort or I know something is happening that is not being brought forth, I usually call it out in a gentle way. Most common for me is to say something like, "I'm noticing something; I'm not sure it's correct, but I'm wondering about…does any of that resonate for you?" I help them explore it, unpack it, make sense out of it, and come to conclusions of their own about what this means for their relationships and what they should do moving forward. I am always listening for how heteronormativity, cisgenderism, and transphobia are internalized and impacting us. I generally externalize all those isms. We explore how they play out, then take a stand on how to challenge them. I make sure they're feeling understood and held enough to step into the scary areas, especially around power dynamics and the need to balance those. When it comes to working with systems outside of the therapy room, I am often writing letters and speaking and standing up on behalf of my clients in the community. Transgender people and their families not only need advocacy around medical interventions, they need us to promote general access to care, safe workspaces, and school settings, and equity in treatment.

Envisioning new stories of resilience is a key part of my work. This is often done with the whole family, but in certain circumstances, if I'm using, say EMDR or IFS for trauma, I always take it to the place where they can rewrite the story with the newfound empowered knowledge of themselves and the connections they've created. From that place, we can create plans to move towards change, even in contexts that may appear hopeless. I'm a bit of a cheerleader towards resilience and transformative change, and tend to hold a very hopeful and positive stance, sometimes holding it for my clients when they can't get there yet.

Power and Subjugation

How we think and talk about power is important. Foucault (1982) argued that power produces, through knowledge claims, what we assume to be real or true. This includes what and who we think of as normal or not normal. The power problem most NF therapists set out to solve is that of being subjects of objective, scientific, or modern knowledge that defines who we are for ourselves and others. This has been revolutionary in the practice of family therapy. At the same time, there is a risk of creating another grand narrative or truth claim by too narrowly and certainly defining what power *is* or *is not.* For example, when we make claims such as "power is everywhere," we run the risk of engaging in the very definitional process Foucault resisted. That is not to say that power isn't everywhere, but that we might be better served by saying something like "when we think of power as being everywhere…" This type of statement suggests a view from somewhere (we) and that there are other perspectives (when we think of power as). This is particularly important in socioculturally attuned NFT as it provides a congruent theoretical perspective by which to acknowledge the lived experience of Foucault's second type of subjugation, such as dependence and control.

By expanding the notion of subject beyond the limits of definition and identity, we are better able to acknowledge the material consequences and lived experience of social and relational processes of oppression. Take, for example, a mother who removes herself and her children from a physically abusive male partner. Her social label and identity may be that of a single mother whose children are being raised in a "broken home." Family members' identities are then deficit-based and determined by divorce. A new narrative might support a family identity as liberated and whose members fought for their freedom. This is a powerful narrative, however, there are still real material consequences to raising children with one income, particularly for females given the gender wage gap, dealing with restraining orders and custody battles, and navigating teacher's biases and perceptions about the children's family and home life.

Foucault (1982) assumed that resistance is present wherever there is power. Deconstructive listening and co-constructing preferred narratives are foundational to resisting the subjugating effects of defining self-as-problem. Socioculturally attuned narrative family therapists pay close attention to the effects of definitional power as well as dynamics of dependence and control. This includes noticing who takes up more space in relational contexts; who gets to talk, who talks most often, whose words have more influence, and whose role in the relationship is most valued. It also includes actively interrupting power-over processes in support of just and equitable relationships.

Let's consider Marvin and Rose, who have been married for nearly 50 years. While they seem to get along well, Marvin frequently teases Rose about what she eats (policing her body and food intake), makes jokes when she gets lost or forgets something (storying her as less competent), and refers to her as his "old girl" (diminishes both her gender and age). Discourses that subjugate women are of course, still present and were particularly dominant during this couple's lifetime. These intimate performances of power both reflect and support dominant discourses about gender, yet are performed by specific people within specific relationships and contexts. Their performance of power is shaped not only by social discourses, but by how the couple's personalities, family of origin backgrounds, independent financial resources, relationships with children and grandchildren, and so on are shaped and impacted by these larger, societal discourses.

Third Order Change

Within the context of the therapeutic relationship, there are varying levels of transformative change that clients experience. As discussed in Chapter 2, therapists often challenge their clients to create second order change rather than first order change, as second order change focuses on altering systems of interactions. Second order change in narrative therapy occurs when clients reclaim their lives from dominant stories, which in turn transforms their narratives and their relationships with those with whom they interact.

•←→•

Third order change raises social awareness helping clients view dominant narratives with a sociopolitical lens. Once clients are able to notice how societal forces perpetuate dominant discourses and contribute to problems, they are better prepared to navigate and resist their effects.

•←→•

Through a socioculturally attuned framework, NF therapists are able to name, explore, and deconstruct the influence of societal structures of oppression, such as racism, heterosexism, sexism, and ableism, with their clients. Questions that aim to deconstruct oppressive societal discourse might include: "How do you think homophobia is influencing the dominant view you have of yourself?" "In what ways has racism played a role in what is bringing you to therapy?," "How does sexism operate in your life?," "If ableism could speak to you, what kind of messages do you think it would say about your worth as a person? A partner? A friend?"—and "If your most empowered, best self were able to stand up to classism, what would you want it to understand about you?" How would you stand up to it?"

Practice Guidelines

The following five practice guidelines help family members recognize the impact of societal systems of power and oppression on not only how they story their lives, problems, and preferred narratives, but also on the material realities of their lives. It is helpful to note that they are not always implemented sequentially and may move fluidly back and forth over the course of the therapy. They are: 1) expand the map to include sociopolitical structures, 2) deconstruct power-embedded relational inequity and name injustices, 3) explore values embedded in narratives, 4) support relational equity and disrupt oppressive power dynamics, and 5) thicken stories of resistance and resilience.

1. Expand the Map to Include Sociopolitical Structures

Socioculturally attuned narrative family therapists **attune** not only to the influence of social discourse but to the impact of societal structures in their clients' lives. They expand the map of the problem to **name** complex, interconnected social, structural, cultural, political, and economic realities that contribute to unequal division of labor, resources, influence, and agency within families and communities. Dominant discourses remain central in the work of deconstructing problem narratives and reconstructing preferred narratives. What is often less clear is the understanding of problems and possibilities within societal contexts and social structures that constrain agency and afford access to opportunities based on the many intersections based on social location/group membership (e.g., race, class, gender, sexual orientation, nation of origin, abilities, religion, etc.). Expanding the map to examine larger social structures such as patriarchy, white privilege, and structures that control and maintain wealth and power helps therapists understand a person's or family's sense of agency and mobility within the larger sociopolitical terrain.

2. Deconstruct Power-embedded Relational Inequity and Name Injustices

Socioculturally attuned narrative family therapists collaborate with clients to deconstruct dominant discourses that are at odds with, or limiting of, their lived experience. Therapists *loosen the grip* of problematic narratives and help *open space* to link discourses to relational dynamics that may give or take away power. This includes identifying how shared narratives support unjust intimate relationships as well as how divergent narratives within families serve to create and maintain problematic power dynamics. There is a recognition that what is "preferred" may be contested across individual, family, and cultural narratives. For example, a narrative supporting male privilege may be preferred by some members of the family, while a narrative supporting gender equity may be optimal for other members of the family or all members some of the time. In other words, narratives, including preferred narratives, serve a role and must be considered relative to negotiating power in intimate relationships.

Additionally, socioculturally attuned narrative therapists would be cognizant of the notion that having a preference is indeed a privilege. For many, having a preferred narrative is facilitated or constrained by the effects of cumulative advantage or disadvantage due to living with the effects of intersecting identities and social locations. A socioculturally attuned narrative family therapist is mindful of bias embedded in the notion of a "preferred narrative," carefully assessing for conflicts and compatibility within and across multiple narratives. These narratives, preferred, beneficial, optimal, or otherwise, may reflect contesting societal discourses and/or be sources of individual struggle and family and community conflict.

3. Explore Values Embedded in Narratives

As problem-supporting discourses are challenged, new narratives emerge that are, in many ways, value-driven propositions. Helping individuals and families identify, clarify, and negotiate **values** is critical to developing preferred narratives that support the well-being of all involved. For example, one parent may value privacy and independence more highly than transparency and collective care. The ways in which they narrate the child's problems and their child's journey through life will be impacted by these values. A father may complain that his son should have launched and been on his own by his early 20s, while a mother appreciates his ongoing concern and care for the family. These are potentially very different storylines to which therapists often add their own valued position, such as launching in early adulthood is healthy, the mother is holding the son back to meet her own needs, the couple cannot stand alone, etc. Additionally, not all values have the same weight and power in society. It may be less apparent for a narrative therapist to determine which narratives reflect values that are supported or not supported by the dominant group in a society. These factors may remain unexamined unless the therapist is carefully attending to the implicit values embedded in the client's and their own narratives.

4. Support Relational Equity and Disrupt Oppressive Power Dynamics

Socioculturally attuned narrative family therapists pay close attention to how power is performed; what people do in relation to others, the types of influence they exert, and the consequences of relational inequity. They are curious about how the performance of power is permitted, accepted, followed, or applauded based on a person's social location. The therapist encourages transparency about these dynamics by asking deconstructive questions, **valuing** each person's voice, and helping clients understand the effects of how power is enacted on each individual, couple, and family. For example, questions that disrupt homophobia, patriarchy, colorism, or sexism would focus on how inequity influences and supports the life of the problem. Clients are invited to deconstruct social and familial narratives that privilege and story unequal adult relationships as being natural, inevitable, or preferred. The therapist intentionally introduces possibilities for co-constructing new narratives that support relational equity, irrespective of culture. In every society in which systemic and culturally sanctioned injustice toward a particular group or person is enacted, there is active resistance. When socioculturally attuned therapists **intervene** by disrupting narratives that fuel oppression, inequity, and relational injustice, we can help clients strengthen **transformative** narratives that amplify voice and resistance.

5. Thicken Stories of Resistance and Resilience

A mistake many therapists make is that we often have a generalized and essentialized view of culture, in which we believe that certain cultures or subcultures will support gender or race oppression and inequality more than others. This is a distorted view of culture. Although patriarchy is embedded in most societies, most would agree that the abuses enacted due to patriarchy, such as violence, femicide, torture, bullying, rape, and victimization in general, should not be supported. It is important to create space for subjugated narratives of resistance in order for clients to **envision** preferred narratives.

In sum, socioculturally attuned therapists do not excuse, validate, or support cultural reasons for oppression, inequity, and inequality. In every place where it is enacted, there are forms of resistance, small and large, internalized or externalized, overt or covert. And when resistance is understood by a therapist, couple, family, or society as problematic, then injustice is likely to be reified in one form or another. For example, if someone resists oppression by becoming withdrawn or depressed, then the problem is oppression, which is feeding the life of the depression. The new narrative will align with the lived experience of the person enacting resistance. Resistance is there, held in the body and relationships, but the **naming** opens one's experience to begin to address the effects of oppression on one's self, body, and relationships.

Sites of power are also sites of resistance. Socioculturally attuned narrative family therapists will excavate these sites to uncover and amplify resilience. These narratives include moments when clients find ways to hold on to their values, strengthen their resolve, and endure despite oppression, and so on. What is often explored only on this personal level is tied to collective resistance and resilience. Discourses of resistance, such as the Black Lives Matter movement, #MeToo movement, women's movements, Pride and queer activism, American Indian Movement, and the fatosphere (an online community for fat acceptance), for example, are introduced as shared narratives that challenge and **transform** dominant oppressive discourses. Likewise, collective resilience among those with whom we identify over time (e.g., Black ancestors, Native communities) thickens individual and family stories of resilience and resistance.

The process of **transforming** oppression and amplifying resilience includes recognizing and enhancing (thickening) the embodied emotional experience associated with the new narrative (Beaudoin & Monk, 2024). In the example of depression as resistance to oppression, depression is the felt embodiment of social injustice. Socioculturally attuned therapists will help clients recognize and amplify what preferred experiences such as agency, hope, or relationship to a greater good feels like in the body and in interactions with others. As suggested by Beaudoin and Monk (2024) and illustrated in the case below, resilience is more able to resist reactivation of dominant narratives when the new, empowered life narratives are affectively embodied and meaningfully experienced within relationships beyond oneself. Prosocial actions, engagement in social causes, or community involvement, can support this embodiment and the ongoing life of the new narrative.

Case Illustration

This case involved family therapy with a mother named Raquel, a father named Aldo, their adult daughter named Ana, and their advocate named Carla. Ana was referred from a center for survivors of sexual abuse to Gabriela at Latino Centered Family Services. Gabriela was a third generation bilingual US citizen of Mexican descent. The family did not speak English, nor read or write in Spanish, and were unauthorized immigrants from Peru. Ana was a young woman in her early 20s, lived at home with her family, and was deaf/hearing impaired. Ana had the support of a loving, cohesive family. She was the oldest of four siblings. Her family cared for her, but she was also responsible for caring for her family by cooking, cleaning, taking care of her siblings, and being a good companion to her mother. She especially had a close relationship with her mother, who was her translator and "voice." Ana had never been in a romantic relationship, had outside friends, or had gone anywhere without her family. Given her inability to communicate with others, she spent most of her time at home and was dependent on her parents. Carla, who accompanied them to therapy, was a bilingual/bicultural Latina who was obtaining her associate's degree in social work and served as a strong support and resource for the family. She would often drive them to the family therapy sessions, women's shelter, police station, and to court. Carla had considerable social capital and was the ideal advocate for the family. Although Ana was facing many challenges, she seemed eager to be in therapy and engaged in the clinical process from the start.

Expand the Map to Include Sociopolitical Structures

Gabriela worked hard to join with Ana and help her feel comfortable. During the first session, much of the time was spent talking to her mother to gather information and find ways to nonverbally connect with Ana, with as much eye contact and signs of empathy as possible. It soon became apparent that Ana and her mother had their own form of sign language. Raquel was Ana's primary support person and translator who effectively relayed the therapist's messages. The therapist would say things like, "Please tell her that I am so glad she is here and that she is so brave for wanting to tell her story and wanting to move forward in her life in a positive way." Then Raquel would tell Ana with a series of signs that were unique to them.

Ana's mother told the therapist (Gabriela) that Ana was sexually assaulted multiple times by a family member who lived near them. Ana's mother, Raquel, was experiencing secondary trauma and would uncontrollably cry when she felt Ana's pain and her own rage toward the abuser, a close relative. Given that Ana could not verbalize or write her story, Gabriela asked her to draw a picture, as a way to stay connected with her during the first session. As she drew, Gabriela would look at Ana and show empathy in response to everything her mother disclosed about what happened and why they were referred to therapy. At the end of the session, it became clear that Ana could express herself through images. Gabriela was relieved and elated that she had a means to communicate with Ana. As a consequence, she decided that, with the use of drawings and enactments, experiential narrative therapy would be the best means of working with Ana and her family.

Deconstruct Power-embedded Relational Inequity and Name Injustices

Art and narrative family therapy can be used as an experiential means to deconstruct problematic narratives, increase a client's sense of agency, and reauthor preferred narratives (Bermúdez & Bermúdez, 2002; Bermúdez et al., 2009; Carlson, 1997; Keeling & Bermúdez, 2006; Simons, 2023). In this case, Gabriela heard of the use of storyboards in the film and animation industry and decided to try to use this as a means to communicate with Ana and help Ana tell her own story. Before beginning, Gabriela met with Raquel and Aldo, Ana's parents, to ask if it was acceptable to proceed in this way of working with Ana. Gabriela told them that she would stop at any point if she assessed that the process was not helpful or harmful for Ana. They both agreed that it would be a good move forward and gave consent for Gabriela to meet with Ana alone, most of the time.

This would afford her privacy and offer support. Raquel (mother) agreed to be a part of the beginning and end of each session. Although Ana did not show any signs of distress when her mother was not in the room, Raquel's presence was important.

The first goal was to **attune** to Ana and her world by demonstrating an attempt to understand and by responding to experience within her societal context. This was done first by learning Ana's signs for her emotions. For example, Ana and her mother explained the signs for sadness; which was a sign of a broken heart with her hands; fear, which was her acting as if she were shivering; joy, which was smiling with her hands on her chest and a thumbs up; peace, which was her pointing to God with prayerful hands or hands on heart; frustrated, overwhelmed and anxious, which was her pointing to her head, shaking it with a sad face; and hopeless, with her hands up in the air, as if not knowing what to do.

This process of intentionally and responsively attuning to Ana led to her naming the events that unfolded that were abusive and unjust. Ana's voice would have been easy to discount or ignore, as none of them knew how to communicate by writing or through American sign language, but as Gabriela communicated her interest, Ana's will to be understood was more powerful than her inability to hear, speak, sign, or write. Through the course of therapy, Ana described what happened with each drawing. She drew a total of 18 drawings, each one representing the sequence of events. The therapist would motion with her finger in a forward circle as if saying, "and then what happened?" and then Ana would draw what happened on a new sheet of paper, which the therapist numbered and kept in order in her file at the clinic. The therapist attempted to honor Ana's language, her ways of knowing, and her ability to tell her own story. Although Ana did not know the names for rape, sexual assault, or abuse, based on the therapist's, mother's, and advocate's empathic responses, Ana was able to **name** the abuse and injustice through her images, expression of emotion, and others' responses.

Explore Values Embedded in Narratives

In the midst of larger familial, social, and cultural systems that may have minimized or discounted Ana altogether, the therapist was able to demonstrate how she **valued** and acknowledged Ana's worth. The social worker also valued Ana and served as a witness to her pain and survival, as well as her telling and retelling of the preferred narrative of strength and courage. The values demonstrated by the therapist, advocate, and her family communicated to Ana that she was loved and that her family was doing all that they could to help her heal and keep her safe. They demonstrated their values of family cohesion, respect, and resilience. As the preferred narrative was thickened by narratives of resilience, they also demonstrated strength and bravery by actively seeking resources for Ana and taking legal action to keep the perpetrator and his wife away from her. Through the course of therapy, the family's narrative of love and cohesion was strengthened, while simultaneously changing Ana's narrative from victim to a young woman who is strong and resilient.

Support Relational Equity and Disrupt Oppressive Power Dynamics

The entire clinical process, which only lasted eight sessions over five months, served to **intervene** and disrupt oppressive power dynamics and support relational equity. Through the course of telling and retelling her story with the images she drew and colored, Ana was able to demonstrate how she claimed her power to disrupt abusive power dynamics. This was especially evident with her reaction toward her family member/abuser, who was their landlord, and had the privileges of being a documented US citizen and a middle-aged man with financial stability. He and his wife threatened to have Ana's family deported if they spoke to authorities about the sexual assaults, which they both denied. With the support of the advocate and the sexual assault center, Ana and her family garnered the courage and support to stand up to violence, threats, and intimidation. The disruption of power dynamics was also reflected in a picture Ana drew of herself when she destroyed the gifts they had given her, which included the flower bushes she pulled up and threw at the front door of their house. This act of resistance, which she initiated on her own, demonstrated her strength and ability to stand up to her abuser/oppressor.

The process of deconstructing the life of the problem and reconstructing the preferred narrative through these drawings was powerful. Halfway through the storyboarding, Ana and her mother were able to co-create space to imagine and envision a better way of life for Ana. At the end of the storyboard, Ana depicted an image of her preferred narrative, with her standing next to her mother, both holding hands and with their arms in the air, as if triumphant. As White and Epston asserted (1990), with every performance of the new narrative, we gain valuable experience in reauthoring our lives. By paying close attention to the aspects of lived experience that fell outside of the dominant story, Ana and her family were able to discover important resources for the generation and re-generation of her preferred narrative to emerge and gain strength and life.

Thicken Stories of Resistance and Resilience

It was important and moving for Ana, her family, the social worker/advocate, and the therapist to **envision** what was possible. **Transformation** took place because they all worked together in collaboration to make what was imagined real. Toward the end of therapy, the therapist asked them to do two family sculptures; one when they were in the grip of fear, grief, and despair, and another one representing how they felt now that Ana and her mother were able to bring to light their courage and strength. The triumphant image was one they sculpted together and brought tears to everyone's eyes. On the day of the last session, the mother stated that she was committed to helping Ana learn American sign language, which would help her make friends and open herself to an adult world of connecting with others. Her parents also created an art space for her at home so Ana could create artwork and give it as gifts or sell it to earn her own money.

Ana, with the support of her family, was able to unite and stand up to the effects of her violence and oppression. Her parents and advocate were committed to renewing the restraining order so that Ana could feel more protected. The therapy process was empowering for everyone involved, even for her younger siblings. As a final ritual, the therapist asked Ana what she wanted to do with the drawings, and with a big smile on her face, she communicated that she was going to bury them in her backyard. She decided to keep the last image of her and her mother feeling triumphant. She also ended the therapy by giving the therapist a gift, which was her very first painting she made with the art supplies her therapist gave her.

Summary: Third Order Change

In this case, first order change occurred when the therapist found ways for Ana to communicate through drawings. This made second and third order change possible. At a second order change level, Ana moved from an unwanted, disempowering narrative of being a victim to that of a survivor. Her father also resisted machismo by supporting his daughter above all else, sharing his feelings, and resisting his desire to cause harm to the abuser. He also stated that he felt as though he failed to protect his daughter; however, his resistance to this dominant discourse led him to have the courage to handle the matter "*con inteligencia y calma*," as he stated in Spanish. He and his wife were able to unite to best support their daughter. Ana's decision to learn sign language would provide ongoing second order change as she would learn to connect with others outside the family for the first time.

Third order change occurred in several ways. Ana had never felt understood by anyone but her mother. The veil of silence that surrounded her left her particularly vulnerable to *hermeneutic injustice* (see Chapter 8). In other words, Ana felt accepted by her family, but not really known, until she had an avenue through which to tell her story. Telling her story also offered her a way to better know herself as she, for the first time, put into pictures what she experienced, thought, and felt. Ana and her family were well versed in narratives of vulnerability and abuse, however, when her family and advocate offered discourses and sites of resistance, such as by going to the sexual assault center, police station, courthouse, and the counseling agency, Ana and her family were able to re-narrate their social experience to one in which allies joined them to help her to reclaim her power and determine how to stand up to the effects of injustice.

Reflexive Questions

- What are some dominant/problematic narratives that have shaped you personally? How have they impacted your work as a therapist?
- What dominant discourses continue to go unnoticed as natural, inevitable, or assumed right due to their widespread support?
- When considering a problem that negatively affects your well-being and interactions with others, what name would you give it? What social forces does it join with to give it the strength to rob you of your joy, health, vitality, and well-being?
- As a socioculturally attuned narrative family therapist, how can you create space to interrupt and loosen the grip of problematic relational dynamics by linking them to larger dominant sociocultural forces? What creative means could you use to do this?
- How would you respond to or manage the conflict of a couple or family members disagreeing on what they deem to be their preferred narrative? What if someone's preferred narrative is unjust or colludes with larger systems of oppression?
- How do we as therapists inadvertently vote in favor, or fail to vote against, what may not align with our values toward equity and relational justice?

References

Agger, B. (1991). Critical theory, poststructuralism, postmodernism: Their sociological relevance. *Annual Review of Sociology*, *17*, 105–131.

Beaudoin, M. & MacLennan, R. (2021). Mindfulness and embodiment in family therapy: Overview, nuances, and clinical applications in poststructural practices. *Family Process*, *60*, 1555–1567.

Beaudoin, M. N. & Monk, G. (2024). *Narrative practices and emotions: 40+ ways to support the emergence of flourishing identities*. Norton.

Berg, S. (2009). The use of narrative practices and emotionally focused couple therapy with first nations couples. In M. Rastogi & V. Thomas (Eds.). *Multicultural Family Therapy* (pp. 371–388). Sage.

Bermúdez, J. M. & Bermúdez, S. (2002). Altar-making with Latino families: A narrative therapy perspective. *Journal of Family Psychotherapy 13*(3/4), 329–347.

Bermúdez, J. M., Keeling, M., & Carlson, T. S. (2009). Using art to co-create preferred problem-solving narratives with Latino couples. In M. Rastogi and V. Thomas (Eds.). *Multicultural couple therapy* (pp. 319–343). Sage.

Blanton, P. G. (2005). Narrative family therapy and spiritual direction: Do they fit? *Journal of Psychology and Christianity*, *24*(1), 68–79.

Boje, D. (2001). Carnivalesque resistance to global spectacle: A critical postmodern theory of public administration. *Administrative Theory & Praxis*, *23*(3), 431–458.

Bourdieu, P. (1986). The forms of capital. In J.G. Richardson (Ed.). *Handbook of theory and research for the sociology of education* (pp. 241–258). Greenwood Press.

Carlson, T. D. (1997). Using art in narrative therapy: Enhancing therapeutic possibilities. *The American Journal of Family Therapy*, *25*, 271–283.

Carr, A. (1998). Michael White's narrative therapy. *Contemporary Family Therapy*, *20*, 485–503.
Chenail, R. J., Reire, M. D., Torres-Gregory, M., & Ilic, D. (2020). Postmodern family therapy. In K. S. Wampler, R. B. Miller, & R. B. Seedall (Eds.). *The handbook of systemic family therapy*, (Vol. 1, pp. 417–440). Wiley.
Combs, G. & Freedman, J. (2016). Narrative therapy's relational understanding of identity, *Family Process*, *55*, 211–224.
Combs, G. & Freedman, J. (2004). A poststructuralist approach to narrative work. In L. Angus & J. McLeod (Eds.). *The handbook of narrative and psychotherapy: Practices, theory, and research* (pp. 137–155). Sage.
Dumaresque, R., Thornton, T., Glaser, D., & Lawrence, A. (2018). Politicized narrative therapy: A reckoning and a call to action. *Canadian Social Work Review*, *35*, 109–129.
Ewing, J., Estes, R., & Like, B. (2017). Narrative neurotherapy (NNT): Scaffolding identity states. In M Beaudoin & J. Duvall (Eds.). *Collaborative therapy and neurobiology: Evolving practice in action* (pp. 87–99). Routledge.
Freedman, J. & Combs, G. (1996). *Narrative therapy: The social construction of preferred realities*. Norton.
Fricker, M. (2007). *Epistemic injustice: Power and the ethics of knowing*. Oxford University Press.
Foucault, M. (1982). The subject and power. *Critical Inquiry*, *8*(4), 777–795.
Gaddis, S. (2016). Poststructural inquiry: Narrative therapy's de-centered and influential stance. In V. Dickerson (Ed.). *Poststructural and narrative thinking in family therapy*. AFTA Springerbriefs in Family Therapy. Springer.
Keeling, M. L. & Bermudez, M. (2006), Externalizing problems through art and writing: Experience of process and helpfulness. *Journal of Marital and Family Therapy*, *32*, 405–419.
Laird, J. (1998). Theorizing culture: Narrative ideas and practice principles. In M. McGoldrick, (Ed.). *Re-visioning family therapy* (pp. 20–36). Guilford.
Madigan, S. (2019). *Narrative therapy* (2nd ed.). American Psychological Association.
McDowell, T. (2015). *Applying critical social theories to family therapy practice*. AFTA Springerbriefs in Family Therapy, Springer.
McGuinty, E., Armstrong, D., Nelson, J., & Sheeler, S. (2012). Externalizing metaphors: Anxiety and high-functioning autism. *Journal of Child and Adolescent Psychiatric Nursing*, *25*(1), 9–16.
McLaren, P. & Farahmandpur, R. (2001). Class, cultism and multiculturalism: A notebook on forging a revolutionary politics. *Multicultural Education*, *8*(3), 2–14.
McNamee, S. J. & Miller, R. K. (2004). *The meritocracy myth*. Rowman & Littlefield.
Merton, R. K. (1988). The Mathew effect in science, II: Cumulative advantage and the symbolism of intellectual property. *Isis*, *79*(4), 606–623.
Miller, L. J. (2000). The poverty of truth-seeking: Postmodernism, discourse analysis and critical feminism. *Theory & Psychology*, *10*, 313–352.
Morgan, A. (2000). *What is narrative therapy?* (p. 116). Adelaide: Dulwich Centre Publications.
Parry, A. & Doan, R. E. (1994). *Story re-visions: Narrative therapy in the postmodern world*. Guilford.
Payne, M. (2006). *Narrative therapy* (2nd ed.). Thousand Oaks, CA: Sage.
polanco, m. (2016). Language justice: Narrative therapy on the fringes of Columbian magical realism. *In International Journal of Narrative Therapy and Community Practice*, (3), 68–76.
Roth, S. & Epston, D. (1996). Consulting the problem about the problematic relationship: An exercise for experiencing a relationship with an externalized problem. In M. F. Hoyt (Ed.). *Constructive therapies 2* (pp. 148–162). Guilford Press.
Salmon, L. (2017). The four questions: A framework for integrating an understanding of oppression dynamics in clinical work and supervision. In: R. Allan & S. Singh Poulsen (Eds.). *Creating cultural safety in couple and family therapy*. AFTA SpringerBriefs in Family Therapy. Springer, Cham.
Sen, S. (2021). Just girls: Conversations on resistance, social justice, and the mental health struggles of women. *International Journal of Narrative Therapy and Community Work, 2021*(1), 60–69.
Simons, S. (2023). Narrative expressive arts therapy. In C. Malchiodi (Ed.). *Handbook of Expressive Arts Therapy* (pp. 170–186). Guilford Press.
Slott, M. (2005). An alternative to critical postmodernist antifoundationalism. *Rethinking Marxism*, *17*(2), 301–318.
Tatum, B. D. (2017). *Why are all the Black kids sitting together in the cafeteria?: And other conversations about race*. Basic Books.
Tilsen, J. (2021). *Queering your therapy practice: Queer theory, narrative therapy, and imagining new identities*. Routledge.

White, M. (2012). Scaffolding a therapeutic conversation. In T. Malinen, S. J. Cooper, and F. N. Thomas (Eds.). *Masters of narrative and collaborative therapies: The voices of Andersen, Anderson, and White* (pp. 121–169). Routledge.
White, M. (2007). *Maps of narrative practice*. Norton.
White, M. (2002). Addressing personal failure. *International Journal of Narrative Therapy and Community Work*, *2*, 17–55.
White, M. (1995). *Re-authoring lives: Interviews & essays*. South Australia Graphic Print Group.
White, M. (1988–1989, Summer). The externalizing of the problem and the re-authoring of lives and relationships. *Dulwich Centre Newsletter*, 3–20.
White, M. & Epston, D. (1990). *Narrative means to therapeutic ends*. Norton.
Zimmerman, J. (2018). *Neuro-narrative therapy: New possibilities for emotion-filled conversations*. Norton.

15 Socio-Emotional Relationship Therapy

An Example of Socioculturally Attuned Couple and Family Therapy

Most clinical models treat social justice as an add-on or special issue (Hardy & McGoldrick, 2019). Socio-emotional relationship therapy (SERT) *begins* with equity at its core. Building on the work of previous feminist and social constructionist researchers and clinicians, Carmen Knudson-Martin and Douglas Huenergardt (2010) with a team of colleagues (Knudson-Martin, Huenergardt et al., 2015, Knudson-Martin, Wells, & Samman 2015, Knudson-Martin et al., 2021; Wells et al., 2017; Williams et al., 2013) developed SERT to detail how therapists can position their work to interrupt and transform the impact of societal inequities in couple and family relationships. Working with the confluence of social discourse, emotion, and power in relational processes, SERT integrates a critical social constructionist conceptualization of human behavior with attention to interpersonal neurobiology and the embodied consequences of societal power in personal and relational health and well-being.

SERT serves as a model of socially responsible practice grounded in the assumption that frames this entire volume—that it is not possible to be clinically "neutral." It may also be used as an overarching umbrella through which to integrate socioculturally attuned principles and ANVIET guidelines with other clinical models and evidence-based practices (e.g., Jenks et al., 2024). The model continues to evolve, with a comprehensive guide detailing the competencies involved in this socially responsible clinical approach (Knudson-Martin, 2024), and a SERT workbook that offers practical ways to create more just, mutually supportive relationships (Knudson-Martin, 2025).

↔

In SERT, third order change is facilitated by an engaged therapist whose clinical decisions take into account how societal power processes impact the moment-by-moment of clinical work, and orient therapy so clients are able to experience relational possibilities outside those constructed by dominant social systems.

↔

Foundational SERT Concepts

SERT therapists view therapy as a social constructionist process and are intentional about their part in it. In the first phase, therapists set the stage by asking questions that frame clinical concerns socio-contextually and invite clients to reflect on their relational ideals. They facilitate a clinical process that experientially interrupts power processes as they present in session. As therapy progresses, clients see themselves through a larger lens and therapists support them to detail and practice the relational values they claim.

DOI: 10.4324/9781003493426-15

•←→•

While dominant social systems across the Western world tend to emphasize independence, competition, and personal achievement, people cannot thrive without mutually supportive relational bonds.

•←→•

SERT's emphasis on shared relational responsibility challenges the individualistic discourse prominent in Western culture and mental health practices (Combs & Freedman, 2016; Mehl-Madrona, 2010). Five concepts organize practice: 1) reciprocally responsive social engagement, 2) socio-emotional experience, 3) societal discourse and felt identities, 4) relational flow of power, and 5) equitable interaction patterns through the Circle of Care.

Reciprocally Responsive Social Engagement

Like attachment theory (Johnson, 2019, see also Chapter 8), SERT emphasizes the role of mutuality and reciprocal engagement in healthy development. For example, when Robert sought therapy because he "felt unhappy and lacked motivation," the therapist explored his engagement with others and learned that Robert kept himself emotionally disengaged from his parents and his partner Raul, and viewed colleagues at work as competitors instrumental to attaining sales goals. Therapy addressed Robert's negative affect in light of these relational encounters and the social contexts that supported his distance from others.

Developmentally, it is critical that one person's mind links with another's (Siegel, 2020). This happens as the neural system of one mutually impacts emotional regulation and the physiologic state of the other (Porges, 2009). When resonance is shared, each person is changed physiologically, psychically, and relationally. As we interact, socially created experience is written into physiology. Though children are most impacted as parents/caregivers and children attune to and adjust to each other, the emotional system and physiology of each evolves (Gerhardt, 2004).

Just, mutually supportive relationships invite neurological "fittedness" that promotes positive adaptation and growth (Fosha, 2009; Knudson-Martin & Kim, 2023). It is not possible when power is unequal or when those with more social power (such as parents, teachers, clergy, therapists) are not accountable for their power by attuning to and responding to others (Knudson-Martin & Huenergardt, 2010, Porges, 2009). In unequal social conditions, the ability to experience responsiveness from others or influence them is not mutual, and the fundamental ethical obligation to support one another is compromised (see also Chapter 10, Contextual Therapy).

As is the case with Robert, when people are not able to, or will not, participate mutually in this social engagement system, optimal development is not possible. Neurochemistry is affected. Robert's body may be experiencing reduced serotonin (associated with feelings of well-being and happiness) and increased cortisol (associated with stress), both of which are associated with depression (Hanna, 2014). Moreover, feelings of discomfort, dissonance, or disquiet are ways socially created differences and power inequities are bodily experienced. It can be helpful to feel and learn from these experiences, rather than disengaging or quickly moving toward only positive feelings (Knudson-Martin & Smoliak, in press).

•←→•

Though not discounting the value of autonomy, SERT positions therapy to counteract societal forces that work against relational engagement and seeks to promote the conditions through which mutual support is accessible.

•←→•

With Robert, this means apprehending how his social location as a relatively affluent, White, cisgender, gay male in the US informs his experiences of vulnerability, power, and openness to reciprocal relational engagement (Knudson-Martin & Kim, 2023; Samman & Knudson-Martin, 2015).

Socio-emotional Experience

Emotions connect the individual and the environment (Knudson-Martin, 2024). People experience emotion personally and physiologically, but its meaning is socio-contextual (Gergen, 2009). For example, across cultures, sadness is demonstrated by turned down lips and squinted eyes and anger involves dilated pupils and pursed lips; these internal responses and the meaning ascribed to them are called forth by interpersonal and sociocultural circumstances (Burkitt, 2014; Siegel, 2020). Thinking, feeling, body, relationship, and sociocultural context are woven into one (Siegel, 2023; Wetherell, 2012).

Emotion alerts us to what is important (Knudson-Martin, 2025). From the first encounter, SERT therapists get to know their clients by attuning to their contextual socio-emotional experience. The therapist's questions and reflections as they seek to "get" how emotionally salient words and actions connect with larger societal contexts also help clients increase contextual awareness of their felt experience. At the same time, *which* words and emotional reactions therapists respond to and how they frame them help create the experiences clients describe. The story that unfolds is not the only possibility (Winslade, 2009), making therapists' inevitable influence an ethical responsibility (Chapter 3, this volume; Knudson-Martin, 2024).

For example, when the therapist asked Robert to say more about his lack of motivation, what it was like for him, she noticed that Robert's body seemed to tighten and his voice took on an edge when he said that he "wants to do better, to work harder." As she imagined what it was like for this relatively affluent White man to "want to do better," she followed this emotional thread outward, asking what doing better meant to him, listening for societal expectations and standards in his responses, and asking questions that helped name these social valuations and make them visible. As she did, the therapist could feel the pressure he felt to always need to achieve more. She could expand the conversation to dominant culture definitions of success, which Robert felt pulled to attain and meet, especially since he felt devalued as a gay man. Though she can not know all the experiences Robert could also have expanded upon, developing the salient emotions around motivation and larger contexts helps them move from an individualistic framing of Robert's concerns to a socio-relational one.

•←→•

Emotional meaning emerges in the context of power and social power works through emotion.

•←→•

Robert's feeling that he needed to keep pushing to achieve illustrates how what is valued socially can color emotional experience. What and who is socially valued affects how parents respond to children and what they expect of them. Social valuation also affects the emotional capital one brings into relationships. In part, Robert keeps emotionally distant from Raul because, as an affluent white male, he does not experience himself needing Raul (or anyone). Feeling his relational needs would challenge his inherent power position. In contrast, Raul feels gratitude that Robert has chosen him, a man with considerably less social standing.

Though Robert does appear very emotional, studies suggest there is no such thing as a "non-affective" thought (Burkitt, 2014, p. 95); that "rational" decision-making requires an internal appraisal based on emotion that is always socioculturally located (Wetherell 2012; Zimmerman, 2018). Helping a client like Robert bring the social context of his emotional experience into awareness gives him more choice regarding the meaning he embodies and the decisions he makes.

Societal Discourse and Felt Identities

Discourse refers to collective ways of thinking and talking that give meaning to experience (Krolokke & Sorensen, 2006). Listening for discourse enables therapists to connect individual identities and relationship patterns to wider sociocultural contexts (Knudson-Martin et al., 2021). Like narrative therapy (see Chapter 14), SERT takes the stance that identity is not fixed, and that discourses are not neutral and reflect only part of the potential values and meanings in any situation (Combs & Freedman, 2012, 2016).

Dominant societal discourses are based on the interests and perspectives of those in power and tend to be generally applied to all. This creates injustice on multiple levels. People internalize standards embedded in the dominant discourse and judge themselves and others by them (Hardy & McGoldrick, 2019). Shared social meaning to understand their experience is less available to those in subordinate groups, making neuro-fittedness and interpersonal attunement less broadly accessible. Persons in oppressed groups may not have words to fully understand or communicate their own experience unless others can receive and share it. Therapists may not recognize dominant discourses in client stories unless they have developed a critical contextual consciousness and apply it in practice (Esmiol et al., 2012; Knudson-Martin, 2024).

Robert's parents have always loved him. When they learned he was gay they "accepted" him, but lacked shared socially constructed meanings to connect with him. They also took dominant cultural constructions of worth and value for granted without knowing they did so. Robert internalized these social messages as well. His feelings of unhappiness and lack of motivation reflect larger dominant discourses that prioritize individual achievement and monetary success as the standard for everyone and support values such as autonomy and independence associated with cisgender masculinity (Loscocco & Walzer, 2013).

Identity validation is related to power. When Robert conformed to dominant cultural discourse he experienced validation. During his upbringing, virtually wherever he went—school, home, and in the media— Robert's competitiveness and personal achievements were recognized and validated. In these moments, he felt a sense of belonging, that he fit and was valued. He was validated when he hid his differences, doubts, and confusion and, instead, presented himself with authority, standing tall, and not showing weakness. His felt identity incorporated these elements of societal success, along with shame regarding those aspects of his experience that were met with disapproval and disconnection (Cozolino, 2016). Robert's identity will necessarily be engaged in the clinical change process.

Robert carries many voices and perspectives within his experience. Which societal discourses become woven into his identity and structured into his body depends on which sociocultural meanings are imbued with emotional salience (Beaudoin & Monk, 2024; Mehl-Madrona, 2010; Zimmerman, 2018). For Robert, this was connected to achievement and "being the best." Gradually, neurobiological physiologies that correspond to these familiar understandings about himself were established (Ewing, et al., 2017). Developing new patterns involves activating the connections between societal discourse, emotion, and identity (Knudson-Martin & Huenergardt, 2010; Knudson-Martin et al., 2021). In Text Box 15.1 Man Tso Wei describes how he applies these principles in his work with Asian immigrants.

Text Box 15.1 Man-Tso Wei 魏满佐, LCSW

Man-Tso Wei 魏满佐 (he/him) is a social work practitioner serving a diverse clientele at Earth Circles Counseling Center in Oakland, California. He previously worked at Asian Health Services, and serving Asian communities continues to be an important focus in his work. Informed by his Taiwanese heritage and queer identity, he is interested in how relational and societal processes impact individual and social belonging and well-being.

I work with many low-income Asian immigrants and their children, insured through Medicaid, facing severe mental health challenges. A common theme among my clients is a sense of "not belonging," often rooted in stigma around mental illness and compounded by being Asian in the US, where many encounter language and cultural barriers, and all are affected by racial stereotypes such as forever foreigner and model minority. Whenever appropriate, I involve family and friends in therapy, recognizing the healing power of relationships and resisting the dominant individualistic mental health system. My work is informed by the Ackerman relational approach (ARA) and socio-emotional relationship therapy (SERT). Both integrative models help me understand clients' experiences and locate their challenges within their relational and sociocultural contexts.

As I listen to my clients' stories, I attend to different aspects of their experience, then expand outward to situate them within their sociocultural contexts, life cycles, and larger societal discourses to capture their felt contextual experience. I also practice location of self (Watts-Jones, 2010) to bring up and explore how our intersecting identities influence the therapeutic relationship and process. I identify the relational and societal power processes around clients' presenting problems, exploring how they contribute to a sense of not belonging, which often triggers and/or exacerbates mental health symptoms. For example, I often see my Asian female clients with psychosis express concerns about their family's safety, but their husbands invalidate their experiences, criticizing them for "worrying too much." The husbands, enacting Confucian patriarchy, also carry anger and frustration from encountering racism and xenophobia outside the home. Adhering to Confucian norms, the wives often suppress their emotions and needs to prioritize and accommodate their husbands, which reinforces their sense of disconnect and not belonging, further exacerbating their symptoms.

I make space for my clients' experiences and concerns—often silenced or negated—to be heard and understood by their families. I explore why these concerns are important to them, highlighting the relational values behind them. I also slow down the process to help clients see how relational and societal power imbalances impact presenting problems and their sense of not belonging in relationships and the community. For example, I help Asian teenagers recognize how they internalize sociocultural expectations, such as the pressure to meet the "model minority" standard and avoid burdening others. These pressures contribute to their sense of not belonging and are often linked to anxiety and depression. I also introduce the new Chinese name for schizophrenia, 思覺失調 (sī jué shī tiáo; imbalance in thoughts and perceptions), replacing the older name 精神分裂 (jīng shén fēn liè; mind splitting disease). This shift in language is liberating for many of my clients, as it reduces stigma and aligns with Chinese medicine ideas, implying the possibility of treatment to address the imbalance between body, mind, and environment.

After locating the client's struggles within broader relational and sociocultural contexts, I invite them to envision preferred ways of relating to others and societal messages and to identify the underlying values of these alternatives. I join with them to co-create experiences that align with their values and resist oppressive societal forces. As clients enact desired changes both in and outside of therapy, I reflect and process these moments with them to strengthen and consolidate new experiential learnings.

I am a visual learner and would like to share the conceptual diagram I drew to help me practice sociocultural attunement. Please see below.

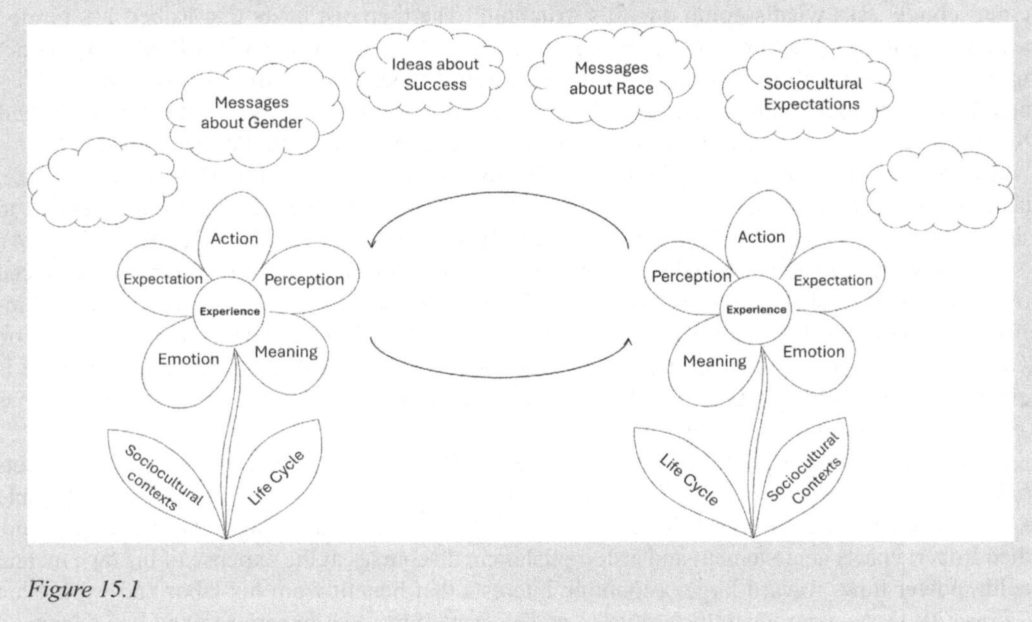

Figure 15.1

Relational Flow of Power

One of the distinctive aspects of SERT is its attention to the flow of power in relationships and how it affects issues such as trust, intimacy, vulnerability, control and influence, conflict resolution, and communication (Knudson-Martin, 2013, 2025; Morrison et al., 2022). SERT defines power as a set of relationally created and structurally embedded social processes "that determine whose experiences, abilities, and interests merit value" (Knudson-Martin et al., 2021, p. 3). From a relational perspective, power is evidenced by whose interests and needs are noticed and attended to (Mahoney & Knudson-Martin, 2009). Those with more social power are usually less aware of or attuned to subordinates (Parker, 2009; Tatum, 1997). They also tend to be less aware of their power positions and may not notice how others attend to and accommodate them. They may not feel powerful (Kimmel, 2016). The flow of power serves as context for emotion and is enacted through social discourses and relationship patterns. Persons in marginalized positions often recognize, and even resist, their minimization, but their voices tend not to be heard or valued in the dominant culture (Smoliak & Knudson-Martin, in review).

↔

Rather than focusing on power as an individual property, SERT focuses on the flow of power from one person or group to another.

↔

SERT therapists are interested in how power imbalances occur, what maintains or transforms them, and how presenting concerns relate to power. Robert's symptoms of unhappiness and lack of motivation could occur in the context of a power imbalance in which power accumulates to him or in one where he holds limited power. Clinical actions will vary depending on this power context. As the therapist gets to know Robert and his concerns, she also begins to track the flow of power in the relationships Robert describes. For example, she asks how Raul responds to him when Robert is feeling low energy. Robert answers with confusion and a blank stare, then says, "I don't know… he gets clingy, asks what's going on—it's irritating." The therapist hears that Robert has limited awareness of Raul's position. To further explore, she asks Robert what he thinks Raul is experiencing when he appears clingy. Robert responds that Raul "needs to get a life" and then says he has enough to worry about with people at work not getting things done. This is an indicator that Robert probably is not well-attuned to Raul or his colleagues, a sign of a potential power imbalance.

Multiple power contexts typically intersect in any relationship, including those related to race, class, gender, sexual orientation, immigration status, abilities, as well as experiences related to trauma, loss, and personal life stories (Knudson-Martin et al., 2021; Young & Seedall, 2024). As part of appraising a situation, human physiology instantaneously emotionally reads the social power context (Cozolino, 2016; Wetherell, 2012). This felt sense organizes relationships and informs how people judge themselves and others, creating boundaries of inclusion and exclusion (Knudson-Martin & Smoliak, in press). An emotional economy actively shapes whose voice is perceived to be credible, feelings of safety and belonging, and expectations regarding what one has a right to expect or ought to fear (Ahmed, 2004; Tate, 2014).

As an affluent White male, social power flows to Robert. He likely experiences a taken-for-granted sense that people around him will accommodate his interests and that he should be able to get or achieve what he wants. When they don't, he is frustrated or angry. On the other hand, when Robert enacts achievement and accomplishment discourses at the expense of his own mental health, power flows toward larger economic interests that benefit from his labor and work ethic (Garcia, 2011). As a gay man, his ability to make sense of his own experience and be understood by others is limited by the imposed silencing he encounters in this social context (Medina, 2013).

•←→•

When SERT therapists talk about powerful or less powerful persons, they are referring to "the outcome of relational patterns that create and maintain differences in who notices and attends to the other, whose needs and goals shape the relationship, and who accommodates or responds to provide care" (Knudson-Martin et al., 2021, p. 3).

•←→•

Equity means that the flow of power in the relationship is relatively balanced across time. Each person is attentive to the other and to the relationship. When power is unequal, emotional connection is compromised and it is difficult to positively respond to conflict, trauma, and life stresses and changes (Baima & Feldhousen, 2007; Jonathan & Knudson-Martin, 2012).

While Robert experiences limited power in some aspects of his life, he appears to be in a power position in relation to Raul. That is, he controls the relational process and his responses drive the emotional climate (Greenberg & Goldman, 2008). The power accruing to him also limits crucial aspects of his emotional and relational well-being, which as described above, require reciprocity and mutual responsiveness. In order to help Robert address his depressive symptoms, the SERT therapist will help Robert shift these power imbalances and invite Raul to participate in the therapy.

SERT therapists emphasize that power processes are subtle and not always easily recognized. They observe and track whose gestures get a response and whose are ignored, who controls the topics of conversation, whose perspectives are perceived as legitimate, and who is available to orient to the other. They note how emotion sustains or disrupts these power processes (Knudson-Martin, 2024, 2025). SERT therapists are also aware that they are embedded in the same larger societal power contexts and reflexively question their own assumptions and reactions as they position their work to interrupt the flow of societal power inequities in interpersonal relationships (Morrison et al., 2022; Smoliak & Knudson-Martin, under review).

Equitable Interaction Patterns through the Circle of Care

Worldwide, people increasingly report egalitarian ideals, but few have an image of how to apply them (Knudson-Martin, 2025; Mahoney & Knudson-Martin, 2009; Sullivan, 2005). SERT thus utilizes the Circle of Care (Figure 15.2), four orienting principles that promote mutually supportive relationships and well-being: mutual vulnerability, mutual attunement, mutual influence, and shared relational responsibility (Knudson-Martin & Huenergardt, 2010). Rather than skills to be taught, they are relational guidelines that clients apply somewhat differently based on their sociocultural backgrounds, situations, and desires. Enacting the Circle of Care involves an equitable flow of power and reciprocal positive impact on one another's neurophysiological and emotional states, which, in line with the SERT model, is the foundation for other clinical change. The Circle of Care guides assessment and clinical decisions.

Mutual Vulnerability

Being emotionally present and engaged requires mutual vulnerability in which people approach one another with openness, curiosity, and willingness to admit mistakes and express needs. Robert has learned not to do this. Like everyone, he experiences vulnerability. His inability to *express* it is shaped by his cultural and gender socialization, as well as his experiences, which, as a gay young

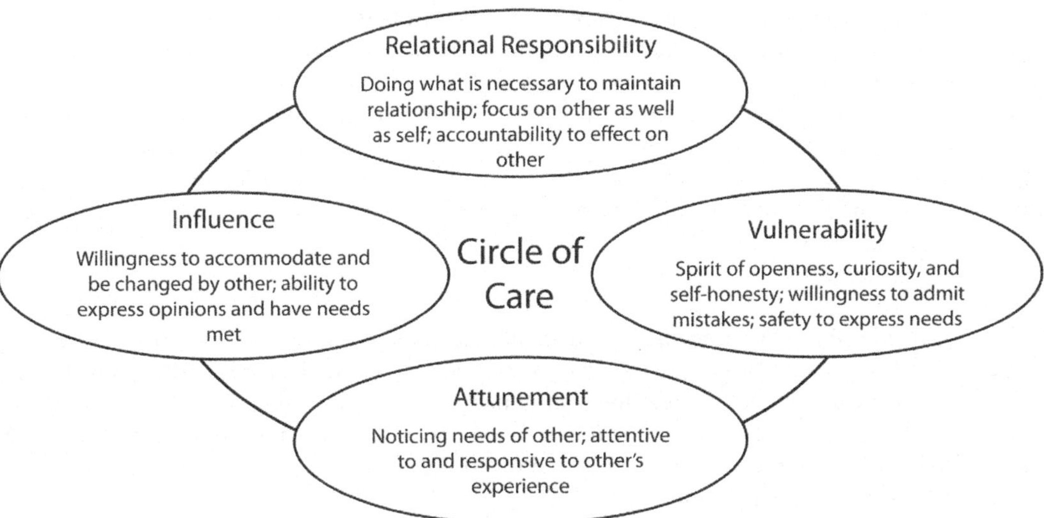

Figure 15.2 Circle of Care

From Knudson-Martin, C. & Huenergardt, D. (2015). Bridging emotion, societal discourse, and couple interaction. In C. Knudson-Martin, M. E. Wells, & S. Samman (Eds.). *Socio-emotional Relationship Therapy: Bridging emotion, societal context, and couple interaction* (p. 6). Springer. Used with permission.

man, he learned that it was often not safe to be emotionally open and vulnerable (Knudson-Martin et al., 2021). On the other hand, when Raul joins the therapy, he repeatedly expresses vulnerability, sharing his worries and asking how he can better approach Robert. In order not to further a power imbalance, SERT therapists will be careful not to place additional vulnerability on Raul without first helping Robert develop the capacity to take a more vulnerable position. In some relationships, neither person can approach the other with vulnerability; however, frequently one is in a more inherently vulnerable position than the other.

To assess for mutual vulnerability, therapists look for the extent to which each is:

- Willing to show weakness, uncertainty, or mistakes
- Safe and willing to share innermost thoughts and feelings
- Seeking relationship repair by expressing a feeling or concern

Mutual Attunement

While also valuing direct communication, SERT therapists emphasize proactive, attuned awareness and responsiveness. In mutual relationships, each person attunes to the other. They notice and respond. Each feels known. When people are not attuned, or when attunement is not mutual, "rather than the relationship being an energizing force for growth and change, the relationship may contribute to stress and symptoms such as depression and anxiety" (Knudson-Martin & Kim, 2023, p. 272).

To assess for mutual attunement, therapists look for the extent to which each person:

- Is interested in knowing and understanding the other
- Listens to the other—about what? In what circumstances?
- Notices and attends to the other's feelings and needs

In observing Robert and Raul, the therapist noted that Robert expected Raul to know his needs and respond to them. When she asked Robert what it might be like for Raul when he emotionally withdraws, Robert said, "he should know I don't like to talk about my feelings." In contrast, Raul responded that he understood that it was especially hard for Robert to talk when he feels like a failure, and went on to explain how that happens for Robert. The SERT therapist will acknowledge the value of Raul's attuned support and persist in helping Robert attune to Raul. This will not only create a more equitable balance of support, it will also help Robert counteract depression (Papp, 2003).

Mutual Influence

Being in a relationship always includes influencing one another. In mutually supportive relationships, each person assumes a disposition to accommodate and be changed. Partners are equally able to express their perspectives and have an impact on the other. On a physiological level, the neurons of one change in response to the other. When power is imbalanced, those with less power accommodate, and those with power do not. Powerful persons may not even be aware of the changes others make in response to them.

To assess mutual influence, therapists look for the extent to which each:

- Can engage the other in addressing issues that concern them
- Feels free to express opinions or make requests
- Shifts their interests/schedule to fit the others' interests and schedule

If Robert needs to change his schedule to accommodate Raul, he feels irritated or controlled. On the other hand, Raul regularly considers what Robert needs and organizes his schedule and personal choices around this awareness. At work, Robert's authoritative style leads many of his team members to follow his lead in ways he does not see or appreciate. Potentially valuable perspectives of other team members get lost. The SERT therapist will be attentive to these imbalances and help Robert more readily open himself to influence. This will require developing awareness of the sociocultural discourses that have framed its meaning.

Shared Relational Responsibility

Shared relational responsibility means that each person attends to what is needed to maintain the well-being of the relationship and is mindful of how their actions affect the other. Those with less power typically make more efforts to safeguard the relationship by doing most of the emotional tending, soothing the other, looking out for their needs, and managing relationship maintenance tasks that more powerful partners may not notice or do not want to handle (Knudson-Martin, 2025).

To assess for shared relational responsibility, therapists look for the extent to which each:

- Focuses on what is needed to maintain or improve the relationship
- Keeps track of what needs to be done for the partner, family, or group
- Is responsible for doing the emotional work in the relationship

Robert's focus has been on personal achievement. He is not used to focusing on what his relationships with others need and is not aware of what Raul and others do to keep his relationships afloat. In the SERT model, transforming the imbalance in relational responsibility will not only support Robert's relationships, it is also necessary for social engagement that will support his well-being as well as that of those around him.

Summarizing SERT's Theory of Change

SERT promotes mutually supportive relationships that help people overcome the damaging effects of a lack of reciprocity, societal inequities, and dominant societal discourses that devalue relationality. Change occurs interpersonally and experientially when something new happens that is viscerally salient and creates and embodies new meaning (Knudson-Martin, 2024). When people enact the Circle of Care, they are reciprocally engaged in relational processes that promote health-affirming connections. Therapists help clients detail and thicken these transformative new experiences into an ongoing awareness of self and other that takes into account the larger societal contexts they navigate.

As Robert comes to see himself sociocontextually and is supported in developing the relational aspects of himself that have previously been societally discounted, he will be able to attune to others and his own emotional experience. He will develop more mutually supportive relationships and have more choice regarding how he responds to societal messages to "do more," all of which will promote his personal and relational health and decrease his depressive symptoms. Raul and others in Robert's life will also benefit.

Principles of Socioculturally Attuned Family Therapy

As an example of a socioculturally attuned practice model, socio-emotional relationship therapy takes into account most of the socioculturally attuned principles discussed throughout this book. Here we highlight some that are especially central to the practice of SERT.

Societal Context

SERT therapists connect personal experiences such as emotion, felt identity, and interaction patterns to larger sociocultural contexts (Knudson-Martin, 2024). When they do, clients are able to have compassion for themselves and others, prioritize their relational interests, and be less constrained by the effects of dominant societal discourses.

Social Context of Emotion

Connecting personal experience to larger social forces becomes much easier when emotions are viewed as a social structuring process that links the personal and the contextual.

As suggested by Bateson (1972), our minds, bodies, and relationships are open systems that both apprehend and have an impact upon our environments. Emotions embody the social meaning of these interconnected systems. Larger forces such as capitalism, patriarchy, and caste extend beyond individual families to schools, workplaces, communities, and media and are reflected not only in discourse and thought, but also construct emotion (Smoliak et al. 2025).

SERT therapists begin to recognize the sociopolitical workings of emotion and attune to it in the initial sessions (Knudson-Martin, 2024). For example, Lena and Samuel sought help following Samuel's disclosure that he had lost $20,000 gambling. The therapist asked Samuel to begin by describing how the gambling fit into his life and what it meant to him. She was especially interested in the words or experiences that seemed most emotionally central to him and how these related to larger societal forces. Samuel said gambling was a way to "unwind," to "relax" before coming home. Knowing he was a 34-year-old African American husband and father starting his own business, the therapist continued to explore what it meant to unwind and relax in light of these social contexts. As Samuel responded to her contextually interested questions, the therapist began to sense the pressure and responsibility he felt to be successful, particularly since his mother sacrificed so much for him to go to college, and Lena's more affluent father was a successful Black businessman in the predominantly White technology field.

With genuine, socioculturally attuned interest on the part of the therapist, Samuel shared the personal autonomy he felt while gambling—being away from all the social demands and expectations. And until this major loss, he felt competent and empowered when gambling. Doing something he was good at stimulated him. "You have to work twice as hard as a Black man," he told the White therapist.

Socio-emotional Expression

Which emotions should be expressed and how they are expressed vary across sociocultural contexts. As described by ChenFeng and colleagues (2017), emotional disclosure in collectivist Asian cultures may feel like a selfish act that places an undue burden on others. Therapists need to extend gentle empathy to emotions from which clients were previously disconnected and/or did not express. It is also important to validate the relational intent of protecting others from distressing emotion and not force a display of emotion (ChenFeng et al., 2017).

Samuel and Lena illustrate another way that limited emotional expression may make sociocultural sense. Lena did not express much emotion in response to Samuel's disclosure about the gambling loss, even though he had previously kept his gambling secret from her. The White therapist wondered why she didn't express more anger. Lena said she knew Samuel worked very hard and was focused on getting his business going; she could understand his need for a release from the pressure. To expand the contextual lens, the therapist shifted the conversation to Lena's experience growing up with professional Black parents in a predominantly White community. She asked how her parents handled pressure and discrimination. Lena said she knew her parents faced those things, but they always kept a positive attitude. They smiled and made home a happy place.

The therapist internally reflected that the pattern Lena described seemed similar to one reported in a study of middle-class Black families, where the emphasis was on "pulling together," which often meant putting aside troubling individual emotions in order to overcome societal injustice (Cowdry et al., 2009). It may also be part of a larger emotional economy that determines whose emotions are important and have a "right" to be expressed (Knudson-Martin & Smoliak, in press). This contextual understanding helped the therapist respond empathically to Lena, "It's really important to you to support Samuel, to be in this together and not let your upset get in the way—you know that as a Black man he has an especially hard path to climb." At the same time, the therapist was attentive to how she may be misconstruing Lena's silence or what she may be missing.

Gender, Vulnerability, and Trauma

In most cultures, men are allowed, perhaps even expected, to display anger while women are not. The gendering of how emotions are expressed and used is one way patriarchy dominates and controls women (Baima & Feldhousen, 2007; Smoliak et al., 2025). Enacting the Circle of Care challenges the societal gender discourse that men should not express vulnerable emotions such as fear or need for relationship and should instead use anger and emotional disconnection as a way to maintain a power position.

Before expecting people who are socialized to avoid "soft" emotions to relationally engage in the Circle of Care, SERT therapists identify and attune to the sociocultural nature of vulnerability. SERT research identified important connections between gender socialization, interpersonal trauma, and marginalized experience in how vulnerability is expressed (Knudson-Martin et al., 2021):

> Socialized expressions of vulnerability tended to reproduce gendered power processes by prescribing expressions of vulnerability as part of female responsibility to preserve relationships and expectations that men appear invulnerable. Reactive responses to vulnerability associated with trauma and/or societal marginalization could further exacerbate power disparities as some women focused even more strongly on preserving the relationship by denigrating themselves and men responded with self-protective stances that further limited their ability to be aware of and accountable for their impact on their partners… [On the other hand,] some women demonstrated self-protective reactive expressions of vulnerability that could look like a powerful position on the surface, with accusations and expressions of anger that also inhibit attunement to their partners, but more likely were expressions of powerlessness that did not increase their limited influence in the relationship. (p. 14)

Sociocultural attunement to vulnerability helps therapists appreciate the conflicts men may experience when their desires to be relational collide with societal pressures to appear invulnerable and all knowing. This is especially complicated when experiences of trauma and marginalization leave them feeling worthless or disempowered (Wells et al., 2017). When examining recordings of couple therapy sessions, Wells and colleagues found that these feelings interacted with gender to incite actions that dominated their partners. Similarly, Smoliak, LaMarre et al. (2022) found that men expressing soft emotions such as vulnerability still tended to organize relationships in ways that maintain male dominance. To counteract this, therapists must attend to both sociocultural vulnerability and accountability (Samman & Knudson-Martin, 2015).

When the therapist asked Samuel what it would be like to share with Lena some of the pressure and doubts he felt as a Black man from a low socio-economic background attempting to "make it" in the dominant culture, he looked at the therapist and said, "You don't do that!" As they explored this socio-emotional discourse, he was able to name his fear that he wasn't good enough for Lena, "What's a poor guy from the farm doing with a woman like her?" This fear embodied and kept in place both a socio-economic hierarchy and a patriarchal one (Knudson-Martin & Smoliak, in press).

Social Valuation of Emotion

When Samuel said, "You don't do that!" he expressed the dominant Western message that emotions, and those who express them, have less worth than "higher" cortical functioning and abstract thought (Knudson-Martin, 2025). In response to the organizing effect of these socio-emotional messages, Samuel had never shared his fears of being less than with Lena or anyone. He did not even let himself think about this fear. In fact, what he typically expressed was just the opposite—that he is on top of everything. Likewise, Lena intuited and attuned to his fears and gave him a pass from expressing them as a way to protect and support him. But this left her feeling lonely and on the outside of Samuel's life, while keeping the White heteropatriarchal structure in place. Intentionally valuing emotion and recognizing and honoring the importance of attending to emotional processes counters heteropatriarchy and discourse that privileges individualism over relationships.

Power

Persistent powerlessness and devaluing cultural stories of self elevate stress hormones, compromise the immune system, and affect genetic expression (Mehl-Madrona, 2010). "Even having memories of 'power-over' comments—which are often experienced as a disregarding voice, and a felt sense of exclusion—can create a nervous system response" (Glaser et al., 2017, p. 3)." In contrast, attuned mutually supportive relationships increase oxytocin and one's ability to reflectively respond to stressful life situations. Simply put, SERT addresses power disparities because they undermine relational engagement and efforts to improve health and well-being. When power is shared, people do better (Knudson-Martin, 2013).

Assessing the Balance of Power

The flow of power in a relationship can be nuanced and is not always apparent at first.

Power is also complex because there are multiple sources and aspects of power (Knudson-Martin, 2024; Young & Seedall, 2024). For example, at first glance, Lena looks quite powerful. She sits tall, appears composed, and speaks clearly. Some of her demeanor represents her upper-middle class background and the cultural capital this affords her, especially in public spaces (McDowell, 2015). Samuel looks down and appears ashamed. He speaks softly at first and does not seem powerful. Assessing the flow of power in this relationship requires looking more deeply and tracking the flow of power in their moment-by-moment interactions, as well as in the history of their relationship. It also involves interactions between their various social identities and latent power built into social roles, as well as how their experiences around power may shift across settings and in public and private spaces.

What is the Balance of Power?

Relative Status

- Whose interests shape what happens in the family?
- To what extent do partners feel equally entitled to express and attain personal goals, needs, and wishes?
- How are low-status tasks like housework handled?

Attention to Other

- To what extent do both partners notice and attend to the other's needs and emotions?
- Does attention go back and forth between partners? Does each give and receive?
- When attention is imbalanced, do partners express awareness of this and the need to rebalance?

Accommodation Patterns

- Is one partner more likely to organize his or her daily activities around the other?
- Does accommodation often occur automatically without anything being said?
- Do partners attempt to justify accommodations they make as being "natural" or the result of personality differences?

Well-being

- Does one partner seem to be better off psychologically, emotionally, or physically than the other?
- Does one person's sense of competence, optimism, or well-being seem to come at the expense of the other's physical or emotional health?
- Does the relationship support the economic viability of each partner?

Figure 15.3 Assessing the balance of power

From Knudson-Martin, C. (2015). When therapy challenges patriarchy: Undoing gendered power in heterosexual relationships. In C. Knudson-Martin, M. E. Wells, & S. Samman (Eds.). *Socio-Emotional Relationship Therapy: Bridging emotion, societal context, and couple interaction* (p. 17). Springer. Used with permission.

Mahoney and Knudson-Martin (2009) developed guidelines for assessing power in relationships, including the four dimensions illustrated in Figure 15.3: 1) relative status of partners, 2) attention to other, 3) accommodation patterns, and 4) well-being. Assessing power can be challenging because it is structured into social roles, making it difficult to recognize or self-report. Power is easier to see when tracking relational processes in session and asking process-oriented questions. Using the Circle of Care as a guide helps make hidden inequities among heterosexual couples visible, and also works well with non-binary and gay persons whose relationships are less likely to include taken-for-granted social power differences (Jonathan, 2009). These assessment guides may also be used to identify power patterns when working with youth and individual adults.

When tracking the flow of power between Lena and Samuel, the therapist noted that although Lena appeared confident and spoke clearly, she tended to stop short of saying what was on her mind when speaking to Samuel. When the therapist explored this pattern as it occurred in session, Lena said she did not want to add to Samuel's pressure—a sign of accommodation. In contrast, even though Samuel internally doubted his status relative to Lena, his responses demonstrated limited willingness to accept influence from her, creating a significant power imbalance in who is open to being influenced by the other. According to Loscocco and Walzer (2013), this gender imbalance in relational responsibility accounts for much of the dissatisfaction in heterosexual relationships in American society.

The flow of power between Samuel and Lena illustrates the complexities involved when macro power processes outside the relationship structure micro processes between partners. As targets of racism and discrimination, Black men have often been unable to meet the gendered expectations of patriarchy and Black women have been portrayed as having power that is seldom actually accessible to them (Hill, 2005). As women and men compensate for these societal perceptions and experiences, women's relative lack of power in relationships is overlooked. Like Lena, women of color may hesitate to push their own issues or concerns since they are aware of the unfairness their partners face in the larger society (Cowdery et al., 2009). Across racial groups, earning more money than their partners or holding a higher status job such as physician seldom translates into a female power imbalance, as partners consciously or unconsciously compensate by finding ways to augment male power (Esmiol Wilson et al., 2014; Tichenor, 2005).

Emotional Expression, Power, and Behavior

Whose emotions have value and what can be expressed are highly dependent on who is doing the emoting (Smoliak et al., 2023; Wetherell, 2012). Emotional expression is one way power imbalances are maintained. Expressions of anger or disappointment on the part of those in powerful positions tend to silence subordinates and lead them to accommodate in order to maintain the relationship and avoid further disruption. Interrupting these power patterns requires remaining socioculturally attuned to the vulnerabilities of both partners while also fostering accountability and mutuality in the Circle of Care (Knudson-Martin et al., 2021).

In the case of Samuel and Lena, the therapist needed to apprehend the vulnerability Samuel felt regarding his masculine position while also identifying and recognizing his relational desires and helping him stay accountable to Lena and the relationship. The therapist had to resist the way in which power was reflected in Samuel's anger, which her body registered, in order to provide leadership that invited alternative responses to this compelling gender discourse (Knudson-Martin, Wells, & Samman, 2015b). When she persisted, Samuel was able to recognize that he was responding to masculine voices that said "don't be a wus," and to give those societal messages less control. Though Lena responded by silencing herself, other women might respond aggressively. When Wells and colleagues (2017) studied heterosexual couples with histories of childhood trauma, they found that men's emotions drove the relational process. This did not mean that women were always submissive; some reacted with anger and actions that served to protect their vulnerability.

SERT therapists understand their clients' behaviors from their context of power. Expressions of rage or disengagement in therapy may follow years in which a partner did not listen, attune, or accept influence from her. Or, as in the earlier example, Robert's irritation and depressed mood helped maintain a power imbalance in which Raul regularly set aside his own needs to soothe Robert. Williams and colleagues (2013) found that the meaning and appropriate clinical interventions for cases involving infidelity depended on whether a partner was unfaithful from a position of power or in response to a relatively powerless position.

Distinguishing Power, Authority, and Responsibility

It can be hard to distinguish between power, authority, and responsibility, especially in more traditional or hierarchical cultures and in generational and workplace contexts. Just because power imbalances are common in a culture does not mean they are healthy or not open to reflection and change. At the same time, hierarchy and mutual support can co-exist (Knudson-Martin & Kim, 2023). People can assign roles hierarchically and respond to each other with the respect accorded to these roles, yet demonstrate mutual attunement and shared relational responsibility.

Some people believe that because a woman makes most of the household decisions, she holds the power in the family, when in fact she is usually responsible for these tasks because they are prescribed by social roles and/or the more powerful partner does not want or need to bother with them (Smoliak, Rice et al., 2022). Therapists need to assess the relational flow of power through the Circle of Care, rather than make assumptions based on stereotypes or ignore power imbalances because they fit within cultural norms.

For example, parenting and intergenerational relationships are inherently hierarchical. Parents are responsible for the safety and well-being of their children. The Typology of Parent-Child Relational Orientations (Tuttle et al., 2012) helps therapists and clients consider how power and relational reciprocity are used in parenting. Like attachment therapists (Siegel & Hartzell, 2004), SERT emphasizes the value of a relational approach to parenting in which "parents listen and respond to the child and teach their children to also be aware of their influence on others, including the parent" (Tuttle et al., p. 81). SERT therapists also consider the social conditions in which parents are preparing their children to live. Working-class parents are likely to emphasize obedience, since it is necessary for survival in environments where others have authority, while professional class parents are more likely to teach their children to speak up and advocate for themselves (Lareau, 2011). Socioculturally attuned practice will take these contexts into account when working with parents and children.

Third Order Change

Knudson-Martin and Kim (2023, p. 284) identified four mechanisms through which SERT promotes third order change:

1 Sociocultural attunement to each partner's felt identities and experience that promotes relational engagement
2 A shift in power imbalances that supports mutual engagement in the Circle of Care
3 Experience engaging with each other from positions of mutual support, and
4 A vision of alternatives to inequitable societal power processes

This enables people to make intentional responses to societal patterns and discourses.

SERT utilizes neurobiological infrastructure to help clients move from cognitive awareness of larger societal patterns in their lives, what narrative theorists call a new story of self and other, to embodied action that "our whole body learns and absorbs" (Mehl-Madrona & Mainguy, 2015, p. 206). This work goes beyond talk toward affective engagement and practice that builds upon new positive experiences (Beaudoin, 2017; Beaudoin & Monk, 2024; Zimmerman, 2018). This process is facilitated by an active and engaged therapist who is aware of societal power processes and uses this to guide clinical decisions.

Guidelines for Practice

Socio-emotional relationship therapy has a well-developed clinical sequence that works in three interconnected phases: Position, Interrupt, and Practice (Figure 15.4). These practices align well with the ANVIET principles described in this text. More detailed guidelines and examples can be found in *A Step-by-Step Guide to Socio-Emotional Relationship Therapy* (Knudson-Martin, 2024).

Phase 1—Position

Phase I positions therapy to counter inequities and orient toward relationality. This phase involves three interconnected processes that help clients connect their personal concerns to larger sociocultural processes and begin to see alternatives. These strategies continue throughout the therapy and can be used in any order.

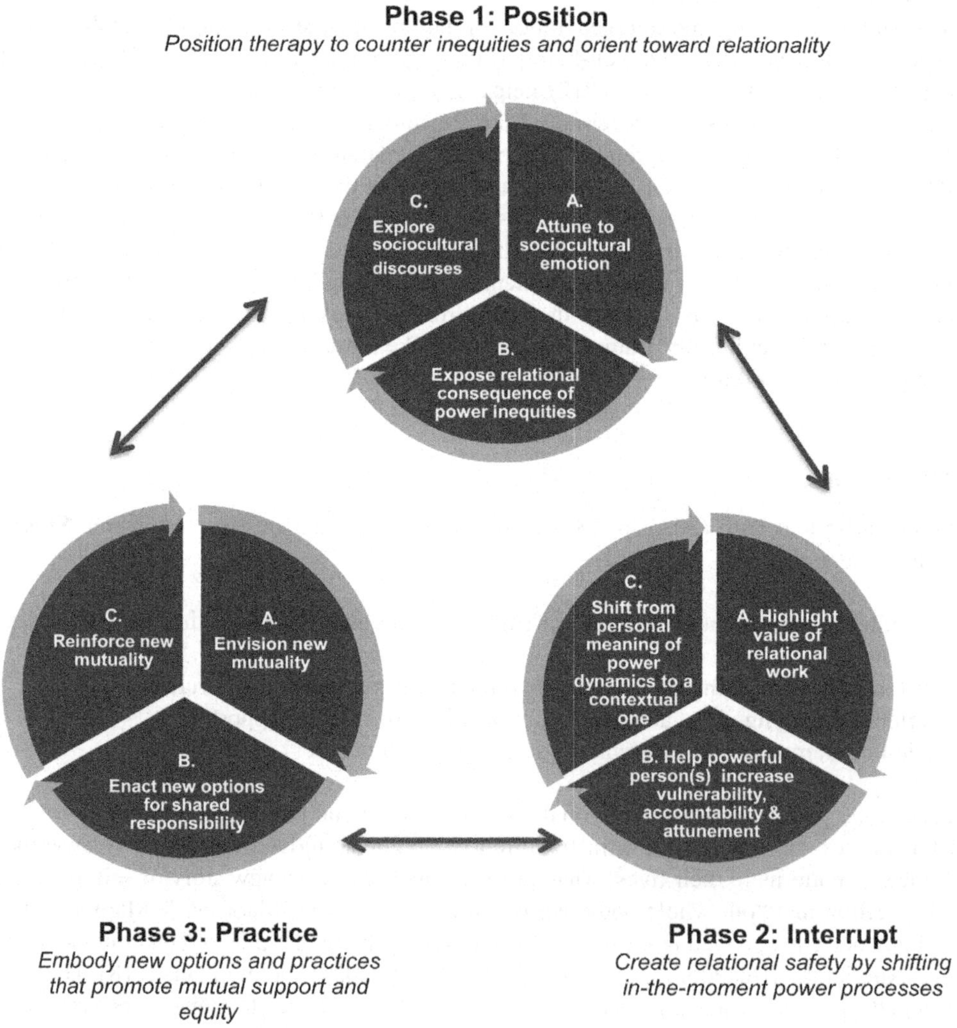

Phase 1: Position
Position therapy to counter inequities and orient toward relationality

C. Explore sociocultural discourses
A. Attune to sociocultural emotion
B. Expose relational consequence of power inequities

C. Reinforce new mutuality
A. Envision new mutuality
B. Enact new options for shared responsibility

C. Shift from personal meaning of power dynamics to a contextual one
A. Highlight value of relational work
B. Help powerful person(s) increase vulnerability, accountability & attunement

Phase 3: Practice
Embody new options and practices that promote mutual support and equity

Phase 2: Interrupt
Create relational safety by shifting in-the-moment power processes

Figure 15.4 SERT clinical sequence

Attune to Sociocultural Emotion

Ongoing socioemotional **attunement** is the foundation for SERT clinical work and helps form the therapeutic alliance. This is a relational process in which therapists seek to take in the felt nature of clients' sociocultural experience. Rather than an objective process in which therapists simply discover what clients feel, sociocultural attunement is an interactive, back and forth process in which therapist and clients begin to evolve a sociocultural understanding of the presenting issues. This can include a visceral awareness of being on the same wavelength as clients demonstrate increased openness about their experience. It can also involve staying with feelings of discomfort or dissonance that arise and attuning to the sociopolitical context of the therapy relationship itself (Knudson-Martin & Smoliak, in press). Attunement to sociocultural vulnerability and relational desires is especially important, and often hidden by dominant societal discourse (Knudson-Martin et al., 2021).

Expose Relational Consequences of Power Differences

Being able to **name** power while also relationally engaging powerful partners is critical to SERT. Therapists track and **name** power differences (such as in who attends, who accepts influence, etc.) and explore the impact of these differences on clients' relationships. Exposing the power dynamic may feel somewhat uncomfortable at first. Successful efforts are socioculturally attuned, validate the powerful partner's relational **values** and interests, and also address the consequences of actions that maintain the power imbalance, such as not listening, minimizing, defining another's "reality," etc. (Samman & Knudson-Martin, 2015). For example, a therapist might say,

> I know how much you love [partner] and want to make her happy. You feel that, as a man, you are supposed to know what to do. And yet she just said that when you make decisions without her, she feels discounted, like you don't really care about her. From what you have said, I don't think that's what you want.

Focusing on power dynamics as they arise in session and linking them to their clinical concerns works best. **Naming** power while highlighting relational **values** creates a therapeutic context that makes it possible to resist dominant societal discourses that perpetuate power inequities. Clients who do not appear open to work within the Circle of Care and/or demonstrate commitment to overt dominance, aggression, or violence should work individually or in a group focused on power issues before considering whether to engage intimate partners or other family members in session (Knudson-Martin & Kim, 2023).

Explore Sociocultural Discourses

SERT therapists listen for societal discourses as clients describe their concerns. Messages about what is valuable and important, how one should carry out their roles, what to expect in relationships, togetherness and independence, the meaning of family and work, and ideas about right and wrong are especially important. As described earlier, knowing that emotions get their meaning from the larger context helps therapists move the conversation from the personal to the contextual. Giving voice to implicit social discourses behind emotion is a good starting point from which to expand the contextual dialogue.

For example, when a mother worries that she should spend more time with her child, a therapist could voice the hidden social message by empathically reflecting, "Good mothers are supposed to prioritize time with their children?" When the client affirms this statement, the therapist can expand the lens to explore this discourse: "What messages do you think women get about being a good mother?" This conversation can be developed to more fully **attune** to her felt sociocultural experience and consider how socially constructed definitions regarding motherhood affect her experience and choices.

Phase 2: Interrupt

In phase 2, therapists create relational safety by using **interventions** that interrupt inequities in the flow of power.

•←→•

Therapists recognize when power imbalances are present and take power into account when deciding which interventions to make and to whom to direct them.

•←→•

The goal is to shift in-the-moment power processes as they arise in client accounts or interactions. This usually means asking different things of each participant, depending on their power positions and based on the following three guidelines.

Help Powerful Partners Take Relational Initiative

Much of phase 2 work involves helping more powerful persons increase their expressions of vulnerability, take accountability for relational engagement and the effect of their actions, and attune to others.

•←→•

Rather than asking an already more vulnerable person in a one-down position to express vulnerability or attune to others, it is important to shift the power dynamic by inviting and supporting those in more powerful positions to engage in these relational actions.

•←→•

This can be surprisingly challenging. Since power processes tend to be invisible to those holding most power, their initial responses may include confusion, deflection, or expressions of helplessness, i.e., "I don't know." Recall that when the therapist asked Robert what Raul might be experiencing (an intervention that interrupts the flow of power), Robert resisted focusing on what Raul might need and instead expressed irritation at his "clinginess." The therapist needed to responsively persist (Knudson-Martin et al., 2021; Sutherland et al., 2013), staying with Robert even when he first declares he doesn't know and encouraging him to attune to what he does know about Raul.

Interventions that suggest each person does or feels the same thing can minimize power differences. For example, saying to a couple, "you both are scared," or "the two of you are avoiding conflict" ignores—and thus reinforces—a power imbalance. Statements such as these should be used cautiously and, if used at all, need to be followed by clinical actions that help distinguish the position each plays. Eventually, each person will be invited to express vulnerability and attune; however, it is important to first create a context in which less powerful persons are likely to be heard and not place the expectation of change on the one already carrying the relational burden.

This principle also applies when working with individuals. If a client is internalizing blame for societal or relational injustices, the SERT therapist will respond with interventions that interrupt this flow of power. For example, if a female client says, "I am not confident enough, I don't express myself well," a response that interrupts power might be, "What happens when you speak? Who listens?" If individual clients in powerful positions seem to be avoiding relational responsibility, the therapist will ask questions that help them attune to others and take relational initiative.

Highlight Value of Relational Work

Relational work tends to be minimized or overlooked in many societies (Knudson-Martin, 2025). To interrupt power imbalances, it is important to recognize, **name**, and expand upon the contributions of those carrying the relationship load. When partners or family members are present, SERT therapists work to increase their awareness of this critical relationship work. In individual therapy, such as the first sessions with Robert in the earlier example, the therapist could ask Robert how Raul's focus on him makes his life better or who in the office is most likely to notice what needs to be done.

↔

Explicitly highlighting the value of relational work is an ongoing focus in SERT.

↔

Shift from Personal to Contextual Meaning of Power

Previously masked power differences become visible when using the Circle of Care. Connecting these interpersonal power processes to larger societal forces reduces blame and makes it easier to help powerful partners share relational responsibility and be accountable for outcomes they may not have intended or do not wish to perpetuate. Relating power processes to sociocultural vulnerabilities associated with marginalization and/or socialization is especially effective in helping a client shift away from a power position (Knudson-Martin et al., 2021). For example, Robert will be more able to attune to Raul if the therapist connects her intervention to Robert's socialization:

> You've learned that people should speak up for what they need—that focusing on others is a sign of weakness. This socialization can make it hard for you to notice or consider what Raul needs. What do you think he needs from you right now?

Phase 3: Practice

As therapy evolves and embodied power dynamics become less entrenched, phase 3 of SERT focuses on helping clients develop and embody new options and practices for mutual support.

↔

Having a more equitable base makes it more possible to address hard issues.

↔

In phase 3, the therapist works as a coach or facilitator to help clients stay in touch with their third order goals and get back on track when old patterns emerge. Therapists may draw upon techniques from a variety of clinical approaches to accomplish the following three clinical tasks.

Envision A New Mutuality

SERT therapists encourage clients to **envision** mutual relational possibilities from the beginning of therapy. Now, to embody these goals, they need to develop a more fully detailed, personalized picture of what enacting them would look like (Knudson-Martin, 2024). For persons like Robert and Samuel, who have resisted engaging in the Circle of Care, this means seeing themselves as wanting and being able to take relational initiative. For those who have been carrying more of the relational weight, like Raul and Lena, it involves envisioning relationships in which the load is shared and in which they are safe to more fully express their perspectives. Narrative (see Chapter 14) and solution-focused (see Chapter 12) practices are helpful. For example, the therapist might ask Robert to **envision** what it will look like when he makes more effort to notice the contributions of his colleagues at work. What will he do? What will he say? What will his colleagues see that tells them he values them? How will his relationships with his colleagues be different?

Enact New Options and Practices for Shared Responsibility

As clients experience new patterns of relational engagement, they begin to neurologically embody these **transformational** relational ideals. The therapist watches their process. When clients fall off track, the therapist "helps them notice and process what happened, with an eye toward what works" (Knudson-Martin & Kim, 2023, p. 283). For example, when she notices that Lena stops expressing herself when Samuel disagrees, the therapist interrupts and says,

> I'm curious about what's happening at this moment. Lena, you seemed to have a lot of energy behind what you were saying, but when Samuel disagreed you stopped talking. I'm wondering what happened to limit your voice?

Then the therapist asks Samuel if he noticed that Lena seemed to be holding back and encourages him to try what he has learned to do to engage her. Enactment promotes the emotional engagement necessary to move from abstract ideals to internalized identity and neurologically accessible felt experience (Zimmerman, 2018). Another example of this is Fatma Arıcı Şahin's use of experiential activities with heterosexual couples in Turkey (see Chapter 7 and Text Box 15.2 below).

Text Box 15.2 Fatma Arıcı Şahin, PhD

Fatma Arıcı Şahin is an assistant professor at Kastamonu University in northern Turkey, with interests in couple and family therapy, feminism and gender studies, art therapy and creativity. She first came across the concepts of "third order thinking" and "sociocultural attunement" while reviewing the literature that would form the basis of feminist and SERT-informed group work that she developed for married heterosexual couples as part of her doctoral dissertation.

In my doctoral research, I developed an 8-session relationship enhancement program based on a feminist perspective. My aim was to address power sharing and equality issues between partners. I applied this program with a group of six married couples and examined the effectiveness of the program in terms of power sharing, self orientations (relational and individualistic orientations), and dyadic adjustment by using a mixed method approach. Beyond a typical relationship enhancement process that only focuses on the couple system, I intended to help partners to critically discuss the sociocultural factors embedded in their relationships and how these affect their interactions, and to develop cooperation with each other to create a shared ideology based on relationship equality (mainly in terms of gender). I also used various fields of art (music, dance, literature, photography, cinema, etc.) as tools/techniques that enable the expression of emotions, and also incorporated Fishbane's Relational Empowerment idea and the Gottman model to address various relational skills (e.g., conflict resolution).

A facilitating and active therapist stance that transforms therapy into a social intervention process, experiential techniques (especially art therapy for me), and relational empowerment are the key elements of this transformative work. I begin to disrupt the unequal flow of power in relationships by inviting the more autonomous partners (mostly male) into a relational position, as in the SERT approach. When they start to speak from their vulnerability with a relational orientation, this can create a basis for cooperation that will enable the partners to resist unjust systems together. Relational empowerment that enables partners to be mutually attuned to each other's vulnerable emotions, to care for each other, and to take responsibility for the relationship together allows them to develop partnerships to resist unfair sociocultural patterns.

Before the last session of the program, I gave the couples homework to write an "Equality Manifesto" in an evening when they could talk about their life ideologies and values with their partners. In the final session, each couple read their equality manifesto to the other group members, as if the group itself represented the society. Other group members reflected their thoughts and feelings to the couple who read their manifesto. I strongly believe that group work accelerates the transformative change in terms of facilitating the transferability of what is experienced in the group to social life.

When scores of the experimental group were compared with the control group, the results showed the program provided a significant increase in power sharing and dyadic adjustment scores that persisted at the three-month follow-up. Quantitative effects on internalizing a relational orientation were not significant; however, qualitative findings showed participants found the program useful by expanding their perspective from an individual focus to a relational and systemic one, examining power distribution, conceptualizing relationship equality, and gaining awareness on the social context.

Reinforce New Mutuality

Third order change that embodies relationality and mutual support needs reinforcement. SERT therapists notice and amplify examples of these changes, accentuating how they achieved them and detailing the impact of these changes on their relationships. For example, when Lena noted in passing that Samuel came home early so she could go out with her friends, the therapist asked how this happened. Did Lena ask Samuel to come home early? When Lena said that she didn't ask, that she had expected she'd need a babysitter, the therapist helped Samuel reflect on what he did to make this act of relational responsibility. Note how the therapist provided leadership in this process:

Therapist: How did you decide to come home early?
Samuel: I knew she had this thing planned with her friends and I thought I should help out.
Therapist: You should help out…this seems different than in the past. How so?
Samuel: (pause) Uhh… I guess I was thinking more about Lena and what it is like for her to do most of the childcare. And I wanted to spend more time with Izzy.

Samuel's response showed that he was beginning to internalize the Circle of Care, which the therapist recognized as a shift in power and challenge to the dominant discourse that had been shaping his actions. To reinforce this change, she continued to help him take in the relational impact of his act:

Therapist: You were thinking more about what doing childcare is like for Lena and your desire to spend time with Izzy. How do you think this focus on Lena and Izzy affected your relationships with them?
Samuel: Well…I feel closer to them. And like I want them to know I care about them.

The therapist also helped Samuel make his challenge to the dominant discourse intentional:

Therapist: It's kind of a break from all that social pressure you felt to always focus and perform at work—that that was the measure of your worth.
Samuel: Yeh. I hadn't realized how much that "money is success" stuff had a grip on me.

The therapist continued to reinforce the new mutuality by asking Lena what it means to her that Samuel appreciates the load she carries and wants to be more connected with her and Izzy.

Over time, clients increasingly relate based on their evolving vision of mutuality and recognize when they are acting counter to inequities. They see their issues through an expanded lens that carries less blame and enables them to be more intentional about how they engage with each other and the world. An example of this may be found in Text Box 15.2, in which Fatma Arıcı Şahin describes her research on a group process she developed to help reinforce couples' evolving mutuality.

Case Illustration

Julia Keller called for therapy saying she was no longer able to cope and didn't know what to do, "Everything is falling to pieces—I just can't hold it together anymore." On the intake form, she checked depressed thoughts, helplessness, and anger. She indicated physical and emotional abuse in a past relationship and occasional thoughts that she did not want to live. Julia identifies as a 45-year-old White, straight woman and has been married to her partner, Michael (55, White) for eighteen years. She and Michael have two sons, Sean (17) and Braden (16), and a 14-year-old daughter, Aubrey. Nate (25), Julia's son from an earlier relationship, is currently in jail. The impetus for her call, Julia said, is that Braden was suspended from his soccer team for coming to practice drunk and Aubrey is at risk of not passing two classes. Julia feels like a failure and hopes someone at the Family Center can help.

Sydney, a 30-year-old newly licensed LMFT, is assigned the case. Sydney identifies as a mixed race (Black/White) cisgender gay male who passes as White. Because Julia appears so distressed, he decides to first meet individually with her to assess safety. He is aware that mothers receive many societal messages that they are singularly responsible for the behavior and well-being of family members, and is mindful that seeing her individually could reinforce this idea. He is curious about her socio-emotional experience and intentional about positioning their work together to counteract these destructive societal discourses and sensitive to potential inequities in the Circle of Care.

Phase 1—Position

Julia opts for an in-person session (rather than virtual), saying she needs to get away from the house. Despite her being upset, Julia presents as a "well-put-together" upper-middle-class woman, with stylish clothes, hair, and nails. Sydney welcomes her and begins to **attune** based on the intake information:

Therapist: It sounds like there is a lot going on in your family [Julia nods] and you're feeling pretty overwhelmed.

Julia begins to cry and describes the relational burden and hopelessness she feels.

Julia: I don't know what to do. I try so hard, but everything I do is wrong. I'm so worried about the kids, but they just ignore me. And Michael doesn't trust me. He says I don't know how to relate to them and should get off their back. [she takes a deep gasp]. I just can't do it anymore.

Sydney expands the lens to get an initial sociocultural sense of her experience of hopelessness and potential suicide risk. He does this by responding to the emotion she appears to carry regarding her roles as wife and mother.

Therapist: (gently) Being a good mother is important to you.
Julia: Yes! That's all I wanted—something I never had. One of the reasons I married Michael was because I could be a stay at home mom.

Sydney has a choice here. He could, and eventually will, explore the family history and those hurts and losses, but at this moment he stays with her experience of societal expectations around being a mother, wife, and woman. Bringing in the larger context will reduce the blame Julia appears to be internalizing and help her feel less alone in her struggles.

Therapist: What does it mean to you to be one of the women who could be a stay at home mom?
Julia: That I'm acceptable. That I'm worth something. That we have the money and resources to do that.
Therapist: (thoughtfully): Being acceptable. To whom? The community? Society?
Julia: To the world. That I'm not trash. That I can take care of my kids.
Therapist: Those are big statements. So in the eyes of the world, women who can't take care of their kids, keep them out of trouble, aren't worth much…are trash? Where do you think that idea comes from?

Inviting Julia to reflect on the larger context of her pain around her identity as a mother set the stage for framing the family's troubles and her own worth through a larger, third order lens that counters injustice and offers more options.

By the end of the first session, Sydney and Julia determined she was not at risk for suicide. They had begun to develop a contextual picture of her situation in which Julia, who had experienced houselessness and foster care as a child, could feel respected and validated. Sydney helped Julia begin to link her current feelings of worthlessness and failure, not simply to a "bad" family background, but also to societal discourses that equate personal **value** with economic resources and place relational burden on women.

Sydney next met with the whole family and with Julia and Michael as a couple. He observed that Michael and the children tended to subtly belittle Julia and discount her opinion. This included teasing Julia that she was a "prude" regarding Braden's alcohol use and suggesting that she was hard on Aubrey because Julia was putting on weight and was jealous of her daughter being so young and beautiful. Sydney **named** these power issues and their effect on Julia and the family.

Therapist: I noticed just now that when Mom spoke about her concerns regarding Aubrey's grades, Sean dismissed her concern as "over-reacting" and Dad suggested she was jealous of Aubrey. When you did that, Mom got angry and you all laughed. What do you think makes it possible for you to respond to her in that way?
Braden: We're just having fun. She's too sensitive.
Therapist: I'm guessing that's hurtful to you, Julia. [Julia nods]. (To the family) How do you think having fun at mom's expense keeps you from addressing important issues?

In this early phase of therapy, Sydney helped the Keller family begin to consider their issues with each other in terms of the larger societal context, while **attuning** to their socio-emotional experience, making the power imbalances between Julia and the rest of the family visible, and **naming** the relational consequences of this inequity. He helped the family validate their relational desires, while observing that societal messages related to prioritizing money and social appearances seemed to get in the way of their well-being and the connection they would like to have with each other. He shared that many people who come to the Center struggle with these concerns, and that these pressures could be especially challenging for White families. This racial statement, which created curiosity and additional discussion among the family members, made sense to them since this observation followed Sydney's careful attunement to their felt experience and connections to their sociocultural contexts.

Phase 2—Interrupt

Subsequent sessions alternated between couple sessions with Michael and Julia and sessions with the whole family. Braden was also referred to a substance abuse group for teens, which Michael agreed to support only because the coach required it before Braden could return to the team. As the therapy began to delve more deeply into the family's issues, Sydney was attentive to power processes and directed his clinical **interventions** to interrupt imbalances. For example, in a couple session, Julia expressed frustration that Michael was not taking Braden's drinking problem seriously. Michael sighed, shook his head, and looked at Sydney:

Michael: She lives in la-la land. What does she want to do, raise a sissy! I know for a fact that all the guys have their beers.

Sydney recognized that Michael was discounting Julia while also attempting to recruit him into societal gender messages that generationally maintain White heterosexual male dominance (Kimmel, 2008). He interrupted that societal power dynamic by challenging it:

Therapist: To be a real guy requires underage beer drinking? This is just what athletes do?
Michael: (pause) well you know…that's how it's always been. It's what guys do!

Sydney seeks to attune to Michael's sociocultural vulnerabilities around masculinity:

Therapist: You're worried that to be a man Braden has to fit into some kind of beer-drinking image? What is your worry for him?
Michael: I don't want people to think he's a mama's boy…he can be a little over-sensitive for a guy.

By interrupting Michael's replication of heteropatriarchy, Sydney opened space for **envisioning** alternatives:

Therapist: When you say Braden can be sensitive, what do you mean?
Michael: He cares a lot about people's feelings. He's always been like that.
Therapist: Braden cares about people's feelings [Michael and Julia both nod]. How do you think that will serve him well as he grows into manhood?

To also intervene in the gendered power dynamic between Michael and Julia, Sydney invited Michael to attune to Julia's frustration:

Therapist: So, earlier when Julia said she was frustrated that you haven't seemed to take Braden's alcohol issues seriously, what do you think it is like for her when you discount her concerns in this way?
Michael: I wasn't really discounting her; I was just trying to tell her like it is.
Therapist: (persisting) and what do you think it is like for her when you "tell her like it is?"
Michael: I don't suppose she likes it very much.
Therapist: (supporting and expanding Michael's move toward Julia's experience) She wouldn't like it because it feels…
Michael: (pause) Belittling, maybe. Like what she thinks is not important.
Therapist: I'm guessing you do care about what she thinks. Is that right? [Michael nods.] So what do you think her concerns for Braden are?

After Michael reflects on Julia's concerns, Sydney encourages him to recognize and express his gratitude to Julia for the caring she gives, an intervention that interrupts their power imbalance and also reinforces relational **values** typically minimized in individualistic Western societies:

Therapist: Julia, you focus a lot on the children's well-being. [Julia nods.] Michael, how does Julia's concern for the kids make their lives better?

During this phase of the therapy, Sydney is actively engaged in interrupting power inequities as they arise in session. This includes helping Michael and the children attune to Julia and respect her, and is facilitated by connecting their personal issues to larger societal processes. For example, Sydney validates Michael's relational interests and then commiserates with him regarding the ways male socialization and societal expectations get in the way:

Therapist: Michael, I see how much you care about your kids, and about Julia too. Other male clients tell us how caring and sensitivity gets washed out of them in our society. It can make it hard to know how to show and express our caring—or how to focus on others and still feel like a man. What has been your experience with this?

Effective **intervention** required that Sydney make sense of the complex intersections of personal and societal power processes. Julia's anger sometimes erupted in ways that masked her limited power and hopelessness. The relationship between Michael and Julia was founded on multiple power differentials based on gender, age, socio-economic status, and perceived need for the relationship. Julia was grateful to Michael for "rescuing" her and her young son. Michael expected her gratitude and subservience and, at the same time, did many things to take care of her. His power was structured into their identities, and his domination was not often overtly expressed. Feeling distant from his own harsh father, Michael tried to maintain a friendship role with the children and left the disciplining to Julia, rather than being accountable as a father and partner. As encouraged by the dominant system, he measured himself by higher socio-economic standards than their current situation and often sacrificed relationships to demonstrate financial success. The children were unaware of their privilege and social capital and were learning that they did not need to work hard or conform to institutional rules to be successful or get what they wanted. In their privileged situation, attunement to others was not valued.

Interrupting these power dynamics took contextual consciousness, self-awareness, and courage on Sydney's part. His internal responses to societal power processes told him that as a young, gay, Person of Color, it may be inappropriate or not safe to actively engage with this relatively affluent White family, especially since Michael was old enough to be his father and exuded an air of superiority. To interrupt power processes despite these vulnerable feelings, he empathically connected with the sociocultural experience of each family member and joined to resist power *with* them (Knudson-Martin, Wells, & Samman, 2015). His peer supervision group, dedicated to socially responsible practice, helped him process his emotional reactions to the family.

Phase 3—Practice

Over time, the Keller family began to incorporate relational themes into their conversations and interactions with one another. Neural pathways supporting trust and mutual support were activated when they experienced each other in emotionally meaningful new ways. With this more equitable foundation beginning to be established, they are now more able to safely deal with unresolved issues between them. Sydney's role is to help the family **envision** and develop what shared responsibility in the Circle of Care looks like for them, keeping them on track when old patterns emerge and reinforcing **transformational** new ones. For example, in a session focused on Aubrey's engagement with school, Aubrey says she isn't worried, that she'll be able to pull it together in the end. When Julia begins to protest, saying Aubrey has to learn to take things more seriously, Aubrey starts to react and then sighs and turns to her mother:

Aubrey: I know you worry about me, Mom. I get it. Just trust me on this OK. I know what it takes to pass.

Sydney reinforces and highlights Aubrey's step toward attuning to her mother, as well as helping flesh out a picture of personal and shared relational responsibility while validating caring work.

Therapist: (leaning in) I wonder if I could interrupt for a moment. Aubrey, I noticed that you began by saying you know your mother worries about you. What did it mean to you to say that to her?

Aubrey: Well, I do appreciate all she does for me, and I get that she worries.

Therapist: It makes sense to you that she worries?

Aubrey: Yeah. I mean, coming here, I've heard her talk about it enough. And I can see why parents worry.

Therapist: What would you want your mom to know about your appreciation of her? Can you please look at her and tell her?

Aubrey: (to Julia) I didn't think about what it's like to be a mother. It's not fair that you should blame yourself for what I do, but I guess that's what mothers are [air quotes] supposed to do. I know I'm lucky to have you to worry about me—even when I don't like it.

Sydney reinforces the effect of Aubrey's demonstrations of caring:

Therapist: (to Julia). What is it like to hear Aubrey say she knows you worry and appreciates it, even though she doesn't always like it?
Julia: (tearfully) I've tried so hard to be a good mom. [looks at Aubrey] Thank you, honey. It really helps to hear that.
Therapist: How does it help?
Julia: It makes me feel not so alone...and better about myself. Like someone notices.

Sydney helped the family broaden and nuance the conversation about their responsibilities to each other, including Michael and the boys. They discussed societal expectations and pressures and how these connect to responsibility for oneself and others. This invited a discussion of what it means to get good grades. It became clear that Aubrey's disengagement from academic expectations was, in part, resistance to automatically falling in line with social standards designed to maintain the dominant socio-economic structure:

Aubrey: I don't even know why you care so much that I get into a good college. What's it for? What's it do for you, Dad? Does it make you happy? I don't think so.

The family was now actively engaged in consciously considering how to enact relational values and life choices previously hidden to them. Similarly to what might happen in contextual therapy (see Chapter 10), Julia was also able to get a broader picture of the intergenerational injustices in her life and be more intentional about how she defined herself and her contributions to others going forward. Michael started to take the lead in demonstrating respect for Julia's caring and reflecting with Sean and Braden through an expanded lens about what it means to be "a guy" and how they want to relate to others. While all the arguments did not go away, and challenges with each other and the larger world are ongoing and not always easily resolved, they now see themselves through the Circle of Care and a broader sociocontextual lens. They have a new framework through which to address old issues, such as how Julia's son Nate fits into the family.

Summary: Third Order Change

As a White family, the Kellers had been socialized to align their internalized identities and parenting practices with the dominant heteropatriarchal capitalist ideals and to expect access to its perceived rewards. The previously unrecognized costs to each person's development and their ability to connect with one another were many. As a consequence, their relationships did not support Julia's emotional well-being or relational responsibility among Michael and the children. As the Keller family began to see their personal struggles in the context of larger systems of systems, they could envision new relational possibilities. Third order change in this case is represented by this new way of seeing themselves and the world around them.

With the therapists' active support, the Kellers used the Circle of Care to help expand upon and begin to enact relational values that mattered to them but had been minimized and masked by dominant social discourses. Julia no longer solely carried the relational load. Michael began to experience the rewards of genuine relationships with his wife and children and obsessed less about financial success. Sean, Braden, and Aubrey also demonstrated more relational responsibility and approached adulthood with more intentionality about their values and broader definitions of success. The family still faced many issues, but were more able to support each other through them.

It would have been easy for a therapist working with this case to get caught in Julia's history of abuse and focus primarily on how she could be less triggered in the present. This first order change, while useful in the context of larger third order change, would have perpetuated the dominant system that put responsibility on her without questioning the larger systems of systems. Family therapists might also have focused on second order change in how the Keller family communicated, which, while also useful, would have left the underlying individualistic material value system unchallenged or implied blame on the family without awareness of the societal context around them. To do third order work, Sydney had to be intentional about how his clinical interventions reinforced or challenged social systems that work against relationships and perpetuate inequalities. Whether working with affluent families like the Kellers or those in marginalized social locations, Sydney always begins by attuning to the effect of their social contexts on their presenting symptoms and felt experiences, and directs his interventions to value what is minimized or overlooked and to counteract social power inequities.

Reflexive Questions

- What is your reaction to this statement: "There is no such thing as a 'non-affective' thought; 'rational' decision-making requires an internal appraisal based on emotion that is always socioculturally located?"
- How can you help clients map the ways in which their emotional responses are structured by contextual social forces? Can you think of examples for yourself?
- If identity is how people know themselves in relation to others, then how is your identity confirmed by a sense of being known, recognized, and validated? How do these processes give or take away your power?
- SERT defines power as a set of relationally created and structurally embedded social processes that determine whose experiences, abilities, and interests merit value. How do these power dynamics affect what and whom you attend to in your clinical practice?
- The Circle of Care uses four orienting principles that promote mutually supportive relationships and well-being: mutual vulnerability, attunement, influence, and shared relational responsibility. How are these relational guidelines aligned or misaligned with your gender and cultural socialization?
- Socio-emotional relationship therapy has a well-developed clinical sequence that works in three interconnected phases: Position, Interrupt, and Practice. When you look at the aspects of these phases carefully, what would it mean for you to practice in this way? How do you think you would personally and professionally be affected by it?

References

Ahmed, S. (2004). Affective economies. *Social Text*, *22*(2), 117–139.

Baima, T. R. & Feldhousen, E. B. (2007). The heart of sexual trauma: Patriarchy as a centrally organizing principle for couple *therapy. Journal of Feminist Family Therapy*, *19*, 13–36.

Bateson, G. (1972). *Steps to an ecology of mind: Collected essays in anthropology, psychiatry, evolution, and epistemology*. Jason Aronson Inc.

Beaudoin, M. (2017). Tapping into the power of the brain–heart–gut axis: Addressing embodied aspects of intense emotion. In M. Beaudoin & J. Duvall (Eds.). *Collaborative therapy and neurobiology: Evolving practice in action* (pp. 75–86). Routledge.

Beaudoin, M. N. & Monk, G. (2024). *Narrative practices and emotions 40+ ways to support the emergence of flourishing identities*. Routledge.

Burkitt, I. (2014). *Emotions and social relations*. Sage.

ChenFeng, J., Kim, L., Knudson-Martin, C., & Wu, Y. (2017). Application of socio-emotional relationship therapy with couples of Asian heritage: Addressing issues of culture, gender, and power. *Family Process*, *56*, 558–573.

Combs, G. & Freedman, J. (2016). Narrative therapy's relational understanding of identity, *Family Process*, *55*, 211–224.

Combs, G. & Freedman, J. (2012). Narrative, poststructuralism, and social justice: Current practices in narrative therapy, *The Counseling Psychologist*, *40*, 1033–1060.

Cowdery, R., Scarborough, N., Knudson-Martin, C., Lewis, M., Shesadri, G., & Mahoney, A. R. (2009). Gendered power in cultural contexts part II: Middle class African American heterosexual couples with young children. *Family Process*, *48*, 25–39.

Cozolino, L. (2016). *Why therapy works: Using our minds to change our brains*. Norton.

Esmiol, E. E., Knudson-Martin, C., & Delgado, S. (2012). Developing a contextual consciousness: Learning to address gender, societal power, and culture in clinical practice. *Journal of Marital and Family Therapy*, *38*, 573–588.

Esmiol Wilson, E., Knudson-Martin, C., & Wilson, C. (2014). Gendered power, spirituality, and relational processes: The experience of Christian physician couples: *Journal of Couple and Relationship Therapy*, *13*, 312–338.

Ewing, J., Estes, R., & Like, B. (2017). Narrative neurotherapy (NNT): Scaffolding identity states. In M Beaudoin & J. Duvall (Eds). *Collaborative therapy and neurobiology: Evolving practice in action* (pp. 87–99). Routledge.

Fosha, D. (2009). Emotion and recognition at work: Energy, vitality, pleasure, truth, desire, and the emergent phenomenology of transformational experience. In D. Fosha, D. J. Siegel, & M. F. Solomon (Eds.). *The healing power of emotion: Affective neuroscience, development & clinical practice* (pp. 172–203). Norton.

Garcia, M. (2011). *Pleasure: The secret ingredient in happiness*. Pink Soda Publishing.

Gergen, K. J. (2009). *Relational being: Beyond self and community*. Oxford University Press.

Gerhardt, S. (2004). *Why love matters: How affection shapes a baby's brain*. Brunner-Routledge.

Glaser, J. E., Ruben, M., Foster, S., & Pearce-McCall, D. (2017). The neurochemistry of power conversations. https://c-suitenetwork.com/news/the-neurochemistry-of-power-conversations/

Greenberg, L. S. & Goldman, R. N. (2008). *Emotion-focused couples therapy: The dynamics of emotion, love, and power*. American Psychological Association.

Hanna, S. (2014). *The transparent brain in couple and family therapy: Mindful integrations with neuroscience*. Routledge.

Hardy, K. V. & McGoldrick, M. (2019). Re-visioning family therapy training. In M. McGoldrick & K. V. Hardy (Eds). *Re-visioning family therapy: Addressing diversity in clinical practice*, (3rd Ed., pp. 477–495). Guildford.

Hill, S. A. (2005). *Black intimacies: A gender perspective on families and relationships*. Alta Mira Press.

Jenks, A., Adams, G., Young, B., & Seedall, R. (2024). Addressing power in couples therapy: Integrating socio-emotional relationship therapy and emotionally focused therapy. *Family process*, *63*(1), 48–63.

Johnson, S. M. (2019). *Attachment theory in practice: Emotionally focused therapy (EFT) with individuals, couples, and families*. Guildford.

Jonathan, N. (2009). Carrying equal weight: Relational responsibility and attunement among same-sex couples. In C. Knudson-Martin & A. Mahoney (Eds.). *Couples, gender, and power: Creating change in intimate relationships* (pp. 79–103). Springer Publishing Company.

Jonathan, N. & Knudson-Martin, C. (2012). Building connection: Attunement and gender equality in heterosexual relationships. *Journal of Couple and Relationship Therapy*, *11*, 95–111.

Kimmel, M. (2016). *The gendered society* (6th ed.). Oxford University Press.

Kimmel, M. (2008). *Guyland: The perilous world where boys become men*. Harper.

Knudson-Martin, C. (2025). *The socio-emotional relationship workbook for couples: Closing the gap between the relationship you want and the relationship you have*. Routledge.

Knudson-Martin, C. (2024). *A step-by-step guide to socio-emotional relationship therapy: A socially responsible approach to clinical practice*. Routledge.

Knudson-Martin, C. (2013). Why power matters: Creating a foundation of mutual support in couple relationships. *Family Process*, *52*, 5–18.

Knudson-Martin, C. & Huenergardt, D. (2010). A socio-emotional approach to couple therapy: Linking social context and couple interaction. *Family Process*, *49*, 369–386.

Knudson-Martin, C., Huenergardt, D., Lafontant, K., Bishop, L., Schaepper, J., & Wells, M. (2015). Competencies for addressing gender and power in couple therapy: A socio-emotional approach. *Journal of Marital and Family Therapy*, *41*, 205–220.

Knudson-Martin, C. & Kim, L. (2023). Socioculturally attuned couple therapy. In J. Lebow & D. Snyder (Eds.). *Clinical handbook of couple therapy* (6th ed., pp. 267–294). Guilford.

Knudson-Martin, C., Kim, L., Gibbs, E., & Harmon, R. (2021). Sociocultural attunement to vulnerability in couple therapy: Fulcrum for changing power processes. *Family Process*, *60*, 1152–1169.

Knudson-Martin, C. & Smoliak, O. (in press). Sociocultural attunement as disquiet: Insights from affect theory. In J. Gaete-Silva, C. Guanaes-Lorenzi, I. Sametband, M. Sesma-Vazquez, & K. Tomm. (Eds.). *Befriending relational disquiet*.

Knudson-Martin, C., Wells, M. A., & Samman, S. (2015). Engaging power, emotion, and context in couple therapy: Lessons learned. In C. Knudson-Martin, M. E. Wells, & S. Samman (Eds.). *Socio-emotional relationship therapy: Bridging emotion, societal context, and couple interaction* (pp. 145–153). AFTA Series in Family Therapy. Springer.

Krolokke, C. & Sorensen, A. S. (2006). *Gender communication theories and analysis: From silence to performance*. Sage.

Lareau, A. (2011). *Unequal childhoods: Class, race, and family life*. University of California Press.

Loscocco, K. & Walzer, S. (2013). Gender and the culture of heterosexual marriage in the United States. *Journal of Family Theory & Review*, *5*, 1–14.

Mahoney, A. R. & Knudson-Martin, C. (2009). Gender equality in intimate relationships. In C. Knudson-Martin & A. Mahoney (Eds.). *Couples, gender, and power: Creating change in intimate relationships* (pp. 3–16). Springer Publishing Company.

McDowell, T. (2015). *Applying critical social theories to family therapy practice*. AFTA SpringerBriefs in Family Therapy. Springer.

Medina, J. (2013). *The epistemology of resistance: Gender and racial oppression, epistemic injustice, and resistant imaginations*. Oxford University Press.

Mehl-Madrona, L. (2010). *Healing the mind through the power of story: The promise of narrative psychiatry*. Bear & Company.

Mehl-Madrona, L. & Mainguy, B. (2015). *Remapping your mind: The neuroscience of self-transformation through story*. Bear & Company.

Morrison, T., Palmgren, E., Ferris Wayne, M., Harrison, T., & Knudson-Martin, C. (2022) Learning to embody a social justice perspective in couple and family therapy: A grounded theory analysis of MFTs in training. *Journal of Contemporary Family Therapy*, *44*(4), 408–421.

Papp, P. (2003). Gender, marriage, and depression. In L. B. Silverstein & T. J. Goodrich (Eds.). *Feminist family therapy: Empowerment in social context* (pp. 211–223). American Psychological Association.

Porges, S. W. (2009). Reciprocal influences between body and brain in the perception and expression of affect. In D. Fosha, D. J. Siegel, & M. F. Solomon (Eds.). *The healing power of emotion: Affective neuroscience, development & clinical practice* (pp. 27–54). Norton.

Parker, L. (2009). Disrupting power and privilege in couples therapy. *Clinical Social Work Journal*, *37*, 248–255.

Samman, S. K., & Knudson-Martin, C. (2015). Relational engagement in heterosexual couple therapy: Helping men move from “I” to “we.” In C. Knudson-Martin, M. A. Wells, & S. K. Samman (Eds.). *Socio-emotional relationship therapy: Bridging emotion, societal context, and couple interaction* (pp. 79–92). AFTA Springerbriefs in Family Therapy. Springer.

Siegel, D. J. (2020). *The developing mind: How relationships and the brain interact and shape who we are* (3rd ed.). Guildford.

Siegel, D. J. (2023). *IntraConnected: Mwe (me = we) as the integration of self, identity, and belonging*. Norton.

Siegel, D. J. & Hartzell, M. (2004). *Parenting from the inside out*. Jeremy P. Tarcher.

Smoliak, O., Al-Ali, K., LeCouteur, A., Tseliou, E., Rice, C., LaMarre, A., … & Henshaw, S. (2023). The third shift: Addressing emotion work in couple therapy. *Family Process*, *62*(3), 1006–1023.

Smoliak, O. & Knudson-Martin, C. (under review). Rethinking sociocultural attunement through a postcolonial lens. *Family Process*.

Smoliak, O., LaMarre, A., Rice, C., Tseliou, E., LeCouteur, A., Myers, M., … & Velikonja, L. (2022). The politics of vulnerable masculinity in couple therapy. *Journal of Marital and Family Therapy*, *48*, 427–446.

Smoliak, O., Rice, C., LaMarre, A., Tseliou, E., LeCouteur, A., & Davies, A. (2022). Gendering of care and care inequalities in couple therapy. *Family process*, *61*(4), 1386–1402.

Smoliak, O., Rice, C., Rudder, D., Tseliou, E., LaMarre, A., LeCouteur, A., … & Henshaw, S. (2025). Emotion regulation as affective neoliberal governmentality. *Family Process*.

Sullivan, O. (2005). *Changing gender relations, changing families; Tracing the pace of change over time*. Rowman & Littlefield.

Sutherland, O., Turner, J, & Dienhart, A. (2013). Responsive persistence part I: Therapist influence in postmodern practice. *Journal of Marital and Family Therapy*, *39*, 470–487.

Tate, S. A. (2014). Racial affective economies, disalienation and "race made ordinary." *Ethnic and Racial Studies*, *37*(13), 2475–2490.

Tatum, B. D. (1997). *Why are all the Black kids sitting in the cafeteria? And other conversations about race*. Basic Books.

Tichenor, V. J. (2005). *Earning more and getting less: Why successful wives can't buy equality*. Rutgers University Press.

Tuttle, A., Kim, L., & Knudson-Martin, C. (2012). Parenting as relationship: A framework for assessment and practice. *Family Process*, *51*, 73–89.

Wells, M. A., Lobo, E., Galick, A., Knudson-Martin, C., Huenergardt, D., & Schaepper, J. (2017). Fostering trust through relational safety: Applying SERT's focus on gender and power with adult-survivor couples. *Journal of Couple & Relationship Therapy*, *16*, 122–145.

Wetherell, M. (2012). *Affect and emotion: A new social science understanding*. Sage.

Williams, K., Galick, A., Knudson-Martin, C., & Huenergardt, D. (2013). Toward mutual support: A task analysis of the relational justice approach to infidelity. *Journal of Marital and Family Therapy*, *39*, 285–298.

Winslade, J. (2009). Tracing lines of flight: Implications of the work of Gilles Deleuze. *Family Process*, *48*, 332–346.

Young, B. & Seedall, R. B. (2024). Power dynamics in couple relationships: A review and applications for systemic family therapists. *Family Process*, *63*(4), 1703–1720.

Zimmerman, J. (2018). *Neuro-narrative therapy: New possibilities for emotion-filled conversations*. Norton.

16 Socioculturally Attuned Praxis

Consciousness in Action

We have contended throughout this text that the broader context impacts families and shapes our practices as we engage in equity-based family therapy. Previous chapters focus on intervening at the level of families and individuals. In this chapter, we focus on the potential impact of, and processes for, intervening at other levels of societal systems (See Figure 16.1), including community engagement, research, teaching, supervision, policy work, and organizational change. These systems are often saturated by the effects of oppression, inequity and injustice. According to Patricia Hill Collins (1990), the work of racial-ethnic feminisms illustrates how theory and social action (praxis) are linked. Similarly, Freire (1970) advocated praxis, "action and reflection upon the world in order to change it" (p. 36). Freire's concept of praxis referred to the resistance expressed by oppressed people and groups to harmful/constraining ideologies and inequitable institutions. Simply put, he argued that praxis is putting consciousness into action. From our perspective, applying ANVIET across social contexts can provide guidance for praxis.

The work of transformative change is certainly not unique to family therapists; however, family therapists are uniquely poised to integrate systemic thinking and critical consciousness across various contexts and are often in positions where we can affect change. So, how can family therapists—along with professionals from all disciplines—use third order thinking to envision transformative change in communities, organizations, governmental systems, and international relationships? How might third order thinking inform knowledge production, shape public policy, and support a healthy, sustainable environment? How might we design and carry out interventions that target third order change at all levels of societal systems? In this chapter, we bring forth the voices of practitioners enacting third order, transformative change across various social systems.

The levels of societal systems shown in Figure 16.1 are not discrete, but overlap and impact each other in complex ways. For example, international dynamics, including wars, sanctions, tariffs, and immigration policies, affect the most intimate aspects of culture, community, and family life. Organizations are positioned in particular places at specific times and rely on governmental and economic/commercial systems and policies. All locations or levels present a variety of constraints and opportunities for relational well-being and equity. For example, judicial systems are in many ways bound by government laws that prescribe minimum sentences regardless of individual circumstances or fairness, yet there are also opportunities to influence court decisions to prioritize rehabilitation over punishment. Public policy and laws are often points of contention as they determine which organizations and public sectors will thrive at what cost to others (e.g., loosening of environmental regulations increases profit and global competition, while risking public health and survival of the environment). This figure also draws attention to the structural and social determinants of health discussed in chapters 1 and 4; broader or more

DOI: 10.4324/9781003493426-16

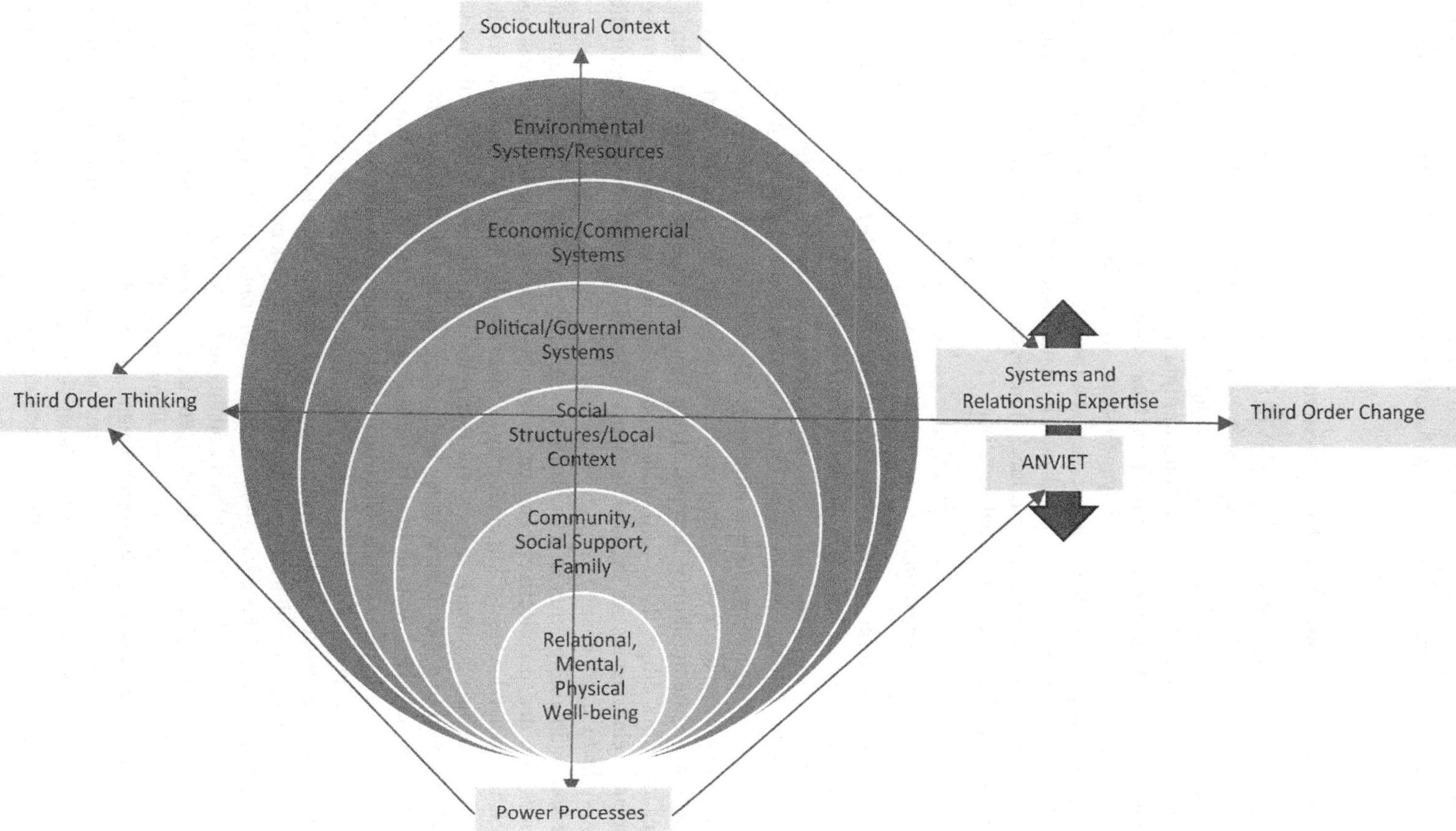

Figure 16.1 Socioculturally attuned praxis across societal systems

"upstream" interventions (e.g., expanding Medicaid coverage) impact lower "downstream" sites (e.g., agency policies, community well-being, educational systems, the health of those living on low income).

Using ANVIET as a Guide for Third Order Systemic Change

A number of core principles, which reflect ANVIET practices, emerge across the many examples of transformation shared by change agents throughout this chapter. Our colleagues describe their work in ways that reflect their abilities to engage in third order thinking across varied contexts. They consistently keep the bigger picture in mind as they navigate, instigate, and solidify change. Just as we do when working with families, these experts pay close attention to the process of change, carefully considering how to engage others, work relationally, generate buy-in and a shared vision, and thoughtfully intervene one step at a time. In line with our ANVIET guidelines, these principles are described below: 1) build and maintain attuned relationships, 2) name without shame, 3) identify and build on collective values, 4) intervene with intention, 5) create a collective vision, and 6) engage in and support transformation.

Build and Maintain Attuned Relationships

Family therapy is first and foremost relational. We are able to apprehend the sociocultural context of others and attune to them, even when we don't share their worldviews or perspectives. Family therapists recognize the importance of engaging all family members, making sure all feel understood, heard, and valued. Boszormenyi-Nagy (1966) referred to the ability to take all family members' views and well-being into account as multidirected partiality. This allows us to hold multiple perspectives in the same space, even when they are in opposition, to stay connected, and to assume the best intentions. Systemic family therapists have long been experts at helping people attune to each other and work diligently toward mutual understanding, growth, and conflict resolution. When therapeutic relationships are stressed, we work efficiently and effectively to repair them. We rely on these skills to create change through relationships.

Building and maintaining attuned relationships necessitates collaboration. It is crucial to develop alliances in order to collectively engage in change efforts within organizations, agencies, communities, and societal systems. Alliances may be intentionally initiated through affirming what is said or named, echoing a remark, a glance of recognition, or a conversation in the parking lot. They often develop around specific initiatives and evolve as organizations transform. Attempting to create change on one's own, without support from others, can lead to being marginalized or even removed from the system. This is particularly true for those who are at the bottom of organizational hierarchies or otherwise at greater risk of being marginalized—those whose identities represent people from minoritized groups within society (e.g., People of Color, women, differently-abled, LGBTQI+ persons). It is also important, whenever possible, to work across social locations toward a common purpose. This collaboration allows for the intentional use of working with allies and accessing others' experience, insights, and positionality to create change.

An important aspect of hope and the ability to envision working toward transformative change is facilitated by seeing ourselves as part of something larger. Building and maintaining attuned relationships can often involve a spiritual component. In Text Box 16.1 William Turner, principal investigator of the HOPE Laboratory, a translational research program that focuses on the application of hope theories, systems theories, and positive psychology principles in systems and organizations at multiple levels, describes the connection between hope, spirituality, and movement toward justice.

Text Box 16.1 William Turner, PhD, LMFT

William Turner serves as Distinguished Professor of Psychology and Family Therapy and Special Counsel to the President at Lipscomb University, Nashville, TN. His teaching and research interests are focused on African American family strengths and the intersections of hope, justice, policy, and faith.

I find more and more as I study hope, the doors are opening for me and other scholars to speak unapologetically about spirituality as a very important ingredient of hope; frankly, I think it is a driver. That doesn't mean that you must be connected to a church, a synagogue, or mosque, or anything like that to experience a greater fullness of being that enables you to access hope. I think particularly for Black and Brown people, if we are trying to do something that doesn't incorporate that sense of hope, we might just as well be talking to the wall. I would like for scientists and clinicians to not be afraid of exploring and acknowledging that reality in the lives of those we are attempting to help.

Clients' clinical presentations are often compounded by feelings of anger, rage, and hopelessness. Thus, fostering hope can be complicated, not only because clients may be subject to one multi-layered, traumatizing experience after another, but also because of therapists' well-intended but often misguided actions. In a nation in which the idea of a "just society" is a vision that we have never really fully embraced, effective intervention requires us as therapists to assess our own social positions of power and privilege and their implications for our work with clients whose everyday lives are colored by inequities in every imaginable way. Hope cannot truly emerge until there is a confrontation of the truths of one's realities and the contexts that have maintained them. Once understood, we can find meaningful ways of moving forward. That is what hope is all about.

Name without Shame

Shaming rarely, if ever, motivates others to engage (McGoldrick et al., 2021). Yet, we sometimes expect that simply pointing out what another is doing—including how they are being oppressive and/or unaware of equity issues—will be transformative. Broadly speaking, we can see this dynamic unfold in "calling out" and "cancel culture" (Brown & Devich-Cyril, 2020; Ross, 2019a, 2019b). As therapists, it is easy to understand that it would be problematic and most likely counterproductive to simply say to a parent, "The way you are going about this is harmful." We would instead make sure we understand and attune to where everyone in the family is coming from, including the parent. We would likely seek out underlying values, help the parent attune to the child, and explore other ways of relating while maintaining a positive relationship with all. We would name the problem from multiple perspectives without shaming the parent. We would call the parent and all members of the family "in" rather than calling them "out." According to Ross (2019b), calling-in is like a call-out done with love and respect:

> Calling-in engages in debates with words and actions of healing and restoration, and without the self-indulgence of drama. And we can make productive choices about the terms of the debate: Conflicts about coalition-building, supporting candidates, or policies, are a routine and desirable feature of a pluralistic democracy. (p. 2)

Engaging with respect is second nature to those of us who work with families day in and day out, yet when we enter our own family and friend systems, places of work or education, and organizations, we sometimes expect a very different outcome when we proclaim, "This is not OK! You're being classist/racist/sexist/homophobic, etc." Direct confrontation surrounding what is just is sometimes appropriate, especially when harm is being done intentionally; however, in most cases, this approach is counterproductive, putting others back on their heels, feeling rejected, defensive, or hurt, and often unwilling to further engage. In fact, speaking out and expecting to be heard is often part of unexamined privilege, i.e., "my voice should and will count." The question in the classroom, boardroom, and meeting room is, How do we call others *into* equity-based work? Naming without shaming is important, especially when creating or building on strengths and collective values.

Identify and Build on Collective Values

Change is most likely to happen when it is in the best interest of all, including those with the greatest power and influence. Derrick Bell (2002) referred to this as interest convergence. When we work with families, we almost intuitively ensure that the proposed change is in the best interest of all and that we have buy-in from as many family members as possible. We work to get family members or community members on board for change, help them come together to fight the problem, not each other. We aspire to help all family members identify how more equitable relationships will help them realize their values and goals. In the first chapter, we discussed political polarization and how it is not uncommon for families to be divided by divergent views and political positions. Exploring collective values can place political differences in perspective as families prioritize mutual support, loving each other through difficult times, and other relational values (Fraenkel & Cho, 2020; Powell, 2024; Ross, 2019a). In other words, identifying and centering core values creates a context in which it is in everyone's best interest to prioritize caring relationships over divergent political ideologies and opinions.

Identifying core values in institutions, communities, and organizations provides a cornerstone for equity-based change. Unjust policies and practices often result in moving away from collective values. For example, an educational institution may value diversity of thought and inclusion, yet has recruiting and hiring practices that result in repeatedly recruiting and hiring conventional thinkers who represent people from the dominant societal group. At times, an institution may be attempting to meet external requirements that are not explicitly tied to its core values, which often reflect the values of the members with the most power and are likely to represent the dominant group's interests within society. Consider a family therapy program that is attempting to accommodate accreditation standards by increasing the number of Students of Color in incoming cohorts without making any other changes to policies, faculty awareness, diversity, or curriculum. The challenge then becomes, "How does increasing racial diversity connect with the program's existing values?" and/or "How do we engage in value building around equity, rather than merely promoting diversity by number of admissions?" Understanding, co-creating, and building on collective values helps us move toward creating intentional systemic change.

Intervene with Intention

The word intervention is complex and has multiple meanings. What does it mean for an educator, administrator, supervisor, student, community member, or client to intervene? What does it mean for a family therapist to intervene? We often tell family therapy trainees that if we randomly stop a recording of a session, they should be able to describe what they are doing and why they are doing it, describing their rationale or intention. When we practice family therapy, we pay close attention to each interaction, making a multitude of decisions about what to do next and why. Contrast this with being in a professional meeting and simply saying whatever is on your mind, loudly repeating a point, or saying nothing at all. When out of the therapeutic context, we can forget to pay attention to relational dynamics and to intervene with the intention to create (often incremental) change.

Deciding how and when to intervene to support equity-based decision-making could be a volume in itself. The best mantra we have found is "it depends." Just as in therapy, there is no "one size fits all" intervention; rather, it depends on carefully reading the situation and examining what might be helpful at any given time. This requires using a systemic lens to consider possible outcomes of any intervention. Consider the power dynamics involved when a colleague with less social influence and institutional status speaks up only to be shut down by a more powerful person in the group. It is not uncommon for someone with a higher status to jump in to "rescue" the lower status colleague, using their own privilege as a form of uninvited leverage or "protection." While this is sometimes necessary and appreciated, it reinforces the dominance structure and is often not experienced as supportive. Contrast this with amplifying what has been marginalized by maintaining composure and stating "I'd like to get back to the point [colleague] made, I am interested in hearing more," or "You know, building off what [colleague] mentioned, I think… [in support of the idea]."

It is vital to consider power dynamics when considering how, when, and where to intervene. This includes analyzing one's designated role and social location, evaluating the impact these have on one's influence, as well as the potential costs of attempting to influence. Role privilege (e.g., positions of organizational leadership, being a teacher or supervisor) may be diminished or enhanced—challenged or supported—within specific systems based on interconnected social identities (e.g., gender, race, abilities, looks, age, ethnicity, sexual orientation, religious affiliation). As we know from therapeutic encounters, power tied to the social location of all involved—including the therapist (change agent)—needs to be factored in when determining how to best intervene.

Create a Collective Vision

Most of us who engage in this work have goals or a vision for what we believe will create greater social equity. A common misstep that many of us have made at some point is to "show all of our cards" before building a collective vision. This can be to our disadvantage when engaging in long-term change initiatives; for example, announcing "The first thing I want to do in my new role as an administrator is to eliminate racism in our organization." This open stance, while authentic and transparent, may serve to polarize a group you need to have working together. Anti-racist initiatives may be at the top of the list, but announcing the plan without first building relationships, attuning to the needs, values, and attitudes of all involved, and creating a collective vision may create undue resistance that sets the initiative back.

Building a collective vision can be painstaking work that requires at least attempting to involve all stakeholders. It is difficult to move a village until everyone is packed and ready to go. Except in the most dire of circumstances, this doesn't occur until (at least most of) those being asked to move/change are invested in the collective vision of an equitable and better future.

Engage in and Support Transformation

Family therapists understand change processes and know that transformation is possible. We recognize the importance of incremental, sequential steps toward change. We persist when change is slow or temporarily moves backward. We don't complain or blame families for not changing. We look for alternatives, try to locate what we have missed, invite greater understanding, expand our creativity, and keep at it. We are often the holders of hope and contributors to the expectation for change, both of which have been noted as being central to client success in therapy. Nonetheless, change can be difficult and complex in any human system, and it rarely works to provide common sense, first-order change interventions. For example, requiring faculty to add readings authored by those from diverse social locations may change the landscape of an institution's syllabi and prompt new conversations in classrooms (i.e., first order change); but it doesn't transform the curriculum (i.e., second order change). Likewise, requiring organizational staff to complete online diversity training may meet legal expectations, but is unlikely to change the organization.

In contrast, being at the table when decisions are made to add diverse voices to the curriculum or to require diversity training may create opportunities for incremental movement toward third order change. For example, one might be in a position to ask, "What are we hoping to change by….", "What are some other ways we might…", "How can we go beyond…", "How does this support our values…," and so on. Purposefully moving into positions that provide opportunities to create change, watching for moments when change interventions are likely to be successful, intentionally intervening in one place to create change in another, and working within one's sphere of influence are all foundational to transformational, third order change.

Third Order Praxis Across Contexts

Third order change involves all levels of societal systems, any of which can be transformed in ways that create and maintain more equitable circumstances and relational dynamics. Those who engage in socioculturally attuned praxis (critical consciousness in action) do so within the contexts they inhabit. In Text Box 16.2, Manijeh Daneshpour describes her work to support social and relational equity across the many contexts in which she lives and works.

Text Box 16.2 Manijeh Daneshpour, PhD, LMFT

Manijeh Daneshpour (she/her) is the Systemwide Director of the Alliant International University Marriage and Family Therapy Programs. She has been working in academic settings since 1996 and has been a clinician, researcher, presenter, and writer while being an administrator for three decades.

I don't have the luxury of not being attuned to the sociocultural contexts I am in. Through my own, at times painful experiences, I have become sensitive and attune to everyone else's intersectionality and social locations. I listen with the ear of my heart and bring my whole humanity to these conversations. I try to contextualize people's experiences and believe in advocacy for the voiceless and challenging the powerful in any setting and capacity. I am familiar with sociopolitical theories of gender and understand the impact of structural and internalized racism. I name and identify these complex issues in every encounter, even at a party with friends and family, and in my conversations with my children.

I believe advocating for the most vulnerable is the most ethical part of socially just family therapy. In my clinical work, I challenge individuals' unfairness and unjust actions and advocate for those with less power, even if they are not part of the therapy process. I interrupt oppressive gendered patterns and challenge the unfair patriarchal hierarchy. I help people with transformative change by providing meaningful and relevant information, tapping into their personal resources, and empowering them to use their sense of agency to challenge themselves and others. I use my knowledge, expertise, and relational skills to help people change their perspectives and become their own agents of change.

In my writings and research, I use topics to directly advocate for those who tend to be more mistreated and misunderstood (family therapy with Muslims, multicultural couple therapy with Muslims, family therapy with immigrants and refugees, third wave feminism, etc.). The topics I choose to write about are culturally, socially, and politically intertwined. For example, I don't try to advocate for Muslims as a religious group. I advocate and write about this group as a misunderstood social group with many relational and familial issues needing the help of mental health professionals.

In the context of my administrative work, I advocate and amplify marginalized voices of students, Faculty of Color, and staff. I personally get involved when a Student of Color gets disciplined on any of our campuses. I go to every faculty meeting, every orientation meeting with students across our multiple campuses, and invite students to directly contact me with any concerns related to experiencing any type of marginalization. I routinely engage in faculty and program directors' training to be more conscious of their implicit biases and conduct culturally sensitive training for our faculty.

I teach alternative ways of thinking and challenge students' perspectives in every class. I blend in the latest articles, images, videos, and news relevant to marginalized people's lives with any topic I cover. In supervision, I use social justice, feminist perspectives, and culturally sensitive perspectives, and ask supervisees to write about their self-of-therapist experiences and bring a tape of a recorded session about how they incorporate social justice perspectives in their work. We read articles, watch the news, and discuss the everyday experiences of people whose lives are impacted by the unfair actions of others.

With the intersections of my identities, my most significant strength is to interrupt unjust relationships loudly. I have met with the presidents and the provosts of different institutions to discuss policies and rules when applied to marginalized students and written letters to other organizations, including AAMFT. I have been told that my authenticity, passion, and recognition of my intersectional self can be a source of transformation and modeling for others in multiple settings and positions. I am bold, kind, considerate, not afraid of being wrong, and learn from my mistakes. I treat every disagreement with my children, spouse, and family members as a professional learning opportunity and believe in human decency and love.

In Text Box 16.3, Dana Stone reflects on how in her context as an educator and supervisor, she supports beginning therapists in developing the capacity to support clients in third order change. She further describes her commitment to engaging in critical intention as an ongoing practice in her professional and personal life.

Text Box 16.3 Dana Stone, PhD, LMFT

Dana Stone (she/her) is an associate professor at California State University in Northridge. She identifies as a multiracial Black-White, cisgender female, hearing, temporarily able bodied, heterosexual, and non-religious. Her work focuses on the multiracial experience and supporting early career therapists with marginalized aspects of identity in navigating the field of marriage and family therapy and counseling (see Stone & ChenFeng, 2019).

My application of third order thinking really starts in the classroom with beginning therapists. In my teaching, I center societal processes such as inequities, power, privilege, and oppression, and embark on a journey beside my students as they consider the impact of these factors in their own lives and in the lives of the people they will serve. As therapists, we can only help our clients and effect third order change if we start first with ourselves.

I have taken guidance from colleagues on how to identify and name these issues (social inequities, the impact of power, privilege, and oppression). My process includes ongoing critical self-reflection. From everything that I read and watch, and the people I turn to for my own learning (through workshops and conferences, etc.) I take time to reflect and think about how my own understanding is achieved and to consider the ways I can integrate the material I am learning. I spend time in conversation with trusted colleagues (from shared and different social locations) to deepen my own understandings, and then collaborate to come up with creative ways to bring the knowledge into the classroom or supervision.

I look for narratives, stories, publications, and media that amplify the marginalized. In my ongoing personal and professional development, I have committed to read with critical intention, to watch with critical intention, and to listen with critical intention. When I engage in this way, I ask: whose voices are telling these stories, whose voices are missing, and where can I go next to learn more from "own voices" perspectives?

I work very hard to provide feedback in ways that will encourage deeper self-reflection when I have observed relational or systemic injustice in the classroom or supervision. I own my mistakes openly and with transparency to lead by example. I continuously talk about individual, interpersonal, and collective responsibility to disrupt inequities and injustice. I often center the conversation in the here and now to promote action at the micro level, especially when students and supervisees feel overwhelmed by the vast injustice that surrounds and wonder how they can affect change as one person.

I guide students in a personal process of self-transformation by encouraging engagement in critical self-reflection regarding intersectional aspects of their own identity. I invite them to name the parts of their identity that are privileged and parts that are not. As students become more attuned to their own intersectional identity and increase their understanding of their power and privilege as well as their experiences of oppression, they begin to recognize how their own experiences may mirror (or not) that of their clients. It is also through sharing of self and identity in group spaces that students begin to understand their experiences in relation to the myriad experiences of their colleagues. This deepens their understanding of themselves as cultural beings and promotes cultural democracy in that it gives voice, value, and respect to diversity and emphasizes the importance of proactive engagement from everyone to dismantle dominant discourses of what is "right" or should be centered.

When students and supervisees engage in a process of critical self-reflection about their intersectional identities and power, privilege, and oppression, it enables them to consider why the sociocultural context of each of their clients matters when considering therapeutic interventions that will promote meaningful change.

Developing Culturally Attuned, Equity-based Community Interventions

Family therapists sometimes extend their work with families to include members of the larger community and may target change in the community itself. The Cultural Context Model (CCM) provides an excellent example of doing so in ways that create third order change (Almeida & Williams, in press; Almeida & Tubbs, 2020; Almeida, 2018). The CCM includes building therapeutic communities of support and accountability, as well as engaging community members as sponsors and stakeholders in the therapeutic process. The model challenges the dominant assumption that therapy is, or should be, a solely private matter by inviting clients and members of the community to join together to build critical consciousness and provide support for liberatory transformation. In fact, the CCM routinely goes beyond impacting individuals or families to making a difference in communities.

Socioculturally attuned practice can be applied in multiple contexts. For example, I (Maria Bermúdez) consider my scholarship, clinical skills, teaching, and activism as forms of praxis that are simultaneously enacted. I had the privilege of being involved as a co-principal investigator in a community-based participatory research project called *Lazos Hispanos* (Hispanic Links). This project was formed to address the challenges and health disparities experienced by members of our Latinx community. Our aim was to enhance the health and well-being of immigrant Latinx people residing in low-income communities by helping them gain knowledge and access to local community services. Theoretically, we aligned with decolonizing and feminist-informed research methods. We asked women regarded as leaders in the local Latinx community to work on our research team as volunteer community health workers/*promotoras*. With their support, and that of colleagues and local community clinics, agencies, and organizations, we formed *Lazos Hispanos*. Our multicultural and interdisciplinary research team enriched every aspect of the program and enhanced culturally responsive community engagement (Matthew et al., 2020).

There are several ways in which third order thinking and ANVIET served to guide third order change with *Lazos Hispanos*. First, we **attuned** to the struggles faced by members of the Latinx community, most of whom are immigrants with mixed legal status. With this awareness, the colleagues conducted a needs assessment to identify and **name** problems within the community (Calva et al, 2020). As scholars invested in equity-based practices, social justice, and immigrants' rights, it was important for us to use our positions of power and social and cultural capital to help members of our community gain access to the community resources they identified. Many suffer the effects of blatant institutionalized and systemic racism and anti-immigrant hostility and xenophobia (Letiecq & Bermúdez, 2023; Vesely et al., 2024; Walsdorf et al., 2020). We listened to them and **valued** what they said is important to them and their families and what they need as a community. We invited a small group of women to be part of our research and outreach team as key stakeholders best positioned to help Latinx families gain access to these resources (**envision**). The program proved to be **transformative** for our community and for all of us who participated in it (Orpinas et al., 2020; 2021). We shared knowledge, information, and gained power from our mutually respectful and beneficial relationships (Bermúdez et al., under review; Letiecq et al., 2022).

Similar to the micro-advocacy work described by Holyoak and colleagues (2021), our program aimed to bridge Latinx families to resources and organizations (**intervene**)—school staff, teachers, and tutoring, free/affordable medical clinics, legal services, employment opportunities, transportation and housing information, food sources and nutrition information, crisis services, financial aid, etc. This community-based work not only helped community members, but our team also felt empowered and afforded the *promotoras* and us greater credibility as knowledgeable and trusted community leaders and advocates (Alvarez-Hernandez et al., 2021). Although our program was sadly truncated due to the effects of the pandemic, it greatly impacted our community and helped Latinx families gain access to community services via their connections with *Lazos Hispanos* and our community-based participatory research team (Orpinas et al., 2020; 2021). We are left with the void of not having this invaluable resource in our community. Latinx people continue to be marginalized, denigrated, and rejected, and live in fear with the real threat of family separation, arrest, detention, and deportation (Diaz McConnell et al., 2023; Letiecq et al., 2023; Walsdorf et al., 2020).

To give perspective, in 2018 the governor of my state (Maria) had a televised campaign ad in which he stated, while holding his rifle and showing staged weapons in the background, "I own guns that no one is taking away… I've got a big truck just in case I need to 'round up criminal illegals and take 'em home myself; yep, I just said that. If you want a politically *incorrect* conservative, that's me." He also addressed the State by declaring that he was going to protect our schools from the dangers of critical race theory. This is the sociopolitical context in which we live and work toward relational and systemic equity and justice. Indeed, the personal is political (Hanisch, 1969).

Creating Third Order Change in Organizations and Institutions

Bartunek and Moch (1987) introduced the idea of third order change in the field of *organizational development* using a cognitive framework that relies on the concept of schemata. They posited that first order, incremental change occurs within organizations when ideas and solutions are developed based on particular shared and accepted schemata. Second order change relies on alterations to existing shared schemata. Third order change requires the ability to change schemata as required when new situations arise. Their work could be expanded to be more akin to what we have referred to as third order thinking and change in family therapy; that is, expanding their definition to include specific attention to an organization's collective values, mission, culture, and structure within the broader sociocultural context to clear a path for understanding, intervening in, and supporting equity within organizations.

We must be able to take a metaview of the organizations in which we ourselves are embedded, as well as those that affect the families with whom we work. Some family therapists engage in systems consultation when invited into organizations to solve problems and help create organizational change (Boverie, 1991; Matheny & Zimmerman, 2001; McDowell, 1999). Likewise, we may be tasked with creating change within our own organizations or institutions, such as improving the quality of care, integrating third order thinking (i.e., spearheading diversity and inclusion efforts), and providing organizational leadership. We are often faced with reconciling organizational and institutional policies and practices with what we believe is fair and just for clients. Unjust policies and practices could include culturally dismissive procedures, race and social class bias, lack of awareness, and/or marginalization of LGBTQ+ clients, among other things. Our own professional organizations are no exception. Furthermore, we ourselves, may be privileged and oppressive and/or marginalized, silenced, and/or oppressed within agencies, community organizations, educational and other institutions, and/or professional networks.

The process of change within organizations is not as simple as sharing our (good) ideas about what is socially and relationally just. As noted above, directly and (sometimes loudly and repeatedly) voicing critiques may be counterproductive. We have witnessed beginning family therapists who are passionate about social justice demand change as newly hired practitioners, only to be fired for "lack of fit" with an agency. The common sense idea that what is right should and will prevail if explained well enough is an example of expecting third order change with a first order intervention. Organizational transformation toward equitable practice requires third order thinking that includes recognizing one's own positionality when considering interventions (McDowell et al., 2019). In Text Box 16.4, Quentin McDowell shares his work, including how he leverages his leadership position and social (White male) privilege to create more equitable practices in an educational organization. Many of his comments are in keeping with McGoldrick, et al. (2021), who argued for the importance of shared values, collective vision, leadership commitment, and collaborative action to create more culturally aware and just organizations.

Text Box 16.4 Quentin R. McDowell, MA, School Administrator

Quentin McDowell (he/his) is the Head of Mercersburg Academy, an independent secondary school. He identifies as White, male, heterosexual, and able-bodied.

As a school leader, I approach my work with a strong sense of optimism and hope. I believe that change is not only necessary but that it is always possible. Social, cultural, and systemic change at the organizational level requires engaging a wide range of stakeholders, including employees, students, and a governing board, as well as alumni and a multitude of parents that we count as key constituents.

Attunement in this context calls for deep listening to those from a wide range of national, cultural, generational, political, and socio-economic backgrounds, as well as a wide spectrum of identities. There is a need to attune to the individual and collective nature of these many constituencies and to facilitate attunement amongst and between them. One of the key challenges is understanding such disparate perspectives and creating opportunities to call all into conversations that promote equity.

I believe it is better to call people into the larger conversation as opposed to calling them out for an act or exchange that may have diminished the dignity of another. While imperative to name an issue so that value can be placed on it, it can be counterproductive to leverage shame as a tool for change. That being said, there are times when a call out is necessary, most specifically when intervening in a moment where harm is occurring or being threatened.

The naming of an issue begins the process of placing value on it. By speaking and acknowledging an issue, it is elevated to a public level where it can then be more intentionally explored and become part of the organizational agenda. Naming what is not just allows the organization to more readily assume the challenge of creating positive cultural change, particularly when tethered to a school's collectively affirmed institutional values.

It can be hard to interrupt unjust relationships and systems without first establishing institutional norms and expectations that are broadly shared and accepted so that when injustice is brought to light, there is an existing framework to reference that illustrates what is, and what is not, expected or permissible. This gives voice, vocabulary, permission, and support necessary to those seeking to interrupt what is unjust. Part of the process for envisioning change requires those with different perspectives within the community to come together and work toward common goals to ensure broader buy-in and support through a sense of democratic engagement.

Key to all of this is support from the very top of the institution. The position I now hold allows me to more effectively encourage third order change because I am in the center of the organization. The inequities within systems are more visible and impacting—as well as more difficult to change—at the margins. As a leader, I must be able to use my social privilege and institutional influence to leverage change, not by demanding or dictating, but by pulling all stakeholders together to ensure equity is a core value in our mission and vision and that we collectively create policies and practices that ensure accountability.

It can be difficult to judge the pace at which we need to move to create lasting change. We have to go fast enough to show progress and to create greater equity for those in the margins, yet slow enough to develop allies with those who have traditional power. At the end of the day, I would rather say we got a long way but moved too slowly than to say we moved too fast and did not get very far.

Our social locations and roles within organizations largely determine how we go about generating and supporting third order change. Where do our social identities place us in organizations? Is our impact minimized in a religious institution if we are not religious or a member of the same religion? What are the organizational dynamics in relationship to race, ethnicity, gender, language, sexual orientation, abilities, etc.? Are we insiders in the organization and an integral part of its mission? Are we outsiders or seen as nonessential? What are the various constraints and opportunities for praxis within specific contexts and how do we strategize accordingly? In Text Box 16.5, Jessica ChenFeng shares some of these dynamics in relation to her efforts to support social and relational equity in a medical school and hospital setting.

Text Box 16.5 Jessica ChenFeng, PhD, LMFT

Jessica ChenFeng (she/her) is a second-generation Taiwanese American therapist and educator who trains licensed clinicians to apply their clinical skills for consultation in diverse contexts. She is interested in social contextual issues such as race, gender, and spirituality.

For a significant season of my career, I worked clinically with resident and attending physicians, along with medical students, to support their well-being while taking into consideration the hierarchical, high stakes environment within which they do their training. As an outsider to the medical community and culture, I tried to understand the power structures and dominant discourses. When supporting individuals—wherever they may be on the medical hierarchy—I considered how they were impacted by the larger discourses, what agency they had within the system, and what were realistic, appropriate, and safe ways for them to engage. I looked for ways I could effect change at various systemic levels through psychoeducation in grand rounds or consultation with directors and deans.

I often worked with physicians and medical students with marginalized identities. I would ask about the various parts of their identity to learn about their experiences within the system. I also spoke to the discourses within and the impact of the medical culture that interacted with these parts of their identity. This often resonated with them as they made these connections for the first time.

I found that the most powerful way for me to amplify those who are silenced or marginalized (Students of Color, queer members of the community) was to address their concerns in faculty meetings when I could speak to deans and program directors who were able to effect change at a larger level. I often needed to fight past my own internalized racism and break model minority stereotypes so that I could speak loudly, clearly, and have these concerns heard.

As is true in many systems, it seems that who says something and how it is said goes a long way in terms of how something is heard, received, and responded to. This awareness leads me to interrupt and challenge in ways that are congruent with my personality and racial/ethnic intersections. I am thinking of Harlene Anderson and Tom Andersen's concept of "appropriately unusual" where I might offer a new perspective that is more easily "digestible" to those in positions of power.

I think of my work as planting seeds—whether in the medical context or in other consultation spaces now. Often, the individuals and departments within which I work are extensions of a larger system with a long history of hierarchy and oppression. Because I interface with most clients and colleagues in multiple capacities, they hear me pose similar questions and offer feedback that speaks to issues of sociocultural context and societal structures. I also use personal examples or past clinical experiences to highlight the significance of having a contextual lens. In most contexts, I find that problems are most often understood at the individual/personal level. When possible, I try to ask questions about relationships, about support systems, about the impact of these on one another. When I am in more of a consultant role, I encourage the person trying to "fix a problem" to consider their personal connection to the change desired.

As I write these reflections, I find that much of how I do my work has to do with my own social location. I am in this interesting position of being both invisible and hypervisible as an Asian American woman in academia. The racialization of Asian Americans has many prongs—proximity to Whiteness, and the expectations associated with the model minority, alongside our forever foreigner status as never fully belonging. This affects how I can or cannot show up in predominantly White contexts.

Public Participation, Politics, and Policies

The majority of this text focuses on what Holyoak and colleagues (2021) refer to as micro-level advocacy; that is, the "client-centered advocacy conducted by CFTs daily in their work with clients" (p. 2). This includes not only socioculturally attuned in-session interventions, but extensions of therapy that involve advocating with and for specific clients in schools, courts, medical systems, and so on. In this section, we explore what Holyoak et al. refer to as macro-level advocacy—political and policy involvement beyond the therapy room.

We agree with Jordan and Seponski (2018) who stated: "given the consequences policies and politics have for therapists, their clients, and their profession…therapists can [should] push beyond the boundaries of therapy into the public arena to transform the social politics that constrain well-being" (p. 19). In many ways, family therapists are well equipped to contribute to the common good through political and policy work because of their expertise in micro-level advocacy and their systemic training (Goodman et al., 2018; Hodgson & Lamson, 2020; Holyoak et al., 2021). Family therapists are on the frontlines, witnessing the needs of clients and the everyday abuse of human rights (Jordan et al., 2021; McDowell et al., 2012). We are well positioned to shed light on seemingly "private" injustices in order to support public change that protects the most vulnerable members of society. We can also use what we witness to inform our research, which in turn can influence public policy (Waldegrave et al., 2016). While details of advocacy and policy work are beyond the scope of this text, we direct readers to Hodgson and Lamson (2020), who offer a primer for how family therapists can engage in advocacy and public policy. According to Hodgson and Lamson (2020), policy and advocacy are critical to the work of systemic family therapists. The importance of this work is inherent in the following description:

> Policies are a series of plans used as a basis for decision making that can either cohere or divide communities; they have the capacity to set a society onto a beneficial or sometimes alarming trajectory. Regardless of individual opinions on policies, they are essential to stimulating change, enforcing boundaries to protect and define, and allocating rights and privileges. (p. 730)

In Text Box 16.6, William Turner describes his role in developing public policy, emphasizing the unique fit between policy work and systemic thinking.

Text Box 16.6 William Turner, PhD, LMFT

William Turner serves as Distinguished Professor of Psychology and Family Therapy and Special Counsel to the President at Lipscomb University, Nashville, TN. He was a Robert Wood Johnson Fellow for Senator Obama and continued to advise President Obama.

I distinguish between politics and policy. My experiences have been primarily in the policy realm. Policies are the rules that govern and guide us. Often, we don't know the origins of our policies, even the ones that most impact us; many have been perpetuated for generations. But if we go back to look at the origins, sadly, many of them were racist at their core. I try to encourage students to think about the genesis of policies that impact families and how these policies either stunt growth or encourage people to develop their fullest potential. Because of their training and expertise as family academicians or therapists, particularly as systems thinkers, they have skills and abilities that very few people have to appreciate the full impact of policies on the lived experiences of families.

Earlier in my career, when I was a professor at the University of Minnesota, I was engaged in a program of research focusing on African American family strengths when I met a director of the Hubert Humphrey Center for Public Policy. He pointed out that by writing academic papers, although important, I was reaching a very small audience in comparison to writing and influencing legislation. He said to me, "I don't know anybody else who is studying the strengths of Black people and families. I know a lot of people who look at pathology and dysfunction. I can guarantee you that there are very few people in the US Congress who are aware that there is that kind of work being done." I realized he was probably right. If I wanted to have a greater impact, I needed to impact the policies that were being written. He suggested that I should explore and consider applying for the Robert Wood Johnson Health Policy Fellowship. If I wanted to make a meaningful difference, I had to affect the policies that are being developed. So, I applied.

An important feature of the Robert Wood Johnson Health Policy Fellowship is that it provides exclusive, hands-on policy experience in the nation's capital, allowing its participants to work hand-in-hand with key players in federal health policy. The goal is to use that leadership experience to improve health, health care, and health policy. After being introduced to the majority of the key health-related players, offices, and organizations in Washington, the fellows are then selected to work hand-in-hand with a member of the US Senate or the US House of Representatives on health policy related matters.

As I applied to work with various senators and representatives, I talked about things I was doing in a modified systems language, in ways I thought they could understand, and they appreciated that. After I was hired by Barack Obama, he said, "one of the reasons I chose you was that you spoke the language of humanity. You looked at things from a broader perspective." I realized that it carried a lot of clout. Even when I got to Washington and was working for Obama, other offices would seek me out because of that kind of understanding.

I believe that our training as systems thinkers gives us the ability to look at things more broadly than the average person. If you're like me, in your earlier career, you probably thought about how to be a great clinician or researcher-clinician. I encourage you to think more broadly than that. We can have a much greater impact than we sometimes realize we can.

Opportunities to engage in public advocacy and policy work may not be as "far away" as they seem. We position ourselves as potential change agents every time we agree to serve on a state advisory board, write a policy and procedures manual, participate in program accreditation efforts, attend a school board meeting or a town meeting focusing on a public concern such as gentrification, volunteer for a public health committee such as a maternal mortality review board, bear witness at a county mental health board meeting, provide professional testimony as part of lobbying efforts, or participate in one of our own professional association meetings.

We may also be positioned to influence organizational policies and practices when we are invited into private and public institutions as consultants or to engage in specific initiatives. This includes, among other things, offering expert testimony, advising municipalities and state departments of health, and serving on local and state mental health advisory boards. Andraé Brown (as cited in McDowell et al., 2023) describes himself as a Black male transformative psychologist and feminist family therapist. Among other things, his work includes serving as a juvenile justice consultant. In his words:

> In my work, I have found transformation can occur in communities and juvenile justice systems when I am able to engage myself and others in ways that attune to and name the impact of family, community, physical, and societal contexts, value the lives of all youth within these contexts, interrupt legal and community systems that maintain unjust treatment of youth, and bring communities as well as professionals together to envision and act on what is possible and just. (p. 347)

Transformative Praxis Across National Contexts

Liberation-based work is itself situated in the contested and uneven territory of societal/global contexts and power dynamics (Daneshpour, 2022). Even though third order thinking invites critical analysis of dominant ideologies and power processes, most of us will fall short of being able to fully recognize how our praxis is impacted by our epistemological lenses and social positions (Bermúdez, et al., 2024). We echo the work of marcela polanco (2016), who urged family therapists to acknowledge and hold themselves accountable for the effects of the internationalization of knowledge produced in prosperous countries that traverse complex cultural borders and circumstances. She aims to disrupt the global expansion of family therapy training within a neoliberal context as she urges family therapists to embrace a decolonizing "multi-lateral fair trade agreement of knowledge" (p. 13) in clinical training and practice. This approach enables transformative cultural alternatives. By doing this work, therapists can honor the legitimacy of all cultures as valid contributors of equity-based knowledge. In the words of polanco (2016),

> I hope to raise a critical perspective to be considered by family therapists when training and practicing in global contexts. This is by cautioning the reader on the importance of situating family therapy theories in the euroamerican geographical and political context in which they belong, along with their values, traditions, and intentions, making visible their foreignness and potential intentions to domesticate or suffocate if not received critically. Rendering foreignness visible may open space for the reader/audience to imagine their own transformative local production of knowledge outside the euroamerican paradigms. (p. 15)

In Text Box 16.7 Mario Fausto Gómez Lamont describes the dangers of wide-spread adoption of therapy models in a non-critical manner, as well as their use of third order thinking and praxis in Mexico.

Text Box 16.7 Mario Fausto Gómez Lamont, PhD

Fausto Lamont is a licensed psychologist, practicing family therapist, and faculty member at the School of Higher Studies Iztacala of the National Autonomous University of Mexico (UNAM). He holds a PhD in Psychological Research from the Iberoamerican University and is part of the network of specialists in Gender Studies and Feminism at the Center for Research and Gender Studies at UNAM. He identifies as a gender-fluid, cisgender gay man, able-bodied, with educational and racial privilege.

Third order thinking has been a breath of fresh air for our practice as systemic family therapy educators at the National Autonomous University of Mexico. In the search for a critical paradigm for our practice, we observed with discouragement the continuous commodification of family therapy models. This has resulted in a lack of critical consciousness as students and faculty adopt models imposed by the Global North without questioning their relevance in the Mexican context (Gómez-Lamont, 2021).

In Mexico, the 2015–2019 National Health Plan emphasized the need for all health care providers, both public and private, to receive multicultural and sociocultural training. This training includes the obligation to recognize Southern epistemologies as a cornerstone of social justice, including Indigenous knowledge and other ways of knowing (Gómez-Lamont, Faudoa Mendoza, & Márquez-Palacios, 2024). In this context, third order systemic therapy and socioculturally attuned intervention have strengthened critical thinking about privilege and social inequality, which are reproduced in our training, practice, and, consequently, in society. The guidelines for transformational practice—attuning, naming, valuing, interrupting, envisioning, and transforming—are aligned with the goal of making visible the power structures that allow inequalities to persist (Gómez-Lamont & Bermúdez, 2023).

A key example of the application of this approach is working with families seeking therapy for gender diversity issues. Consider the case of a traditional family seeking therapy because their 11-year-old daughter has identified as transgender. The mother, a working-class, cis-heterosexual woman, comes to therapy expecting her child to "stop being confused." Additionally, she shares that their Christian community will not accept her child's gender identity. From a utilitarian or postmodern perspective, it could be argued that the therapist must respect all realities as valid. However, third order systemic therapy demands that the therapist not only validate narratives but also recognize and challenge the structural oppression experienced by the transgender girl.

Cultural relativism becomes problematic when it prevents us from denouncing discriminatory practices that perpetuate injustice. In Mexico, the application of social constructionism in family therapy has stagnated social change, inclusion, and access to justice for minorities (Gómez-Lamont & Bermúdez, 2023). This leads us to ask:

What are the limits of postmodern interpretation in systemic therapy?

How can Mexican family therapists integrate third order thinking and feminist critique into their practice?

How can we incorporate Global South epistemologies to resist the neoliberal model that turns therapy into a business and excludes families without financial resources?

Third order thinking in family therapy is a humble, socially just approach that resonates with Latin American concerns, particularly in Mexico. Recent studies have demonstrated its relevance in the treatment of chronic anxiety disorders (Gómez-Lamont, Faudoa Mendoza, & Márquez-Palacios, 2024) and in addressing family violence from a gender perspective (Gómez-Lamont, Sánchez Mora, & Pérez Sánchez, 2024). The Virtual Clinic for Family Therapy at UNAM has been a key space for applying these ideas, providing access to families who might otherwise lack psychological care. In this context, third order systemic therapy has facilitated the recognition of structural inequalities within family narratives and has promoted the construction of new relational dynamics based on social justice. Through work with families and couples, a reduction in the impact of anxiety on relational dynamics has been observed, along with greater agency among women who are victims of gender-based violence (Gómez-Lamont, Sánchez Mora, & Pérez Sánchez, 2024).

For me, third order systemic therapy represents a critical evolution of therapeutic thought in Mexico. Its application in spaces such as the Virtual Clinic for Family Therapy at UNAM is an example of the transformative potential of this approach. It is essential for family therapists and researchers to continue to explore ways to integrate Global South epistemologies into their practice, recognizing intersectionality and power dynamics that influence human relationships.

In the text box above, Fausto described a critical perspective that he and his colleagues were longing to have. It is also important to acknowledge, however, that these ideas are recursive and developed and shared across many people and contexts. While many have co-constructed these ideas, not everyone is credited or rewarded in the same manner. Who gets acknowledged for particular ideas is significant to note. Questions to consider are: Who is credited? Which ideas are privileged and seen as valuable? Whose ideas are subjugated and whose are brought forth and elevated as being "cutting edge," "brilliant," "scientific," and "novel?" Although we have applied critical/contextual frameworks to family therapy, many of the ideas foundational to socioculturally attuned family therapy stem from the work of scholars who came before us from South America and other parts of the world. For example, we have applied Martin-Baró's work in liberation psychology and Paulo Freire's concept of conscientization, and many others, to socially just family therapy practices. In doing so, we are acutely aware of balancing the tension of honoring and applying those perspectives and not culturally appropriating them. We are also aware that the reader will interpret these ideas as either liberatory, colonizing, or a combination of both. Our approach, which is significantly based on the work of those from the Global South, is now seen as new or a breath of fresh air. This indeed is a colonizing paradox.

Engaging in Equity-based Knowledge Production

All research and professional knowledge is produced, evaluated, and assumed to be true or untrue based on our epistemological lenses (see Chapter 3). We separate what we believe from what we don't believe by determining whether or not legitimate proof has been offered that fits within our worldviews. Consider a Western medical doctor who views traditional Chinese medicine as unproven even though its healing qualities have been recognized and its use has been perfected over two thousand years. In this case, the dominance of Western scientific epistemology (Harding, 1998, 2008) prevails over how and what is considered to be proven as effective.

The evidence-based practice movement in behavioral health has followed the Western medical model in an attempt to prove that a treatment of one type or another is effective or more effective than an alternative treatment. While this is certainly useful in determining best practices and what is most helpful for solving specific types of problems, this stance often discounts that which has not undergone an evidence-based research process. Furthermore, there is a tendency to view evidence of effectiveness as an overall stamp of approval, rather than carefully reviewing the usefulness of outcome criteria, study limits, and other sociopolitical, economic, and contextual factors inherent in the industry of knowledge production and research processes.

The modern scientific agenda prioritizes research that leads to knowledge that describes, explains, and allows us to predict and control. The preoccupation with generalizability and validity makes sense when a phenomenon is viewed from an essentialist perspective—that is the belief that what is being studied can be known and understood from a single objective vantage point (Harding, 2006). The assumption that modern scientific methods ensure the objectivity of truth claims delimits what questions get asked, which research projects get funded, and what types of analyses are considered legitimate. The association between numbers and truth further creates a false dichotomy when applied to research. Both positivist and non-positivist approaches to knowledge production can have numbers associated with results.

Critical theorists, Indigenous scholars, and those writing about decolonizing methods have long advocated for the need to dismantle positivist, elitist approaches to research (Denzin et al., 2008). These approaches include methods that are not conducive to evidence-based trials. The wisdom that extends beyond manualized treatment and diverse forms of knowledge that originate from nondominant epistemologies are at risk of losing credibility as a result of the rush toward scientific knowledge at the expense of all else. In recent years, there has been increasing interest in creating knowledge from critical and social constructionist frameworks. Critical research aims to question truth claims created through dominant scientific methods that obscure the politics of knowledge production behind a veil of (non-existent) objectivity. Critical researchers consider who benefits from knowledge claims, whose voices are being marginalized, what experiences are being rendered silent, and whose perspectives dominate the process (Bermúdez et al., 2016; Brown & Strega, 2015). Critical scholars and social constructionists consider questions such as who is telling the story, how are truth claims influenced by the questions being asked, and how does the research open and/or close possibilities for multiple truths and previously silenced narratives?

The answers to these questions often determine whose research gets funded or is considered legitimate. Empirically supported treatments are necessary and important in terms of advancing scientific knowledge, clinical practice, and the field of family therapy; however, we limit our knowledge when we assume empirical research is the only form of research that is rigorous, valuable, and legitimate. In Text Box 16.8, Iva Košutić describes her work as a social researcher who pays close attention to how knowledge is constructed and the potential impact of research to both obscure and expose social inequities.

Text Box 16.8 Iva Košutić, PhD

Iva Košutić (she/her) is a scholar and social researcher. She is the author of numerous publications that support social equity in, and beyond, family therapy. Much of her current work involves the evaluation of social and health programs.

Having inhabited different national and local contexts, I have learned that the valuation of a wide range of attributes is a function of social agreement. What is deemed beautiful, important, or successful within one local or national context may not be deemed so within another. And similarly, what is silenced and marginalized in one setting may not be so elsewhere. As I operate within any one reality, I bear in mind memories of other realities and I maintain awareness of the fact that attributions of value are, in most instances, relative. I have experienced being more intelligent, more interesting, more attractive in some contexts than in others, and I imagine that the same would be true of others. There is often (if not always?) another way to look at things, and the collective perception of reality may be just as flawed as individual perceptions often are.

Interruption of injustice within professional contexts is challenging for me because I tend to operate in fits and bursts, and experience disappointment when change doesn't happen quickly. Support from like-minded colleagues and a focus on the process—a steady progression of tiny contributions—helps me continue to work in the face of injustice.

I try to avoid thinking that my perception is correct, and I maintain openness to the possibility that there are errors in my thinking. These days, the chief way in which I influence others is through my way of being, with the hope that I am making a positive contribution to their lives.

Applied to social research, this approach involves considering how programs, interventions, and people fit within local and national contexts and how they contribute to or detract from health equity. Such considerations inform all aspects of research, from planning and data collection to interpretation of findings and reporting. For example, the finding of an absence of difference in health outcomes between two groups may be prematurely celebrated as a sign of health equity. Considering such findings within the sociocultural context, and triangulating it with other data sources, often points to the shifting form of inequity as an alternate explanation.

Over the past two decades, there has been much emphasis in social science on evidence-based programs and interventions. The evidence-based designation rests on evidence from randomized controlled trials (RCTs), which are considered the gold standard for effectiveness research, and quasi-experimental comparison group designs. Such evidence most often pertains to isolated, narrowly defined outcomes that in real life typically manifest as but a few symptoms of a bigger problem.

The reduction of complex phenomena to their constituent elements is consistent with the scientific approach, as often understood and implemented, but is inconsistent with people's lived realities. Interventions that are validated through the evidence-based designation may indeed have a positive effect on the outcomes of interest, and they may, at the same time, do little for the underlying problem. For example, sexual health programs are deemed evidence-based if they are backed by "rigorous evaluations" (RCTs) that show an improvement in outcomes such as abstinence, consistent condom use, absence of disease, or absence of mistimed pregnancy. That a program may be successful in addressing one or a handful of these outcomes does not say anything about its ability to promote sexual health, the broader concept of relational health, or an even broader concept of community health.

To be clear, I am not discounting the value of RCTs and quasi-experimental designs. Rather, I am advocating for an expansion in our collective view of what counts as knowledge to include research approaches that draw from a contextual perspective and bring the voices and the lived experiences of research participants to the fore.

As mentioned, science is not neutral nor objective. Kathrine Allen (2022) and colleagues (2009) suggested socially just family scholars engage in critically reflexive methods and consciousness that leads to praxis. Given the urgency of social change, feminism offers a framework for epistemology (knowledge), methodology (production of knowledge), ontology (the subjective way in which we live in the world), and praxis (how we translate knowledge into action that creates social change) (Allen, 2022). Allen asserted that feminist family science, in particular, is vital for advancing critical, intersectional, and queer approaches to examine inequity, injustice, and abuses of power among individuals and families in diverse contexts.

Socioculturally attuned researchers hold the tensions of multiple epistemologies and research methodologies in ways that provide access to the opportunity to do research and to disseminate knowledge that supports social equity. We must attend to the politics and ideologies embedded within every facet of the research process, as well as within the self-of-the-researcher (Brown & Strega, 2015). The Critical Methodologies Collective (2022) pointed out that qualitative research is always political as researchers seek to represent those being studied in ways that can further oppress, maintain unjust situations, and/or resist social structures that are unjust. We take this a step further, suggesting all research is political, whether using quantitative, qualitative, or other methods.

McDowell and Fang (2007) identified six fundamental assumptions for engaging in feminist-informed, critical multicultural, equity-based research. These include 1) holding ourselves accountable as researchers to be aware and accountable for our own positionality and social awareness, 2) interrogating the politics of knowledge production itself, 3) carefully attending to culture and context prior to and throughout the research process, 4) making certain the efforts of the researcher amplify marginalized voices, 5) ensuring the research serves to benefit those in the center of the analysis, and 6) using diverse methodologies and methods to support social equity.

Socioculturally attuned researchers might ask themselves a number of questions, including: Am I the right person to do this research? What do I need to understand about the sociocultural context I am asking to enter? In what ways am I an insider or an outsider to the group I am hoping to research? Who will own the results of the research and have the right to disseminate the knowledge produced by this study? Who will benefit from this research and how? What epistemological lens am I proposing for this research, and what effect will that have on the production of knowledge? How will research methods affect participants and study outcomes? And so on. Researchers might also apply ANVIET to their work, as suggested by the questions in Table 16.1.

In Text Box 16.9 Sally St. George and Dan Wulff (St. George et al., 2015; Wulff & St. George, 2014, 2020) share their approach to Research As Daily Practice and how this approach broadens possibilities by challenging what we think we know, including what we believe qualifies as research.

Table 16.1 Applying ANVIET to equity-based research

Attune	How do I make certain I am attuned as a researcher to the sociocultural experience of participants? How will the research increase attunement?
Name	In what ways will this research help name what is unjust?
Value	How do I design and report research in ways that optimize the likelihood of marginalized experiences being valued and participants feeling valued?
Intervene	How does the research aim to intervene in what is unjust? How do I ensure that dominant power dynamics of knowledge production don't misshape or silence results?
Envision	How does the research and the way I present results encourage participants and others to see greater possibilities for liberation? How might the research process itself help participants envision pathways for equity and transformation?
Transform	What is the aim of this research? How is it designed, implemented, and shared in ways that are transformative? What potential does the research process have to transform the lives of participants?

Text Box 16.9 Sally St. George, PhD and Dan Wulff, PhD

Sally St. George (she/her) describes herself as a "pracademic." Sally is developing a new phase of professional life primarily focused on supporting others as they develop their work.

Dan Wulff (he/him) is a retired professor who is now investing in reading all those books he intended to for many years and writing about the things he most wants to write about.

What we value most about a systemic/relational/social constructionist stance is working in the areas of connection. Therefore, we as "pracademics" (practitioners and academics), developed ways to attend to the mutual influence across our research, therapy practices, service, and teaching. In an era of increasing specialization, we prefer focusing on the intersections between practices and issues. We propose a way of re-imagining and conducting research that is already contained within family therapy practice itself, with "research" part of everything else and no longer a stand-alone practice. Using established methodological practices, or parts of them, or developing new ways, we systematically examine what we are doing in ways that make common or intuitive sense to us while trying to improve our work as we are engaged in it. We call this Research As Daily Practice.

Research As Daily Practice is predicated on partnering with others and capitalizing on a variety of viewpoints. For example, when we are feeling unsuccessful in working with certain situations in therapy (e.g., high-conflict families living in multiple households), we gather with our colleagues to compare our various understandings of what is happening and what could happen. We examine how to understand our situations by systematically looking across cases and therapists with the aim of envisioning alternative approaches.

In our Research As Daily Practice, we ask ourselves "What are we missing?" or "What else could we know?" and seek a wide range of perspectives. Our aim is to stretch our thinking about the issues we are attending to rather than to affirm or confirm current understandings. We deliberately and persistently inquire about ideas or viewpoints that are not currently present in our thinking or practice. One question could be, "What are various ways in which this situation could make 'perfect sense'?"

Research As Daily Practice is our attempt to loosen the grip of standardized regimes of locating and determining truth, thereby opening opportunities to talk about and imagine people's lives differently. Other questions could include, "Who benefits and who does not as we work in the current situation?" What does this family feel entitled to?" "Who is not present in our conversation and who could be?" "What ideas have been dismissed as irrelevant?" "How might practitioners in other fields or disciplines understand this situation?" We would consider inviting representatives of opinions that are most distant from our current understandings about the issue in therapy. We reach for understandings from other cultural locations, languages, or times that might shake our confidence in our traditional ways of knowing and practicing.

This way of working varies markedly from utilizing so-called "evidence-based practice" or "best practices." We believe there is an endless supply of ways to respond to families in therapy. We embrace variety and special cases. We search to see what problems look like as they present in differing families and contexts. Examining how unfairnesses present and are articulated, performed, and responded to in different families extends our understanding and responses that are more attuned to the specific context within and outside of the family in therapy.

Research As Daily Practice allows us to entertain the question of transformative change with fewer limitations or boundaries. Values, relationships, and inclusiveness have room to flourish. Equity, for example, can become the primary framework for our therapeutic work/response. We can build our practices around positions of value or commitment whereas with the traditional forms of research, we subscribed to ideas and practices that professed value-neutrality. Now we can bring values or interpersonal commitments into the center.

Conclusion

Many voices have joined together in this text to encourage third order change in our work with individuals, families, communities, agencies, institutions, governments, and beyond. We have been encouraged to do our best to influence public policy and support environmental justice in ways that support social and relational equity, as well as the environment itself. We have been called to work together across national borders while using a global framework in our local contexts. As systems thinkers and relationship experts, we are in the unique position of being able to take transformative action that is connecting rather than polarizing. Thinking from a third order perspective helps us avoid attempting first order solutions; thinking strategically and collaboratively to create systemic change rather than expecting change to occur when we simply point out when we believe something is not right or others are not socially aware.

It is difficult to end a book such as this. Even as we write, we experience endless urges to further investigate, analyze, cite more authors, reorganize our ideas, and rethink what we "know." The ideas and ways of applying third order thinking are fluid and continuously evolving. Our work will need to be critiqued, expanded, and revised by others in response to societal changes and collective movement in the field toward equity-based praxis. The work itself is rewarding, yet arduous, messy, contradictory, painful, and often carried out in stressful, perilous, and liminal spaces. The pace of change can be excruciatingly slow, and the costs are often high, particularly for those at the margins.

We have come to believe that socioculturally attuned family therapists must balance courage with discernment, knowledge and awareness with humility, and realism with hope. Looking back over the years and our careers in the field of family therapy, we have witnessed uneven, hard-won, yet persistent movement toward socially just practice. Systemically, movements that disrupt the status quo tend to experience setbacks and backlash. Though painful, they are not unexpected. Experiencing small "wins" and witnessing transformation gives us hope for the future; hope that collectively, family therapists will continue to move the field toward relationally just, equitable practices that support all people and families, and develop new and creative ways to do this work.

Reflexive Questions

- What alliances have you developed to collectively engage in change efforts within organizations, agencies, communities, and/or societal systems?
- How can you actively rally support for collective values instead of focusing on political differences and divides?
- How can calling people in with care and compassion (instead of calling out) help create a context in which everyone can grow, learn, and be held accountable while prioritizing mutual respect, health, and well-being?

- When building a collective vision, what strategies can you use to involve all stakeholders? How can you engage in socioculturally attuned praxis within the various contexts you inhabit (e.g., clinical, research, personal, political, community, etc.)?
- What is your vision for your own praxis (consciousness in action)?

References

Allen, K. R. (2022). Feminist theory, method, and praxis: Toward a critical consciousness for family and close relationship scholars. *Journal of Social and Personal Relationships*, *40*(3), 899–936.

Allen, K. R., Lloyd, S. A., & Few, A. L. (2009). Reclaiming feminist theory, method, and praxis for family studies. In S. Lloyd, A. Few, & K. Allen (Eds.). *Handbook of feminist family studies* (pp. 3–17). Sage.

Almeida, R. V. (2018). *Liberation based healing practices*. Institute for Family Services.

Almeida, R. & Tubbs, C. (2020). Intersectionality: A liberation-based healing perspective. In K. S. Wampler, R. B. Miller, & R. B. Seedall (Eds.). *The handbook of systemic family therapy*, (Vol. 1, pp. 227–249). Wiley.

Almeida, R., & Williams, J. C. (2026). Postmodernism, decolonial critiques, and liberatory praxis. In O. Smoliak et al. (Eds.). *The Routledge international handbook of postmodern therapies* (pp. 86–99). Routledge.

Alvarez-Hernandez, L. R., Cardenas, I., & Bloom, A. (2021). COVID-19 pandemic and intimate partner violence: an analysis of help-seeking messages in the Spanish-speaking media. *Journal of Family Violence*, 1–12.

Bartunek, J. M. & Moch, M. K. (1987). First-order, second-order, and third-order change and organization development interventions: A cognitive approach. *The Journal of Applied Behavioral Science*, *23*(4), 483–500.

Bell, D. 2002. *Ethical ambition: Living a life of meaning and worth*. Bloomsbury.

Bermúdez, J. M., McDowell, T., & Knudson-Martin, C. (2024). Socioculturally attuned family therapy: Third order thinking in a global context. In K. Hertlein (Ed.) *International handbook of couple and family therapy (*pp. 83–97*)*. Routledge.

Bermúdez, J. M., Muruthi, B. A., Alvarez-Hernandez, L., Machado, Y., & Lamont-Gomez, F. (equal authors) (under review). Decolonizing approaches to family science as intersectional Latinx and Caribbean scholars working toward third order change, *Invited Paper. Journal of Family Theory and Review.*

Bermúdez, J. M., Muruthi, B. A., & Jordan, L. S. (2016). Decolonizing research methods for family science: Creating space at the center. *Journal of Family Theory & Review*, *8*(2), 192–206.

Boszormenyi-Nagy, I. (1966). From family relationships to a psychology of relationships: Fictions of the individual and fictions of the family. *Comprehensive Psychiatry.*

Boverie, P. E. (1991). Human systems consultant: Using family therapy in organizations. *Family Therapy*, *18*(1), 61.

Brown, A. M. & Devich-Cyril, M. (2020). *We will not cancel us: And other dreams of transformative justice*. AK Press.

Brown, L. A. & Strega, S. (2015). *Research as resistance: Revisiting critical, Indigenous, and anti-oppressive approaches* (2nd ed.). Canadian Scholars' Press.

Calva, A., Matthew, R. A., & Orpinas, P. (2020). Overcoming barriers: Practical strategies to assess Latinos living in low-income communities. *Health promotion practice*, *21*(3), 355–362.

Collins, P. H. (1990). Black feminist thought in the matrix of domination. *Black feminist thought: Knowledge, consciousness, and the politics of empowerment*, *138*(1990), 221–238.

Critical Methodologies Collective, The (2022). *The politics and ethics of representation in qualitative research: Addressing moments of discomfort*. Routledge.

Díaz McConnell, E., Sheehan, C. M., & Lopez, A. (2023). An intersectional and social determinants of health framework for understanding Latinx psychological distress in 2020: Disentangling the effects of immigration policy and practices, the Trump Administration, and COVID-19-specific factors. *Journal of Latinx Psychology*, *11*(1), 1.

Daneshpour, M. (2022). *Gender, power, and global social justice: The healing power of psychotherapy*. Routledge.

Denzin, N. K., Lincoln, Y. S., & Smith, L. T. (Eds.). (2008). *Handbook of critical and Indigenous methodologies*. Sage.

Fraenkel, P. & Cho, W. (2020). Reaching up, down, in, and around: Couple and family coping during the coronavirus pandemic. *Family Process*, *59*, 825–831.

Freire, P. (1970). Cultural action and conscientization. *Harvard Educational Review*, *40*(3), 452–477.
Gómez- Lamont, M. F. (2021). El Pensamiento de Tercer Orden en la Terapia Breve Estratégica para Parejas que vivieron una infidelidad. *Revista Digital Internacional de Psicología y Ciencia Social*, *7* (2), 290–298.
Gómez-Lamont, M. F., Faudoa Mendoza, L. C., & Márquez-Palacios, J. H. (2024). *Abordando los trastornos crónicos de ansiedad en México: La importancia de la atención a las familias y parejas desde la terapia sistémica de tercer orden*. In J. I. Uribe Alvarado, C. I. Huerta Solano, L. Pérez Sánchez, A. M. Méndez Puga, & K. I. Martínez Martínez (Eds.). Investigación social, experiencias y metodologías en psicología desde una perspectiva interinstitucional (pp. 85–111). Universidad de Guadalajara.
Gómez-Lamont, M. F., Sánchez Mora, M. I., & Pérez Sánchez, L. (2024). Consecuencias psicológicas de la violencia familiar en mujeres: Un análisis sistémico de tercer orden con perspectiva de género. *Regiones y Desarrollo Sustentable*, *24*(Número especial), ISSN electrónico: 2594-1429, ISSN impreso: 1665-9511.
Gómez-Lamont, M. F. & Bermúdez, J. M. (2023). *La Terapia Familiar Sistémica y El Pensamiento de Tercer Orden: Teoría crítica y política con perspectivas de género, multiculturalidad e interseccionalidad*. México: UNAM. EE.UU. Universidad de Georgia.
Goodman, J., Morgan, A., Hodgson, J., Caldwell, B. (2018). From private practice to academia: Integrating social and political advocacy into every MFT identity. *Journal of Marital and Family Therapy*, *44*(1), 32–45.
Hanisch, C. (1969). The personal is political. The original feminist theory paper at the author's website. Carol Hanisch of the Women's Liberation Movement.
Harding, S. (2008). *Sciences from below: Feminisms, Postcolonialities, and Modernities*. Duke University Press.
Harding, S. (2006). *Science and social inequality: Feminist and postcolonial issues*. University of Illinois Press.
Harding, S. (1998). *Is science multicultural? Postcolonialisms, feminisms, and epistemologies*. Indiana University Press.
Hodgson, J. & Lamson, A. L. (2020). The importance of policy and advocacy in systemic family therapy. *The handbook of systemic family therapy*, *1*, 727–751.
Holyoak, D., McPhee, D., Hall, G., & Fife, S. (2021). Microlevel advocacy: A common process in couple and family therapy. *Family Process*, *60*(2), 654–669.
Jordan, L. S. & Seponski, D. M. (2018). "Being a therapist doesn't exclude you from real life": Family therapists' beliefs and barriers to political action. *Journal of Marital and Family Therapy*, *44*(1), 19–31.
Jordan, L. S., Seponski, D. M., Armes, S. E., & Young, S. S. (2021). A sociopolitical response to vicarious witnessing: testimonial therapy. *Journal of Ethnic & Cultural Diversity in Social Work*, 1–5.
Letiecq, B. & Bermúdez, J. M. (2023). Situating Latinx immigrant romantic relationships in the context of illegality: Using a socioculturally attuned lens. In B. G. Ogolsky (Ed.). *The socio-cultural context of romantic relationships* (chapter 12, pp. 226–246). Cambridge University Press.
Letiecq, B. L., Davis, E., Vesely, C. K., Goodman, R. D., Zeledon, D., & Marquez, M. (2022). Central American immigrant mothers' narratives of intersecting oppressions: A resistant knowledge project. *Journal of Marriage and Family*, *84*(5), 1291–1313.
Matheny, A. C. & Zimmerman, T. S. (2001). The application of family systems theory to organizational consultation: A content analysis. *American Journal of Family Therapy*, *29*(5), 421–433.
Matthew, R., Orpinas, P., Calva, A., Bermúdez, J.M., Darbisi, C. (2020). *Lazos Hispanos*: Promising strategies and lessons learned in the development of a multisystem, community-based *promotoras* program. *Journal of Primary Prevention*, *41*(3), 229–243.
McDowell, T. (1999). Systems consultation and Head Start: An alternative to traditional family therapy. *Journal of Marital and Family Therapy*, *25*(2), 155–168.
McDowell, T. & Fang, S. (2007). Feminist-informed critical multiculturalism: Considerations for family research. *Journal of Family Issues*, *28*(4), 549–566.
McDowell, T., Libal, K., & Brown, A. L. (2012). Human rights in the practice of family therapy: Domestic violence, a case in point. *Journal of Feminist Family Therapy*, *24*(1), 1–23.
McDowell, T., Knudson-Martin, C., & Bermúdez, J. M. (2023). *Socioculturally attuned family therapy: Guidelines for equitable theory and practice* (2nd ed.). Routledge.
McDowell, T., Knudson-Martin, C., & Bermúdez, J. M. (2019). Third-order thinking in family therapy: Addressing social justice across family therapy practice. *Family process*, *58*(1), 9–22.
McGoldrick, M., Hynes, P., Preto, N., & Petry, S. (2021). Reflections on our efforts to help mental health agencies become more "culturally competent." *Family Process*, *60*, 116–132.

Orpinas, P. Matthew, R. A., Alvarez-Hernandez, L. R., Calva, A., & Bermúdez, J. M. (2021). *Promotoras* voice their challenges in fulfilling their role as community health workers. *Health Promotion Practice, 22*(4), 502–511.

Orpinas, P., Matthew, R. A., Bermúdez, J. M., Alvarez-Hernandez, L. R., & Calva, A. (2020). A multi-stakeholder evaluation of Lazos Hispanos: An application of a community-based participatory research conceptual model. *Journal of Community Psychology, 48*(2), 464–481.

polanco, m. (2016). Knowledge fair trade. In L. Charlés & Samarasinghe, G. (Eds.). *Family therapy in global humanitarian contexts: Voices and issues from the field* (pp. 13–25). AFTA Springerbriefs in Family Therapy, Springer.

Powell, J. A. (2024). *The power of bridging: How to build a world where we all belong*. Sounds true.

Ross, L. J. (2019a). Speaking up without tearing down: A veteran human rights educator explains the value of teaching students to call each other in rather than out. *Learning for Justice, 61* Retrieved on Feb 18, 2022, from https://www.learningforjustice.org/magazine/spring-2019/speaking-up-without-tearing-down.

Ross, L. J. (2019b). I'm a Black feminist. I think call-out culture is toxic. There are better ways of doing social justice work. *The New York Times*, Aug 17, 2019 https://www.nytimes.com/2019/08/17/opinion/sunday/cancel-culture-call-out.html.

St. George, S., Wulff, D., & Tomm, K. (2015). Research as daily practice. *Journal of Systemic Therapies, 34*(2), 3–14.

Stone, D. J. & ChenFeng, J. L. (2019). *Finding your voice as a beginning marriage and family therapist*. Routledge.

Vesely, C. K., Letiecq, B., Davis, E., Goodman, R., DeMulder, E., Marquez, M., & Amigas de la Comunidad. (2024). "The spirit of a fighter": Mixed-status Latine immigrant families' experiences during COVID. *Family Relations, 73*(3), 1483–1500.

Waldegrave, C., King, P., Maniapoto, M., Tamasese, T. K., Parsons, T. L. and Sullivan, G. (2016). Relational resilience in Māori, Pacific, and European sole parent families: From theory and research to social policy. *Family Process, 55*, 673–688.

Walsdorf, A. A., Machado, Y., & Bermúdez, J. M. (2020). Undocumented and mixed-status Latinx families: Sociopolitical considerations for systemic practice. *Journal of Family Psychotherapy, 30*(4), 245–271.

Wulff, D. & St. George, S. (2020). We are all researchers. In S. McNamee, M. M. Gergen, C. Camargo-Borges, & E. F. Rasera (Eds.). *The Sage handbook of social constructionist practice* (pp. 68–76). Sage.

Wulff, D. & St. George, S. (2014). Research as daily practice. In G. Simon & A. Chard (Eds.). *Systemic inquiry: Innovations in reflexive practice research* (pp. 292–308). Everything is Connected Press.

Index

Note: Page references in *italics* denote figures and in **bold** tables.

accountability 1, 3, 62–63, 65–66, 78, 111, 126, 336, 338; collective 3; for communication 141; encourage 223, 229; relational 48, 223; shared 179
Afuape, T. 129
Agbai, C. O. 82
Ainsworth, Mary 163
Allen, Kathrine 375–376
Almeida, Rhea V. 41–43
alternative relationship models 246
alternative schemas 251
American Association for Marriage and Family Therapy (AAMFT) Code of Ethics 49
Anderson, H. 275, 280, 288
Anderson, S. R. 11
Anderson, Tom 275
ANVIET (attunement, naming, valuing, envisioning, and transforming) 13, 36–43, *37*, 63, **64–65**, 358–362, **376**
assess/assessment: differentiation through relational lens 200; as foundation for third order change 93; impacts of power on clinical issues 87–89; for mutual vulnerability 332; socioculturally attuned 70–94, *71*
attachment-based family therapies (ABFTs) 163–164; case illustration 179–182; emotional connection 167; interdependence and responsiveness 166; intersubjective emotional regulation 166; power 174–175; relational process 164–165; relational security and trust 166–167; societal context 168–174; sociocultural attunement 167–176; third order change 175–176
attune/attuning: cultural 149–151; sociocultural 124–130, 167–176, 277–289, 300–321
attuned relationships: building 358–359; maintaining 358–359
authority: and power 339; and responsibility 339
awareness of power 53
awareness of self 154–155, 158–159
Bagharamian, M. 48
Baima, Timothy 147–148, 177–178
balance of fairness 212–213
balance of power 336–338
Barbetta, Pietro 128
Bartunek, J. M. 366
Bateson, Gregory 22, 334
Bava, Saliha 278–279
behavior 338; abusive or harmful 222; change 246, 251–252; disruptive 72, 91, 124, 194; energetic 238; impulsive 238; law-breaking 26; relational patterns of 235–236; symptomatic 122
Bell, Derrick 360
Berg, Insoo Kim 255, 257
Bermudez, J. M. 51, 174
Bidwell, D. R. 265
Boszormenyi-Nagy, I. 54, 211, 358
Bourdieu, P. 27, 105, 106, 107
Bowen, Murray 187
Bowen Family Systems theory (BFST) 187–208; assessing differentiation through relational lens 200, 204; case example 202–207; client observing own part in system 201, 205–206; critical consciousness 200–201, 204–205; differentiation and societal power processes 195–197; differentiation in societal context 191–195; differentiation of self 188; emotional engagement 189–190; empowerment 197–199; equity/flexibility in system 201, 206; family therapy concepts 188–199; flow of anxiety 189; planning meetings with family/community 202, 207; practice guidelines 199–202; presenting problem to larger contexts 199, 202–203; sociocultural attunement 191; stabilize immediate situation 200, 203–204; therapist's family of origin work 191; third order change 197–199, 207; transgenerational patterns/transmission 188–189
Bowlby, John 163, 168

brief and strategic family therapies: case illustration 133–136; concepts 118–124; power 127–130; practice guidelines 130–132; sociocultural attunement 124–130; third order change 136–137
Brief Family Therapy Center (BFTC) in Milwaukee, Wisconsin 255
Brooks, Stephanie 220–221
Brown, Andraé 157, 371
Brown, J. 131
Buber, Martin 212
Bumberry, W. 143

capital: cultural 107; economic 107; and power 107–108; social 107; and structural family therapy 107–108; symbolic 107
case illustration: attachment-based family therapies 179–182; brief and strategic family therapies 133–136; collaborative-dialogic family therapy 291–296; contextual family therapy 223–229; counter-intuitive thinking 134–135; equity-based attunement and connection 160; experiential family therapy 157–160; narrative family therapy 317–320; socio-emotional relationship therapy 346–351; solution-focused family therapy 270–272
Chappelle, N. 105
ChenFeng, Jessica 10, 150, 368–369
Circle of Care 325, 331, 333, 335, 337–339, 341, 343–344, 346, 350–352
circular questioning 119–120, 131
class and attachment 172–173
client goals: co-constructing 269, 271–272; equity in 269, 271–272; focusing on 261–263
co-constructing client goals 269, 271–272
cognitive behavioral family therapy: case example 246–252; mutual behavioral reinforcement 234–243; practice guidelines 243–246; primary enduring family therapy concepts 233–234; socioculturally attuned 233–253; third order change 252
cognitive distortion/incongruent thinking 235
collaborative-dialogic family therapy: case illustration 291–296; conversational partners 276–277; critically informed stance 289, 292–294; culture/power differences 290–291, 295–296; enduring and foundational concepts 276–277; humility and uncertainty 277; participate with transparency 290, 294; possibilities 277; power 285–287; practice guidelines 289–291; social construction of meaning 276; societal context 278–284; sociocultural attunement 277–289; sociocultural experiences 290, 294–295; third order change 287–289, 296–297; using inquiry to promote equity 291, 296
collaborative therapeutic relationships 260–261
collective values 154, 360
collective vision 361, 366, 379
Collins, Patricia Hill 173–174, 356
colonialism 311–312
colonization 28, 311–313
communication: and experiential family therapy 141–142; experiential therapists 141
communities of practice 63
Connell, G. 143, 144
consciousness 356–379
constructive entitlement 213, 216
contexts: circularity in 125–126; justice across 218; sociocultural 72–76; and sociocultural attunement 37–38
contextual differentiation 10
contextual family therapy 40, 211–230; accountability 223, 229; assume people want to give 222, 228; balance of fairness 212–213; case illustration 223–229; due crediting 222–223, 229; entitlement 213; intergenerational loyalty 213–214; interpersonal consequences 212; multidirected partiality 214–215; multidirected sociocultural attunement 221, 224–225; practice guidelines 221–223; primary enduring concepts 211–221; principles of socioculturally attuned 215; societal power 218–219; societal systems 215–218; socio-historical context/background 221, 225–226; third order change 219–221, 229–230; unfairness 222, 226–228
contextual meaning of power 343
contextual nature of schema 237–239
contextual self-in-relationship 48–65; awareness of power 53; myth of neutrality 54; relational engagement 56–57; self-disclosure 56–57; therapist social location 52–53; use of power in practice 54–56
conversational partners 276–277
coping questions 258, 260
counter-intuitive thinking: brief and strategic therapies 121–122; case illustration 134–135; to counter hegemony 131
COVID-19 pandemic 58
critical postmodernism 308
cultural attunement 149–151
cultural capital 27, 107
Cultural Context Model (CCM) 364–365
cultural democracy 149–151
culturally attuned/equity-based community interventions 364–366
culturally sensitive/personal agency 59–60
cultural paradigms 32
culture 27–30, 311–313; case illustration 158; in dialogical processes 290–291; experiential family therapy 154; justice across 218; and power 128–129
cultures of connection 5

Daneshpour, Manijeh 362–363
D'Aniello, C. 10
D'Arrigo, Justine 12, 282–283
D'Arrigo-Patrick, J. 282, 289
Deatrick, J. 6
de-colonization 311–313
definitional ceremonies 308
de Shazer, S. 121, 255
destructive entitlement 213, 216, 223, 226, 230
developmentally appropriate relational equity 110, 115
Diagnostic and Statistical Manual of Mental Disorders (DSM-5-TR) 78
dialogical processes: culture in 290–291; power differences in 290–291, 295–296
differentiation: of self 188; in societal context 191–195; and societal power processes 195–197
distant other 4, 5
dominant cultural assumptions/contexts 168–170
dominant societal discourses 327
due crediting 214, 222–223, 229

economic capital 107
emotional connection 167, 171, 178, 188, 194, 330
emotional engagement 189–190
emotional expression 103, 140–141, 189, 194, 338
emotional fusion 188, 190–191, 195, 197, 207
emotionally focused family therapy (EEFT) 163
emotionally focused therapy (EFT) 163, 171
emotions: case illustration 159; and expression 156; negative 151; positive 151; and power 151–152, 156, 174; relational patterns of 235–236; social construction of 170; social context of 334; social valuation of 336; sociocultural nature of 177, 180
empowerment 197–199
entitlement 213, 215–216; constructive 213, 216; contextual family therapy 213; destructive 213, 216, 223, 226, 230
environmental justice 217–218
envision/envisioning 179, 223, 242, 246, 251, 267–269, 303–304, 320, 350–351, 365, 371, 372; acceptance and support 157; change 71, 91, 93, 115, 201; just alternatives 40; new mutuality 344; new realities 291; possibilities 93, 241; preferred narratives 317
epistemic injustice 8, 50, 79
epistemology 50–51, 310, 375; ecosystemic 2; temporal 311; Western scientific 51, 373
Epston, David 300
Equal Pay Act of 1963 26
equitable relational patterns 179, 182
equity 201, 206; -based attunement and connection 156–157, 160; -based knowledge production 373–378; -based relationships 110, 114; -based research **376**; -based therapists 57, 60; in co-constructing client goals 269, 271–272; use inquiry to promote 291, 296
Erikson, Milton 121
ethics, ethical: defined 48; relational 50; third order 48–65
everyday resistance 58–59; symptoms as forms of 129–130
exoneration 214, 215
expectancy for change 11–12
experiential family therapy 140–160; case illustration 157–160; and communication 141–142; cultural attunement 149–151; cultural democracy 149–151; and experiential interventions 143–144; and neurobiology 145–146; power 151–153; practicing 154–157; and sharing emotions 142–143; societal context 146–149; therapist's use of self 144–145; third order change in 141, 153–154
experiential interventions: and experiential family therapy 143–144; and experiential therapists 144
exploitative oppression 216
expression: case illustration 159; and emotions 156; and power 156

fairness 1, 196, 211–214, 216, 219–222, 228–230, 282, 287, 356
family: cartography 148, **149**; development 98–99; power dynamics 110, 113; projection process 189; revisioning the definition of 109, 111; sculpting 144; and societal structures 109–110, 112–113; structure and hierarchy 99–100
family schemas 245, **245**, 250–251
family therapy: individualism and distant other 5; models 89–91, **90**; in our current societal context 4–7; polarization 7; social inequities 5–7; social isolation 4–5; and societal context 2–4
Farrall, S. 25–26
Fausto Gomez Lamont, Mario 371–373
first order change 23–24
Fisch, R. 121
flexibility 201, 206
flow of anxiety 189, 191
Foucault, Michel 34, 300, 314
Fraenkel, Peter 288–289
Freire, Paulo 20, 198, 356
Fricker, M. 8, 50, 173
function, defined 4
Furrow, James 168
Fürst, M. 50

Galveston Declaration 62
Garcia, M. 152
Garcia-Westburg, Marisol 60
gender 335–336; equity 24, 307, 316; inequalities 234; and relational needs 170–171; schemas 238; stereotypes 40, 115, 171
general systems approach 19
general systems theory 19
Gergen, K. 50

Giammattei, Shawn V. 312–313
GI Bill 81–82
Goodrich, T. 125
Goolishian, H. A. 275
Greenberg, Les 171
group relational systems 106–107

habitus 106
Haley, J. 123–124, 125
Hare-Mustin, R. 277–278
Hecker, L. 50
hermeneutical justice 173–174
hermeneutic injustice 50, 173–174
heteronormativity 33, 57, 128, 205, 238, 283, 310, 313
historical injustices and trauma 217
Hoa Nguyen 41
Hoffman, Lynn 275
hope 264
Huenergardt, D. 216, 324
Huft, J. 146
humility 37, 54, 277, 287, 292, 378

incongruent hierarchies 122–123
individualism 4, 5, 7, 39, 73, 150, 200, 336
individual schemas 245, **245**, 250–251
influence: decisions about using 35; mutual 332–333; and societal schemas **244**
injustice: epistemic 8, 50, 79; hermeneutical 50, 173–174, 321; name/naming 315–316; testimonial 50
institutions 366–369
interaction patterns 97–98
interdependence and responsiveness 166
intergenerational loyalty 213–214
International Family Therapy Association 193
interrupt/interrupting 19–20, 33, 37, 40, 342–343, 348–350; microaggressions 157; power patterns 338; processes 50; societal power dynamics 179; typical dynamics 104
intersubjective emotional regulation 166
intimate partner violence (IPV) 19
invisible loyalty 214

Johnson, L. N. 11
Johnson, S. M. 164, 171
Jonathan, N. 146
Jordan, L. S. 33
justice 215–216; across cultures and contexts 218; environmental 217–218; hermeneutical 173–174
just relationships 132, 136
just solutions 269–270, 272

Kabura, Paschal 127
Kim, Lana 8–9, 339
Knudson-Martin, C. 33, 153, 216, 324, 337, 339
Košutić, Iva 152, 374–375
Krasner, B. 54

language 266–267
Larner, G. 49, 286
Latino Health Access (LHA) 175–176
Lazos Hispanos (Hispanic Links) 365
ledgers of merits 215
levels of learning 22; Learning I 22; Learning II 22; Learning III 22

Madanes, Cloé 122, 136
Mahoney, A. R. 337
Man-Tso Wei 328–329
Maton, K. 106
McDowell, Quentin R. 367
McDowell, T. 54–55, 148, 152
McGoldrick, Monica 190, 199
meaning 266–267; social construction of 276; socially constructed 301–303
metamodernism 32, 308
Minuchin, Salvador 97, 100–101
miracle questions 258
Mitten, T. 143
Moch, M. K. 366
Morrison, T. 63
multi-directed partiality 54, 214–215
multidirected sociocultural attunement 221, 224–225
Murphy, M. 50
mutual attunement 332
mutual behavioral reinforcement 234–243; behavior, relational patterns of 235–236; cognitive distortion/incongruent thinking 235; contextual nature of schema 237–239; emotion, relational patterns of 235–236; power and social schemas 239–241; schemas 234–235; sociocultural attunement 237; therapist as coach 236–237; third order change 242–243; thought, relational patterns of 235–236
mutual influence 332–333
mutual vulnerability 331–332

name/naming 38; injustices 315–316; without shame 359–360
Nardone, G. 122, 123
narrative family therapy (NFT) 300–321; case illustration 317–320; co-create preferred narratives 307–308; (de)colonization 311–313; culture 311–313; deconstruct life of the problem 306–307; name injustices 315–316, 318–319; oppressive power dynamics 316–317, 319–320; people and problems 304–305; power and subjugation 314; power-embedded relational inequity 315–316; practice guidelines 315–317; primary enduring concepts 301–308; relational equity 316–317; socially constructed

meaning 301–303; socially constructed reality 301–303; societal context and discourses of resistance 310–311; sociocultural attunement 300–321; sociopolitical structures 315, 318; thicken stories of resistance/resilience 317, 320; third order change 314–315, 320–321; time-oriented/generative therapy 303–304; values embedded in narratives 316, 319
Narrative Means to Therapeutic Ends (White and Epston) 300
narratives: explore values embedded in 316, 319; preferred 307–308
neurobiology: and experiential family therapy 145–146; interpersonal 145–146
neutrality 54
new mutuality: envisioning 344; reinforcing 345–346

ontology 50–51, 128, 375
oppression 59–60
oppressive power dynamics 316–317, 319–320
organizations 366–369

parentified child 213
Parker, Elizabeth Oshrin 242–243
participation with transparency 290, 294
patriarchal gender systems 238
Penn, Peggy 275
People of Color 26, 28; societal constraints 57
personal agency: challenging oppression 59–60; culturally sensitive 59–60; everyday resistance 58–59; perspectives 59–60; societal constraints on 57–61
personal meaning of power 343
place/placing: defined 80; families and therapy 80–82
polanco, marcela 28, 29, 311, 371
polarization 7–8, 36, 54, 360
policies 369–371
politics 369–371
Porges, S. W. 166
poststructural/social constructionist language 257–260
power 32–36, 266–267, 285–287, 336–339; attachment-based family therapies 174–175; and authority 339; awareness of 53; brief and strategic family therapies 127–130; and capital 107–108; case illustration 159; contextual meaning of 343; contextual self-in-relationship 53; and culture 128–129; decisions about using 35; defined 32; differences in dialogical processes 290–291, 295–296; dynamics 40; effects on relational safety 176; and emotions 151–152, 156, 174; experiential family therapy 151–153; imbalances 218–219; impact on clinical issues 87–89; personal meaning of 343; in practice of family therapy 33–34; and resistance 35–36, 152–153; and responsibility 339; and social schemas 239–241; societal 218–219; and sociocultural attunement 37–38; and structural family therapy 107–108; and subjugation 314; therapist power 219; use of 54–56, 61
power-embedded relational inequity 315–316, 318–319
power processes 33
praxis: ANVIET as guide for third order systemic change 358–362; socioculturally attuned 356–379; third order praxis across contexts 362–378
preferred narratives 307–308
privilege 215–216
problematic schemas: identify 244; identifying 248
psychotherapy 41, 163, 281
public participation 369–371

quality, defined 4–5

Rastogi, Mudita 30–31
reciprocally responsive social engagement 325–326
reflexive praxis 61–63
relational: alternatives 40; consequences of power differences 341–342; engagement 56–57; equity 316–317, 319–320; ethics 50, 214; flow of power 329–331; initiative 342–343; patterns of thought/emotion/behavior 235–236; process 164–165; security and trust 166–167; work, value of 343
relational needs: and attachment-based therapies 178, 181; and gender 170–171
relationships: attuned 358–359; between species 31
resilience 35, 43, 59, 71, 86–87, 93, 129–131, 154, 165, 168, 260, 263, 269, 288, 296, 315; amplifying 317; collective 317; emotional 173; family 31; individual 31; relational 7, 80; thicken stories of 317, 320
resistance: everyday 58–59, 129–130; and power 35–36, 152–153; thicken stories of 317, 320
responsibility: and authority 339; and power 339
responsibly position therapy 76–79
Robbins, Rocky 51
Roberts, J. 144

Şahin, Fatma Arıcı 155, 344–345, 346
Salmon, Laurel 309
Satir, Virginia 140, 141, 143
scaffolding 302–303
scaling questions 258–259
Scarborough, Norma 53
schemas 234–235; contextual nature of 237–239; create behavioral change based on new 246, 251–252; problematic 244, 248; social 239–241
"sealed-off" sex 171
second order change 23–24

second order thinking 19–20
self-disclosure 56–57
shared relational responsibility 333
shared responsibility 344–345
Shaw, A. 48
Siegel, D. J. 145–146, 168
social capital 107
social construction of meaning 276
social context of emotion 334
social determinants of health (SDOH) 5–6, 82–86
social isolation 4–5
social location 4, 10–11, 43, 50, 52–53, 62, 76–77, 83, 105–106, 113, 183, 216, 234, 237, 283, 287–288, 302, 315–316, 326, 352, 358, 361–362
social schemas 239–241, **250**, 250–251
social structures 25–27
social valuation of emotion 336
societal context 2–7, 24–32, 334–336; AFBTs 168–174; brief and strategic family therapies 125–126; collaborative-dialogic family therapy 278–284; culture 27–30; and discourses of resistance 310–311; experience and broader 146–148; experiential family therapy 146–149; relationships between species 31; social structures 25–27; structural family therapy 105–107; taking a superposition 31
societal discourse and felt identities 327
societal power 131–132, 135, 218–219
societal schemas 245, **245**; and influence **244**; sources of **244**
societal structures 109–110, 112–113
societal systems 215–218; environmental justice 217–218; historical injustices and trauma 217; justice, privilege, and entitlement 215–216; justice across cultures and contexts 218; values 216
sociocultural attunement 44, 48–49, 191; ANVIET 37–38; attachment-based family therapies 167–176; brief and strategic family therapies 124–130; defined 8; integrating principles of 237, 264–268; SFT 104–109; socioculturally attuned family therapy 10–12; tensions in 57
sociocultural context: attune to 72–76; client's 74–76; of this therapy 72–74
sociocultural discourses 341–342
socioculturally attuned assessment: attune to sociocultural context 72–76; elements 71–91; family therapy models 89–91, **90**; impacts of power on clinical issues 87–89; responsibly position therapy 76–79; socio-relational determinants of health 82–86, *84*
socioculturally attuned family therapy (SCAFT): application of models 12; client and extratherapeutic factors 10; conceptual framework for *21*; defined 8; expectancy for change 11–12; guiding principles for 19–44; limitations 14; overview 2–4; practice 36; principles of 24–36; therapeutic relationship 10–11; therapist characteristics 10–11; third order thinking 1–2
socioculturally attuned/sociocultural attunement: praxis 356–379; therapeutic relationships 70–71
socio-emotional experience 326–327
socio-emotional expression 334–335
socio-emotional relationship therapy (SERT) 324–352; case illustration 346–351; equitable interaction patterns 331–333; foundational SERT concepts 324–333; guidelines for practice 340–346; phase I positions therapy *340*, 340–341; power 336–339; principles of 333–339; reciprocally responsive social engagement 325–326; relational consequences of power differences 341–342; relational flow of power 329–331; societal context 334–336; societal discourse and felt identities 327; socio-emotional experience 326–327; theory of change 333; third order change 339, 351–352
Socio-Emotional Relationship Workbook (Knudson-Martin) 246
The Socio-Emotional Relationship Workbook for Couples: Closing the Gap Between the Relationship You Want and the Relationship You Have (Knudson-Martin) 62
socio-relational determinants of health 82–86, *84*
Socio-relational determinants of health
solid self 188
solution-focused family therapy (SFFT): case illustration 270–272; client goals 261–263; clients and societal context 269, 271; collaborative therapeutic relationships 260–261; equity in co-constructing client goals 269, 271–272; exceptions, discovering/amplifying 263–264; hope 264; just solutions 269–270, 272; language, meaning, and power 266–267; poststructural/social constructionist language 257–260; practice guidelines 268–270; primary enduring family therapy concepts 256–264; search for solutions 269, 272; sociocultural attunement 255–273; solutions in societal/cultural context 265–266; third order change 267–268, 272–273
space 80, 91–92, 105–107, 148–149
split loyalty 214
Stabilize immediate situation 200, 203–204
A Step-by-Step Guide to Socio-Emotional Relationship Therapy (Knudson-Martin) 340
Stevenson, Bryan 196
St. George, S. 38, 376–378
Stone, Dana 56, 363–364
structural determinants of health 6
structural family therapists 97–98, 100–102, 104–105, 108–111, 119, 122
structural family therapy (SFT) 97; challenging assumptions 101–103; concepts core to

practicing 97–104; family development 98–99; family structure and hierarchy 99–100; joining 100–101; patterns of interaction 97–98; restructuring 103–104; societal context and structure 105–107; sociocultural attunement 104–109
structure, defined 4
superposition 31
symbolic capital 107
symbolic violence 107–108
symptom-free resistance 132, 136
Systemic Integrative Framework (SIF) 30

Tadros, E. 105
Tamura, Takeshi 193
Tatum, Beverly 287, 301
Telfener, Umberta 128
testimonial injustice 50
theory of change 333
therapeutic alliance 10–11, 13, 70, 145, 341
therapeutic relationship 10–11
therapists: as agent of change 123–124; characteristics 10–11; as coach 236–237; equity-based 57, 60; family of origin work 191; first order change 23–24; power 219; role and language 78–79; second order change 23–24; social location 52–53; sociocultural position and values 77–78; structural family 97–98, 100–102, 104–105, 108–111, 119, 122; third order change 23–24; use of power in practice 54–56; use of self 144–145
third order change 23–24, 40, 108, 207, 242–243, 267–268, 272–273, 287–289, 296–297, 314–315, 320–321, 339, 351–352; attachment-based family therapies 175–176, 182–183; brief and strategic family therapies 130, 136–137; and empowerment 197–199; in experiential family therapy 141, 153–154; in institutions 366–369; in organizations 366–369; structural family therapy 115–116
third order ethics 48–65; practicing 50–51
third order praxis: equity-based community interventions 364–366; equity-based knowledge production 373–378; policies 369–371; politics 369–371; public participation 369–371; third order change in organizations/institutions 366–369; transformative praxis 371–373
third order thinking 1–2, 19–23
thought, relational patterns of 235–236
Tilsen, J. 306
tracking patterns 244–245, 248–250
transformative praxis across national contexts 371–373
transforming/transformation 14, 37, 39, 108, 157, 179, 183, 201, 215, 223, 267, 270, 287, 291, 320, 340, 350, 361–362, 365–366, 378
transgenerational patterns and transmission 188–189
transtheoretical socioculturally attuned practices 36–43
trauma 335–336
triangulation 189
trust 159, 164–168, 199, 214
Turner, William 108–109, 359, 369–370

uncertainty 277
unfairness 222, 226–228

value/valuing 39, 216; collective 360; explore, embedded in narratives 316, 319; of relational work 343
vulnerability 335–336

Watson, M. 1, 239
Watzlawick, P. 121, 122, 123
Weakland, J. 121
Whitaker, Carl 140
White, Michael 300
Williams, A. E. 104
Wilson, Elisabeth Esmiol 171–172
within-system alliance 11
withness 275–276
Wulff, Dan 38, 376–378

Zimmerman, Toni Schindler 267–268

Made in the USA
Coppell, TX
15 April 2026